AVOIDING COMMON
ICU ERRORS

AVOIDING COMMON ICU ERRORS

LISA MARCUCCI, MD
Assistant Professor of Surgery
Division of Critical Care and Trauma Surgery
Department of Surgery
Thomas Jefferson University, Philadelphia, Pennsylvania

ELIZABETH A. MARTINEZ, MD, MHS
Cardiac Sciences
Assistant Professor
Anesthesiology/Critical Care Medicine and Surgery
Johns Hopkins University
Medical Director
Adult Post Anesthesia Care Units
The Johns Hopkins School of Medicine, Baltimore, Maryland

ELLIOTT R. HAUT, MD
Surgery
Assistant Professor of Surgery and Anesthesiology and Critical Care Medicine
Division of Critical Care and Trauma Surgery
The Johns Hopkins University School of Medicine
The Johns Hopkins Hospital, Baltimore, Maryland

ANTHONY D. SLONIM, MD, DrPH
Medicine
Executive Director, Center for Clinical Effectiveness
Children's National Medical Center
Associate Professor and Vice Chairman
Department of Pediatrics
The George Washington University School of Medicine
Washington, District of Columbia

JOSE I. SUAREZ, MD
Neurosciences
Associate Professor
Department of Neurology/Neurosurgery
Case Western Reserve University
Director, Neurosciences Critical Care
Department of Neurology/Neurosurgery
University Hospitals of Cleveland, Cleveland, Ohio

Wolters Kluwer | Lippincott Williams & Wilkins
Health
Philadelphia · Baltimore · New York · London
Buenos Aires · Hong Kong · Sydney · Tokyo

Drs. Shah, Barochia, Janka, and Altaweel contributed to this book in their personal capacity. The views expressed are their own and do not necessarily represent the views of the National Institutes of Health or the United States Government.

Acquisitions Editor: Brian Brown
Managing Editor: Nicole T. Dernoski
Marketing Manager: Angela Panetta
Production Editor: Bridgett Dougherty
Senior Manufacturing Manager: Benjamin Rivera
Design Coordinator: Risa Clow
Compositor: TechBooks
Printer: R. R. Donnelley

Library of Congress Cataloging-in-Publication Data
Avoiding common ICU errors / Lisa Marcucci ... [et al.].
    p. ; cm.
  Includes bibliographical references and index.
  ISBN-13: 978-0-7817-6739-2 (alk. paper)
  ISBN-10: 0-7817-6739-3 (alk. paper)
  1. Intensive care units. 2. Medical errors. 3. Critical care medicine.
4. Medication errors.   I. Marcucci, Lisa.
  [DNLM: 1. Intensive Care Units–organization & administration.
2. Medical Errors–prevention & control. 3. Intensive Care–methods.
4. Safety Management–organization & administration.   WX 218
A961 2007]
  RA975.5.I56A96 2007
  362.17′4068–dc22   2006031128

   The publishers have made every effort to trace the copyright holders for borrowed material. If they have inadvertently overlooked any, they will be pleased to make the necessary arrangements at the first opportunity.
   To purchase additional copies of this book, call our customer service department at (800) 638-3030 or fax orders to (301) 824-7390. International customers should call (301) 714-2324.
   Visit Lippincott Williams & Wilkins on the Internet: http://www.LWW.com. Lippincott Williams & Wilkins customer service representatives are available from 8:30 AM TO 6:00 PM, EST.

To
Brett, for his support, love, and inspiration
and
Jayne and Arenal, the best little family ever
and
Mariana and Ana Maria

PREFACE

In the six years since the Institute of Medicine released its landmark report "To Err is Human," progress toward improving patient safety has been slow and arduous. Clinicians and researchers struggle to advance the science of patient safety, understand its epidemiology, clarify priorities, implement scientifically sound yet feasible interventions, and develop measures to evaluate progress. As Robert Frost said, ". . . we have miles to go before we sleep."

As errors have become more visible and our patients continue to suffer preventable harm, patients, regulators, accreditators, and caregivers have grown frustrated. While there is broad consensus that faulty systems rather than faulty people cause most errors, healthcare workers struggle to find practical and sound ways to address and mitigate hazards.

Intensive care units provide life-sustaining therapies, but are also a place where harm lurks. ICUs are highly complex environments in which clinicians make time-pressured decisions for patients with limited physiological reserves. This combination of conditions makes ICU care at times hazardous for vulnerable patients.

To make progress toward reducing this harm, we need to expose the mistakes, develop strategies to reduce them, and evaluate our progress. This book moves us in that direction. It includes a broad array of commonly-made ICU errors and expert review regarding strategies to mitigate them. These reviews are written by practicing clinicians who understand the science of improving patient safety. The information contained in this book is timely, accurate, and practical. Imagine what ICU care would look like if we could eliminate all the hazards identified in this book. As such, reading this well-written book is a first step on a journey to improve patient safety.

PETER PRONOVOST, MD, PhD
BALTIMORE, MARYLAND

The editors welcome comments and suggestions regarding this book and request that they be sent to: lisa.marcucci@gmail.com

CONTRIBUTORS

YASIR M. AKMAL, MD
Resident
Department of Surgery
Geisinger Medical Center
Danville, Pennsylvania

LAITH R. ALTAWEEL, MD
Critical Care Fellow
Department of Critical Care Medicine
National Institutes of Health
Bethesda, Maryland

RAHUL G. BAIJAL, MD
Resident, Departments of Anesthesia and
    Critical Care Medicine
Johns Hopkins
Baltimore, Maryland

**AMISHA V. BAROCHIA, MD,
CCMD**
Post Graduate Fellow
Critical Care Medicine
National Institutes of Health
Bethesda, Maryland

M. CRAIG BARRETT, PHARMD
Surgery Clinical Specialist
Department of Pharmacy
Carolinas Medical Center
Charlotte, North Carolina

MAZEN I. BEDRI, MD
Plastic Surgery Resident
Department of Surgery
The Johns Hopkins University School
    of Medicine,
Johns Hopkins Hospital
Baltimore, Maryland

**SEAN M. BERENHOLTZ, MD,
MHS, FCCM**
Assistant Professor
Anesthesiology & Critical Care Medicine
Johns Hopkins School of Medicine
Baltimore, Maryland

LAUREN C. BERKOW, MD
Assistant Professor
Anesthesia & Critical Care Medicine
The Johns Hopkins School of Medicine
Staff Anesthesiologist
Director of Difficult Airway Education,
    Anesthesia & Critical Care Medicine
Johns Hopkins Medical Institution
Baltimore, Maryland

ADAM R. BERLINER, MD
Fellow in Nephrology
Department of Medicine
Johns Hopkins University School of
    Medicine
Baltimore, Maryland

ERIC M. BERSHAD, MD
Fellow
Neurosciences Critical Care
Department of Neurology
Case Western Reserve University
University Hospitals of Cleveland
Cleveland, Ohio

**RACHEL BLUEBOND-LANGNER,
MD**
Resident
Plastic & Reconstructive Surgery
The Johns Hopkins University School
    of Medicine
Johns Hopkins Hospital
Baltimore, Maryland

AARON BRANSKY, MD
Critical Care Fellow
Department of Surgery
University of Texas, Southwestern
Parkland Hospital
Dallas, Texas

BENJAMIN BRASLOW, MD
Assistant Professor
Department of Surgery
University of Pennsylvania School of
    Medicine
Division of Traumatology/Surgical
    Critical Care
Department of Surgery
Hospital of the University of Pennsylvania
Philadelphia, Pennsylvania

E. DAVID BRAVOS, MD
Resident
Department of Anesthesiology and Critical
    Care Medicine
Johns Hopkins University
Johns Hopkins Hospital
Baltimore, Maryland

BENJAMIN S. BROOKE, MD
Postdoctoral Fellow
Department of Surgery
Johns Hopkins University
Resident
Department of Surgery
The Johns Hopkins Hospital
Baltimore, Maryland

**DANIEL R. BROWN, MD, PHD,
FCCM**
Assistant Professor
Chair
Division of Critical Care Medicine
Department of Anesthesiology
Mayo Clinic
Rochester, Minnesota

BRANDON R. BRUNS, MD
Surgery Resident
Department of General Surgery
University of Texas Southwestern
Parkland Hospital
Dallas, Texas

WILLIAM R. BURNS, MD
Resident
Department of Surgery
Johns Hopkins University
The Johns Hopkins Hospital
Baltimore, Maryland

**CHRISTINA L. CAFEO, RN,
MSN**
Nurse Manager, Department of Surgery,
Johns Hopkins Hospital
Cardiac Surgical Intensive Care Unit
Cardiac Progressive Care Unit
Baltimore, Maryland

MELISSA S. CAMP, MD
Resident
Department of Surgery
Johns Hopkins
Baltimore, Maryland

**MOLLY B. CAMPION, MS,
CCC-SLP**
Speech-Language Pathologist
Physical Medicine & Rehabilitation
Johns Hopkins Hospital
Baltimore, Maryland

DAVID J. CAPARRELLI, MD
Resident
Division of Cardiac Surgery
The Johns Hopkins University School of
    Medicine
The Johns Hopkins Medical Institutions
Baltimore, Maryland

BRENDAN G. CARR, MD, MA
Fellow
Division of Trauma and Surgical
    Critical Care
Department of Surgery
Instructor
Department of Emergency Medicine
Hospital of the University of Pennsylvania
Philadelphia, Pennsylvania

BRETT M. CASCIO, MD
Chief Resident, Orthopedic Surgery
Johns Hopkins
Baltimore, Maryland

ALAN CHENG, MD
Assistant Professor of Medicine
Department of Medicine-Cardiovascular
    Electrophysiology
Johns Hopkins University School of
    Medicine
Baltimore, Maryland

SARA E. COSGROVE, MD, MS
Assistant Professor of Medicine
Division of Infectious Diseases
Johns Hopkins University School of
    Medicine
Director, Antibiotic Management Program
Associate Hospital Epidemiologist
Johns Hopkins Hospital
Baltimore, Maryland

BRYAN A. COTTON, MD
Assistant Professor
Department of Surgery
Vanderbilt University School of Medicine
Trauma & Surgical Critical Care Attending
Department of Surgery
Vanderbilt University Medical Center
Nashville, Tennessee

**PETER F. CRONHOLM, MD,
MSCE**
Assistant Professor
Family Medicine and Community Health
University of Pennsylvania
Hospital of the University of Pennsylvania
Philadelphia, Pennsylvania

GREGORY DALENCOURT, MD
Resident, Department of Surgery
Geisinger Medical Center
Danville, Pennsylvania

**CONSTANTINE A.
DEMETRACOPOULOS, BS**
Medical Student
The Johns Hopkins School of Medicine
Baltimore, Maryland

CAMERON DEZFULIAN, MD
Clinical Fellow
Critical Care Medicine Department
National Institutes of Health
Bethesda, Maryland
Clinical Fellow
Pediatric Anesthesia and Critical Care
Medicine Division
Johns Hopkins Hospital
Baltimore, Maryland

**J. CHRISTOPHER
DiGIACOMO, MD**
Director of Trauma
Department of Surgery
Jersey City Medical Center
Jersey City, New Jersey

MICHAEL J. DORSI, MD
Resident, Neurosurgery
Johns Hopkins School of Medicine
Baltimore, Maryland

LESIA K. DROPULIC, MD
Assistant Professor of Medicine,
Department of Medicine
Johns Hopkins University School of
    Medicine
Co-Director, Transplant & Infectious
    Diseases
Department of Medicine
Johns Hopkins Hospital
Baltimore, Maryland

MUHAMMAD I. DURRANI, MD
Fellow, Cardiac Anesthesiology
The Johns Hopkins Hospital
Baltimore, Maryland

DAVID T. EFRON, MD
Assistant Professor of Surgery
Department of Surgery
Johns Hopkins School of Medicine and
  Nursing
Johns Hopkins Hospital
Baltimore, Maryland

MICHAEL J. FAULKNER, MD
Division Chief, Cardiac Anesthesiology
Department of Anesthesia and Perioperative
  Medicine
William Beaumont Hospital,
Royal Oak, Michigan

ELIAHU S. FEEN, MD
Fellow, Neurosciences Critical Care
Department of Neurology
Case Western Reserve University
University Hospitals of Cleveland
Cleveland, Ohio

DEREK M. FINE, MD
Assistant Professor
Department of Medicine
Division of Nephrology
The Johns Hopkins School of Medicine
The Johns Hopkins Hospital
Baltimore, Maryland

HEIDI L. FRANKEL, MD
Associate Professor of Surgery
Department of Surgery
UT Southwestern
Chief, Surgical Critical Care
Parkland Memorial Hospital
Dallas, Texas

FRANK J. FRASSICA, MD
Robert A. Robinson Professor and Chair
Department of Orthopaedics
Johns Hopkins University
Baltimore, Maryland

IOSIFINA GIANNAKIKOU, MD
Anesthesiologist
Department of Cardiac Anesthesia
Metropolitan Hospital
Athens, Greece

B. ROBERT GIBSON, MD
Postdoctoral Fellow
Anaesthesia–Critical Care Medicine
The Johns Hopkins Hospital
Baltimore, Maryland

ASHITA GOEL, MD
Resident
Anesthesiology and Critical Care Medicine
The Johns Hopkins University
Baltimore, Maryland

**SHERITA HILL GOLDEN, MD,
MHS**
Assistant Professor of Medicine and
  Epidemiology
Department of Medicine
Division of Endocrinology and Metabolism
The Johns Hopkins School of Medicine
Chairperson, Glucose Control Task Force
The Johns Hopkins Hospital
Baltimore, Maryland

KELLY L. GROGAN, MD
Assistant Professor, Department of
Anesthesiology and Critical Care Medicine
Johns Hopkins Hospital
Baltimore, Maryland

**MICHAEL D. GROSSMAN, MD,
FACS**
Associate Clinical Professor
Department of Surgery
University of Pennsylvania School of
  Medicine
Chief, Division of Trauma/Surgical
  Critical Care
St. Luke's Hospital
Bethlehem, Pennsylvania

RAJAN GUPTA, MD
Assistant Professor
Department of Surgery
Dartmouth Medical School
Department of Surgery
Dartmouth Hitchcock Medical Center
Lebanon, New Hampshire

JACOB T. GUTSCHE, MD
Fellow, Surgical Critical Care
Department of Anesthesiology and
    Critical Care
University of Pennsylvania School of
    Medicine
Philadelphia, Pennsylvania

BARBARA HAAS, MD
Resident
Department of Surgery
University of Toronto
Toronto, Ontario, Canada

ALA' S. HADDADIN, MD
Attending Anesthesiologist
Assistant Professor
Department of Anesthesia
Yale University School of Medicine
New Haven, Connecticut

DAVID N. HAGER, MD
Fellow
Departments of Pulmonary and Critical
    Care Medicine
Johns Hopkins Medical Institutions
Baltimore, Maryland

**NANCY SOKAL HAGERMAN,
MD**
Fellow, Pediatric Anesthesiology
Department of Anesthesia
Cincinnati Children's Hospital
Medical Center
Cincinnati, Ohio

NADIA N. HANSEL, MD, MPH
Instructor of Medicine
Department of Medicine
The Johns Hopkins School of Medicine
Baltimore, Maryland

ELLIOTT R. HAUT, MD
Assistant Professor of Surgery and
Anesthesiology and Critical Care Medicine
Division of Critical Care and
    Trauma Surgery
Department of Surgery
The Johns Hopkins School of Medicine
The Johns Hopkins Hospital
Baltimore, Maryland

MICHAEL JOEL HAUT, MD
Clinical Professor
Department of Medicine
University of Pennsylvania School of
    Medicine
Hematologist/Oncologist
Department of Medicine
Pennsylvania Hospital
Joan Karnell Cancer Center
Philadelphia, Pennsylvania

AWORI J. HAYANGA, MD
Resident, General Surgery
Department of General Surgery
University of Michigan Health Systems
Ann Arbor, Michigan

**EUGENIE S. HEITMILLER, MD,
FAAP**
Associate Professor
Anesthesiology and Critical Care Medicine
The Johns Hopkins School of Medicine
Vice Chairman for Clinical Affairs
Anesthesiology and Critical Care Medicine
Johns Hopkins University Hospital
Baltimore, Maryland

J. GREGORY HOBELMANN, MD
Fellow, Department of Anesthesiology and
   Critical Care Medicine
Johns Hopkins
Baltimore, Maryland

DEBORAH B. HOBSON, BSN
Surgical Intensive Care Nurse
Coach for Center for Innovation in Quality
   Patient Care
Johns Hopkins Hospital
Baltimore, Maryland

WILLIAM S. HOFF, MD
Clinical Associate Professor of Surgery
University of Pennsylvania Medical Center
Philadelphia, Pennsylvania
Trauma Program Medical Director
St. Luke's Hospital
Bethlehem, Pennsylvania

JAMES H. HOLMES, IV, MD
Assistant Professor of Surgery
Department of Surgery
Wake Forest University School of Medicine
Medical Director, Burn Center
Department of Surgery
Wake Forest University Baptist Medical
   Center
Winston-Salem, North Carolina

**EDWARD T. HORN, PHARMD,
BCPS**
Clinical Associate Professor
University of Maryland School of
   Pharmacy
Clinical Pharmacy Specialist
Surgical Intensive Care
Department of Pharmacy Services
The Johns Hopkins Hospital
Baltimore, Maryland

LEO HSIAO, DO
Housestaff, Department of Anesthesiology
   and Critical Care
Johns Hopkins University
The Johns Hopkins Hospital
Baltimore, Maryland

DAVID G. HUNT, RN, BSN
Clinical Nurse Educator
Department of Cardiac Surgery
The Johns Hopkins Hospital
Baltimore, Maryland

**ELIZABETH A. HUNT, MD,
MPH**
Assistant Professor, Anesthesiology &
   Critical Care Medicine
The Johns Hopkins School of Medicine
Director, Johns Hopkins Simulator Center
Baltimore, Maryland

JACQUELINE JANKA, MD
Infectious Diseases and Critical Care
National Institutes of Health
Bethesda, Maryland

PRAVEEN KALRA, MD
Assistant Professor
Department of Anesthesia
Oklahoma University Health Science
   Center
Oklahoma City, Oklahoma

ANDREW J. KERWIN, MD,
Assistant Professor of Surgery
Medical Director
Surgical Intensive Care Unit
Department of Surgery
University of Florida Health Sciences
Center – Jacksonville
Jacksonville, Florida

SUNEEL KHETARPAL, MD
Assistant Professor
Department of Surgery
University of Florida Health Sciences
    Center – Jacksonville
Jacksonville, Florida

PATRICK K. KIM, MD
Assistant Professor of Surgery
Department of Surgery
University of Pennsylvania School of
    Medicine
Attending Surgeon
Department of Surgery
Hospital of the University of Pennsylvania
Philadelphia, Pennsylvania

BENJAMIN KRATZERT, MD
Resident, Anesthesiology
Department of Anesthesiology
University of California, San Diego
San Diego, California

LEE ANN R. LAU, MD
Chief Resident
Department of Surgery
University of Texas Southwestern
Dallas, Texas

NOAH LECHTZIN, MD, MHS
Assistant Professor
Department of Medicine
The Johns Hopkins School of Medicine
Baltimore, Maryland

**JOHN J. LEWIN, III, PHARMD,
BCPS**
Clinical Assistant Professor
University of Maryland School of
    Pharmacy
Clinical Specialist, Neurosciences
Critical Care
Department of Pharmacy Services
The Johns Hopkins Hospital
Baltimore, Maryland

JAYME E. LOCKE, MD
Resident, Department of Surgery
The Johns Hopkins Hospital
Baltimore, Maryland

YING WEI LUM, MD
Resident, Department of Surgery
The Johns Hopkins Hospital
Baltimore, Maryland

**SHELLEY SYLVESTER
MAGILL, MD**
Assistant Professor
Department of Medicine
The Johns Hopkins University School
    of Medicine
Active Staff, Division of Infectious
    Disease
Department of Medicine
The Johns Hopkins Hospital
Baltimore, Maryland

WARREN R. MALEY, MD
Associate Professor, Department
    of Surgery
Division of Transplantation
The Johns Hopkins School of Medicine
Baltimore, MD

D. JOSHUA MANCINI, MD
Resident, Department of General Surgery
Dartmouth Hitchcock Medical Center
Lebanon, New Hampshire

BENJAMIN A. MANDEL, MD
Resident, Department of Surgery
University of Wisconsin
University of Wisconsin Hospital and
    Clinics
Madison, Wisconsin

GARY T. MARSHALL, MD
Instructor of Surgery
Trauma and Critical Care
Vanderbilt University Medical School;
Instructor of Surgery
Trauma and Critical Care
Vanderbilt University Medical Center
Nashville, Tennessee

ELIZABETH A. MARTINEZ, MD, MHS
Assistant Professor
Anesthesiology/Critical Care Medicine
    and Surgery
The Johns Hopkins School of Medicine
Medical Director
Adult Post Anesthesia Care Units
Johns Hopkins Medicine
Baltimore, Maryland

SUSANNA LOVELL MATSEN, MD
Halsted Resident, Department of Surgery
Johns Hopkins University
The Johns Hopkins Hospital
Baltimore, Maryland

MADHAVI MEKA

CHRISTIAN MERLO, MD, MPH
Instructor, Department of Medicine
The Johns Hopkins School of Medicine
Baltimore, Maryland

WILLIAM G. MERZ, PHD
Professor of Pathology (Microbiology)
Department of Pathology
The Johns Hopkins School of Medicine;
Director of the Mycology Lab
Co-Director of The Molecular
Epidemiology Lab
Department of Pathology
The Johns Hopkins Hospital
Baltimore, Maryland

ROBERT K. MICHAELS, MD, MPH
Resident
Anesthesiology and Critical Care Medicine
The Johns Hopkins Hospital
Baltimore, Maryland

JENNIFER MILES-THOMAS, MD
Postdoctoral Fellow, Department of Urology
The Johns Hopkins University
Baltimore, Maryland

STEPHEN M. MILNER, MD, FACS
Director, Department of Burn Surgery
Johns Hopkins Medical Institution
Baltimore, Maryland

ANUSHIRVAN MINOKADEH, MD
Assistant Clinical Professor
Department of Anesthesiology
University of California
San Diego Medical Center
San Diego, California

ARDALAN MINOKADEH, BS
Tulane University Health Sciences
    Center
MD/PhD Candidate
New Orleans, Louisiana

TIMOTHY M. MOORE, MD, PHD
Resident
Departments of Anesthesiology and Critical
    Care Medicine
Johns Hopkins Medical Institutions
Baltimore, Maryland

MICHAEL J. MORITZ, MD
Chief, Section of Transplantation Services
Lehigh Valley Hospital
Allentown, Pennsylvania

DANA Y. NAKAMURA, OT, CLT, CLMC
Occupational Therapy Clinical
   Specialist—Burns
Department of Rehabilitation Medicine
University of Washington, Burn Center
Harborview Medical Center
Seattle, Washington

HARI NATHAN, MD
Research Fellow, Department of Surgery
The Johns Hopkins School of Medicine
House Staff, Department of Surgery
The Johns Hopkins Hospital
Baltimore, Maryland

BEVERLY J. NEWHOUSE, MD
Resident, Department of Anesthesiology
UCSD Medical Center
San Diego, California

SHAYTONE NICHOLS, MD

KELLY ORLINO, MD
Resident, Department of Surgery
Johns Hopkins Hospital
Baltimore, Maryland

LAWRENCE OSEI, MD
Clinical Fellow
Critical Care Medicine
National Institutes of Health
Bethesda, Maryland

MEHMET S. OZCAN, MD
Assistant Professor
Department of Anesthesiology
University of Oklahoma
Attending Anesthesiologist
Department of Anesthesiology
Oklahoma University Health Sciences
   Center
Oklahoma City, Oklahoma

DEREK F. PAPP, MD
Resident Physician, Orthopaedic Surgery
The Johns Hopkins School of Medicine
The Johns Hopkins Hospital
Baltimore, Maryland

B. LAUREN PATON, MD
Resident, General Surgery
Carolinas Medical Center
Charlotte, North Carolina

RONALD W. PAULDINE, MD
Assistant Professor
Anesthesiology and Critical Care Medicine
Johns Hopkins University
Vice Chair, Anesthesiology and Critical
   Care Medicine
Johns Hopkins Bayview Medical
   Center
Baltimore, Maryland

TRAVIS L. PERRY, MD
Surgery Critical Care Fellow
Department of Surgery
The University of Texas Medical Branch
Burn Surgery Fellow
Department of Burn Surgery
Shriners Hospital for Children
Galveston, Texas

JULIUS CUONG PHAM, MD
Assistant Professor
Department of Anesthesia/Critical Care
   Medicine
Department of Emergency Medicine
The Johns Hopkins School of Medicine
The Johns Hopkins Hospital
Baltimore, Maryland

MYRON S. POWELL, MD
General Surgery Resident
Department of General Surgery
Wake Forest University
Baptist Medical Center
Winston-Salem, North Carolina

PETER J. PRONOVOST, MD, PhD
Professor
Department of Anesthesiology and Critical
  Care Medicine
The Johns Hopkins School of Medicine
Baltimore, Maryland

JUAN N. PULIDO, MD
Chief Resident Associate
Resident
Department of Anesthesiology
Mayo Clinic College of Medicine
Rochester, Minnesota

JEREMY W. PYLE, MD
Resident
Department of Plastic and Reconstructive
  Surgery
Wake Forest University
Baptist Medical Center
Winston-Salem, North Carolina

MELVIN K. RICHARDSON, MD
Resident
Department of Anesthesia and Critical Care
  Medicine
The Johns Hopkins Hospital
Baltimore, Maryland

JOSE MANUEL RODRIGUEZ-PAZ, MD
Assistant Professor
Anesthesiology and Critical Care Medicine
Johns Hopkins University
Johns Hopkins Medical Institutions
Baltimore, Maryland

FRANK ROSEMEIER, MD
Assistant Professor
Department of Anesthesiology
Perioperative Medicine, and Pain
  Management
University of Miami Miller School of
  Medicine
Jackson Memorial Hospital
Miami, Florida

ANDREW L. ROSENBERG, MD
Assistant Professor
Chief, Division of Critical Care
Departments of Anesthesiology, Critical
  Care, and Internal Medicine
University of Michigan Medical Center
Ann Arbor, Michigan

TUHIN K. ROY, MD, PhD
Assistant Professor of Anesthesiology
Department of Anesthesiology
Mayo Clinic College of Medicine;
Consultant
Department of Anesthesiology
Mayo Clinic
Rochester, Minnesota

DEBA SARMA, MD
Resident
Johns Hopkins University
Baltimore, Maryland

PRASERT SAWASDIWIPACHAI, MD
Instructor
Department of Anesthesiology
Mahidol University
Instructor
Department of Anesthesiology
Siriraj Hospital
Bangkok, Thailand

PATRICK SCHANER, MD
Jefferson Medical College, General Surgery
Resident
Department of Surgery
Thomas Jefferson University Hospital
Philadelphia, Pennsylvania

DORRY L. SEGEV, MD
Instructor, Surgical Staff
Department of Transplant Surgery
The Johns Hopkins Hospital
Baltimore, Maryland

ASHISH S. SHAH, MD
Assistant Professor of Surgery
Division of Cardiac Surgery
The Johns Hopkins School of Medicine
The Johns Hopkins Hospital
Baltimore, Maryland

NIRAV GOPAL SHAH, MD
Critical Care Fellow
Critical Care Medicine Department
National Institutes of Health
Bethesda, Maryland

RICHARD WONG SHE, MHB (HONS), MBCHB, FRACS (PLASTICS)
Consultant Burn and Plastic Surgeon
National Burn Centre and Regional Centre
    for Reconstructive Plastic Maxillofacial
    and Hand Surgery
Middlemore Hospital
Auckland, New Zealand

KRISTIN SHIPMAN, MD
Assistant Instructor of Surgery
UT Southwestern Medical Center
Trauma/Surgical Critical Care Fellow
Parkland Hospital
Division of Burns, Trauma, Critical Care
Dallas, Texas

ANGELA D. SHOHER, MD
Resident, Department of Surgery
Johns Hopkins University
Baltimore, Maryland

CARRIE A. SIMS, MD, MS
Assistant Professor
Division of Surgery
University of Pennsylvania
Division of Trauma and Surgical
Critical Care
Hospital at the University of Pennsylvania
Philadelphia, Pennsylvania

RONALD F. SING, DO
Associate Professor of Surgery
Department of Surgery
University of North Carolina at Chapel Hill
Faculty, Department of Surgery
Carolinas Medical Center
Charlotte, North Carolina

HARJOT K. SINGH, MD
Clinical Fellow
Department of Infectious Disease
The Johns Hopkins Hospital
Baltimore, Maryland

VIJAY ANAND SINGH, MD
Burn Fellow
Department of Burn Surgery
Johns Hopkins Medical Institute
Baltimore, Maryland

TAMMY SLATER, CRNP
Acute Care Nurse Practitioner
Department of Surgery
The Johns Hopkins Hospital
Baltimore, Maryland

ANTHONY D. SLONIM, MD, DRPH
Executive Director, Center for Clinical
Effectiveness
Children's National Medical Center
Associate Professor and Vice Chairman
Department of Pediatrics
The George Washington University School
    of Medicine
Washington, DC

CHRISTOPHER J. SONNENDAY, MD, MHS
Clinical Lecturer
Department of Surgery
The University of Michigan
Fellow in Transplantation
Department of Surgery
The University of Michigan Hospital
Ann Arbor, Michigan

KONSTANTINOS SPANIOLAS, MD
Research Fellow
Department of Surgery
Harvard Medical School
Research Fellow
Department of Surgery
Massachusetts General Hospital
Boston, Massachusetts

JASON L. SPERRY, MD
Trauma Critical Care Fellow
Department of Surgery
University of Texas Southwestern Medical
    Center
Dallas, Texas

DIMITRIS STEFANIDIS, MD, PhD
Fellow, General Surgery
Carolinas Medical Center
Charlotte, North Carolina

JOSEPH B. STRATON, MD, MSCE
Assistant Professor, Family Medicine and
    Community Health
University of Pennsylvania
Philadelphia, Pennsylvania

MICHAEL B. STREIFF, MD
Assistant Professor of Medicine
Departments of Medicine and Hematology
Johns Hopkins Medical Institutions
Assistant Professor, Attending Physician
Department of Medicine
The Johns Hopkins Hospital
Baltimore, Maryland

JOSE I. SUAREZ, MD
Associate Professor
Department of Neurology/Neurosurgery
Case Western Reserve University
Director, Neurosciences Critical Care
Department of Neurology/Neurosurgery
University Hospitals of Cleveland
Cleveland, Ohio

ARUNA K. SUBRAMANIAN, MD
Assistant Professor
Division of Infectious Diseases
Johns Hopkins University
Co-Director, Transplant Infectious Diseases
Department of Medicine
The Johns Hopkins Hospital
Baltimore, Maryland

SANDRA M. SWOBODA, RN, MSN
Senior Research Program Coordinator
Department of Surgery
The Johns Hopkins School of Medicine
Baltimore, Maryland

MEGHAN C. TADEL, MD
Resident Physician, Anesthesiology and
    Critical Care Medicine
Johns Hopkins University
Baltimore, Maryland

PETER G. THOMAS, DO
Trauma and Surgical Critical Care Fellow
Department of Surgery
University of Pennsylvania
Philadelphia, Pennsylvania

GLEN TINKOFF, MD
Clinical Associate Professor
Department of Surgery
Thomas Jefferson Medical College
Philadelphia, Pennsylvania
Medical Director, Trauma Program
Christiana Care Health System
Newark, Delaware

MEREDITH S. TINTI, MD
Fellow, Departments of Trauma and
    Surgical Critical Care
Hospital of the University of Pennsylvania
Philadelphia, Pennsylvania

OLIVER A. VARBAN, MD
Resident
Department of Surgery
Wake Forest University
Winston-Salem, North Carolina

GEORGE C. VELMAHOS, MD, PHD, MSED
Professor of Surgery
Harvard Medical School
Chief, Trauma, Emergency Surgery,
    and Surgical Critical Care
Massachusetts General Hospital
Boston, Massachusetts

PATRICIA M. VELOSO, MD
Instructor
Department of Anesthesiology & Critical
    Care Medicine
The Johns Hopkins School of Medicine
Baltimore, Maryland

TONYA N. WALKER, MD
House Staff
Emergency Department
New York Presbyterian Hospital, Cornell
    and Columbia
New York, New York

ERIC S. WEISS, MD
Resident in General Surgery
Department of Surgery
The Johns Hopkins School of Medicine
The Johns Hopkins Hospital
Baltimore, Maryland

MATTHEW J. WEISS, MD
Resident
Department of Surgery
The Johns Hopkins Hospital
Baltimore, Maryland

JAMES F. WELLER, MD
Staff Anesthesiologist
Department of Anesthesiology
Bethesda North Hospital
Cincinnati, Ohio

KATHLEEN A. WILLIAMS, RN, MSN CRNP
Inpatient Diabetes Nurse Practitioner
Department of Medicine
Division of Endocrinology
The Johns Hopkins Hospital
Baltimore, Maryland

BRADFORD D. WINTERS, MD, PHD
Assistant Professor, Anesthesiology and
    Critical Care Medicine
The Johns Hopkins School of Medicine
Baltimore, Maryland

JOHN ZANNIS, MD
Resident, Plastic & Reconstructive Surgery
Wake Forest University
Winston-Salem, North Carolina

FARAMARZ ZARFESHANFARD, RPH
Pharmacist
Department of Pharmacy
The Johns Hopkins Hospital
Baltimore, Maryland

CONTENTS

MEDICATIONS

DEVICES/LINES/TUBES/CATHETERS/DRAINS/PROCEDURES

VENTILATORS/AIRWAY/INTUBATION/ EXTUBATION

INFECTIOUS DISEASE

SHOCK/FLUIDS/ELECTROLYTES

NEURO

LABORATORY

RENAL

BLOOD

IMAGING AND TESTS

PREGNANCY

BURNS

MISCELLANEOUS

MEDICATIONS

MONITOR PATIENTS WHO HAVE RECEIVED INTRATHECAL PRESERVATIVE-FREE MORPHINE

MELVIN K. RICHARDSON, MD

The intrathecal administration of opioids has emerged as a popular and effective form of postoperative pain control. Intrathecal opioids are able to provide long-lasting analgesia after a single injection. They work by binding to the μ opioid receptors, which are located in the substantia gelatinosa of the dorsal horn of the spinal cord. These receptors are concentration dependent and are typically not activated by systemic doses of opioids. Unlike intrathecal local anesthetics, intrathecal opioids provide analgesia without disrupting sensory, motor, or sympathetic functions.

Because of its hydrophilic properties and potent receptor affinity, preservative-free morphine (i.e., Duramorph or Astramorph) is the ideal opioid for intrathecal use. The onset of analgesic effects is directly proportional to the lipid solubility of the opioid. Preservative-free morphine (along with hydromorphone and meperidine) has a relatively low lipid solubility and its onset of action is delayed for typically 20 to 40 minutes after administration. The hydrophilic nature of the opioid also determines its duration of action. Preservative-free morphine is very hydrophilic and poorly lipid soluble, which extends its duration of analgesic effect up to 12 to 24 hours. Because of its poor lipid solubility, intrathecal morphine remains in the cerebrospinal fluid (CSF) for a prolonged period of time. It is circulated through cerebral spinal bulk flow and eventually rises rostrally to supraspinal levels. Intrathecal morphine, therefore, has bimodal analgesic effects. The first peak is soon after administration and is due to spinal opiate receptor binding. The second peak occurs 12 to 24 hours later and is due to supraspinal binding as the drug is circulated.

Compared with systemic dosing of morphine, intrathecal administration is effective in providing analgesia at a fraction of the systemic dose (0.25–0.5 mg) and thus has a much lower side-effect profile. The side effects, however, are important to recognize and treat. Respiratory depression can be delayed up to 24 hours after administration and is due to the cephalad spread of intrathecal morphine to the opioid receptors in the medullary centers of the brain stem. Thus, patients receiving intrathecal morphine must be closely monitored for up to 24 hours afterward for signs of respiratory depression.

WHAT NOT TO DO

Patients with postoperative pain despite having received intrathecal morphine present a management dilemma. Giving the patient additional systemic opioids must be done cautiously, as it may increase and potentiate the risk of respiratory depression. Generally, patients who have received intrathecal morphine should not be placed on a patient-controlled analgesia machine and should be given only intermittent doses of short-acting narcotics until the intrathecal morphine analgesic effect occurs. Nonopioid analgesics can also be considered if not contraindicated after surgery.

Other potential side effects of intrathecal morphine are similar to side effects of systemic morphine and include pruritus, nausea, vomiting, and urine retention. These effects are dose related and may be reversed with naloxone.

SUGGESTED READINGS

Raj PP, ed. Practical Management of Pain. 3rd Ed. St Louis: Mosby; 2000:180.
Rathmell JP, Lair TR, Nauman B. The role of intrathecal drugs in the treatment of acute pain. Anesth Analg 2005;101:S30–S43.
Waldman SD, ed. *Interventional Pain Management*. 2nd Ed. Philadelphia: WB Saunders; 2001: 621–622.

KNOW THE CHARACTERISTICS OF THE NARCOTICS YOU PRESCRIBE

NIRAV G. SHAH, MD

Pain control is an important aspect of critical care medicine and the use of opiate medications has typically been an important method of achieving control in the intensive care unit (ICU) setting. The brain has four opiate receptors that include the mu, kappa, delta, and sigma receptors. Currently used opioid analgesics bind to the mu receptor and initiate the pharmacological effects of analgesia, miosis, respiratory depression, euphoria, and physical dependence.

The route of opiate administration is often intravenous, with bolus administration for mild to moderate pain, continuous infusion for moderate to severe pain, and patient-controlled analgesia for the postsurgical patient who can participate in his or her care. Like other ICU interventions where benefits must be balanced against risks, adequate analgesia must carefully be balanced with the side effects of opiate therapy, particularly in the critically ill patient. These include respiratory depression, hypotension, emesis, flushing, bronchospasm, and constipation.

WHAT TO DO

The three most commonly prescribed analgesics in the ICU are morphine, hydromorphone, and fentanyl. While morphine is widely used in the ICU setting, fentanyl has additional benefits for the critically ill patient because of its increased potency, lipid solubility, and hemodynamic stability. Morphine dosing usually begins at 2 mg and is then titrated up by 1 mg to 2 mg every few hours if given in intermittent bolus form and 1 mg/hour if given continuously. Morphine metabolism occurs in the liver with excretion occurring in the kidney. Therefore, the dose should be reduced if the patient has a glomerular filtration rate less than 30 mL/min in order to prevent accumulation of its active metabolite.

Hydromorphone, a semisynthetic opiate agonist, is markedly more potent and quicker in onset than morphine. Dosing begins at 0.2 to 0.6 mg with repeated doses every 2 to 3 hours. This dose may need to be increased in patients who have had marked exposure to opiates in the past. In addition, if given as an intravenous continuous infusion, the dose should be 0.5 to 1 mg per hour after the bolus dose. Like morphine, hydromorphone is metabolized by the liver. In contrast to morphine, however, the metabolites are all inactive. Therefore, dose adjustment should be considered for hepatic failure.

Fentanyl is a synthetic opiate agonist and is 100 times more potent than morphine. Many ICUs have increasingly used fentanyl as the analgesic of choice because of its rapid onset and potency. When administered in intermittent boluses, the dose is usually 25 to 75 mcg every hour. However, it is more effectively used to prevent pain if given continuously at a rate of 25 to 50 mcg/hour after the bolus dose. Fentanyl accumulates in adipose tissue and if administered for longer than 5 days may have prolonged sedation effects upon its discontinuation. Fentanyl is metabolized to inactive compounds by the liver and excreted by the kidneys; thus the dose may need to be adjusted for liver failure, but not renal failure.

Physical dependence can occur with any of these medications and will result in withdrawal if stopped abruptly. In addition, many patients develop tolerance to the opiates and require increasing dosages to achieve the same level of pain control. One method of overcoming tolerance is to use adjuvant therapies that enhance the effect of opiates. For example, the concomitant use of benzodiazepines will assist with anxiolysis and improve the response to analgesia. However, it will also contribute to the side effect of respiratory depression already seen with opiate medications.

SUGGESTED READINGS

Hamill-Ruth RJ. Evaluation of pain in the intensive care unit. Crit Care Clin 1999;15: 35–54.

Joranson DE, Ryan KM, Gilson AM, et al. Trends in medical use and abuse of opioid analgesics. JAMA 2000;283:1710.

3

CONSIDER CLONIDINE TO COMBAT EFFECTS OF DRUG WITHDRAWAL

MELVIN K. RICHARDSON, MD

Clonidine is an alpha-2 receptor agonist that down regulates the sympathetic nervous system. By stimulating alpha-2 adrenergic receptors in the brain stem, clonidine activates inhibitory pathways in the central nervous system (CNS), which results in reduced catecholamine release and reduced sympathetic outflow from the CNS. This effectively causes a decrease in blood pressure, heart rate, peripheral resistance, and renal vascular resistance.

Clonidine's mechanism of action makes it a useful antihypertensive agent but also enables it to combat effects of drug withdrawal, especially nicotine and opioids (including heroin and methadone). Both nicotine and opioid withdrawal typically involve catecholamine release with such varied symptoms as pupillary dilatation, lacrimation, rhinorrhea, piloerection, yawning, sneezing, anorexia, nausea, vomiting, and diarrhea. Clonidine has been found to be effective in counteracting these sympathetic-mediated symptoms through its CNS inhibitory mechanisms.

WHAT TO DO

For withdrawal, clonidine should be started via the oral route. Clonidine is typically given at 0.1 mg by mouth (PO) 2 to 4 times per day. An alternate approach for rapid detoxification, using clonidine in conjunction with naltrexone, is clonidine 6 mcg/kg/day PO divided into 3 doses the first day, increased to 11 mcg/kg/day PO divided into 3 doses on day two, then tapered to 0.6 mcg/kg/day PO divided into 3 doses on the third day. Increased side effects of clonidine use are likely with higher doses, and include orthostatic hypotension, sedation, dry mouth, and constipation.

Clonidine can be continued PO and gradually tapered over a 10-day period or converted to a 7-day transdermal patch, using the following conversion protocol:

Day 1: Place transdermal clonidine. Additionally, administer 100% of oral dose.

Day 2: Patch remains; administer 50% of oral dose.

Day 3: Patch remains; administer 25% of oral dose.

Day 4: Patch remains; no further oral clonidine necessary.

Abrupt discontinuation of clonidine may cause a hypertensive rebound and symptoms of sympathetic overactivity. Severe hypertension can be seen 12 to 36 hours after the last dose, especially in patients receiving higher doses. Clonidine, therefore, should be tapered gradually over several days with close monitoring for the signs and symptoms of clonidine withdrawal. It should be remembered that during clonidine withdrawal, concomitant beta blockade may worsen rebound hypertension.

SUGGESTED READINGS

Davison R, Kaplan K, Fintel D, et al: The effect of clonidine on the cessation of cigarette smoking. Clin Pharmacol Ther 1988;44:265.

Franz DN, Hare BD, McCloskey KL: Spinal sympathetic neurons: Possible sites of opiate-withdrawal suppression by clonidine. Science 1982;215:1643.

Gold MS, Pottash AC, Sweeney DR, Klever HD: Opiate withdrawl using clonidine. A safe, effective, and rapid nonopiate treatment. JAMA 1980;243:343.

Hughes JR: Clonidine, depression, and smoking cessation. JAMA 1988;259:2901.

4

STRONGLY CONSIDER PROPHYLAXIS FOR ALCOHOL WITHDRAWAL

BRADFORD D. WINTERS, MD, PHD

Withdrawal from alcohol is a serious and common complication associated with hospitalization that can result in the condition known as delirium tremens. Many patients who consume alcohol cease drinking on or prior to admission for both voluntary and involuntary reasons. A patient does not need to be an alcoholic by medical definition to be at risk for this alcohol withdrawal syndrome. Patients who drink as little as two drinks per day have been known to develop delirium tremens. Additionally, chronic benzodiazepine users are also at risk for the same syndrome, since this class of drugs affects the same receptors in the brain.

SIGNS AND SYMPTOMS

Delirium tremens is a constellation of signs and symptoms that include confusion, agitation, delirium, combativeness, hallucinations (commonly visual changes involving bright lights and color), and potential seizure activity. These responses put patients at risk for self-injury as well as injury to staff and others. Additionally, these patients exhibit surges of sympathetic output resulting in tachycardia, hypertension, profuse sweating, and mydriasis. Patients with concomitant cardiovascular disease are at risk for myocardial infarction, intracerebral hemorrhage, and stroke. Even with treatment, delirium tremens carries a mortality risk of approximately 10%.

WHAT TO DO

One way to prevent delirium tremens is to have the patient continue alcohol consumption. While it is desirable to treat someone for alcoholism, abrupt cessation is not the answer in the acute hospitalization period when other medical or surgical concerns are paramount. If the patient is able to drink liquids or has an enteral feeding tube (e.g., nasogastric tube, orogastric tube, percutaneous endoscopic gastronomy tube) and there are no other contraindications to enteral feeding, the easiest way to prevent delirium tremens is simply to give the patient alcohol. Many hospitals stock beer or spirits either in their pharmacy or as part of their food service system and these may be prescribed for the patient deemed at risk of developing delirium tremens. Limited amounts will suffice, generally one to two beers or the equivalent in spirits or wine (one 12-ounce beer is equal to 5.5 ounces of wine or 1.5 ounces of spirits such as vodka or whiskey assuming a proof of 80) with meals. This will not lead to overt intoxication, particularly in someone who normally consumes much larger amounts. Blood alcohol levels can be measured, however, if there is such a concern. If enteral feeding is not an option, ethanol can be infused intravenously. It is usually ordered as 10% ETOH to be run at a rate of 20 to 40 cc/hr. Like enteral alcohol, this in most cases will prevent withdrawal and delirium tremens without leading to overt intoxication.

Alternatively, if the pharmacy cannot or will not make an ethanol infusion and enteral ethanol is not an option, benzodiazepines are the preferred alternative method of preventing ethanol withdrawal. These may be given enterally or intravenously. Lorazepam is commonly employed because of its lack of active metabolites and an intermediate duration of action, but most drugs in this class will work effectively. Benzodiazepines may be given on an around-the-clock (ATC) or as needed (prn) basis. Doses commonly used are 2 to 4 mg every 4 to 8 hours or prn. Recent literature suggests that while the ATC method is most commonly employed, treating the emergence of symptoms prn with benzodiazepines is just as effective at preventing and treating delirium tremens and will minimize complications while at the same time reducing length of stay.

Despite prophylaxis, a certain percentage of patients may still progress to withdrawal and delirium tremens. Once this has occurred, any ethanol being given enterally or by intravenous infusion should be abandoned (ethanol is not effective in treating the symptoms of delirium tremens) and benzodiazepines substituted. The intravenous form is preferred to ensure administration since withdrawal may include symptoms of nausea and vomiting, impeding enteral absorption. Once the delirium tremens has started, doses of benzodiazepines equal to or higher than prophylaxis are used. Sometimes, very large doses or continuous infusions are necessary. Once the withdrawal syndrome is under control, these should be weaned slowly so as to avoid re-emergence of withdrawal.

Additional agents to consider are clonidine and haloperidol. Clonidine 0.1 mg orally every 8 hours is very effective in blunting the sympathetic surge associated with ethanol withdrawal and as such may help prevent complications such as myocardial infarction in those at risk. Beta-1 specific blockers may also be used to block end-organ responses if tachycardia is a threat but this may have little effect on blood pressure secondary to alpha-1 agonism, which may need to be treated with separate agents. Haloperidol is effective in providing sedation and ameliorating some of the hallucinations that occur. An electrocardiogram should be checked each day to watch for long QT syndrome when the patient is getting haloperidol. Treatment for this is cessation of haloperidol and magnesium supplementation.

One final note is that many patients hide or do not admit to their alcohol use and their families may not be aware of the extent of their use. Delirium tremens should be in the differential for any patient experiencing mental status change, especially when coupled with signs of sympathetic activity.

SUGGESTED READINGS

Ebell MH. Benzodiazepines for alcohol withdrawal. Am Fam Physician 2006;73:1191.

McIntyre J, Hill KR, Woodside J Jr. Alcohol withdrawal syndrome. Am Fam Physician 2004;69:1443.

Sanouri I, Dikin M, Soubani AO. Critical care aspects of alcohol abuse. South Med J 2005;98:372–381.

Avoid Concomitant Use of Steroids, Neuromuscular Blockade, and Aminoglycosides to Lessen the Risk of Critical Illness Myopathy

Timothy M. Moore, MD, PhD

Acute myopathy has been increasingly recognized as a significant complication of patients cared for in the intensive care unit (ICU). The term *critical illness myopathy* (CIM) is now used to describe a general syndrome of muscle dysfunction occurring in the critically ill patient, with subtypes of CIM also being defined. The major feature of CIM is diffuse, flaccid weakness of limb, neck, and facial muscles, as well as the diaphragm. Ophthalmoplegia may be present and tendon reflexes are often depressed. The timing of onset of CIM is difficult to determine, but by definition weakness must present after the onset of critical illness. Currently, the overall occurrence of CIM is unknown because of nonuniformity in studies' patient case mixes, diagnostic criteria used, and timing of evaluation for CIM.

SIGNS AND SYMPTOMS

It is only during a systematic workup for generalized weakness and ventilatory failure in the critically ill patient that a diagnosis of CIM can be reached. A combination of electrophysiologic studies and histopathologic findings is required. Criteria for the diagnosis of CIM include sensory nerve action potential amplitudes >80% of the lower limit of normal; needle electromyogram (EMG) with short-duration, low-amplitude motor unit potentials with early or normal full recruitment (with or without fibrillation potentials); absence of a decremental response on repetitive nerve stimulation; muscle biopsy findings of myopathy with myosin loss; and compound muscle action potential amplitudes <80% of the lower limit of normal in two or more nerves without conduction block. Elevated serum creatinine kinase and demonstration of muscle inexcitability are also diagnostic features when taken together with the other findings. Further identification of the subtype of CIM (thick filament myosin loss, rhabdomyolysis, necrotizing myopathy of intensive care, or cachectic myopathy) may aid in prognostication, since only necrotizing myopathy of intensive care is associated with a poor prognosis for return of muscle strength.

The definitive pathophysiology of CIM is still elusive, but most clinicians and scientists to date agree that the systemic inflammatory response syndrome (SIRS) accounts for the muscle organ failure, with CIM similar to other organ failures seen in patients with SIRS. This is due to the increased cytokine burden having a strong potential for mediating sepsis-induced proteolysis of myofibrillar proteins in muscle. In addition to cytokine mediation, external factors can trigger the onset of CIM, with the most important being high-dose glucocorticoids. Additionally, the protein degradation potency of steroids is increased by impaired neuromuscular transmission, which can be induced by surgical stress, drugs, or an underlying critical illness neuropathy. Taken together, sepsis, steroids, and impaired neuromuscular transmission act synergistically to stimulate muscle proteolysis characteristic of CIM. The defined subtypes of CIM may therefore reflect the balance of proteolytic inputs in a dose-dependent manner, exposure-dependent manner, or both, and the severity of CIM may be controlled through limiting these inputs.

In terms of altering neuromuscular transmission, more than 50 drugs, notably neuromuscular blocking agents (i.e., pancuronium and vecuronium), aminoglycosides, clindamycin, and colistin cause pharmacologic muscle denervation. In addition, denervation also causes a rise in glucocorticoid receptors in the cytosol of skeletal muscle resulting in increased sensitivity of muscle to steroids. Thus, the potential exists for a vicious cycle to develop when neuromuscular blockade, aminoglycosides, and steroids are administered simultaneously in the critically ill ICU patient.

There is no current treatment for CIM, although intensive physiotherapy seems promising. The current mainstay of CIM management is directed at prevention through judicious use of drugs associated with the development of the myopathy. It should be noted, however, that other mytotoxic factors responsible for producing myopathies in the critically ill have been identified, independent of sepsis or glucocorticoids or neuromuscular blocker administration. Most subtypes of CIM still carry a good prognosis for recovery of muscle strength over time, with the exception of necrotizing myopathy.

Suggested Readings

Bolton CF. Neuromuscular manifestations of critical illness. Muscle Nerve 2005;32: 140–163.

Friedrich O, Fink RHA, Hund E. Understanding critical illness myopathy: approaching the pathomechanism. J Nutr 2005;135:1813S–1817S.

Latronico N, Peli E, Botteri M. Critical illness myopathy and neuropathy. Curr Opin Crit Care 2005;11:126–132.

Latronico N, Shehu I, Seghelini E. Neuromuscular sequelae of critical illness. Curr Opin Crit Care 2005;11:381–390.

6

USE PROPHYLAXIS FOR THE IMMEDIATE SIDE EFFECTS OF STEROIDS

D. JOSHUA MANCINI, MD
RAJAN GUPTA, MD

Glucocorticoids are most commonly used to mitigate an inflammatory response. They are used in a wide variety of patient populations seen in the intensive care unit (ICU). Unfortunately, these agents have many side effects, which often limit their use. In the ICU setting, the functions most commonly affected are endocrine regulation, immune response, and gastrointestinal (GI) integrity, as well as skin and wound healing.

WATCH OUT FOR

Derangement in glucose metabolism can be caused by glucocorticoids through decreased insulin production, increased insulin resistance, and altered glucose synthesis. Steroid-induced diabetes should be managed similarly to glucose control used for other patients in the ICU. Insulin infusion therapy to control hyperglycemia is often necessary. Hyperglycemia secondary to glucocorticoid treatment typically recedes within 48 hours of discontinuation of the glucocorticoids.

The immune-modulating effects of glucocorticoids are central to their therapeutic effects as well as one of their greatest limitations. They can cause a leukocytosis in the absence of systemic infection. Immune suppression occurs from effects on inhibition of inflammatory cells as well as inhibition of the release of cytokines and proinflammatory modulators. Some have suggested that systemic fungal infection is a contraindication to the institution of steroid therapy.

Steroids impair wound healing by inhibiting the early inflammatory phase and the attraction of cells central to the process of wound healing. They also inhibit new protein synthesis, leading to decreased collagen deposition by fibroblasts. Wounds eventually heal with the same tensile strength but take longer to do so. Limited case reports suggest that vitamin A administration can help ameliorate some of these deleterious effects on wound healing, and supplementation may be considered in these patients.

Within the gastrointestinal system, glucocorticoid therapy can result in increased acid secretion, decreased gastric mucous production, and parietal cell hyperplasia. This leads to an increased incidence of peptic ulcer disease and upper GI bleeding in patients receiving this therapy. ICU patients often carry other risk factors for gastrointestinal stress ulceration as well. Patients receiving steroids should have stress ulcer prophylaxis in the form of H2-blockers or proton pump inhibitors (PPIs). Studies have not shown a clear benefit of PPIs over H2-blockers. Early enteral feeding may also help reduce the incidence of stress ulcers in the ICU patient population.

Long-term glucocorticoid therapy may lead to suppression of the hypothalamus-pituitary-adrenal axis. Sudden withdrawal of steroid therapy can cause severe adrenal insufficiency and hemodynamic instability. Adrenal insufficiency can also result after a patient experiences increased stress from inflammation, surgery, or trauma without an increase in the exogenous dose of steroids. Thus, stress-dose therapy should be considered for patients on previous steroid therapy undergoing surgery. Similarly, a patient suffering from the stress of surgery, trauma, or inflammation who is not receiving exogenous steroid therapy is also at risk to develop relative adrenal insufficiency. This is usually due to an inability of the hypothalamus-pituitary-adrenal axis to appropriately respond to the increased need for circulating corticoids, resulting in a physiologic deficiency. Thus, the dosing for replacement therapy in such patients is significantly lower than stress or therapeutic dosing, and it remains unclear if the side effects of this lower dosing are as pronounced. Adrenal insufficiency should also be a part of the differential diagnosis in ICU patients with hypotension and hemodynamic instability refractory to fluid and vasopressor management.

SUGGESTED READINGS

Britt RC, Devine A, Swallen KC, et al. Corticosteroid use in the intensive care unit: at what cost? Arch Surg 2006;141:145–149.

Daley RJ, Rebuck JA, Welage LS, et al. Prevention of stress ulceration: current trends in critical care. Crit Care Med 2004;32:2008–2013.

Schacke H, Docke WD, Asadullah K. Mechanisms involved in the side effects of glucocorticoids. Pharmacol Ther 2002;96:23–43.

7

SPECIFICALLY QUERY FOR PREVIOUS STEROID USE

LISA MARCUCCI, MD
PRASERT SAWASDIWIPACHAI, MD

Human steroids are produced by the adrenal gland and are under the direct or indirect control of the hypothalamus, pituitary, and adrenal glands. The two major classes of steroids that have significant clinical metabolic effects are the glucocorticoids (mainly cortisol), which regulate glucose and other anabolic cascades, and the mineralocorticoids (mainly aldosterone), which handle Na–K equilibrium.

Patients can become deficient in steroid production through primary Addison's disease (e.g., adrenal cortex destruction, hemorrhage) or secondary Addison's disease (e.g., through a deficiency of corticotropin or adrenocorticotropic hormone [ACTH] or through exogenous steroid administration). Primary Addison's disease is rare, but secondary Addison's disease is not uncommon. Exogenous glucocorticoids are used in a variety of diseases including organ and bone transplants, rheumatoid arthritis, systemic lupus erythematosus and other collagen vascular disorders, psoriasis, chronic obstructive pulmonary disease, inflammatory bowel disease, and many hematological diseases such as idiopathic thrombocytopenic purpura (ITP).

WHAT TO DO

Although the indications and dosages of stress-dose steroids for these patients undergoing surgery is an area of active discussion, it is imperative that the astute clinician knows steroid history so that an informed decision can be made. Acute adrenal insufficiency is a morbid and sometimes fatal condition that can be manifested by circulatory collapse, fever, hypoglycemia, and depressed mental status. Because of the seriousness of this condition and the relative ease of adequately treating it prophylactically, all patients should be specifically queried as to whether they have ever been on steroids and if so, how much and when. Some experienced clinicians feel the level of adrenal functioning remains decreased if an equivalent of 5 mg of prednisone was administered for at least 2 weeks in the previous year.

One final note is that 1 mg of dexamethasone equals 5 mg of prednisone, which equals 25 mg of hydrocortisone (which is similar to natural cortisol).

SUGGESTED READINGS

Annane D. Effect of treatment with low doses of hydrocortisone and fludrocortisone on mortality in patients with septic shock. JAMA 2002;288:862–871.

Cooper MS. Corticosteroid insufficiency in acutely ill patients: current concepts. N Engl J Med 2003;348:727–734.

Salem M. Perioperative glucocorticoid coverage: a reassessment 42 years after emergence of a problem. Ann Surg 1994;219:416–425.

8

DO NOT USE SUCCINYLCHOLINE IN PATIENTS WITH BURNS, PARALYSIS, OR OTHER HIGH POTASSIUM STATES

EUGENIE S. HEITMILLER, MD

Succinylcholine is a depolarizing muscle relaxant used for urgent endotracheal intubation in the operating room, intensive care unit (ICU), and emergency department. The intravenous (IV) dose is 0.5 to 1.5 mg/kg. Time to effect is 1 minute and duration of action in patients with normal pseudocholinesterase activity is approximately 2 minutes with complete recovery in 5 minutes. If a working IV catheter is not available, succinylcholine may be given 3 to 4 mg/kg intramuscularly (IM) (maximum dose 150 mg) with an onset of 2 to 3 minutes. Muscle fasciculations will often be seen prior to complete muscle relaxation. Known side effects of succinylcholine are bradycardia and muscle pain.

Succinylcholine is indicated when rapid sequence induction is needed to quickly secure the airway with an endotracheal tube. Although succinylcholine may increase intracranial pressure, it can be used in patients with acute head trauma because the rapid onset, superior intubating conditions, and reversibility outweigh the risk associated with its use. Succinylcholine in lower doses is also used to treat laryngospasm.

WHAT NOT TO DO

Succinylcholine is contraindicated in patients after the acute phases of major trauma or burns, extensive denervation of skeletal muscle, upper or lower motor neuron injury, and severe infections, particularly clostridia, botulism, and tetanus, because succinylcholine in these patients may result in severe hyperkalemia and cardiac arrest. The risk of hyperkalemia in these patients increases over time and usually peaks at 7 to 10 days after the injury, although the precise time of onset and the duration of the risk period are unknown. It is also contraindicated in patients with a personal or family history of malignant hyperthermia or skeletal muscle myopathies and in patients with disuse atrophy because acute severe rhabdomyolysis may occur with subsequent hyperkalemia, ventricular arrhythmias, and cardiac arrest resulting.

The mechanism by which succinylcholine use results in hyperkalemia is related to its effect on muscle nicotinic acetylcholine receptors. In the conditions at risk for hyperkalemia listed previously, there is an increase of muscle nicotinic acetylcholine receptors, which when depolarized by succinylcholine leads to efflux of intracellular potassium into the plasma, leading to acute hyperkalemia.

Alternative agents are nondepolarizing agents such as vecuronium and rocuronium, but these do not result in as rapid a relaxation.

SUGGESTED READINGS

Koenig KL. Rapid-sequence intubation of head trauma patients: prevention of fasciculation with pancuronium versus minidose succinylcholine. Ann Emerg Med 1992;21:929–932.

Martyn JAJ, Richtsfeld M. Succinylcholine-induced hyperkalemia in acquired pathologic states. Anesthesiology 2006;104:158–169.

Naguib M, Samarkandi AH, El-Din ME, et al. The dose of succinylcholine required for excellent endotracheal intubating conditions. Anesth Analg 2006;102:151–155.

9

Consider Using Cisatracurium for Neuromuscular Paralysis in Patients with Hepatic and Renal Failure

Muhammad I. Durani, MD

The ideal neuromuscular blocking (NMB) drug would be rapid in onset, have a predictable offset, be nontoxic, lack deleterious cardiovascular or autonomic effects, undergo a defined means of metabolism and excretion preferably independent of end-organ function, and be inexpensive. Many of these characteristics are found in clinically available drugs like cisatracurium.

To briefly review, neuromuscular blockade occurs via one of two different pharmacologic modes. Drugs that act as a prolonged agonist at the nicotinic acetylcholine (nACh) receptor are called depolarizing agents (e.g., succinylcholine). Succinylcholine attaches to each of the alpha subunits of the nACh receptor and mimics the action of acetylcholine, thus depolarizing the postjunctional membrane. Neuromuscular blockade develops because a depolarized postjunctional membrane cannot respond to subsequent release of acetylcholine.

A second group of WMB agents that bind noncovalently and competitively to nACh receptors and inhibit neuromuscular transmission are called nondepolarizing NMB drugs. In high doses, these drugs may act by blocking the ion receptor channels. Occupation of as many as 70% of the nACh receptors does not produce evidence of neuromuscular blockade. Neuromuscular transmission, however, fails when 80% to 90% of the receptors are blocked.

Nondepolarizing NMB drugs may be classified on the basis of their structure and duration of action. Clinically available nondepolarizing drugs can be grouped into two basic structural categories. The benzylisoquinolinium drugs (atracurium, cisatracurium, mivacurium, tubocurarine) tend to be potent (and therefore slower in onset) NMB drugs that are eliminated by the kidneys or by Hofmann elimination and may trigger histamine release. Conversely, the aminosteroid compounds (pancuronium, vecuronium, rocuronium) are less potent, have a faster onset of action, are eliminated by the liver with active metabolites, and lack significant histamine release or autonomic interactions.

NMB drugs also may be classified as short (succhinylcholine, mivacurium), intermediate (atracurium, cisatracurium, vecuronium, rocuronium), or long- acting (tubocurarine, pancuronium) on the basis of their duration of action.

CISATRACURIUM

This is the purified form of one of the ten stereoisomers of atracurium. Cisatracurium has an ED95 of 50 μg/kg and has an onset of action of 3 to 5 minutes and duration of neuromuscular blockade lasting 20 to 35 minutes. Neuromuscular blockade is easily maintained at a stable level by infusion at a constant rate and does not diminish over time. In contrast to vecuronium, the rate of spontaneous recovery from cisatracurium-induced neuromuscular blockade is not influenced by length of infusion in patients requiring mechanical ventilation.

Cisatracurium undergoes spontaneous nonenzymatic degradation at normal body temperature and pH by a base-catalyzed reaction termed *Hofmann elimination*, to form laudanosine and monoquaternary acrylate. Hofmann elimination represents a chemical mechanism of elimination accounting for 77% of the clearance of cisatracurium, whereas renal clearance is responsible for another 16%. The organ-independent clearance of cisatracurium means that this nondepolarizing NMB drug can be administered to patients with hepatic or renal dysfunction without a change in its neuromuscular blocking profile. The pharmacokinetics of cisatracurium is only marginally influenced by advanced age.

The metabolites of cisatracurium by Hoffman elimination are inactive at the neuromuscular junction (NMJ). In contrast to atracurium, plasma concentrations of laudanosine after administration of 2 × ED95 dose of cisatracurium are fivefold less than that present after a 1.5 × ED95 dose of atracurium (Lien et al., 1996). Cisatracurium, in contrast to atracurium, is devoid of histamine-releasing effects such that cardiovascular changes do not accompany the rapid intravenous (IV) administration of even large doses (8 × ED95) of cisatracurium. Cisatracurium administered to adult neurosurgical patients produces less cerebral hemodynamic changes compared with equipotent doses of atracurium.

PANCURONIUM

This is a long-acting aminosteroid nondepolarizing NMB drug with an ED95 of 70 μg/kg that has an onset of action in 3 to 5 minutes and a duration of neuromuscular blockade lasting 60 to 90 minutes. An estimated 80% of a single dose of pancuronium is eliminated unchanged in the urine. In renal failure, the plasma clearance is decreased 33% to 50%. An estimated 10% to 40% undergoes hepatic deacetylation. The 3-desacetylpancuronium metabolite is approximately 50% as potent as pancuronium at the NMJ. Patients with total biliary obstruction and hepatic cirrhosis have an increased volume of distribution, decreased plasma clearance, and prolonged elimination half-time of pancuronium.

VECURONIUM

This is an intermediate-acting aminosteroid nondepolarizing NMB drug with an ED95 of 50 μg/kg that produces an onset of action in 3 to 5 minutes and a duration of neuromuscular blockade lasting 20 to 35 minutes. Vecuronium undergoes both hepatic metabolism and renal excretion. The 3-desacetylvecuronium metabolite is approximately one half as potent as the parent compound. The elimination half-time is prolonged in patients with renal failure. In patients with cholestasis, hepatic cirrhosis, or alcoholic liver disease, the administration of vecuronium, 0.2 mg/kg, results in a prolonged elimination half-time and increased duration of action.

　　Rocuronium is an intermediate-acting aminosteroid with an ED95 of 0.3 mg/kg that has an onset of action in 1 to 2 minutes and a duration of neuromuscular blockade lasting 20 to 35 minutes. Rocuronium is largely excreted unchanged (up to 50% in 2 hours) in the bile. Liver disease increases the volume of distribution of rocuronium and could result in a longer duration of action, especially with repeated doses or prolonged IV administration. Renal excretion of rocuronium may be >30% in 24 hours, and administration of this drug to patients in renal failure may produce a modestly prolonged duration of action.

SUGGESTED READINGS

Lien CA, Schmith VD, Belmont MR, Abalos A, Kisor DF, and Savarese JJ. Pharmacokinetics of cisatracurium in patients receiving nitrous oxide/opioid/barbiturate anesthesia. *Anesthesiology* 84:300–308, 1996.

Murray MJ, Cowen J, DeBlock H, Erstad B, Gray AW, Jr., Tescher AN, McGee WT, Prielipp RC, Susla G, Jacobi J, Nasraway SA, Jr., and Lumb PD. Clinical practice guidelines for sustained neuromuscular blockade in the adult critically ill patient. Crit Care Med 30:142–156, 2002.

Stoelting RK, ed. Pharmacology and Physiology in Anesthetic Practice. 3rd Ed. Philadelphia: Lippincott Williams & Wilkins; 1999:182–223.

10

REMEMBER THAT THERE ARE TWO "NEOS"

NANCY SOKAL HAGERMAN, MD

In our current culture of patient safety, it is important to avoid commonly used medical abbreviations so that medical errors can be prevented. For example, the term *neo* is often used in the operating room and intensive care unit (ICU) to refer to the drug Neo-Synephrine; however, it could also reasonably be interpreted as neostigmine, another commonly used drug in the operating room and ICU. To avoid this confusion and to decrease the risk of a medication error, the use of the brand name Neo-Synephrine should be abandoned.

NEO-SYNEPHRINE

Neo-Synephrine is the trade name for phenylephrine. It is a pure alpha receptor agonist and has both venous and arterial constrictive effects. Because α_1 receptors have been discovered in the myocardium, it is also possible that it has positive inotropic effects. Acutely, phenylephrine causes an increase in venous return (preload) due to its venous constrictive effects; it increases afterload as well. In normal individuals, it does not affect cardiac output. However, in patients with ischemic heart disease, it can decrease cardiac output. Other uses for phenylephrine include reversing right-to-left shunt flow in patients with tetralogy of Fallot and terminating supraventricular tachycardias (SVTs) as it can cause reflex vagal stimulation in response to elevated blood pressure. In this last circumstance, phenylephrine is particularly useful as it treats both the arrhythmia and the hypotension.

Phenylephrine is given as either an intravenous (IV) bolus or infusion; bolus doses are 1 to 10 mcg/kg, or in 50- to 100-mcg boluses in adults. As an IV infusion, it is usually mixed as 10 to 15 mg in 250 mL and dosed as 0.15 to 0.75 mcg/kg/min. For use in pediatric patients with tetralogy of Fallot, IV bolus doses are 5 to 50 mcg/kg.

NEOSTIGMINE

Neostigmine (marketed under the trade name Prostigmin) is a reversible acetylcholinesterase inhibitor. It is used clinically in the treatment of myasthenia gravis, glaucoma, and atony of the gastrointestinal and urinary tracts. In the operating room and ICU settings, it is commonly used to reverse nondepolarizing neuromuscular blockade.

Although it antagonizes neuromuscular blocking agents at nicotinic receptors, it has muscarinic effects as well. Its adverse effects result from its action at these receptors: bradycardia and bradyarrhythmias; increased salivation; increased bowel motility; and possibly bronchospasm. To counteract these adverse effects, neostigmine is typically given in conjunction with an anticholinergic agent – either atropine or glycopyrrolate.

The dose of intravenous neostigmine required to reverse neuromuscular blockade is greater in long-acting neuromuscular blockers than short-acting blockers. For example, 40 to 50 mcg/kg of neostigmine is required to reverse a 90% block produced by pancuronium or d-tubocurarine, whereas 20 to 30 mcg/kg is needed for atracurium, vecuronium, and rocuronium, and 5 mcg/kg is needed for mivacurium. Because neostigmine dosage has a ceiling effect, administering greater than 0.07 mg/kg has little benefit.

SUGGESTED READINGS

Barash PG, Cullen BF, Stoelting RK, ed. Clinical Anesthesia. 4th Ed. Philadelphia: Lippincott Williams & Wilkins; 2001:296–297,439–441.
Hensley FA Jr., Martin DE, Gravlee GP, ed. *A Practical Approach to Cardiac Anesthesia*. 3rd Ed. Philadelphia: Lippincott Williams & Wilkins; 2003:43.

11

Treat Neuroleptic Malignant Syndrome as an Emergency and Remember its Presentation May Not Be Dose Dependent

ELIAHU S. FEEN, MD
JOSE I. SUAREZ, MD

Neuroleptic malignant syndrome (NMS) is a clinical syndrome consisting of four primary features: rigidity, altered mental status, hyperthermia, and autonomic instability. It occurs in the setting of the use of dopamine-blocking agents or the withdrawal of dopamine-enhancing medications.

EPIDEMIOLOGY

Incidence of NMS is estimated at 0.1% to 2%. There is a preponderance of young men with NMS, but this may be because of the increased frequency of schizophrenia and affective disorders in this group and the subsequent increased use of neuroleptics. Other risk factors may include neuroleptic-induced catatonia, dehydration or malnutrition as a precipitating cause, and a history of elevated serum creatinine kinase (CK) during psychotic episodes not in association with NMS.

CLINICAL PRESENTATION

The motor symptoms consist most commonly of parkinsonian-type symptoms such as "lead-pipe" rigidity, but other symptoms include a tremor superimposed on the rigidity ("cogwheel rigidity"), akinesia, bradykinesia, and dystonia (e.g., blepharospasm, opisthotonus, oculogyric crises, trismus, and orobuccal dyskinesia). The altered mental status ranges from delirium to stupor or even coma. A fever is seen in almost all cases (unlike malignant hyperthermia) and is usually greater than 38°C and often greater than 41°C. Arrhythmias, blood pressure fluctuations, and respiratory abnormalities constitute the main, potentially life-threatening autonomic features of NMS. Rare clinical manifestations include seizures, ataxia, and nystagmus. NMS usually evolves over 24 to 72 hours. Occasionally there can be a slower progression over days, but in the case of depot neuroleptics (e.g., intramuscular form of fluphenazine), progression over a couple of weeks has been reported. The clinical course lasts 7 to 10 days, with a longer time if the inciting agent was depot neuroleptics, because of slower clearance. Laboratory abnormalities found in association with NMS are leukocytosis in the range of 10 to 40,000 cells/μL and elevated serum creatinine kinase (CK) in the range of 200 to several thousand IU/L.

Cases of NMS with prominent medical complications and fatalities are widely described. Some of the causes for the morbidity and mortality of NMS relate to its secondary complications. Because of the associated rhabdomyolysis, severe dehydration and prerenal acute renal failure can occur. This is predictive of mortality, with aggressive hydration absolutely necessary (urine alkalinization is controversial). Because of rigidity and consequent immobility, as well as activation of the coagulation cascade to metabolic conditions created by the rhabdomyolysis, venous thromboembolism has been reported. Pulmonary embolism has been reported to cause almost one quarter of fatalities. In severe cases, aspiration pneumonia, respiratory failure, cardiac arrhythmias, and dysautonomia have been reported.

Some important clinical syndromes with a similar clinical picture form a differential for NMS. Malignant hyperthermia appears in the setting of exposure to certain anesthetic agents such as halothane, isoflurane, sevoflurane, and desflurane, and depolarizing muscle relaxants like succinylcholine. Acute lethal catatonia involves hyperthermia, akinesia, and rigidity, but this is usually preceded in the previous couple of weeks by behavioral changes. The serotonin syndrome occurs in the setting of an overexposure to selective serotonin reuptake inhibitors (SSRIs) or the combination use of SSRIs together with monoamine oxidase inhibitors, tricyclic antidepressants, or meperidine.

PRECIPITATING FACTORS

NMS is clearly medication related *(Table 11.1)*. For the neuroleptic medication-related cases, the onset is not dose related and can occur many months after initiation of therapy. For patients who have been on dopamine agonists (most typically Parkinson patients), NMS typically occurs in the setting of a sudden withdrawal of the agonist agent or the change of dosage or change to a different agonist altogether. Most of the Parkinson patients have had symptoms of their disease for more than 8 years. The perioperative period is a classic scenario for onset of NMS because of the alterations in serum levels of the agonist related to changes when patients take their medications or to metabolic alterations. For patients who have been on dopamine-blocking agents, such as haloperidol, NMS can occur even after initial exposure. Increased dosages of,

TABLE 11.1 MEDICATIONS ASSOCIATED WITH THE DEVELOPMENT OF NMS	
DOPAMINERGIC/DOPAMINE AGONISTS WITHDRAWAL	**DOPAMINE ANTAGONIST/ NEUROLEPTIC ADMINISTRATION**
Levodopa COMT inhibitors: tolcapone, entacapone Dopamine agonists: bromocriptine, pergolide, ropinirole, pramipexole, cabergoline, apomorphine Amantadine	Neuroleptics: phenothiazines, butyrophenones, thiothixanes Atypical antipsychotics: clozapine, olanzapine, risperidone, quetiapine Antiemetics: metoclopramide,droperidol, prochlorperazine, promethazine Others: reserpine, carbamazepine Rare reported cases in: overdose of some tricyclic and SSRI antidepressants, overdose of citalopram, loxapine, diatrizoate, lithium Rare reported cases in drug abuse: cocaine, amphetamines

changes in the particular agent, or parenteral administration of the neuroleptic are risk factors for the development of NMS in this group of patients. The etiology of NMS is consequently thought to be related to the acute blockade of the nigrostriatal and hypothalamic dopamine pathways in the brain.

MANAGEMENT

Treatment involves first and foremost reversing the inciting cause—either discontinuing the neuroleptic/dopamine-mediating agent or reinstituting the dopaminergic therapy that may have been stopped. Supportive care is essential and possibly lifesaving, because of the secondary complications. Aggressive cooling, careful monitoring of cardiovascular functions, and high-volume intravenous fluid therapy necessitate intensive care hospitalization for all but the mild cases. Pharmacologic therapy includes bromocriptine (a dopamine agonist) and/or dantrolene (a skeletal muscle relaxant) in addition to supportive care. These two medications are used independently or together. Pharmacologic therapy improves the prognosis of NMS, decreasing time of resolution of symptoms from 16 days with supportive therapy alone to about 9 days. Medication administration is started immediately and continued for 10 days after the resolution of symptoms. However, residual parkinsonian or catatonic symptoms can persist for weeks after the acute episode resolves. Electroconvulsive therapy (ECT) has been reported to be beneficial in cases of NMS refractory to other therapies. For such cases ECT has been reported to resolve symptoms after three to four treatments and is generally used for 6 days total.

Recurrence of NMS has been reported. Some of the risk factors for recurrence when neuroleptics are restarted include higher potency of neuroleptics, restarting within 2 weeks of an episode of NMS, higher initial dose, and use of concomitant lithium.

SUGGESTED READINGS

Bhanushali MJ, Tuite PJ. The evaluation and management of patients with neuroleptic malignant syndrome. Neurol Clin 2004;22:389–411.

Chan TC, Evans SD, Clark RF. Drug-induced hyperthermia. Crit Care Clin 1997;13:785–808.

Sachdev PS. Neuroleptic-induced movement disorders: an overview. Psychiatr Clin North Am 2005;28:255–274.

REMEMBER THAT MALIGNANT HYPERTHERMIA MAY NOT HAVE HYPERTHERMIA

NANCY SOKAL HAGERMAN, MD

Malignant hyperthermia (MH) is a hypermetabolic disorder of skeletal muscle that is triggered in susceptible individuals by several inhalation anesthetic agents (sevoflurane, desflurane, isoflurane, halothane, enflurane, and methoxyflurane) and succinylcholine. These anesthetic triggers cause intracellular hypercalcemia in skeletal muscle by decreasing the uptake of calcium by the sarcoplasmic reticulum. The intracellular hypercalcemia activates metabolic pathways that result in adenosine triphosphate (ATP) depletion, acidosis, membrane destruction, and ultimately cell death. Susceptibility to MH is inherited as an autosomal dominant disorder and most susceptible individuals are completely asymptomatic until exposed to triggering agents.

Episodes of MH occur most often, but not exclusively, in children. The mean age for MH is 15 years, although cases have been reported in infants as well as the elderly. The incidence of MH ranges from approximately 1 in 10,000 to 1 in 50,000 individuals who are exposed to the triggering agents.

SIGNS AND SYMPTOMS

In most cases, the first signs and symptoms of the disorder are evident in the operating room. However, MH can also occur in the recovery room or even after the patient has been transferred to the patient floor. It is important to remember that none of the signs and symptoms occur in all cases. Initial signs usually include tachycardia (90% of cases) and tachypnea (80% of cases) due to the sympathetic nervous system response to the underlying hypermetabolism and hypercarbia (80% of cases). In the paralyzed patient under general anesthesia, the first sign of MH can be hypercarbia that is resistant to adjustments in the ventilator setting. Next, an increase in blood pressure, cardiac dysrhythmias, and muscle rigidity (80% of cases) are often seen. Patients may then become hyperthermic (70% of cases), with a rise of 1 to 2 degrees Celsius every 5 minutes. An arterial blood gas will usually show respiratory and metabolic acidosis. Other lab abnormalities include hyperkalemia, hypercalcemia, lactic acidemia and myoglobinuria. Creatinine kinase levels rise to 20,000 or more within 12 to

24 hours, putting the patient at risk for myoglobinuric renal failure. Isolated myoglobinuria in the early postoperative period should make the anesthesiologist and surgical team suspicious for MH. Masseter muscle rigidity shortly after the administration of succinylcholine has also been associated with MH as well.

MH is a treatable disorder. With early diagnosis and appropriate treatment, the mortality rate approaches zero. If MH is suspected, all triggering agents should be discontinued immediately. In the operating room, the patient should be ventilated with 100% oxygen at a flow of 10 L/minute. If a general anesthetic must be continued, it is safe to administer barbiturates, benzodiazepines, opioids, and propofol. The patient should be intubated as soon as possible. Cardiac dysrhythmias, hyperkalemia, acidosis, and other medical problems should be managed appropriately. The patient should be given dantrolene as soon as possible. Dantrolene acts by inhibiting the release of calcium from the sarcoplasmic reticulum. The initial dose is a 2.5mg/kg intravenous (IV) bolus followed by 1 mg/kg IV every 6 hours for at least 24 hours. Dantrolene's side effects include nausea, phlebitis, and weakness for approximately 24 hours after the drug is discontinued. Each vial of dantrolene contains 20 mg of dantrolene and 3 mg of mannitol and must be mixed with 60 mL of sterile water. The initial dose for a 70-kg adult is 175 mg or 9 vials. Assistance should be sought in mixing the dantrolene as it is poorly soluble. Dantrolene 2.5 mg/kg should be given every 5 to 10 minutes until there is a fall in heart rate, normal cardiac rhythm, a reduction in muscle tone, and a decline in body temperature. Maintenance of normal volume status is essential in the setting of rhabdomyolysis. Hyperkalemia may require treatment with insulin and glucose. Caution should be excercised with potassium-losing diuretics as hypovolemia should be avoided. Furthermore, administration of calcium should be avoided unless there is symptomatic hypocalcemia because of the expected hypercalcemia during the recovery phases of rhabdomyolysis. Dysrhythmias can be treated with beta-blockers and lidocaine. Calcium channel blockers should be avoided. The patient's temperature should be managed with ice packs, cold IV fluids, and cold water down the nasogastric tube. Patients should recover in the intensive care unit (ICU) to receive monitoring of arterial blood gas, electrolytes, creatinine kinase, myoglobin, and lactate levels. Patients should also be monitored for a recrudescence of MH that can occur within hours of the initial episode, as well as disseminated intravascular coagulation (DIC) and myoglobinuric renal failure, for which the patients should receive ample volume replacement.

The Malignant Hyperthermia Association of the United States (MHAUS) is a nonprofit organization that was created to educate the public, to counsel MH patients and their relatives about their condition, and to educate anesthesia and operating room personnel about the management of MH. A hotline is available to advise clinicians in the acute management of MH. Additional educational materials can be obtained by calling the hotline number, 1-800-MHHYPER (1-800-644-9737).

SUGGESTED READINGS

Barash, Paul G., Cullen Bruce F., Stoelting, Robert K. ed. *Clinical Anesthesia* 4th ed. Lippincott Williams and Wilkins, Philadelphia, 2001 pp. 521–530.

Collins, Chad P., Beirne, O. Ross. Concepts in the Prevention and Management of Malignant Hyperthermia. *Journal of Oral and Maxillofacial Surgery* 61:1340–1345; 2003.

McCarthy, E. Jane. Malignant Hyperthermia: Pathophysiology, Clinical Presentation, and Treatment. *American Association of Critical-Care Nurses* 15:231–237; 2004.

13

Remember that Amiodarone Causes Hypothyroidism

Benjamin S. Brooke, MD

Amiodarone has become a popular drug in the intensive care unit (ICU) because of its utility in the management of a broad spectrum of ventricular and atrial arrhythmias. As a class III antiarrhythmic agent, its mechanism of action is to delay repolarization and increase the duration of the action potential through inhibition of myocardial potassium ion channels. While very effective as an antiarrhythmic, amiodarone therapy is also associated with a wide array of adverse side effects involving the cornea, lungs, liver, skin, and thyroid. Although the majority of amiodarone's adverse effects on these organs result from deposition of the drug in the parenchyma, its effect on the thyroid gland is quite unique.

WATCH OUT FOR

Amiodarone bears a structural resemblance to the thyroid hormones thyroxine (T_4) and triiodothyronine (T_3), while containing approximately 37% iodine by weight. Metabolism of amiodarone causes deiodination, which results in the release of up to 50- to 100-fold excess iodine compared with normal daily intake. Amiodarone-induced thyroid dysfunction results from this massive increase in total iodine, as well as alterations in hormone metabolism caused by the drug. While amiodarone can cause either hyper- or hypothyroidism, it typically induces hypothyroidism in iodine-sufficient areas such as the United States where the incidence is estimated to range up to 30%. In particular, patients with preexisting thyroid autoimmunity are at increased risk for the development of hypothyroidism while receiving the drug. The acute effects observed after initiating therapy is an increase in thyroid-stimulating hormone (TSH) levels by 20% to 50%, with a decrease in serum T_3 levels by 15% to 20% within the first 2 weeks of therapy. Amiodarone blocks the peripheral conversion of T_4 to T_3 and inhibits the entry of these hormones into peripheral tissue. The resulting symptoms of hypothyroidism include cold intolerance, dry skin, weight gain, and fatigue. In the ICU, signs of hypothyroidism may also manifest when a patient is having difficulty weaning from mechanical ventilation. Once patients are diagnosed, treatment with levothyroxine should be initiated and amiodarone may be continued if a suitable replacement antiarrhythmic is not available.

Before starting patients in the ICU on amiodarone therapy, a careful examination of the thyroid should be performed along with baseline measurements of serum TSH, free T_4, T_3, and thyroid peroxidase and thyroglobulin antibodies. This will help detect underlying thyroid dysfunction and identify patients who may be more predisposed to develop thyroid dysfunction while on amiodarone. Thyroid function should thereafter be checked every 3 to 6 months while patients are continued on therapy.

SUGGESTED READINGS

Basaria S, Cooper DS. Amiodarone and the thyroid. Am J Med 2005;118:706–714.
Martino E, Bartalena L, Bogazzi F, et al. The effects of amiodarone on the thyroid. Endocr Rev 2001;22:240–254.

14

DO NOT USE AMIODARONE TO RATE CONTROL CHRONIC ATRIAL FIBRILLATION

BRADFORD D. WINTERS, MD, PHD

Chronic atrial fibrillation (A fib) has an incidence of 0.4% in the general population (approximately 10% of those more than 60 years of age) and many of these patients are admitted to intensive or intermediate care units for reasons unrelated to this diagnosis. Chronic A fib needs to be clearly differentiated from new-onset A fib since the treatment and management strategies will differ.

Since chronic A fib or paroxysmal A fib has a very low likelihood of converting to sinus rhythm and remaining in sinus, the primary strategy is rate control with agents that slow conduction through the atrioventricular (AV) node so that the patient does not experience a rapid ventricular response that may severely compromise cardiac output. Patients with A fib already have lost approximately 20% of their diastolic filling secondary to the loss of coordinated "atrial kick" at end diastole. A rapid heart rate that compromises diastolic filling time further can thus compromise cardiac output to the point of shock. This may especially be true with patients who have diastolic dysfunction secondary to aortic stenosis and chronic hypertension. Commonly used agents include beta-blockers or calcium channel blockers. Digoxin was a mainstay of treatment in the past but is much less commonly used currently.

WHAT NOT TO DO

Pharmacological rhythm control, that is, converting A fib to sinus rhythm, is not desirable in chronic A fib. Patients with chronic A fib may develop clot in the fibrillating atria, particularly in the atrial appendage. Sudden conversion to sinus may lead to an embolus that can result in a stroke, myocardial infarction, gut ischemia, or limb infarction. For this reason, patients with chronic A fib, especially if it is paroxysmal in nature, are usually on anticoagulation therapy to reduce the risk of developing atrial clot. Agents that promote conversion to sinus rhythm such as amiodarone and procainamide are not used to acutely treat chronic A fib.

Treatment and management of new-onset A fib falls into two primary approaches and practitioners vary as to which they subscribe to. The first, like chronic A fib, is rate control and the second is rhythm control. So long as the patient has not been in A fib for an extended period of time (generally more than 48 hours), the risk of having developed clot is judged to be low and conversion may be desirable. This may be achieved electrically with synchronized cardioversion or pharmacologically with amiodarone or other agents. However, the natural history of new-onset A fib is such that most patients (80%) will spontaneously convert on their own, usually within 2 weeks.

Several factors contribute to this, most notably the reasons most patients develop new-onset A fib. Postcardiac surgical patients have some of the highest rates of new-onset A fib (reportedly as high as 60%), presumably secondary to tissue damage associated with cannulation of the atrium during surgery. General surgical patients also have a high incidence of this condition (as high as 40% in noncardiac thoracic patients) secondary to a variety of factors including atrial stretch induced by hypervolemia and circulating catecholamines. Once these perturbations have resolved, so mostly does the A fib. Because of this, many advocate that rate control is perfectly adequate in new-onset A fib since it is usually a self-limiting phenomenon. Amiodarone, beta-blockers, and calcium channel blockers are good choices. Rate control may be the goal (amiodarone will slow the rate) but conversion, whether spontaneous or pharmacological, is likely to be sustained at which time the drug may be weaned off. For the unusual patient who remains in A fib, one must then determine whether to switch to chronic rate control with long-term anticoagulation or consider electrophysiological studies and possibly ablation therapy.

SUGGESTED READINGS

De Denus S, Sanoski CA, Carlsson J, et al. Rate vs rhythm control in patients with atrial fibrillation: a meta-analysis. Arch Intern Med 2005;165:258–262.
Nattel S, Opie LH. Controversies in atrial fibrillation. Lancet 2006;367:262–272.

15

EXERCISE CARE IN THE USE OF AMIODARONE AND ALTERNATIVE ANTIARRHYTHMICS FOR THE TREATMENT OF ATRIAL FIBRILLATION

MUHAMMAD I. DURRANI, MD
ALAN CHENG, MD

Atrial fibrillation is a common arrhythmia in the intensive care unit (ICU) setting. The mainstay of therapy is rate control, with beta-blockers being the first-line agent. However, frequently the decision is made to use rhythm-converting agents, such as amiodarone. Amiodarone is a complex antiarrhythmic agent (predominantly class III) that shares at least some of the properties of each of the other three Vaughn-Williams classes of antiarrhythmics. Amiodarone is commonly used for the treatment and prevention of persistent atrial and ventricular tachyarrhythmias, although it is only FDA approved for management of ventricular arrhythmias. It is one of the few agents that can be used safely in individuals with congestive heart failure. Contraindications to amiodarone include severe sinus node dysfunction with marked sinus bradycardia or syncope, second- or third-degree heart block, known hypersensitivity to its contents, cardiogenic shock, possibly severe chronic lung disease.

Amiodarone is highly lipid soluble, extensively distributed in the body, and highly concentrated in many tissues, especially in the liver and lungs. After variable (30% to 50%) and slow gastrointestinal absorption, amiodarone is very slowly eliminated, with a half-life of about 25 to 110 days. The onset of action after oral administration is delayed and a steady-state drug effect may not be established for several months unless large loading doses are used. It undergoes extensive hepatic metabolism to the pharmacologically active metabolite desethylamiodarone (DEA). Amiodarone is not excreted by the kidneys but rather by the lacrimal glands, the skin, and the biliary tract. Neither amiodarone nor DEA is dialyzable.

Amiodarone is both an antiarrhythmic and a potent vasodilator. Amiodarone lengthens the effective refractory period by prolonging the action potential duration in all cardiac muscles, including bypass tracts (class III activity). It also has a powerful class I antiarrhythmic effect that works by inhibiting inactivated sodium channels at high stimulation frequencies. Amiodarone slows phase 4 depolarization of the sinus node as well as conduction through the atrioventricular (AV) node. It also decreases Ca^{2+} current (class IV effect) and transient outward delayed rectifier and inward rectifier K^+ currents. Amiodarone noncompetitively blocks α- and β-adrenergic receptors (class II effect); this effect is additive to competitive receptor inhibition by beta-blockers.

There is a risk of hypotension with intravenous amiodarone administration, which is more common with rapid administration. Other notable acute effects include bradycardia, hypokalemia, interactions with medications such as warfarin (Coumadin) and digoxin, and rarely *torsades de pointes*. There is a risk of pulmonary toxicity with high doses starting with pneumonitis and leading to pulmonary fibrosis. Other organ systems affected by amiodarone therapy include thyroid (hypothyroidism or hyperthyroidism), central nervous system (proximal muscle weakness, peripheral neuropathy, and neural symptoms), gastrointestinal (nausea 25%, elevated liver functions), testicular dysfunction, corneal microdeposition, and photosensitive slate-gray or bluish skin discoloration.

Agents that can be considered as alternatives to amiodarone for the treatment of atrial fibrillation depend upon the patient's cardiac history, as individuals with reduced left ventricular systolic function are especially prone to the proarrhythmic effects of certain antiarrhythmic agents. Some commonly used alternatives include ibutilide, dofetilide, and sotalol. Strong consideration should be made for obtaining consultation with a cardiac electrophysiologist prior to initiating these agents.

Ibutilide prolongs repolarization by inhibition of the delayed rectifier potassium current (Ikr) and by selective enhancement of the slow inward sodium current. This drug is efficacious in the termination of atrial fibrillation (AF) and flutter with both single and repeated intravenous infusions. It is as effective as amiodarone in cardioversion of atrial fibrillation. The proarrhythmic effect resulting in *torsades de pointes* is higher in individuals with heart failure, those with bradycardia, nonwhite subjects, women, and those given the drug for atrial flutter rather than atrial fibrillation. The risk of this is greatest during or shortly after the infusion of the drug (within 1 hour) and rapidly wanes after administration since the half-life (2 to 12 hours) of this agent is short. The patient should be monitored for at least 4 hours after the start of the infusion.

Dofetilide prolongs the action potential and QT_C in a concentration-related manner. Dofetilide exerts its effects solely by inhibition of the rapid component of the delayed rectifier potassium current Ikr. Dofetilide has stronger evidence in its favor for acute cardioversion of atrial fibrillation than for maintenance thereafter, according to a meta-analysis. It can be given to patients with depressed function but needs to be initiated while being continuously monitored on telemetry for the first 3 days of therapy since this too has a risk of proarrhythmia-like ibutilide. The risk of *torsades de pointes* can be reduced by normal serum potassium and magnesium levels, predose adjustment of renal function, and postdose reduction based on QT_C (ideally baseline QT_C below 429 milliseconds). Administration of dofetilide requires that the hospital and the prescriber be trained as confirmed administrators.

Sotalol has combined class II and class III properties and is active against a variety of arrhythmias and has the ability to produce profound bradycardia or prolongation of the QT interval. Of the many indications, sotalol is most commonly used for maintenance of sinus rhythm after cardioversion for atrial fibrillation and reducing ventricular tachyarrhythmias. Despite its ability to prevent tachyarrhythmias, sotalol can also be proarrhythmic (as with any other antiarrhythmic) through its ability to profoundly prolong the QT interval. As a result, initiation of this drug should occur while the patient is closely monitored. Sotalol is contraindicated in patients with reduced creatinine clearance (below 40 mL/minute) and asthma. It should be avoided in patients with serious conduction defects, in bronchospastic disease, and when there are evident risks of proarrhythmia.

SUGGESTED READINGS

Miller MR, McNamara RL, Segal JB, et al. Efficacy of agents for pharmacologic conversion of atrial fibrillation and subsequent maintenance of sinus rhythm: a meta-analysis of clinical trials. J Fam Pract 2000;49:1033–1046.

Opie LH, Gersh BJ, eds. Drugs for the Heart. 6th Ed. Philadelphia: Elsevier; 2005:218–274.

Tikosyn. Pfizer. http://www.tikosyn.com

16

BE AWARE THAT FUROSEMIDE CONTAINS A SULFA MOIETY

ARDALAN MINOKADEH, BS
ANUSHIRVAN MINOKADEH, MD

Furosemide (Lasix) is a member of the general class of *loop diuretics* that inhibit the $Na^+/K^+/2Cl^-$ cotransport carrier within the ascending limb of the loop of Henle. The decrease in sodium and chloride reabsorption seems to come from the fact that furosemide competes for the chloride position on the carrier. Although all loop diuretics have the same primary mechanism of action, furosemide has been shown to additionally inhibit sodium and chloride reabsorption in the distal renal tubule. It is important to note the additional decrease in calcium reabsorption because calcium transport in the loop of Henle is directly related to the gradient established by the movement of sodium and chloride. It has a wide range of clinical uses including treatment of hypertension, congestive heart failure, and hyperkalemia.

SIGNS AND SYMPTOMS

Clinically, a controversial issue in the administration of furosemide is the incidence of cross-reactivity with sulfonamide-containing antibiotics because of the sulfonamide moiety that furosemide contains (*Fig. 16.1*). The clinical issue centers on the administration of furosemide to a patient with documented sulfa allergy. Opinions differ on the believed hypersensitivity cross-reaction that may manifest itself as anaphylaxis, dermatitis, urticaria, eczema, Stevens-Johnson syndrome, rash, or fever within 30 days, but current literature states that the lack of published clinical evidence for the allergic reactions is noteworthy. The authors of a recently published review of the literature on this topic state that much of the evidence used to provide support for the theory is in fact not conclusive and does not implicate appropriate causation. Detractors of the belief of a legitimate cross-reactivity also cite that sulfonamide nonantibiotics lack the aromatic amine group at the N4 position of sulfonamide-containing antibiotics, believed to be the cause of sulfonamide antibiotic hypersensitivity.

A retrospective study was performed to determine if furosemide produced allergic cross-reactions in patients who reported sulfa allergies. The authors did not find sufficient evidence to implicate a reported sulfa allergy in producing severe reactions. It is also the opinion

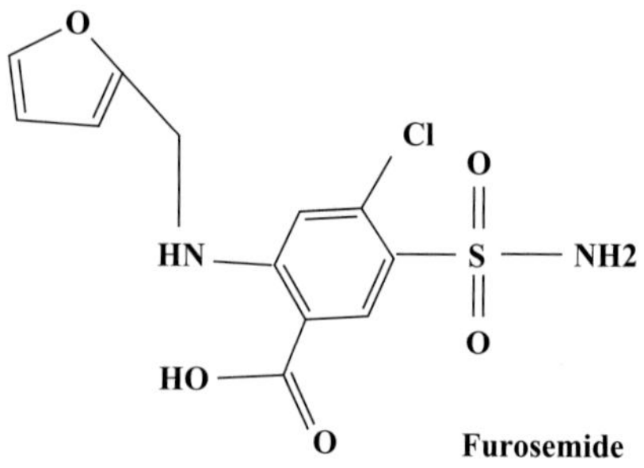

FIGURE 16.1. Chemical Structure

of some authors that the risk of reactions is so low that if alternative nonsulfa treatments are unavailable, administration of a drug such as furosemide with monitoring is warranted. Physicians who wish to provide an alternate drug to patients about whom they may be concerned could consider ethacrynic acid, a loop diuretic that does not contain a sulfa moiety.

SUGGESTED READINGS

Lee A, Anderson R, Kardon R, et al. Presumed "sulfa allergy" in patients with intracranial hypertension treated with acetazolamide or furosemide: cross reactivity, myth or reality? Am J Ophthal 2004;138:114–118.

Johnson K, Green D, Rife J, et al. Sulfonamide cross-reactivity: fact or fiction? Ann Pharmacother 2005;39:290–301.

Sullivan TJ. Cross-reactions among furosemide, hydrochlorothiazide, and sulfonamides [Letter]. JAMA 1991;265:120–121.

17

CAREFULLY OBSERVE THE CLINICAL RESPONSE TO INTERMITTENT FUROSEMIDE DOSING WHEN DECIDING ON ADDITIONAL DOSES

MELISSA S. CAMP, MD

Furosemide is a loop diuretic that acts by inhibiting the reabsorption of sodium and chloride (via the $Na/K/2Cl$ cotransporter) in the thick ascending limb of the loop of Henle. It enhances the excretion of sodium, potassium, calcium, chloride, and water. Furosemide is used frequently in the intensive care unit (ICU) setting for diuresis.

Intravenous furosemide begins to work in 5 minutes, peaks at 30 minutes, and lasts for about 2 hours. The elimination half-life is approximately 30 to 120 minutes. A dosing interval of 6 hours allows for four to five half-lives of elimination. Typically, with the appropriate dose of IV furosemide, a maximal response will be seen within the first hour and the increased urine output will continue in a tapering fashion for up to 6 hours. A large initial response followed by a rapid tapering of urine output may be an indication that the patient is not quite ready for diuresis.

The dose of furosemide is titrated to effect, but the dose depends on renal function. Higher doses are needed with worsening renal function. Furosemide acts in the loop of Henle, so the effect seen after a dose of furosemide depends on the rate at which blood is filtered through the glomerulus. As creatinine clearance decreases (implying lower glomerular filtration rate [GFR] and worse renal function), a higher dose of furosemide is needed to achieve a timely response. If the dose of furosemide administered is too low for a given creatinine clearance, then a delayed diuretic response can be seen.

WATCH OUT FOR

The main toxicities of furosemide include ototoxicity, electrolyte abnormalities, and allergic reactions. Ototoxicity is more common with very high doses of furosemide and the mechanism is thought to be due to the presence of a similar $Na/K/2Cl$ cotransporter in the inner ear. Electrolyte abnormalities from the diuresis induced by furosemide include hypokalemia, hyponatremia, and metabolic alkalosis. Overly aggressive diuresis can lead to elevated blood urea nitrogen (BUN) and creatinine as well as hypotension. The presence of allergic reactions to furosemide do occur; however, many clinicians doubt the existence of a true sulfa allergic reaction. Purported allergic reactions can be as mild as a rash or as serious as anaphylaxis or Stevens-Johnson syndrome.

One final note is that when thinking about the clinical effects of furosemide, the astute clinician will remember that the brand name was chosen in part based on the duration of the medication lasting six hours; hence, the name _La-six_.

SUGGESTED READINGS

Micromedex. Martindale—The Complete Drug Reference: Furosemide. USP DI Drug Information for the Health Care Professional: Diuretics, Loop http://www.thomsonhc.com/hcs/librarian.

Rose B. Optimal dosage and side effects of loop diuretics. UpToDate. 2005. http://www.uptodate.com/physicians/pulmonology_toclist.asp

18

DO NOT ADMINISTER METHYLENE BLUE IF THERE IS POSSIBLE GASTROINTESTINAL ABSORPTION

BEVERLY J. NEWHOUSE, MD
ANUSHIRVAN MINOKADEH, MD

Methylene blue is a water-soluble blue thiazine dye used most commonly as a treatment for methemoglobinemia or as an indicator dye. Its utility as an indicator dye has been applied to several clinical situations including identification of aspiration or placement of nasogastric tubes in critically ill patients; localization of parathyroid adenomas; testing of the integrity of the biliary system during hepatic surgery; and testing of the integrity of ureteral or bladder anastomoses. Additional applications of methylene blue include its use as a urinary antiseptic, reversal for chemotherapy-induced encephalopathy, a topical agent to photoinactivate viruses, an experimental cytotoxic agent for tumor cells, and a vasopressor in patients with septic or anaphylactic shock or for patients undergoing the reperfusion phase of liver transplantation.

Treatment of methemoglobinemia is the most common clinical use of methylene blue. Methemoglobin is the oxidized form of hemoglobin, created when the iron moiety changes from Fe^{2+} to Fe^{3+}. This form of hemoglobin cannot bind O_2 or CO_2 and therefore loses its oxygen-carrying capacity and transport function, predisposing the patient to hypoxemia. Drug-induced causes of methemoglobinemia include local anesthetics (e.g., prilocaine and benzocaine) and nitrates (e.g., nitroglycerin and nitroprusside). Methylene blue, administered slowly at a dose of 1 to 2 mg/kg intravenously (IV) with a maximum dose of 7 mg/kg, is converted in vivo to leukomethylene blue, which reduces methemoglobin back to hemoglobin. Nicotinamide adenine dinucleotide phosphate (NADPH) is essential in the conversion to leukomethylene blue and thus, IV methylene blue administration is contraindicated in those with low endogenous NADPH (i.e., glucose-6-phosphate dehydrogenase [G6PD] deficiency). Without this NADPH-dependent conversion, the use of methylene blue can lead to hemolytic anemia and exacerbation of methemoglobinemia. Similarly, if too high a dose of methylene blue is given or it is given too quickly, high concentrations can accumulate and saturate the reducing pathway such that methylene blue will act as an oxidizing agent and paradoxically create more methemoglobin.

SIGNS AND SYMPTOMS

Although the risks of IV administration of methylene blue were well known, the use of this substance enterally was thought to be relatively benign. However, the U.S. Food and Drug Administration (FDA) has recently become concerned about enteral exposure to methylene blue and has issued a warning against using it in this situation. This is based, in part, on the reported cases of toxicity (including death) associated with enteral exposure of a very similar dye, FD&C Blue No.1 (Blue 1). In most of these cases, the patients had a history of sepsis. The FDA concluded that patients at risk of increased intestinal permeability (e.g., patients with cancer, sepsis, burns, renal failure, celiac sprue, or inflammatory bowel disease) were at risk for mitochondrial toxicity. Signs and symptoms of mitochondrial toxicity include nausea, vomiting, abdominal pain, fever, sudden weight loss, dizziness, headache, precordial pain, tachycardia, hypertension, dyspnea, profuse sweating, restlessness, tremors, and confusion. Untreated, mitochondrial toxicity can result in myopathy, neuropathy, lipoatrophy, hemolytic anemia, hypoxemia, arrhythmias, hepatic steatosis, liver failure, lactic acidosis, and refractory hypotension.

SUGGESTED READINGS

Clifton J, Leikin JB. Methylene blue. Amer J Ther 2003;10:289–291.

FDA Public Health Advisory: Reports of blue discoloration and death in patients receiving enteral feedings tinted with the dye, FD&C Blue No. 1. U.S. Food and Drug Administration; 2003. http://www.cfsan.fda.gov/~dms/col-ltr2.html

Nguyen ST, Cabrales RE, Bashour CA, et al. Benzocaine-induced methemoglobinemia. Anesth Analg 2000;90(2):369–371.

Reed DN, Vitale GC, Wrightson WR, et al. Decreasing mortality of bile leaks after elective hepatic surgery. Am J Surg 2003;185(4):316–318.

19

BE ALERT FOR METABOLIC ACIDOSIS IN PATIENTS ON LORAZEPAM DRIPS

YASIR M. AKMAL, MD

Lorazepam (Ativan) is a frequently used sedative in the intensive care unit (ICU). It is a benzodiazepine that can be administered enterally, as intermittent parenteral doses, or as a continuous infusion. The beneficial effects include anterograde amnesia and an opioid-sparing effect via a moderation of the anticipatory pain response. However, it is not a benign drug and side effects include respiratory depression, tolerance, withdrawal, paradoxical agitation, and prolonged elimination.

SIGNS AND SYMPTOMS

One of the carrier molecules of lorazepam is propylene glycol. This has been implicated as the cause of hyperosmolar metabolic acidosis in ICU patients on continuous infusions of lorazepam. About 12% to 45% of propylene glycol is excreted unchanged in the urine, with the remainder metabolized by the liver. Therefore, caution should be exerted when administering lorazepam in patients with renal or hepatic dysfunction. Toxicity from propylene glycol has also been seen with administration of other drugs that use it as a carrier or solvent such as phenytoin, etomidate, nitroglycerin, and diazepam (*Table 19.1*). Other effects of propylene glycol include renal dysfunction, intravascular hemolysis, cardiac arrhythmias, seizures, and central nervous system (CNS) depression. Fortunately, these metabolic derangements appear to correct after discontinuing the infusion of lorazepam.

It is important to note that the upper limit of lorazepam dosing is 0.1 mg/kg/hr, which is about 7 to 10 mg/hr as an infusion for a 70- to 100-kg patient. Each milliliter of lorazepam contains about 0.8 mL (830 mg) of propylene glycol, which has a recommended daily allowance of 25 mg/kg/day. The dose of propylene glycol required for toxicity has not been well established and accumulation has been described over a wide range of lorazepam doses. Also, toxicity has been seen with serum propylene glycol concentrations of 12 to 130 mg/dL and infusion periods ranging from 2 to 24 days. The main factors that appear to be related to toxicity are rate of infusion, length of infusion, and degree of osmolar gap (*Table 19.2*).

| TABLE 19.1 | PROPYLENE GLYCOL CONTENT IN SELECTED DRUGS | |

DRUG	AMOUNT OF PROPYLENE GLYCOL (% V/V)
Lorazepam, 2 mg/mL	80
Phenobarbital, 30–130 mg/mL	67.8–75
Diazepam, 5 mg/mL	40
Phenytoin, 50 mg/mL	40
Trimethoprim-sulfamethoxazole, 16:80 mg/mL	40
Etomidate, 2 mg/mL	35
Nitroglycerin, 5 mg/mL	30

Modified from Arroliga AC, Shehab N, McCarthy K, et al. Relationship of continuous infusion lorazepam to serum propylene glycol concentration in critically ill adults. *Crit Care Med*. 2004; 32(8):1709–1714. Table 1.

| TABLE 19.2 | CALCULATION OF OSMOL GAP |

Osmol gap = (measured osmolality) – (calculated osmolality)
Calculated osmolality = (12 × sodium) + (glucose/18) + (blood urea nitrogen/2.8)

| TABLE 19.3 | DOSING AND HALF-LIFE OF ACTION OF SELECTED SEDATIVES | | | |

DRUG	ONSET AFTER IV DOSE	HALF-LIFE OF PARENT COMPOUND	INTERMITTENT IV DOSE	INFUSION DOSE RANGE
Lorazepam	5–20 min	8–15 hr	0.02–0.06 mg/kg q 2–6 hr	0.01–0.1 mg/kg/hr
Diazepam	2–5 min	20–120 hr	0.03–0.1 mg/kg q 0.5–6 hr	—
Midazolam	2–5 min	3–11 hr	0.02–0.08 mg/kg q 0.5–2 hr	0.04–0.2 g/kg/hr
Propofol	1–2 min	26–32 hr	—	5–80 μg/kg/min
Haloperidol	3–20 min	18–54 hr	0.03–0.15 mg/kg q 0.5–6 hr	0.04–0.15 mg/kg/hr

Modified from Jacobi J, Fraser GL, Coursin DB, et al. Clinical practice guidelines for the sustained use of sedatives and analgesics in the critically ill adult. *Crit Care Med*. 2002;30(1):119–141. Table 3.

Alternative sedative drugs to lorazepam include midazolam, propofol, and haloperidol. The half-life and dosing regimens of some of these drugs are shown in *Table 19.3*. Because of the side effects and often unpredictable wake-up time associated with benzodiazepines and other sedatives, the agent used should be tailored to each individual patient.

SUGGESTED READINGS

Arroliga AC, Shehab N, McCarthy K, et al. Relationship of continuous infusion lorazepam to serum propylene glycol concentration in critically ill adults. Crit Care Med 2004; 32(8):1709–1714.

Jacobi J, Fraser GL, Coursin DB, et al. Clinical practice guidelines for the sustained use of sedatives and analgesics in the critically ill adult. Crit Care Med 2002;30:119–141.

Wilson KC, Reardon C, Theodore AC, et al. Propylene glycol toxicity: a severe iatrogenic illness in ICU patients receiving IV benzodiazepines: a case series and prospective, observational pilot study. Chest 2005;128:1674–1681.

20

BE ALERT FOR THE DEVELOPMENT OF CYANIDE TOXICITY WHEN ADMINISTERING NITROPRUSSIDE.

E. DAVE BRAVOS, MD

Hypertension is commonly seen in the perioperative setting as well as the intensive care unit (ICU). There are many agents to lower blood pressure with different mechanisms of action. One of the most potent vasodilators is sodium nitroprusside, which causes arteriolar and venous smooth muscle relaxation via nitric oxide–mediated mechanisms. It has a rapid onset and relatively short duration of action, making it a readily titratable agent. However, its dose must be limited because of its potential toxic side effects.

Toxicity from sodium nitroprusside is due to the cyanide groups released from metabolism of the nitroprusside molecule. After gaining an electron from the iron moiety of hemoglobin, the sodium nitroprusside produces an unstable radical and methemoglobin. The unstable nitroprusside radical produces five cyanide ions, which can have one of three fates. They can interact with methemoglobin to produce cyanomethemoglobin. They can produce thiosulfate and its end product thiocyanate. Additionally, cyanide ions can bind cytochrome oxidase and ultimately inhibit oxidative metabolism, leading to cyanide toxicity. Organs most susceptible to the effects of loss of oxidative metabolism are the heart and brain.

Clinically, patients with cyanide toxicity may exhibit altered mental status, cardiovascular instability, and an anion gap metabolic acidosis. Initially, patients may present with sinus tachycardia that may progress to sinus bradycardia or ventricular dysrhythmias and even asystole. Patients begin to have restlessness and agitation when the central nervous system is affected. With worsening toxicity, convulsions may occur and can ultimately lead to encephalopathy and coma. With loss of aerobic metabolism there is an increase in lactate, leading to an anion gap metabolic acidosis.

WHAT TO DO

Treatment of cyanide toxicity begins with discontinuation of nitroprusside administration. Patients should concomitantly be placed on supplemental oxygen and may even require mechanical ventilation. Additionally, thiosulfate and sodium nitrate (to convert hemoglobin to methemoglobin) can be given to increase the kinetics of the other two metabolic pathways, resulting in less cyanide to bind to cytochrome oxidase. Prevention of cyanide toxicity can be achieved by limiting the dose of nitroprusside to less than 8.0 micrograms/kg/min over 1 to 3 hours. Additionally, thiosulfate can be given concomitantly with the nitroprusside.

It is important to note that nitroprusside has multiple effects on organ systems. Given that nitroprusside relaxes arteriolar venous smooth muscle, there is a decrease in afterload as well as preload. This can reflexively cause an increase in heart rate and contractility. However, cardiac output is usually not affected given the decrease in preload as well. An intracoronary steal syndrome may occur in areas where there is coronary artery disease and inability to further dilate these diseased vessels compared with nondiseased vessels. Effects on the cerebral vasculature can cause an increase in cerebral blood flow and ultimately in intracranial pressure. Dilatation of the pulmonary vasculature also occurs. This can increase shunt fraction by preventing hypoxic pulmonary vasoconstriction. Renal activation of the renin-angiotensin system and catecholamine release can occur with a decrease in arterial blood pressure, which can cause rebound hypertension with discontinuation of nitroprusside.

Finally, alternate agents to nitroprusside include other vasodilators such as nitroglycerin and hydralazine. Additionally, other classes of agent such as ACE inhibitors, alpha-blockers, or calcium channel blockers may be used to control hypertension.

SUGGESTED READINGS

Morgan GE. Clinical Anesthesiology. 3rd Ed. New York: Lange/McGraw-Hill; 2002: 225–227.
Stoelting RK, ed. Pharmacology and Physiology in Anesthetic Practice. 4th Ed. Philadelphia: Lippincott-Raven; 2006:321–337.

21

ADMINISTER BETA-BLOCKADE INITIALLY BEFORE ADMINISTERING "OTHER" ANTIHYPERTENSIVES WHEN TREATING AORTIC DISSECTION

ERIC S. WEISS, MD

ERIC S. WEISS, MD

SIGNS AND SYMPTOMS

CASE

A 44-year-old man whose only past medical history consists of hypertension and unilateral cataracts presents to his local emergency department with the acute onset of severe "tearing" chest pain radiating to his back. On exam the physician notes that the patient is 6 feet 8 inches tall with long, lanky fingers. The patient states that everyone in his family has been tall and lanky like him. His initial pulse rate is 105 and his blood pressure reads 185/95. His electrocardiogram shows no ST-segment changes and initial laboratory tests show no abnormalities with a blood urea nitrogen level of 11 mg/dL and creatinine of 0.8 mg/dL. A computed tomography (CT) with intravenous contrast shows a 6-cm dilated descending thoracic aortic aneurysm with a dissection flap present. He is immediately transported to the surgical intensive care unit (SICU) for management. In the SICU, the on-call resident orders hydralazine for blood pressure control. His heart rate climbs to 126 and his systolic blood pressure drops to 145 mm Hg. Over the next 6 hours, despite these maneuvers, his pain does not improve and he becomes progressively tachycardic and hypotensive, initially responding to fluid but then requiring vasopressor support. Repeat laboratory analysis shows a serum lactate of 5.0 and a rising serum creatine to 1.8 mg/dL. During this time he stops making urine and his abdomen becomes tender and progressively distended. He also develops a metabolic acidosis with a pH of 7.20, requiring intubation and mechanical ventilation for his increased work of breathing. Immediate abdominal CT shows propagation of the dissection to involve the abdominal aorta with visceral vessel involvement and pneumatosis of the small intestine. He is immediately taken to the operating room but at this point requires massive vasopressor support and is profoundly acidotic. Direct visualization inside the abdomen shows diffusely necrotic bowel. Approximately 45 minutes into the operation the patient suffers a cardiac arrest and despite cardiopulmonary resuscitation and administration of code drugs, the patient expires on the operating room table.

DISCUSSION

The preceding case illustrates the necessity of treating acute aortic dissections with beta-blockade concomitantly with vasodilatory antihypertensives. The patient described had the inherited connective tissue disorder Marfan syndrome with the classic presentation of an acute aortic dissection heralded by the acute onset of chest or back pain. The patient received adequate antihypertensive therapy but continued to deteriorate because of the failure to initiate beta-blockade.

To briefly review, aortic dissections can be classified according to the Stanford classification as type A (those involving the ascending aorta) and type B (those involving only the descending aorta).

Elective operative repair is preferable as mortality rates from urgent operative procedures for aortic dissection range between 2% and 21%. Indications for operative repair include type A dissections with or without ulcers and type B dissections with visceral involvement or large, open free-flowing false lumens. When urgent surgery is not indicated, management consists of pain control and blood pressure lowering to a target of 110 mm Hg systolic. This is usually accomplished with sodium nitroprusside, but beta-blockade is *imperative* because the pulsatile force must also be minimized with appropriate beta-blockade so as to not propagate the dissection, and beta-blockers decrease wall stress. Vasodilators by themselves can lead to reflex tachycardia, which can increase shear stress and propagate the intimal tear.

SUGGESTED READING

Mukherjee D, Eagle KA. Aortic dissection: an update. Curr Probl Cardiol 2005;30:287–325.

22

DO NOT USE VASOPRESSIN IN PATIENTS WITH HEART FAILURE OR MESENTERIC ISCHEMIA

BENJAMIN S. BROOKE, MD

Vasopressin is the exogenous, parenteral form of antidiuretic hormone (ADH) that may be used for several conditions in the intensive care unit (ICU), including the treatment of central diabetes insipidus and as a vasopressor agent in shock. Endogenous vasopressin is an important stress hormone and plays a critical role in maintaining volume hemostasis. However, its beneficial physiological effects may be offset when there is excess hormone in the circulation. It is important to understand vasopressin's mechanism of action and to be able to recognize which ICU patients may suffer adverse effects from the use of this drug.

Endogenous vasopressin is synthesized in neurosecretory cells of the hypothalamus and excreted by the posterior pituitary gland in response to decreases in blood volume and increases in serum osmolality. Receptors for vasopressin are primarily located in vascular smooth muscle (V_1) and the renal collecting duct (V_2) and act to stimulate vasoconstriction and increase free water reabsorption, respectively. These are normal compensatory mechanisms designed to maintain vascular tone and circulatory homeostasis during periods of low cardiac output.

WATCH OUT FOR

In patients with congestive heart failure, however, chronic activation of this neurohormonal axis contributes to the progression of disease through an increase in afterload and water retention. Moreover, giving vasopressin infusions to patients with existing heart failure will cause an acute increase in systemic vascular resistance and pulmonary capillary wedge pressure, possibly resulting in a further decrease in cardiac output. Therefore, caution should be used when administering exogenous vasopressin in patients with known heart failure in the ICU.

Another adverse effect of excessive vasopressin in the circulation is the potential for mesenteric hypoperfusion. When vasopressin stimulates the contraction of vascular smooth muscle, this effect is often most prominent in the capillaries and small arterioles or venules of the splanchnic circulation. This vasoconstriction can cause a major redistribution of blood flow away from the bowel mucosa that can result in ischemia and produce its associated signs, including hyperlactatemia. Along with the concurrent decrease in cardiac output and global oxygen delivery, high doses of exogenous vasopressin may produce or exacerbate mesenteric ischemia and has been shown to increase gut pCO_2 in tonometry studies.

In order to avoid detrimental reductions in mesenteric blood flow associated with vasopressin, other vasopressors should be considered first-line agents in shock. This includes norepinephrine, epinephrine, and dopamine, which do not compromise regional blood flow or tissue oxygenation at normal levels. Vasopressin should be used only as a supplementary vasopressor to these agents at a continuous low-dose infusion (≤ 0.04 U/min) and should not be titrated as a single agent.

One final note is that vasopressin analogue desmopressin (DDAVP) is the treatment of choice for central diabetes insipidus, given that it has a longer duration of action and causes less stimulation of smooth muscle than vasopressin.

SUGGESTED READINGS

Chatterjee K. Neurohormonal activation in congestive heart failure and the role of vasopressin. Am J Cardiol 2005;95:8B–13B.
Holmes CL, Walley KR. Vasopressin in the ICU. Curr Opin Crit Care 2004;10:442–448.

23

REMEMBER THAT CARDIAC PRESSORS DO NOT WORK IN A LOW-pH ENVIRONMENT

BRADFORD D. WINTERS, MD, PhD

Critically ill patients often require inotropic and/or pressor support to maintain adequate cardiac output and adequate blood pressure to sustain end-organ perfusion. Because end-organ perfusion has already likely been compromised and may continue to be problematic despite use of these agents, anaerobic metabolism rather than aerobic metabolism is likely to be generating a limited amount adenosine triphosphate (ATP) in the hypoperfused tissues. The consequence is lactic acid production and acidosis. Additionally, critically ill patients may have other causes of acidosis contributing to the overall acidotic state including renal failure, hyperchloremia, or ketoacidosis. The acidosis may be severe with pH values well below 7.0.

Binding of the inotropic or pressor agents to their receptors is influenced by pH, along with other factors such as temperature and concentration. Presumably, the greater the deviation in either direction from the optimal pH for the drug-ligand interaction, the less binding that will occur and hence, the less the effect of the drug. This has led to the widely held opinion that inotropes and vasopressors don't work at the acidic pH values often encountered in critically ill patients. The actual relationship is much more complex since the target of the inotropes and vasopressors, the alpha and beta adrenergic receptors, includes several subtypes whose individual responsiveness to these agents is quite variable under acidic conditions.

WATCH OUT FOR

The variability in responsiveness stems from not only changes in affinity for binding to the receptors but also because acidic conditions have been shown to change receptor numbers on cell surfaces as well as alter the downstream regulation mediated by G-coupled proteins. Some receptors are upregulated while their binding affinity may drop. Others exhibit no change in their affinity or overall responsiveness to inotropes and vasopressors. Still others increase their responsiveness. Different blood vessels in different tissue beds also are highly variable in their responsiveness since the predominant population of the receptor subtype present varies with the site and even caliber of the vessel. The degree of pH change influences these results dramatically. Mild acidemia actually stimulates the sympathetic nervous system output, increasing ventricular function and vasomotor tone. As the acidemia becomes more severe, changes in ligand binding and pharmacological effect of circulating catecholamines may become more prominent. The final clinical effect will be a balance between the two competing phenomena. Overall, pH values as low as 7.15 do not have an appreciable clinical effect on the activity of these drugs. Below this value, however, reductions in overall effectiveness may become clinically apparent.

It is often noted that when bicarbonate is given, blood pressure improves and vasopressors can be titrated. One explanation for this benefit is that an ampule of sodium bicarbonate acts as a hypertonic fluid bolus expanding plasma volume. Additionally, the change in pH alone can have effects on vasomotor tone separate from any effects on drug binding and this may be prominent when a certain pH threshold is crossed. Treatment of an acidotic pH with bicarbonate, with the goal of improving inotrope and vasopressor effectiveness, should be reserved for when the pH is below 7.1. Other reasons for wanting to correct the acidosis when the pH is above this value may exist (such as facilitating weaning from a mechanical ventilator) but significant improvement in the effectiveness of inotropes and vasopressors with bicarbonate administration should not be expected at less acidotic pH values. As always, simply relying on bicarbonate infusion to correct pH should not alter an aggressive search for and treatment of the underlying cause of the acidosis.

SUGGESTED READINGS

Cooper DJ, Walley KR, Wiggs BR, et al. Bicarbonate does not improve hemodynamics in critically ill patients who have lactic acidosis: a prospective controlled clinical study. Ann Intern Med 1990;112:492.

Hall JB, Schmidt GA, Wood LD. Principles of Critical Care Medicine. 3rd Ed. New York: McGraw-Hill; 2005:1954–1965.

24

CONSIDER THROMBOLYTICS IN ST-ELEVATION MYOCARDIAL INFARCTION IF PERCUTANEOUS CORONARY INTERVENTION IS NOT AVAILABLE OR DELAYED

JULIUS CUONG PHAM, MD

CASE

Mr. AMI is a 66-year-old male who is postoperative day number one after hip replacement surgery and complains of acute onset of chest pain and shortness of breath. An electrocardiogram (ECG) is performed that shows new ST-segment elevation in leads II, III, and aVF. You are alone in Community General Hospital, which does not have a percutaneous coronary intervention (PCI) team. As you begin treatment, you recall that Good Heart University Hospital has a PCI team and that door-to-catheterization-table time from your hospital to theirs is 90 minutes. You administer oxygen, nitroglycerin, morphine, aspirin, metoprolol, and heparin and contemplate your next step.

DISCUSSION

ST-elevation myocardial infarction (STEMI) is a myocardial infarction usually associated with acute plaque rupture and occlusion of a coronary artery. In addition to the therapies described earlier, patients with STEMI require immediate reperfusion therapy. This can be achieved with either thrombolytic therapy or percutaneous coronary intervention. Upon identification of STEMI, the practitioner should consider the following.

General Guidelines

1. Generally, thrombolytics are more effective if given earlier. If presentation is within 3 hours from symptom onset, there is no preference between thrombolytic or percutaneous coronary intervention therapy. After 3 hours PCI (when available) is preferred over thrombolytics.
2. Generally, when the risk of mortality is high, PCI is preferred over thrombolytics.
3. The higher the patient's risk of bleeding with thrombolytic therapy, the more strongly the decision should favor PCI.
4. When the differences in time for door to balloon and door to needle is less than 1 hour, PCI is preferred.

Indications for Thrombolytic Therapy (All Required)

1. Symptoms of myocardial ischemia
2. ST elevation greater than 0.1 mV in at least two contiguous leads or new left bundle branch block on presenting ECG
3. Onset of symptoms within 12 hours
4. Presentation in a facility without capability of percutaneous coronary intervention within 90 minutes or prolonged transport (>1 hour) to such a facility

Contraindications to Thrombolytics

1. Any prior intracranial hemorrhage
2. Known cerebral vascular lesion
3. Known malignant intracranial neoplasm
4. Ischemic stroke within 3 months
5. Suspected aortic dissection
6. Active bleeding or bleeding diathesis (except menses)
7. Significant closed head or facial injury within 3 months

Relative Contraindications to Thrombolytics

1. History of chronic, severe, or poorly controlled hypertension
2. Severe uncontrolled hypertension on presentation (systolic blood pressure >180 mm Hg or diastolic blood pressure >110 mm Hg)
3. History of prior ischemic stroke greater than 3 months, dementia, or known intracranial pathology not covered in contraindications
4. Recent traumatic or prolonged cardiopulmonary resuscitation or major surgery (<3 weeks)
5. Recent (2 to 4 weeks) internal bleeding
6. Noncompressible vascular punctures
7. For streptokinase or anistreplase: prior exposure (>5 days ago) or prior allergic reaction
8. Pregnancy
9. Active peptic ulcer
10. Current use of anticoagulants: the higher the international normalized ratio (INR), the higher the risk of bleeding

Choice of Agents. Thrombolytic agents are all plasminogen activators. They function enzymatically to produce the active compound plasmin from plasminogen. Plasmin functions in the breakdown of thrombus. Three agents are approved for treatment of STEMI. Both reteplase and tenecteplase have the advantage of being bolus administered.

1. Altepase: 100 mg over 90 minutes

2. Reteplase: 10 units × 2, each over 2 minutes
3. Tenecteplase: 30 to 50 mg (depending on weight) bolus

After administration of thrombolytic therapy, the pattern of ST elevation should be monitored over the next 60 to 90 minutes. If signs and symptoms of reperfusion do not occur (relief of symptoms, maintenance or restoration of hemodynamic stability, electrical stability, reduction in initial ST-segment elevation), rescue PCI should be considered.

Before hospital discharge, patients who have had a STEMI and thrombolytic therapy require further risk stratification. This includes structural evaluation echocardiography (ECG) and functional evaluation (stress testing) to determine the need for catheterization and revascularization.

SUGGESTED READINGS

Antman EM, Anbe DT, Armstrong PW, et al. ACC/AHA guidelines for the management of patients with ST-elevation myocardial infarction: executive summary. A report of the American College of Cardiology/American Heart Association Task Force on Practice Guidelines (Writing Committee to revise the 1999 guidelines for the management of patients with acute myocardial infarction). J Am Coll Cardiol 2004;44:671–719.

Tintinalli J, Kelen G, Stapczynski S, eds. Emergency Medicine: A Comprehensive Study Guide. 5th Ed. New York: McGraw-Hill; 2000:366–374.

25

CONSIDER THE USE OF GLYCOPROTEIN IIb/IIIa INHIBITORS IN UNSTABLE CORONARY SYNDROMES

ANDREW L. ROSENBERG, MD

Current treatments for acute coronary syndromes including unstable angina and non–ST-elevation myocardial infarction now include agents aimed at inhibiting platelet activation, adhesion, and aggregation with fibrinogen cross-linking. Two classes of drugs exist that inhibit these platelet effects at the level of the glycoprotein (GP) IIb/IIIa receptor on the platelet surface membrane. The first group are the thienopyridines (clopidogrel and ticlopidine). These drugs block GP IIb/IIIa complex activation by inhibiting adenosine diphosphate (ADP) binding to the platelet receptor. These oral agents have a slower onset and longer-term treatment duration. The CURE, TARGET, CREDO, and STAIG trials have demonstrated a 21% to 46% improvement in primary cardiac end points attributed to the addition of a thienopyridine. Significant benefits were demonstrated with the addition of clopidogrel to aspirin among patients undergoing percutaneous coronary interventions (PCI) (4.5 % versus 6.4% cardiovascular death, myocardial infarction, or urgent revascularization).

The second group of drugs are the direct GP IIb/IIIa antibodies or receptor antagonists (abciximab, tirofiban, and eptifibatide). These drugs inhibit the final pathway of platelet aggregation via fibrinogen cross-linking. Abciximab is a monoclonal antibody with a high affinity for both activated and resting platelets, whereas eptifibatide and tirofiban are nonantibody receptor inhibitors with less affinity for resting platelets and much faster dissociation rates (shorter half-lives) than abciximab. Meta-analysis of several large clinical trials (PRISM, PURSUIT, PARAGON, CAPTURE, and GUSTO-IV) has suggested only a modest 12% overall survival benefit attributable to the use of direct GP IIb/IIIa inhibitors when added to other therapeutics in acute coronary syndromes. Several subpopulations of high-risk patients, however, may have significantly improved outcome due to these agents. These include patients receiving emergent percutaneous interventions (34% reduction in primary end points versus 7% without GP IIb/IIIa), patients with raised troponin levels (58% reduced mortality versus 5% increase), and diabetic patients, in whom the greatest increase in survival was demonstrated. Of interest to physicians is

TABLE 25.1 DRUG DOSING

DRUG	PHARMACOKINETICS AND DYNAMICS	DOSE	SIDE EFFECTS
THIENOPYRIDINES			
Clopidogrel (Plavix)	Max antiplt effect after 600 mg load within 3 hours. Extensive hepatic metabolism, renal excretion, 8 hr t1/2	300 mg to 600 mg po load, 75 mg/day.	9% vs. 5% major and minor bleeding, sig ↑ bleeding after CABG. Stop 5 days prior to CABG.
Ticlopidine (Ticlid)	24- to 48-hour onset, 24 hr t1/2, extensive hepatic metabolism.	250 mg/BID po.	2% neutropenia in first 3 months of rx.
GP IIB/IIIA INHIBITORS			
Abciximab (ReoPro)	30 min t1/2, 10-day platelet bound state, 80% plts inhibited in 2 hrs. Sustained inhibition after 12 to 24 hr of infusion.	0.15 to 0.3 mg/kg IV bolus, then 10 mcg/min to maintain ACT 300–500s.	Twofold increase in bleeding. ↓Plt . 14% incidence of ↓BP with infusion.
Eptifibatide (Integrilin	15 min t1/2, 75% renal clearance, 25% hepatic clearance.	180 mcg/kg IV bolus, then 1 mcg/kg/min infusion.	5% to 11% major bleeding (same as controls), 3% ↓Plt.
Tirofiban (Aggrastat)	2 hour t1/2, 65% renal clearance, 25% reduced clearance in elderly.	0.4 mcg/kg/min IV bolus, then 0.1 mcg/kg/min infusion for 24 hr.	2% major bleeding, possible reversible ↓Plt. Renal insuf prolongs effect.
Lamifiban (phase III)	85 min t1/2, 50% return of plt function 6 hr after terminating infusion.	150 to 600 mcg IV bolus, 1 to 5 mcg/min infusion for 120 hr.	Concomitant heparin infusion significantly ↑s bleeding from 0.8% to 3%.

that women who receive GP IIb/IIIa inhibitors appear to have a 14% increase in combined end points as compared with men.

WHAT TO DO

The American College of Cardiology and American Heart Association guidelines and the Seventh American College of Chest Physicians (ACCP) Consensus Conference on antithrombotic therapies suggest that the thienopyridines are as effective as aspirin alone and recommend clopidogrel as an alternative in patients with aspirin insensitivity because of its lower side effects. It is preferable to delay giving clopidogrel to patients who may undergo coronary artery bypass graft surgery (CABG) because of excessive postoperative bleeding. GP IIb/IIIa inhibitors are of most benefit in patients undergoing or likely to undergo PCI and may be of little benefit in patients who do not receive PCI. Eptifibatide is used more often because it costs less and there is more experience with its dosing (*Table 25.1*).

SUGGESTED READINGS

Braunwald E, Antman EM, Beasley JW, et al. ACC/AHA guidelines for the management of patients with unstable angina and non–ST-segment elevation myocardial infarction. A report of the American College of Cardiology/American Heart Association Task Force on Practice Guidelines (Committee on the Management of Patients with Unstable Angina). J Am Coll Cardiol 2000;36:970.

Moustapha A, Anderson V. Contemporary view of the acute coronary syndromes. J Invasive Cardiol 2003;15:71–79.

Simons M. Antiplatelet agents in unstable angina and acute non–ST elevation (non-Q-wave) MI. In: Rose BD, ed. UpToDate. Waltham, MA: UpToDate; 2006.

26

STRONGLY CONSIDER LOW-MOLECULAR-WEIGHT HEPARIN IN THE TREATMENT OF UNSTABLE ANGINA AND NON–ST-ELEVATION MYOCARDIAL INFARCTION

JULIUS CUONG PHAM, MD

CASE

Mrs. ACS is a 74-year-old female who is admitted to the intensive care unit (ICU) for an acute coronary syndrome. She presents to the emergency department with substernal chest pain with radiation to the neck, diaphoresis, and dizziness. Her electrocardiogram (ECG) shows T-wave flattening in the inferior leads (II, III, and aVF). No ST-segment elevations are noted. The patient is started on aspirin, nitroglycerin, and metoprolol. As you write for a heparin drip, the nurse asks, "Why don't we do Lovenox [enoxaparin], that way I don't have to start a drip."

DISCUSSION

Acute coronary syndrome is a relatively new classification term for a set of acute coronary diseases. Causes of acute coronary syndrome include ST-elevation myocardial infarction (STEMI), non–ST-elevation myocardial infarction (NSTEMI), and unstable angina. *STEMI* is defined as myocardial infarction involving ST-segment elevation of 0.1 mV in two or more consecutive leads or a new left bundle branch block. *NSTEMI* refers to acute myocardial damage from atherosclerotic disease that results in release of cardiac biomarkers without causing ST-segment elevation. *Unstable angina* refers to myocardial damage that does not result in release of cardiac biomarkers or ST-segment elevation. These definitions are important because they relate to the pathogenesis, severity of disease, and management strategy of the affected patients.

In the treatment of acute coronary syndrome, anticoagulant therapy is indicated to minimize further thrombus formation. Heparin is the recommended parenteral anticoagulant in treatment of acute coronary syndrome. Heparin accelerates the action of antithrombin. This leads to inactivation of factors IIa (thrombin), IXa, and Xa. This leads to decrease thrombus formation. Unfractionated heparin is a mixture of different weights of heparin (5 to 30k) that have varying effects on factors IIa, IXa, and Xa. Low-molecular-weight heparin (LMWH) is a subset of heparin (weight ~5k) that has activity on factor Xa, but not on IIa. LMWH has the advantage of less binding to protein and dose-independent clearance. This leads to more predictable dosing and a longer half-life (3 to 6 hours). Because of the longer half-life, LMWH can be administered subcutaneously twice a day as opposed to a continuous infusion for unfractionated heparin (half-life 1 to 2 hours).

In patients with unstable angina or NSTEMI, enoxaparin (Lovenox) is preferable to unfractionated heparin in patients not scheduled for a coronary artery bypass graft within 24 hours. Four trials have evaluated the benefits of low-molecular-weight heparin over unfractionated heparin in the treatment of unstable angina or NSTEMI. The two trials that used enoxaparin each showed a reduction in the composite end point of death, myocardial infarction, and recurrent ischemia when compared with unfractionated heparin. The TIMI 11B trial showed a 12% relative risk reduction (19.6% unfractionated heparin vs. 17.3% LMWH). The ESSENCE trial showed a 19% relative risk reduction (23.3% unfractionated heparin vs. 19.8% LMWH). The two trials that used another form of LMWH (dalteparin and nadroparin) demonstrated a trend toward increased risk of the composite end point, although this was not statistically significant.

The advantages of LMWH are the ease of administration, absence of need for monitoring, and lower association with heparin-induced thrombocytopenia. In all trials, there was an increased risk of minor bleeding, but no difference in risk of major bleeding. Unfractionated heparin is preferred in patients who have a planned percutaneous coronary intervention and coronary artery bypass graft because LMWH is less effectively reversed with protamine and does not allow monitoring to adjust the level of anticoagulation.

SUGGESTED READINGS

Antman EM, McCabe CH, Gurfinkle EP, et al. Enoxaparin prevents death and cardiac ischemic events in unstable angina/non-Q-wave myocardial infarction; results of the thrombolysis in myocardial infarction (TIMI) 11B trial. Circulation 1999;100:1593–1601.

Braunwald E, Antman EM, Beasley JW, et al. ACC/AHA guideline update for the management of patients with unstable angina and non-ST-segment elevation myocardial infarction: 2002. Summary article from the Committee on the Management of Patients with Unstable Angina. Circulation 2002;106:1893–1900.

Cohen M, Demers C, Gurfinkle EP, et al. A comparison of low-molecular-weight heparin with unfractionated heparin for unstable coronary artery disease. Efficacy and Safety of Subcutaneous Enoxaparin in Non-Q-Wave Coronary Events Study Group. N Engl J Med 1997;337:447–452.

Comparison of two treatment durations (6 days and 14 days) of a low molecular weight heparin with a 6-day treatment of unfractionated heparin in the initial management of unstable angina or non-Q wave myocardial infarction: FRAX.I.S. Eur Heart J 1999;20:1553–1562.

Klein W, Buchwald A, Hillis SE, et al. Comparison of low-molecular-weight heparin with unfractionated heparin acutely and with placebo for 6 weeks in the management of unstable coronary artery disease. Fragmin in Unstable Coronary Artery Disease Study (FRIC). Circulation 1997;96:61–68.

27

Strongly Consider Using Glycoprotein IIb/IIIa Inhibitors as an Added Treatment to Stenting in Acute Myocardial Infarction

Nirav G. Shah, MD

Percutaneous coronary intervention (PCI) with stenting has revolutionized the care for patients with acute myocardial infarctions. Intracoronary stent placement reduces the long-term recurrence of stenosis. In addition, the combination of stenting with administration of glycoprotein IIb/IIIa (GP IIb/IIIa) inhibitor agents, which prohibit the binding of fibrinogen and proteins to platelets, has reduced the frequency of ischemic complications following percutaneous coronary interventions.

WATCH OUT FOR

GP IIb/IIIa therapy is indicated in patients undergoing coronary angioplasty, in particular those patients with unstable angina or with other clinical characteristics of high risk. Contraindications to GP IIb/IIIa inhibitors include active bleeding, a bleeding diathesis in the past 30 days, intracranial tumors, intracranial hemorrhage, arteriovenous malformation, recent stroke, major surgery or trauma in the preceding month, thrombocytopenia, severe hypertension, and aortic dissection. The agents in this class include eptifibatide, tirofiban, and abciximab. Eptifibatide and tirofiban are preferred in patients with unstable angina and non–ST-elevation myocardial infarction (NSTEMI) managed medically, while abciximab is preferred in those undergoing PCI. The dose of abciximab as an adjunct in PCI is 0.125 mcg/kg/minute and when used for unstable angina the dose is 10 mcg/minute for 18 to 24 hours. Tirofiban is dosed at 0.1 mcg/kg/minute and should be continued for 12 to 24 hours after PCI. Eptifibatide is dosed at 2 mcg/kg/minute after a 180-mcg/kg bolus for acute coronary syndromes. The side effects of these medications include intracranial hemorrhage, gastrointestinal bleeding, thrombocytopenia, hematuria, retroperitoneal bleeding, and other severe bleeding diatheses.

It is important to note that stent technology has also improved over the past few years. The initial technology of stents has now been replaced by stents with better clinical outcomes. The various types of stents include bare metal, self-expandable, balloon expandable, covered, small vessel, and drug eluting. Current practice uses mostly drug-eluting stents, which are coated with an antistenotic drug that is released over 14 to 30 days after implantation. The two that are approved by the Food and Drug Administration are sirolimus- and paclitaxel-coated stents. Drug-eluting stents should be used preferentially in lesions involving the left-anterior descending artery and for left main disease.

SUGGESTED READINGS

Fischman DL, Leon MB, Baim DS, et al. A randomized comparison of coronary-stent placement and balloon angioplasty in the treatment of coronary artery disease. N Engl J Med 1994;331:496–501.
Schomig A, Neumann FJ, Kastrati A, et al. A randomized comparison of antiplatelet and anticoagulant therapy after the placement of coronary-artery stents. N Engl J Med 1996;334:1084–1089.

28

CONSIDER NESIRITIDE IN ACUTELY DECOMPENSATED HEART FAILURE

JACQUELINE JANKA, MD

In patients with cardiogenic pulmonary edema due to acute decompensated heart failure, plasma brain natriuretic peptide (BNP) measurements can guide the diagnosis, distinguishing this etiology of dyspnea from pulmonary causes. Plasma BNP concentration is elevated in both asymptomatic and symptomatic heart failure (left ventricular dysfunction) and is useful for both diagnosis and prognosis.

BNP is a hormone abundantly found in the heart (especially the ventricles) but initially identified in the brain. It is released from myocardial cells in response to wall stress, volume expansion, and high filling pressures. Physiologically, endogenously produced BNP targets the heart, blood vessels, and kidneys to reduce preload and afterload through vasodilatation, diuresis, and natriuresis (sodium excretion). BNP also counters neurohormones such as endothelin, aldosterone, and angiotensin II. Murine studies further suggest that BNP may protect against the progressive cardiac fibrosis associated with chronic heart failure. In whole, BNP reduces the workload on the heart to improve cardiac performance.

A rapid BNP fluorescence immunoassay was approved in 2000 and can be rapidly performed in 10 to 15 minutes at the bedside. Patients with heart failure have significantly higher levels of plasma BNP than those with dyspnea due to other causes. Remarkably, plasma BNP is more accurate for predicting heart failure than classic parameters such as rales, cardiomegaly, or the National Health and Nutrition Examination Survey (NHANES) or Framingham criteria. BNP also correlates with the New York Heart Association functional class. A value >100 pg/mL makes the diagnosis of heart failure with a sensitivity of 90%, specificity of 76%, and a predictive value of 83%. Conversely, low BNP has a strong negative predictive value to rule out heart failure. The rapid assay costs approximately $20 per test.

Despite having elevated levels of cardioprotective BNP, patients with heart failure are generally paradoxically vasoconstricted and sodium avid. Of interest to the clinicians is that, while appearing minimally responsive to endogenous BNP, heart failure patients will effectively respond to exogenously administered BNP (nesiritide).

WHAT TO DO

Nesiritide is a recombinant form of human B-type natriuretic peptide (hBNP), approved in 2001 for the intravenous (IV) treatment of patients with acutely decompensated congestive heart failure. Nesiritide is given as an initial IV bolus of 2 mcg/kg, followed by a continuous infusion at 0.01 mcg/kg/min. The dose may be increased to a maximum rate of 0.03 mcg/kg/min. There is no dose adjustment for renal insufficiency. Nesiritide promotes sodium excretion, reduced cardiac filling pressures (reduced pulmonary capillary wedge pressures), and improved cardiac indices and clinical status (e.g., dyspnea, fatigue) in patients with heart failure. These positive hemodynamic effects are seen within the first hour of administration and are maintained throughout the infusion period and up to 6 to 24 hours after discontinuation.

WATCH OUT FOR

The most common side effect of nesiritide is dose-related hypotension, which may be enhanced when given with other vasodilators, such as angiotensin-converting enzyme (ACE) inhibitors. While nesiritide appears fairly safe and is well tolerated, there are data that have prompted questions about its effects on renal function and survival. For example, one analysis suggested that patients treated with nesiritide may have been more likely to develop progressive renal insufficiency, although this may be due to hypoperfusion rather than direct renal toxicity. Another retrospective analysis suggested a trend (nonsignificant) toward a higher 30-day mortality in patients treated with nesiritide.

In summary, nesiritide is an effective therapy for patients hospitalized with acute decompensated heart failure, especially those requiring inotropic support. It may be particularly useful in heart failure patients with tachycardia or arrhythmias, which would otherwise limit the use of traditional agents such as dopamine or dobutamine. Nesiritide may be used in combination with other heart failure medications (e.g., diuretics, ACE inhibitors, dopamine, dobutamine, or milrinone) when tolerated. Close monitoring of hemodynamics, urine output, and renal function is essential.

SUGGESTED READINGS

Colucci WS, Elkayam U, Horton DP, et al. Intravenous nesiritide, a natriuretic peptide, in the treatment of decompensated congestive heart failure. Nesiritide Study Group. N Engl J Med 2000;343:246.

Mills RM, Hobbs RE. How to use nesiritide in treating decompensated heart failure. Clev Clin J Med 2002;69:252.

Nesiritide for decompensated congestive heart failure. Med Lett Drugs Ther 2001;43:100.

29

BE AGGRESSIVE IN CONSIDERING REPERFUSION THERAPY IN ACUTE MYOCARDIAL INFARCTION

ANTHONY D. SLONIM, MD, DrPH

Cardiovascular disease is a dominant cause of morbidity and mortality in the United States and acute myocardial infarction (MI) is one of the major underlying etiologies. Acute MI is a medical emergency that is precipitated when coronary occlusion leads to ischemia and then necrosis of cardiac myocytes. The necrosis will often precipitate a cardiac arrhythmia (e.g., ventricular fibrillation), which is a major cause of death for patients presenting in the acute phase. The diagnosis of an acute MI is based on the patient's history and diagnostic testing, including an electrocardiogram (ECG) and serum enzymes. The faster the diagnosis can be made and the occlusion reversed, the more likely the patient is to salvage myocardial tissue and benefit from improved outcomes.

WATCH OUT FOR

In nondiabetic patients, the major symptom of acute MI is pain. This pain is usually described as severe. It is located in a retrosternal area and may radiate to either the arms or neck. The characteristic quality of the pain is described as pressurelike or bandlike; however, other descriptions including burning, aching, and crushing have also been used. The pain usually lasts beyond 20 to 30 minutes and does not dissipate. Associated symptoms include nausea, vomiting, shortness of breath, dizziness, and diaphoresis.

In the setting of a possible acute MI, the ECG is a readily available, noninvasive, easy-to-obtain diagnostic test that has excellent sensitivity and specificity. The ECG provides information on the distribution of changes and the impact on cardiac rhythm. The pattern of ST-segment elevation representing a "current of injury" is usually associated with acute MI and implies a coronary occlusion. This is helpful for triaging for strategies of reperfusion.

In addition to the ECG, cardiac enzymes are particularly sensitive for detecting myocardial damage. These proteins are released from the myocardial cells that have sustained damage. Troponins are particularly important for the diagnosis of acute MI since under normal conditions, they are not found in the serum. These enzymes first become detectable from 2 to 4 hours after injury and persist for days. Creatine kinase (CK) and the MB subtype have for many years dominated the clinical arena as the major cardiac marker in the setting of acute MI now being supplanted by troponins. These tests are important early markers of myocardial necrosis but take longer to be detected and disappear from the serum more rapidly than troponins. It must be noted that in postoperative patients, creatine phosphokinase (CPK) and troponin have not been shown to be as sensitive markers for cardiac damage as they are in nonsurgical patients.

WHAT TO DO The management of patients presenting with chest pain suggestive of acute MI should trigger a number of immediate events. The longest delay in therapy is usually related to the patient's delay in seeking care. Denial of the pain and the hope that it will go away are important underlying reasons for this phenomenon. When the patient presents to the emergency department with chest pain, a focused history, physical examination, and electrocardiogram should be obtained. If the appropriate clinical symptoms and ECG findings suggest an acute MI, aggressive management should include intravenous access, oxygen, sublingual nitroglycerin, morphine, and beta-blocker therapy. If the patient presents within 12 hours of symptoms, aggressive methods to achieve reperfusion should be considered.

The recommended strategy for achieving reperfusion is cardiac catheterization with angioplasty if the institution is capable of achieving a door-to-balloon time of <90 minutes. This strategy begins with the administration of glycoprotein IIb/IIIa inhibitors in addition to the more generic therapies described previously. This strategy has the advantage of achieving higher recanalization rates, reducing residual stenosis, and improving the outcomes in the setting of cardiogenic shock. When an institution is unable to provide primary angioplasty strategies, thrombolytic therapy can be attempted. A number of contraindications to thrombolytic therapy need to be considered before providing this intervention and include bleeding, a history of stroke, severe hypertension, recent trauma or surgery, pregnancy, aortic dissection, and intracranial or spinal cord neoplasms.

SUGGESTED READINGS

Goldman L, Ausiello D, eds. *Cecil Textbook of Internal Medicine*. 22d ed. Philadelphia: WB Saunders; 2004:410–424.

Keely EC, Boura JA, Grines CL. Primary angioplasty versus intravenous thrombolytic therapy for acute myocardial infarction. A primary review of 23 randomized trials. Lancet. 2003; 3612:13–20.

30

STRONGLY CONSIDER STARTING AN ANGIOTENSIN-CONVERTING ENZYME INHIBITOR OR ANGIOTENSIN RECEPTOR BLOCKER AFTER MYOCARDIAL INFARCTION

YING WEI LUM, MD

The renin-angiotensin-aldosterone system (RAAS) regulates aldosterone release in the body via the action of angiotensin II on angiotensin I receptors. Angiotensin II by itself is also a potent vasoconstrictor (even more than norepinephrine), leading to hypertension (*Fig. 30.1*). Its other harmful effects include the promotion of atherosclerosis and hypertrophic changes in the blood vessels and left ventricle. Angiotensin-converting enzyme (ACE) inhibitors, by blocking the conversion of angiotensin I to angiotensin II, are believed to attenuate ventricular dilatation and remodeling. Furthermore, ACE inhibitors block the degradation of bradykinin, which is thought to have antihypertensive effects. The accumulation of bradykinin is believed to be the cause of the chronic cough associated with use of ACE inhibitors. Angiotensin II receptor blockers (ARBs), on the other hand, work further downstream in the RAAS by blocking angiotensin II at the receptor site.

In general, patients initiated on ACE inhibitors during myocardial infarction (MI) have demonstrated a reduction in overall mortality by about 20% to 30%. This benefit is most profound in patients with symptomatic congestive heart failure and their therapy should be continued indefinitely. However, therapy in patients without evidence of left ventricular dysfunction may be ceased after 4 to 6 weeks. These patients should then be re-evaluated in 4 to 6 months to reassess ventricular function. Patients who are intolerant to ACE inhibitors (because of severe cough, etc.) may take an ARB as a suitable alternative. Valsartan was recently compared with captopril and found to be as effective at reducing mortality, heart failure hospitalizations, and reinfarction.

Of interest to clinicians is that patients taking chronic ACE inhibitor therapy have demonstrated circulating angiotensin II levels similar to that prior to initiating therapy. This "ACE escape" syndrome is incompletely understood but thought to be associated with other synthetic pathways for angiotensin II. Hence, maximal blockade of the RAAS would encompass blocking both the formation of angiotensin II and action of angiotensin II on the angiotensin I receptor.

ACE-I   ARB

$\downarrow$ $\downarrow$

Angiotensinogen → Angiotensin I → Angiotensin II → Aldosterone release

Vasoconstriction

Increased sympathetic activity

FIGURE 30.1. Mechanism of Action

In congestive heart failure patients, this combination therapy has been shown to decrease the incidence of hospitalizations for heart failure. However, combination therapy has yet to show any survival benefit in patients during myocardial infarction, with or without heart failure.

WHAT TO DO

Barring hypotension (systolic blood pressure <100 mm Hg), treatment with an ACE or ARB should be commenced on the first post–MI day (as early as the first 12 hours). Therapy should be initiated only after the routine recommended administration of thrombolytic therapy, aspirin, and beta-blockers. Captopril offers the advantage of being the drug whose use within the first 24 hours has been best studied (SAVE and ISIS-4 trial). However, various ACE inhibitors including lisinopril (GISSI-3 trial), ramipril (AIRE trial), and trandolapril (TRACE trial) have also received FDA approval for treatment of heart failure after myocardial infarction. Enalapril (CONSENSUS-II trial) and zofenopril (SMILE trial), though not currently FDA approved for treatment during myocardial infarction, are also felt to be equivalent in their beneficial effect on mortality. Currently, valsartan (VALIANT trial) is the only ARB that has been FDA approved for use during myocardial infarction.

WATCH OUT FOR

The most common cause for discontinuing therapy in the acute peri-MI period is hypotension. This is unusual, but it can occur in up to 2% of heart failure patients who have undergone vigorous intravascular depletion from diuretic use. Intravascular volume depletion can in turn cause decreased renal perfusion and azotemia. In general, renal insufficiency Cr >2.5 mg/dL is a contraindication in initiating or continuing therapy, as is renal artery stenosis. Hyperkalemia (K >5.5 mEq/mL) can occur as a result of decreased aldosterone levels. Other rare adverse reactions include dry cough, rash, and angioedema.

SUGGESTED READINGS

Pfeffer MA. ACE inhibition in acute myocardial infarction. N Engl J Med 1995;332:118–120.

Voors AA, van Veldhuisen DJ. Role of angiotensin receptor blockers in patients with left ventricular dysfunction: lessons from CHARM and VALIANT. Int J Cardiol 2004;97;3:345–348.

31

USE PROPHYLAXIS FOR EROSIVE GASTRITIS IN THE APPROPRIATE PATIENT

RACHEL BLUEBOND-LANGNER, MD

Gastrointestinal (GI) prophylaxis in the intensive care unit (ICU) is important in the prevention of stress gastritis. The incidence of clinically significant bleeding in critically ill patients is 2% to 15%. However, it is important to understand the actual indications for prophylaxis. Most experienced clinicians feel it should be limited to patients at high risk for stress-related mucosal diseases, which include the following conditions: mechanical ventilation longer than 48 hours; coagulopathy; endoscopic or radiographic diagnosis of peptic ulcer or gastritis; history of an upper GI bleed less than 6 weeks prior to admission; significant burns (greater than 15% of total body surface area); traumatic brain injury; and large doses of glucocorticoids (e.g., >50 mg hydrocortisone/day).

Prophylactic medications to prevent stress gastritis include antacids, sucralfate, histamine-2 receptor antagonists (H2-blockers), and proton pump inhibitors (PPIs). Cook et al., in a multicenter randomized double-blind controlled trial, demonstrated that H2-blockers (ranitidine) compared with sucralfate decreased clinically significant bleeding with no difference in ventilator-associated pneumonia. To date there are no studies that have prospectively evaluated the ability of intravenous PPIs to reduce clinically significant bleeding in high-risk critically ill patients; however, PPIs have been shown to raise and maintain an elevated gastric pH. When deciding between H2-blockers and PPIs, side effects and cost should be considered. If the patient requires intravenous medications, H2-blockers are the most cost-effective. However, if the patient is able to tolerate oral medications, PPIs are a good choice given their ability to maintain gastric pH for a sustained period of time. The overall need for prophylaxis should be assessed when patients are able to meet their nutritional requirements by mouth.

WATCH OUT FOR

Side effects of both drugs should be kept in mind. H2-blockers have been associated with tachyphylaxis (i.e., tolerance and thus decrease in gastric pH), interstitial nephritis, confusion, inhibition of the cytochrome oxidase enzyme system (cimetidine only), and dose adjustment in patients with creatinine clearance of less than 50 mL/min. PPIs are generally safe but rare side effects include diarrhea, nausea, and pruritus.

SELECTED READINGS

Cook D. A comparison of sucralfate and ranitidine for the prevention of upper gastrointestinal bleeding in patients requiring mechanical ventilation. N Engl J Med 1998;338:791–817.

Cook DJ, Fuller HD, Guyatt GH, et al. Risk factors for gastrointestinal bleeding in critically ill patients. N Engl J Med 1994;330:377–381.

Steinberg K. Stress related mucosal disease in the critically ill patient: Risk factors and strategies to prevent stress-related bleeding in the intensive care unit. Crit Care Med 2002;30: S362–S364.

32

BEWARE OF METABOLITES

BRADFORD D. WINTERS, MD, PhD

Many drugs are metabolized to active metabolites. This is usually carried out by the liver in the form of reductions, oxidations, and the addition of methyl, acetyl, and other groups. While metabolites are usually a fraction as potent as the parent compound, in some situations they may be more potent and may accumulate to significant concentrations under the right conditions. Often the metabolites of lipophilic drugs are made more water soluble to facilitate renal excretion. However, intensive care unit (ICU) patients often have renal and/or hepatic impairment altering the clearance of the drugs and their metabolites. Thus, while a particular drug may be hepatically metabolized, renal insufficiency may impair its excretion and lead to buildup of an active metabolite. Other metabolites may not be active in terms of the original effect of the drug but are actually more toxic than the parent compound. Both of these situations may have dire consequences.

Meperidine is a prime example of this problem. This is a commonly used narcotic in anesthesiology and other settings including the ICU and its half-life is approximately 3 hours. It is hepatically metabolized to normeperidine (half-life of 15 to 20 hours), which can build up in the face of renal impairment and promote seizure activity when it reaches high enough concentrations. These seizures are not reversed by naloxone, which is usually used to reverse the deleterious effects of most narcotics.

Morphine is another very commonly used narcotic in the ICU that is metabolized to two active metabolites, 3- and 6-glucuronides. The half-life of morphine is usually 2 to 3 hours. The 3-glucuronide is not active as an analgesic but does cause sedation and can precipitate seizures. The 6-glucuronide is active as an analgesic, in fact, more so than morphine itself. Both of these metabolites are dependent on renal excretion and may build up in critically ill patients with renal insufficiency, leading to prolonged sedation and/or respiratory depression or possibly seizures like normeperidine.

Benzodiazepines are very commonly used in the ICU for sedation, to assist with mechanical ventilation, and to provide anxiolysis during painful procedures and critical illness. Many of the drugs in this class are hydroxylated to active metabolites, including midazolam and diazepam. Midazolam is normally a short-acting drug (duration of action is approximately 1 hour), but this is dependent on normal excretion of the hydroxylated metabolite. While this metabolite has only about 10% of the activity of the parent drug, renal impairment may lengthen the effect of the drug. Thus a short-acting drug may become a longer-acting drug especially when used in large doses. A long-acting benzodiazepine such as diazepam (duration of action is 3 to 5 hours) can become very long acting when its active metabolite is not cleared. Diazepam has several active metabolites, some of which are prepared and marketed as separate drugs, including temazepam and oxazepam.

It should be noted that the accumulation of active metabolites secondary to hepatic and/or renal insufficiency is often compounded by the act of repetitive dosing and continuous infusions of the parent drugs. As a result a patient may not awaken from sedation for prolonged periods of time, leading to more time spent on a ventilator and an unnecessary battery of tests being performed to assess the patient's decreased mental status. These problems are additionally compounded by the fact that many of these drugs are not used in isolation. Many patients are on several drugs at the same time, especially the benzodiazepines and narcotics. If careful attention to dosage is maintained in the face of potentially impaired clearance, these problems may be minimized. Better yet, drugs that have no active metabolites may be the preferred choice assuming all other characteristics (side effects, etc.) are equal. Instead of using diazepam or midazolam, one may choose lorazepam, which has no active or toxic metabolites. While this drug has a long duration of action (6 hours), paradoxically its effect may be shorter in ICU patients compared with the ones with active metabolites. Similarly, Fentanyl may be used as the preferred narcotic since its metabolites are not toxic or active.

SUGGESTED READINGS

Horn E, Nesbit SA. Pharmacology and pharmacokinetics of sedatives and analgesics. Gastrointest Endosc Clin N Am 2004;14:247–268.

Shafer A. Complications of sedation with midazolam in the intensive care unit and a comparison with other sedative regimens. Crit Care Med 1998;26:947–956.

33

DO NOT USE ERYTHROMYCIN AS A PROKINETIC AGENT IN PATIENTS ON TACROLIMUS (OR CYCLOSPORINE)

MATTHEW J. WEISS, MD

Erythromycin is a macrolide antibiotic that inhibits bacterial protein synthesis and is effective against the same organisms as penicillin G. The drug is commonly used to treat community-acquired pulmonary infections in penicillin-allergic patients. Erythromycin also has prokinetic effects on the gastrointestinal system. At low doses, erythromycin induces activity in the gastric antrum, which propagates to the small intestines. At higher doses, erythromycin induces a prolonged period of antral activity by stimulating motilin receptors to accelerate gastric emptying. Although transplant recipients frequently suffer from opportunistic bacterial infections and/or gastrointestinal dysmotility, erythromycin should not be given to recipients taking FK506 (tacrolimus, Prograf) or cyclosporine.

FK506 is structurally similar to erythromycin. It is a macrolide that exhibits strong immunosuppressive properties by inhibiting the transcription of interleukin-2 during T-cell activation. Like FK506, cyclosporine is a calcineurin inhibitor and both drugs are routinely given for prophylaxis of organ rejection. Both FK506 and cyclosporine have narrow therapeutic windows and both require daily lab draws in the perioperative period to ensure efficacious drug levels. Both drugs are metabolized by the liver's P450 CYP 3A4 enzyme pathway (the most common pathway for drug metabolism). Erythromycin is a strong inhibitor of this pathway and concurrent administration of erythromycin and FK506 (in particular) or cyclosporin can result in elevated immunosuppression drug levels and severe toxicity even after one or two doses of erythromycin. This toxicity can manifest as severe renal dysfunction, tremors, seizures, brittle diabetes, or corneal ulcerations.

Other common intensive care unit medications can also induce the P450 CYP 3A4 system and thus decrease serum levels of FK506 and cyclosporine. These include phenobarbital, carbamazepine, phenytoin, and rifampin. Drugs metabolized through this pathway should always be double-checked for drug interactions.

Suggested Readings

Padhi D, Long P, Basha M, et al. Interaction between tacrolimus and erythromycin. Ther Drug Monit 1997;19:120–122.

Shaeffer MS, Collier D, Sorrell MF. Interaction between FK506 and erythromycin. Ann Pharmacother 1994;28:280–281.

34

Consider use of enoxaparin over unfractionated heparin in trauma patients

Suneel Khetarpal, MD
Barbara Haas, MD

Trauma patients are at high risk of deep venous thromboembolism, with the majority of patients exhibiting no symptoms. Although meta-analyses report the overall incidence of deep vein thrombosis (DVT) in trauma patients to be approximately 12%, the incidence of DVT in patients receiving no prophylaxis has been reported to be as high as 58%. Although a number of factors have been purported to increase the incidence of DVT, including long bone fractures, pelvic fractures, and head injuries, meta-analysis suggests that only spinal fractures and spinal cord injuries independently increase the incidence of DVT among trauma patients. Specifically, spinal cord injury has been shown to increase the risk of DVT threefold.

Various modalities have been used in an attempt to decrease the incidence of DVT and associated pulmonary embolism (PE) in trauma patients, including both low-dose unfractionated heparin and low-molecular-weight heparin (LMWH). Unfractionated heparin acts by binding to antithrombin III, which accelerates its ability to inactivate several molecules in the coagulation cascade, including factor Xa and thrombin. LMWH acts primarily by inhibiting factor Xa and its activity is correlated to factor Xa levels. LMWH has improved bioavailability and decreased incidence of bleeding as compared with unfractionated heparin.

Although low-dose unfractionated heparin has been shown to be very effective in reducing the incidence of DVT among patients undergoing elective surgery, a number of studies suggest that its effect in trauma patients is limited and that this intervention may not decrease the incidence of DVT in this population. In contrast, having originally been shown to decrease the incidence of DVT in patients undergoing orthopedic procedures, LMWH has been shown to be safe following trauma, and several reports suggest it is effective in reducing the occurrence of DVT and associated complications in the trauma population. One landmark study demonstrated a decrease of 30% in the incidence of DVT and a decrease of 58% in the incidence of proximal vein thrombosis with the use of LMWH. Suggested dosage for enoxaparin is 30 mg injected subcutaneously twice a day. It is important to note, however, that a recent review of published studies examining LMWH suggests that even this therapy may not offer significant benefit, and better quality studies are required to settle this debate.

WHAT NOT TO DO

Certain subgroups of trauma patients cannot receive either heparin or LMWH prophylaxis because of ongoing risk of hemorrhage. Generally, most clinicians avoid the use of heparin in the presence of brain and spinal cord injuries, solid organ injuries that are being managed non-operatively, and retroperitoneal bleeding requiring transfusion. Nevertheless, patients with these contraindications to heparin therapy can still form thrombi in the extremities and require an alternative mode of PE prevention. In these patients, inferior vena caval (IVC) filters are frequently considered an acceptable alternative. While there is convincing evidence for the use of IVC filters in patients who have known DVTs and either cannot receive heparin or have DVTs or PE despite full anticoagulation, the timing and target population of filters inserted for prophylaxis remain debatable. IVC filters can cause significant complications, including caval penetration, and the evidence for the use of these filters as prophylaxis in the general trauma population is equivocal. Their use is supported in specific patterns of injury, including spinal cord injury, pelvic fracture combined with long bone fracture, severe head injury combined with long bone fracture, and complex long bone injuries. More recently, temporary filters have been studied in the trauma population and the literature suggests they are a safe option in these patients. However, reported retrieval rates are as low as 35%, and long-term follow-up is required to assess the proportion of these devices that is ultimately retrieved.

One final note is that the use of enoxaparin in the setting of renal failure is problematic. The manufacturer's package insert recommends the dose of enoxaparin to be 30 mg sq qday if the creatinine clearance is <30. However, many experienced ICU pharmacists and clinicians recommend a dose of unfractionated heparin q8 hours for patients receiving hemodialysis or continuous venovenous hemodialysis.

SUGGESTED READINGS

Geerts WH, Jay RM, Code KI, et al. A comparison of low-dose heparin with low-molecular-weight heparin as prophylaxis against venous thromboembolism after major trauma. N Engl J Med 1996;335:701–707.

Knudson MM, Ikossi DG, Khaw L, et al. Thromboembolism after trauma: an analysis of 1602 episodes from the American College of Surgeons National Trauma Data Bank. Ann Surg 2004;240:490–496; discussion 496–498.

35

MAINTAIN TIGHT GLUCOSE CONTROL IN THE INTENSIVE CARE UNIT

MICHAEL J. MORITZ, MD

Hyperglycemia and insulin resistance are common in critically ill patients even if they did not have diabetes before their illnesses. Hyperglycemia in the intensive care unit (ICU) setting has been shown to be associated with an increased mortality, and restoration of normoglycemia using intensive insulin therapy has decreased mortality for the following populations: myocardial infarction, burn, and stroke. Specifically, in the surgical ICU setting, the use of intensive insulin therapy to achieve normoglycemia has resulted in a lower incidence of nosocomial infections.

The most compelling study by Van den Berghe et al. showed that, for hyperglycemic patients in the surgical ICU setting on the ventilator, intensive insulin therapy to achieve normoglycemia (80 to 110 mg/dL = 4.4 to 6.1 mmol/L) resulted in a 43% reduction in mortality (8% compared with 4.6%) when compared with patients treated with sliding scale insulin with the aim of achieving a glucose level between 180 and 200 mg/dL (10.0 to 11.1 mmol/L). The lowered mortality was largely accounted for in the group with an ICU stay of more than 5 days whose mortality from multiple organ failure was lowered. Additional outcomes associated with normoglycemia included fewer bacteremias, reduced requirement for hemodialysis, fewer transfusions, and shorter duration on the ventilator and in the ICU. Although their ICU population was skewed toward postoperative cardiac surgery patients, the-ICU-stay population in whom the mortality reduction was more striking, and therefore a better balanced group.

Accordingly, the currently available evidence favors aiming for normoglycemia (blood glucose level of less than 110 mg/dL = 6.1 mmol/L) through intravenous insulin infusion in adult surgical ICU patients. It has not been proven that the same improved outcomes will be found in nonadult or nonsurgical ICU patients. The use of intensive insulin infusion can result in hypoglycemia either from excess insulin or from improvement in the patients' conditions (with a fall in insulin resistance). Many ICUs counteract this risk of hypoglycemia by also placing the patient on an infusion of dextrose during insulin administration. Frequent blood glucose monitoring (on the order of hourly) is an important part of the treatment protocol in insulin infusion to avoid hypoglycemia.

SUGGESTED READINGS

Coursin DB, Connery LE, Ketzler JT. Perioperative diabetic and hyperglycemic management issues. Crit Care Med 2004;32:S116–S125.

Van den Berghe G, Wouters P, Weekers F, et al. Intensive insulin therapy in the surgical intensive care unit. N Engl J Med 2001;345:1359–1367.

DO NOT USE SUBCUTANEOUS INSULIN IN THE INTENSIVE CARE UNIT POPULATION

KRISTIN SHIPMAN, MD
HEIDI L. FRANKEL, MD

Regular insulin should be administered intravenously and not subcutaneously in the intensive care unit (ICU). This is because the rate of subcutaneous insulin absorption is highly variable. Insulin absorption is slower with high insulin concentrations and in the typically high dose volumes that are often required to control blood glucose in the critically ill. In addition, decreased capillary surface area decreases insulin absorption; because of poor perfusion, critically ill patients often experience this condition secondary to cardiogenic shock, hypotension, or vasopressor therapy. Lastly, poor perfusion of the subcutaneous tissues may lead to slow or erratic absorption of subcutaneous insulin with resulting poor glucose control.

In contrast to subcutaneous administration, intravenous insulin administration leads to reliably effective absorption and prompt treatment of elevated blood glucose levels. Intravenous insulin has an onset of action in 10 to 30 minutes with a duration of action of 1 hour; subcutaneous insulin has an onset of action of 30 to 60 minutes and peaks at 2 to 4 hours and lasts up to 8 hours.

It cannot be overstated that strict glucose control reduces mortality. Intensive insulin therapy is recommended for critical care patients to maintain blood glucose between 80 and 110 mg/dL. The risk reduction for mortality has been shown to be as high as 45%. Intensive insulin therapy reduces overall hospital mortality by 34%, bloodstream infections by 46%, acute renal failure requiring dialysis or hemofiltration by 41%, median number of red blood cell transfusions by 50%, and critical illness polyneuropathy by 44%. This is best achieved with insulin infusion and titrated for blood glucose levels between 80 and 110 mg/dL.

SUGGESTED READINGS

Mizock BA. Alterations in carbohydrate metabolism during stress: a review of the literature. Am J Med 1995;98:75–84.

Van den Berghe G, Wouters P, Weekers F, et al. Intensive insulin therapy in critically ill patients. N Engl J Med 2001;345:1359–1365.

Van den Berghe G, Wilmer A, Hermans G, et al. Intensive insulin therapy in the medical ICU. N Engl J Med 2006;354:516–518.

DO NOT USE INSULIN GLARGINE IN THE INTENSIVE CARE UNIT WITHOUT ALSO GIVING A SHORTER-ACTING INSULIN FORM

KRISTIN SHIPMAN, MD
HEIDI L. FRANKEL, MD

Lantus is a long-acting insulin analogue also known as insulin glargine. Similar to human insulin, it is produced using recombinant DNA techniques. Insulin glargine substitutes glycine for asparagine at position A21 of the insulin molecule and adds two arginine molecules at position B30. The isoelectric point of insulin glargine is close to a pH of 7.0. Altering these amino acids makes insulin glargine precipitate in subcutaneous tissue. Zinc is added to stabilize intrahexamer contact to prolong activity.

Lantus is given subcutaneously as a depot injection. The onset of action is 2 to 4 hours. There is no peak action. The duration of action is 20 to 24 hours. With a long duration of action, Lantus lends itself to once-a-day dosing in the morning—an attractive formulation for those not critically ill.

Lantus should be used only as a basal insulin replacement. Prandial insulin requirements should be covered with short-acting insulin and the patient should be followed closely as insulin needs often decrease as patients become less ill.

Lantus should not be used in those in whom blood glucose levels may vary greatly (e.g., critically ill patients whose levels may fluctuate as pressors are titrated and sepsis occurs) or in whom interruption of parenteral nutrition and tube feeds may occur (as it does in virtually all ICU patients for many reasons). It should be noted that in critically ill patients, the long duration of Lantus can cause profound hypoglycemia without concomitant administration of glucose calories.

SUGGESTED READINGS

Hirsch I. Insulin analogues. N Engl J Med 2005;352:174–183.
Yki-Jarvinen H, Ziemen M, Dressler A. Less nocturnal hypoglycemia and better post-dinner glucose control with bedtime insulin glargine compared with bedtime NPH insulin during insulin combination therapy in type 2 diabetes. Diabetes Care 2000; 23:1130–1136.

38

REMEMBER THAT PATIENTS WITH INSULIN DEFICIENCY REQUIRE BASAL INSULIN EVEN WHEN THEY ARE NIL PER OS

KATHLEEN A. WILLIAMS, RN, MSN CRNP
SHERITA HILL GOLDEN, MD, MHS

Maintaining euglycemia (defined as glucose <110 mg/dL in intensive care unit settings and <180 mg/dL in non–intensive care unit settings by American College of Endocrinology Consensus Guidelines) has been shown to greatly reduce morbidity and mortality. This has created a paradigm shift in the inpatient setting where the goal is now to prevent hyperglycemia rather than treat hyperglycemia after it develops. Insulin, in both intravenous and subcutaneous regimens, is being used in the inpatient setting to achieve optimum glucose control. The clinical challenge with the use of insulin includes recognizing when to hold or decrease insulin and in which type of diabetic patient insulin should be adjusted in the nil per os (NPO) setting.

Considerable confusion has been caused by the previous diabetes classifications of insulin-dependent diabetes mellitus (IDDM) and non–insulin-dependent diabetes mellitus (NIDDM). Because of the obesity epidemic, NIDDM patients often progress to requiring insulin, causing health care providers to then refer to these patients as having IDDM. Yet, the NIDDM patient who progressed to requiring insulin is physiologically very different from the patient who was diagnosed initially as an IDDM patient. While both patients require insulin, the physiological cause of their insulin requirement and the response to exogenous insulin is significantly different.

In response to this issue, diabetes is now classified based on the etiology of the respective disease process. These classifications are as follows:

a. Type I Diabetes: Characterized by absolute insulin deficiency. The patient is physiologically unable to make endogenous insulin. This inability is due to either an immune-mediated process or severe injury or resection of the pancreas. In rare cases, there is an idiopathic process leading to beta cell destruction.

b. Type II Diabetes: Varying degree of insulin resistance and relative insulin deficiency. This can occur in both children and adults and is most often associated with obesity. It is often treated initially

---

TABLE 38.1   FEATURES OF INSULIN DEFICIENCY

Features of insulin deficiency include the following:
- Type I diabetic patients
- Type II diabetic patients who have required insulin therapy for >5 years
- Type II diabetic patients or who have been diagnosed as a type II diabetic for >10 years
- Patients who have undergone a total pancreatectomy

---

with oral agents but will usually progress to requiring insulin for adequate glucose control.

It is recommended that patients who are insulin deficient (*Table 38.1*) must be given some form of basal insulin either as an insulin infusion or as a subcutaneous intermediate (NPH) or long-acting (glargine) insulin to prevent diabetic ketoacidosis, even in the patient who is NPO.

It is often difficult to ascertain which patients are insulin deficient. If it is unclear which type of diabetes a patient may have, the following physiological indictors of insulin deficiency should be considered:

- Positive serum or urine ketones
- Wide fluctuations in glucose values
- History of requiring insulin therapy to control blood sugar since initial diagnosis
- Previous admissions for diabetic ketoacidosis (DKA) or hyperosmolar hyperglycemia nonketotic syndrome (HHNK)

SUGGESTED READINGS

Clement S, Braithwaite SS, Magee MF, et al. Management of diabetes and hyperglycemia in hospitals. Diabetes Care 2004;27:553–591.

Coursin DB. Perioperative diabetic and hyperglycemia management issues. Crit Care Med 2004;32:S116–S125.

Dagogo-Jack S. Management of diabetes in surgical patients. Diabetes Spect 2002;15:44–48.

39

LOOK FOR MEDICATION-INDUCED CAUSES OF HYPERGLYCEMIA IN INTENSIVE CARE PATIENTS

EDWARD T. HORN, PHARMD

Hyperglycemia, defined as blood glucose levels >110 mg/dL, has been shown in multiple studies to adversely impact outcomes in critically ill patients. Patients who are diabetic are at an increased risk for developing hyperglycemia postoperatively. With the harm of hyperglycemia now known, it is important to search out patient factors that can contribute to this. Patients need to have their intravenous (IV) fluids assessed. For example, infusing fluids that contain dextrose 5% in water (D5W) at 125 cc/hr can deliver as much as 150 grams of dextrose, or more than 500 kcal of carbohydrate fuel. The IV fluids that are used to administer medications also need to be examined. For example, sulfamethoxazole-trimethoprim (Bactrim) requires a large amount of D5W to be infused (at least 250 mL per dose). Hyperglycemia can also be seen with peritoneal dialysate solutions that contain high (>2.5%) concentrations of dextrose. Intolerance to parenteral nutrition can manifest as hyperglycemia.

In addition to intravenous fluids, many medications that are used in the critically ill can exacerbate hyperglycemia. Medications can interfere with glucose metabolism through multiple mechanisms, including increased insulin resistance, decreased insulin secretion, and increased glucagon production. The major organs that are influenced by medications are the pancreas, liver, and skeletal muscle. Medications can inhibit insulin secretion from the beta cells of the pancreas (e.g., gatifloxacin), as well increase glycogen breakdown in the liver (e.g., diazoxide), and cause peripheral insulin resistance in the skeletal muscle (pentamidine). Octreotide inhibits both glucagon and insulin secretion, resulting in either hypo- or hyperglycemia, but the latter is more common clinically. Other medications (e.g., protease inhibitors, atypical antipsychotics) can cause weight gain and fat redistribution, which can lead to type II diabetes mellitus. *Table 39.1* contains examples of medications that can cause glycemic dysregulation.

Management strategies include avoiding (if possible) these agents in patients at risk for the development of hyperglycemia (diabetics, obese patients) and monitoring serum glucoses closely. Insulin should be initiated for agents that affect insulin secretion and cause an increase

TABLE 39.1	MEDICATION EFFECTS ON GLUCOSE HOMEOSTASIS	
SITE OF DYSREGULATION	MECHANISM	MEDICATION IMPLICATED
Pancreas	Inhibition of insulin secretion	Thiazide diuretics Beta-agonists Diazoxide Glucocorticoids Cyclosporine Tacrolimus Pentamidine Epinephrine Gatifloxacin
Liver	Increased glycogenolysis	Thiazide diuretics Beta-agonists Diazoxide Glucocorticoids Ethanol
Peripheral tissues	Decreased insulin sensitivity	Thiazide diuretics Beta-agonists Diazoxide Glucocorticoids Cyclosporine Pentamidine

in glycogen breakdown. Insulin-sensitizing agents (metformin, thiazolidinediones) can be started in patients who will require therapy for hyperglycemia as outpatients, although these agents carry their own risks (lactic acidosis, exacerbation of peripheral edema) and should not be routinely started in the critically ill. Metformin should especially be avoided if the patient is in renal failure or is going to have procedures done that require IV dye because of the risk of life-threatening lactic acidosis. Insulin therapy, with regular insulin, may be preferred while patients are in the intensive care unit.

SUGGESTED READINGS

Luna B, Feinglos MN. Drug-induced hyperglycemia. JAMA 2001;286:1945–1948.

Pandit MK. Drug induced disorders of glucose tolerance. Ann Intern Med 1993;118:529–539.

Van Den Berghe G, et al. Intensive insulin therapy in the critically ill patients. N Engl J Med 2001;345:1359–1367.

40

DO NOT USE MIDAZOLAM AND LORAZEPAM INTERCHANGEABLY IN THE INTENSIVE CARE UNIT

M. CRAIG BARRETT, PHARMD
RONALD F. SING, DO

A common misconception regarding benzodiazepines used in the intensive care unit (ICU) is that they are interchangeable agents producing the same effects. This approach does not acknowledge the pharmacologic differences between midazolam and lorazepam, which is primarily in their lipophilic properties. Lipophilicity directly affects the onset and duration of action of a drug. In addition, it is important to note that the pharmacokinetics of each drug changes considerably when they are given as a single bolus versus an infusion.

As a single bolus, midazolam has a shorter onset and duration of action than lorazepam, which makes it optimal for acute agitation or sedation prior to a procedure. The reason is that midazolam undergoes a transformation to a highly lipid state after administration. The highly lipophilic benzodiazepines, such as midazolam and diazepam, are able to cross the blood–brain barrier rapidly, causing a quick onset of action; midazolam has an onset of action of 0.5 to 5 minutes. In contrast, lorazepam is less lipophilic, which delays the crossover into the blood–brain barrier after a single bolus; lorazepam has an onset of action of 15 to 20 minutes. Being highly lipophilic also results in short duration of action after a single bolus. Agents like midazolam are able to readily leave the central nervous system (CNS) and move back into the plasma compartment (midazolam duration is 2 hours), whereas the more polar lorazepam is trapped in the CNS, resulting in a longer duration of action (6 to 10 hours).

WATCH OUT FOR

However, this time course of action is reversed in the setting of continuous infusions. It is important to note that a continuous infusion of midazolam results in drug accumulation in peripheral tissues. The general rule is that the longer the midazolam infusion and the higher the dose, the longer it will take for the patient to awaken once the infusion has been discontinued. In essence, the prolonged and/or high–dose infusions create a midazolam depot in the peripheral compartment. Once the infusion has been discontinued, peripheral tissues begin to release midazolam into plasma, where it reaches the CNS and crosses the blood–brain barrier. The clinical effect that occurs is a delayed and unpredictable wake time. As discussed earlier, lorazepam is less lipophilic, resulting in minimal peripheral accumulation with constant infusion. The clinical effect is a more predictable, although still prolonged, wake time, which is proportional to the dose administered.

The clinical relevance of this information is that midazolam should be the preferred benzodiazepine for patients who need to be sedated for less than 48 to 72 hours while lorazepam should be reserved for those patients requiring sedation longer than 72 hours. One strategy is to initiate sedation with midazolam for the first 48 to 72 hours and to switch to lorazepam if therapy is prolonged. There is no consensus on equivalent doses for lorazepam and midazolam, but an easy-to-remember rule of thumb is a 2:1 dose of midazolam to lorazepam. Converting back to midazolam in preparation for extubation should be a consideration.

Another common error in the ICU is the misconception that patients receiving lorazepam infusions should receive lorazepam boluses for acute agitation. Midazolam should be the agent of choice for acute agitation for patients receiving either midazolam or lorazepam infusions because of midazolam's more rapid onset of action. In addition, bolus doses need to be given with each infusion rate increase. The bolus is intended to alleviate acute agitation until the infusion reaches its new steady state (five drug half-lives).

One final note is that prolonged high-dose infusions of lorazepam have been reported to cause reversible acute tubular necrosis, lactic acidosis, and hyperosmolar states. The lorazepam solvents polyethylene glycol (PEG) and propylene glycol (PG) have been suggested as the cause of these effects and these high doses should be avoided if possible.

SUGGESTED READING

Jacobi J, Fraser GL, Coursin DB, et al. Society of Critical Care Medicine, American Society of Health-System Pharmacists, American College of Critical Care Medicine. Clinical practice guidelines for the sustained use of sedatives and analgesics in the critically ill adult. Crit Care Med 2002;30:119–141.

41

TRY TO AVOID USING BENZODIAZEPINES FOR SLEEP IN THE INTENSIVE CARE UNIT, ESPECIALLY IN THE ELDERLY

BRYAN A. COTTON, MD

During hospitalization, repeated arousals disrupt sleep continuity. These awakenings are secondary to laboratory draws, daily chest radiographs, vital sign recording, and numerous awakenings by nursing staff, ancillary personnel, medical students, and varying levels of physicians in training. Several studies have noted the frequency of sleep interruptions to be as often as every 20 minutes. In addition, the absence of diurnal light cycles is a major source of intensive care unit (ICU) sleep disruption and frequently results in cognitive disturbances. Almost 50% of sleep experienced by patients in the ICU occurs in the daytime. This form of sleep, however, lacks delta wave (deep) and rapid eye movement (REM) sleep, which are the "restful" and physiologically stable forms of sleep. In addition, sleep disruption is associated with many frequently used ICU medications such as beta-blockers, diuretics, benzodiazepines, and opiates.

WATCH OUT FOR

Sleep disruption results in numerous deleterious effects on an already fragile and disturbed physiology. Pulmonary consequences include decreased functional vital capacity, blunted hypercapnic and hypoxic responses, and decreased respiratory muscle endurance. As a result of the autonomic imbalances that follow sleep deprivation, increased hypertensive episodes, more frequent arrhythmias, and increased risk of acute myocardial ischemia have been described. In addition, sleep deprivation promotes a negative nitrogen balance, increased resting-energy expenditure, and immunological depression via suppression of antibody and cell-mediated responses. Most obvious to the physician, however, are the neurocognitive sequelae. Delirium, anxiety, hallucinations, and mood disorders have been associated with sleep deprivation in the ICU. In fact, healthy volunteers subjected to ICU-like sleep disturbances develop irritability, disorientation, and slurred speech.

Nonpharmacologic options to improve sleep hygiene include placing patients in private or single rooms with several windows, minimizing nighttime conversations by hospital personnel, placing alarms outside of patient rooms, and scheduling baths, linen changes, routine laboratory draws, and radiographs during the daytime. Studies that have evaluated the impact of noise reduction in the ICU have noted marked improvement in sleep quality. Improved REM sleep has been demonstrated with the implementation of earplugs in ICU patients. Additionally, lights should be turned off or dimmed at night to maintain circadian light cycles. Conversely, keeping the lights on during the daytime has been shown to reset circadian cycles and improves sleep at night, specifically in the elderly. In the high-risk population of elderly ICU patients, physical therapy and increased activity have been shown to promote sleep with shorter latency and deeper levels achieved.

Pharmacological agents are often used to improve sleep in the ICU. The ideal hypnotic would have a short half-life, have few drug-drug interactions, have few cardiac or pulmonary effects, and maintain sleep architecture. Although this drug has yet to be created, several agents currently available come close and should be considered for the critically ill patient with sleep disturbances. One of the oldest and least expensive medications available for sleep in this population is chloral hydrate. It is frequently used to initiate sleep for polysomnography studies, sedate children for procedures and diagnostic evaluations, as well as induce deeper levels of sleep in the pediatric ICU setting. Chloral hydrate induces sleep without changes in respiratory rate, $PaCO_2$, PaO_2, or tidal volumes. This is particularly safe and useful in the elderly in the induction and maintenance of sleep.

Other drugs sometimes used are zolpidem, trazodone, and mirtazapine. Although zolpidem is chemically unrelated to the benzodiazepines, it binds to omega receptors in the brain and has been shown to preserve the deep stages of sleep, as well as REM. This agent (or similar drugs in its growing class) may prove to be the ideal hypnotic, but it has yet to be studied in the ICU. Two other agents worthy of consideration are the antidepressants trazodone and mirtazapine. With the increasing recognition of mood disorders associated with prolonged ICU stays, these agents have seen increased utilization in those critically ill patients with sleep disturbances and posttraumatic stress disorder (PTSD) or situational-appropriate mood disorders. Trazodone has been identified as a very effective agent for sleep in depressed patients and those with PTSD. In addition, trazodone is well tolerated and associated with decreased awakenings and deeper levels of sleep achieved. Mirtazapine has a superior effect on the symptoms of insomnia, poor appetite, and anxiety. It has been shown to improve sleep latency, increase deeper stages of sleep, and increase total time of sleep.

Several drugs should be avoided in the ICU patient, especially when used as hypnotics. Benzodiazepines have been previously prescribed for sleep promotion and are frequently the only option known to many house officers, as well as attendings. However, this class of drugs may have deleterious effects on the respiratory system (increased hypercapnia, upper airway hypotonia) and on sleep architecture. Benzodiazepines are associated with a significant hangover effect and cognitive disturbances, especially in the elderly. Benzodiazepine use in the elderly has been associated with increased incidence of delirium, likely as a result of increased susceptibility to cognitive decline, as well as less predictable plasma drug levels. Moreover, the apolipoprotein E (APOE) 4 allele, which is associated with increased risk of development of Alzheimer disease, has been identified as a potential explanation as to why many elderly patients respond to benzodiazepines with a paradoxical agitation and/or confusion following exposure. However, diphenhydramine, an antihistamine and sedating drug with strong anticholinergic properties, is the agent most likely to result in adverse events following its use as a sleep agent. Paradoxical excitement, visual disturbances, and delirium are a result of its anticholinergic properties. The frequency of these events, especially in the elderly, should limit the use of diphenhydramine in the ICU to anaphylactic reactions.

One final note is that although potentially effective in the outpatient setting, melatonin has failed to show improvement in sleep in the ICU patient.

SUGGESTED READINGS

Gabor JY, Cooper AB, Hanly PJ. Sleep disruption in the intensive care unit. Curr Opin Crit Care 2001;7:21–27.

Parthasarathy S, Tobin MJ. Sleep in the intensive care unit. Intens Care Med 2004;30:197–206.

Peruzzi WT. Sleep in the intensive care unit. Pharmacotherapy 2005;25:34S–39S.

42

REMEMBER THAT ACTIVATED PROTEIN C IS NOT AS USEFUL FOR SEPSIS AS ONCE HOPED

RONALD W. PAULDINE, MD

Activated protein C (APC) exerts a number of biological effects including anti-inflammatory, antithrombotic, and profibrinolytic properties. Profibrinolytic effects include inactivation of plasminogen activator inhibitor. Antithrombotic effects include inactivation of factor Va and VIIIa. These effects are thought to aid in restoration and maintenance of microcirculatory blood flow, re-establishment of coagulation homeostasis, and preservation of the microcirculation. Tissue injury and organ dysfunction is thought to be attenuated by anti-inflammatory properties including decreasing thrombin-related inflammation, inhibiting tumor necrosis factor (TNF) and macrophage migration inhibitory factor production, blocking adhesion of leukocytes to selectins, and decreasing nuclear factor–$\kappa\beta$ activation.

The initial optimism associated with recombinant human activated protein C (rhAPC), (drotrecogin alfa [activated]) has been tempered by subsequent clinical trials. Data from the Recombinant Human Activated Protein C Worldwide Evaluation in Severe Sepsis (PROWESSS) trial demonstrated an absolute reduction of death from all causes at 28 days of 6.1%. The trial observed an increase in serious bleeding from 2.0% in the placebo group to 3.5% in the APC group. However, this effect was not statistically significant (it must be noted that this study was not powered to detect significance). Subgroup analysis revealed that the greatest risk reduction occurred in patients with the greatest severity of disease as assessed by APACHE II scores. Subsequently the drug was approved by the Food and Drug Administration (FDA) for use in patients with APACHE II scores >25. The recommendation to limit therapy to the sicker group of patients was confirmed in a trial of APC in patients with APACHE II scores <25 or with single organ failure. This trial, the Administration of Drotrecogin Alfa (Activated) in Early Stage Severe Sepsis (ADDRESS), was discontinued after enrolling 2,640 patients because of an inability to demonstrate reduced mortality in this less severely ill group with APC. Adding further to the argument against using APC is that the risk of serious bleeding with APC may be greater than originally reported in PROWESS. An uncontrolled open label trial (ENHANCE) reported incidence of serious bleeding at 6.5%. Other open-label trials have also demonstrated lack of benefit in pediatric patients.

| | Contraindications to treatment with RhAPC in-
| **WATCH OUT FOR** | clude conditions associated with risk of bleed-
| | ing such as active bleeding, recent hemorrhagic

stroke (within 3 months), recent intracranial or spinal surgery or recent severe head trauma (within 2 months), trauma with increased risk of life-threatening bleeding, presence of an epidural catheter, or intracranial neoplasm, mass lesion, or cerebral herniation. An FDA warning was added early in 2005 noting higher all-cause mortality in patients with recent surgery (within 30 days) and single organ dysfunction based on data from patients enrolled in the PROWESS trial. The ADDRESS trial also found higher all-cause mortality in patients with recent surgery and APACHE II score <25 with single organ dysfunction. Based on this data, many experts recommend consideration of rhAPC for surgical patients only if two or more organ failures are present.

One final note is that a 4-day course of rhAPC costs approximately $6,800. Using data from PROWESS, the cost per quality-adjusted life year for patients with APACHE II scores >25 is $27,400. rhAPC is administered via a continuous infusion at 24 mcg/kg/hr for 96 hours based on actual body weight.

SUGGESTED READINGS

Abraham E, Laterre PF, Garg, R, et al. Drotrecogin alfa (activated) for adults with severe sepsis and a low risk of death. N Engl J Med 2005;353:1332–1341.

Bernard GR, Vincent JL, Laterre PF, et al. Efficacy and safety of recombinant human activated protein C for severe sepsis. N Engl J Med 2001;344:699–709.

Fourrier F. Recombinant human activated protein C in the treatment of severe sepsis: an evidence-based review. Crit Care Med 2004;32:S534–S541.

Rice TW, Bernard GR. Drotrecogin alfa (activated) for the treatment of severe sepsis and septic shock. Am J Med Sci 2004;328:205–214.

Vincent JL, Bernard GR, Beale R, et al. Drotrecogin alfa (activated) treatment in severe sepsis from the global open-label trial ENHANCE; further evidence for survival and safety and implications for early treatment. Crit Care Med 2005;33:2266–2277.

43

KNOW THE ALTERNATE ROUTES FOR ADMINISTRATION OF CARDIOPULMONARY RESUSCITATION MEDICATIONS

ERIC M. BERSHAD, MD
JOSE I. SUAREZ, MD

In a cardiac arrest, pharmacologic support may be needed to help restore spontaneous circulation. These medications may include atropine, epinephrine, lidocaine, vasopressin, dopamine, naloxone, and others. In some patients, a central line or peripheral IV are not readily available, thus other methods of drug delivery must be used. The alternative methods include intraosseous (IO) and endotracheal (ET) administration.

WHAT TO DO

The American Heart Association recommends the use of intraosseous (IO) cannulation before resorting to endotracheal (ET) administration of cardiopulmonary resuscitation (CPR) medications. This is based on multiple studies in children and adults documenting safe and effective fluid resuscitation, drug delivery, and blood sampling with the IO approach. Furthermore, IO cannulation enables drug delivery comparable with that achieved by using a central line. This may be in part related to the noncollapsible venous plexus accessed in the IO approach. Any drug that can be given for resuscitation intravenously can also be given IO. In adults the sternum or proximal tibia has been successfully used for IO drug delivery. There are commercially available kits that facilitate IO access in adults.

If IV or IO access is not available, the ET route should be used. The medications that can be given ET include the NAVEL drugs: *n*aloxone; *a*tropine; *v*asopressin; *e*pinephrine; and *l*idocaine (*Table 43.1*). Additionally, vasopressin may be administered via the ET route. Blood levels of drugs given the ET route are lower than comparable blood levels when drugs are given intravenously. The optimal dose of ET-administered medications is unknown, but generally should be given at least 2 to 2.5 times greater than the IV dose, with two studies suggesting the required dose of epinephrine given ET should be 3 to 10 times higher than the equipotent IV dose. The administered endotracheal medications should be given in 5 to 10 mL of water or normal saline and then flushed with several brisk ventilations with a bag-mask valve. Some published studies examining ET-administered

TABLE 43.1	STANDARD DOSES OF CPR DRUGS	
DRUG	**IV OR IO**	**ET (EXACT DOSING UNKNOWN)**
Lidocaine	1 to 1.5 mg/kg, can repeat 0.5 to 0.75 mg/kg q 5 to 10 minutes to a maximum dose of 3 mg/kg	Multiply IV/IO dose by 2.5 to get ET dose.
Atropine	1 mg q 3 to 5 minutes up to maximum dose of 0.04 mg/kg	Same
Naloxone	0.4 to 2.0 mg initially, can repeat q 2 to 3 minutes up to 10 mg	Same
Epinephrine	1 mg q 3 to 5 minutes	2 to 2.5 mg q 3 to 5 minutes
Vasopressin	40 units × 1 dose	

epinephrine and lidocaine showed that dilution with water, rather than normal saline, may achieve better absorption.

SUGGESTED READINGS

American Heart Association. 2005 American Heart Association guidelines for CPR and ECC. Circulation 2005;112:IV-1–IV-203.

Iserson K. Intraosseous infusions in adults. J Emerg Med 1989;7:587–591.

Macnab A, Christenson J, Findlay J, et al. A new system for sternal intraosseous infusion in adults. Prehosp Emerg Care 2000;4:173–177.

44

Alkalinize the Urine in Tricyclic Antidepressant Overdose

Eliahu S. Feen, MD
Jose I. Suarez, MD

Tricyclic antidepressants (TCAs) are three-ringed organic compounds that have been used for decades in the treatment of depression and certain other psychiatric conditions. Other common conditions for which TCAs are used include chronic pain syndromes and migraine prophylaxis. Currently, TCAs are less commonly used for the treatment of depression and other mood disorders and psychiatric conditions because of the rise of newer therapies, especially the introduction of selective serotonin reuptake inhibitors (SSRIs).

Mechanism of Action

The mechanism of action of TCAs relates to the inhibition of the reuptake of both serotonin and norepinephrine from the synaptic cleft of neurons in the central nervous system. Inhibition of reuptake has an acute onset; however, the desired clinical effects can take weeks. Thus, TCAs likely induce postsynaptic neuron regulatory changes that ultimately provide their clinical benefits. In addition, TCAs have anticholinergic effects and inhibitory effects at histamine and α_1-adrenergic receptors, which explains the TCA side-effect profile.

Clinical Manifestation of TCA Overdose

Compared with other antidepressants (SSRIs or monoamine oxidase inhibitors [MAOIs]), TCAs carry a greater risk of death due to overdose. TCAs have more than twice the risk of death associated with overdoses of MAOIs and more than five times the risk associated with SSRIs and atypical antidepressant medications. Of TCA overdoses, 2% to 3% result in death, and most of these are due to cardiac complications. The clinical manifestations of TCA overdose include psychomotor depression, seizures, tachycardia, and cardiac conduction defects (specifically, prolonged PR, QRS, and QT intervals). In addition, the anticholinergic properties of TCAs will induce dry skin and mucous membranes, blurred vision, flushing, urinary retention, constipation, and potentially autonomic instability—most notably hypotension.

Management of TCA Overdose

Treatment of TCA overdose, like any poisoning, necessitates immediate attention to the patient's ABCs (airway, breathing, and circulation) and prompt contact with a local poison control center, if available. Gastric lavage using a nasogastric tube may be helpful if the patient presents within 12 hours of ingestion. Activated charcoal administration is highly recommended. However, syrup of ipecac is not recommended because of aspiration risk, since patients are usually lethargic. Hemodialysis and similar methods (charcoal hemoperfusion, peritoneal dialysis, and exchange transfusion) are not known to be significantly effective in removing TCA from the serum and tissues.

A central tenet of treatment of TCA overdose is that all patients should be alkalinized. It must be noted that while alkalinizing the urine in order to prevent renal reabsorption of certain ionic substances is helpful in some poisonings, it does not specifically assist with inhibition of renal reabsorption in TCA. *However*, the reason for urine alkalinization in TCA overdose is because of the cardiovascular toxicity of TCAs. Administration of intravenous (IV) sodium bicarbonate and/or hyperventilation (in intubated patients) can reverse toxic effects on the myocardium due to TCAs. Alkalinization has been shown to decrease QRS prolongation and repress arrhythmias. Typically 1 to 2 mEq per kg of sodium bicarbonate in normal saline (or D5W, if avoiding a saline load is desired) is given as a bolus, followed by 150 mEq in a liter of normal saline (or D5W) as a continuous infusion. The goal is to achieve an arterial pH of between 7.45 and 7.55. Patients with persistent QRS prolongation may be bolused with sodium bicarbonate to achieve a QRS duration of less than 0.16 seconds.

Suggested Readings

Henry JA, Alexander CA, Sender EK. Relative mortality from overdose of antidepressants. BMJ 1995;310:221–224.

Pimentel L, Trommer L. Cyclic antidepressant overdoses. Emerg Med Clin North Am 1994;12:533–547.

Sarko J. Antidepressants, old and new: a review of their adverse effects and toxicity in overdose. Emerg Med Clin North Am 2000;18:637–654.

45

CHECK TRIGLYCERIDE LEVEL IN PATIENTS ON PROPOFOL DRIPS

AMISHA BAROCHIA, MD

Propofol is a lipid–soluble alkylphenol agent that is frequently used to sedate mechanically ventilated patients in the intensive care unit (ICU). It has many desirable properties of an ideal sedative. It crosses the blood–brain barrier rapidly and has a rapid onset of action. It is metabolized quickly to inactive metabolites, giving it a short duration of action. It is easy to titrate and no dose adjustment is necessary for hepatic or renal insufficiency. It is not associated with tolerance or withdrawal symptoms. Propofol decreases cerebral metabolism and cerebral blood flow, which results in a decrease in intracranial pressure. It has been used with benefit in trauma patients with brain injury. It has also been used for seizure control in status epilepticus when other therapeutic agents have failed. In addition, propofol can be used as a general anesthetic at higher doses and can provide some antegrade amnesia. However, it does not have analgesic properties and its amnestic properties are not reliable, so it is often used in conjunction with benzodiazepines or opiates.

In comparison with midazolam, propofol seems to be a better sedative in many ICU patients. It is more easily titratable, it can be reversed more quickly without the development of withdrawal or tolerance, and its use may decrease the need for muscle relaxants when propofol is used as a first-line agent for sedation. Of note, a reduced time to weaning from the ventilator has been shown with propofol use as compared with midazolam. Propofol and midazolam have also been used together (with or without narcotics) to minimize the shortcomings of each agent used alone.

WATCH OUT FOR

As with most other sedatives, there are some drawbacks to using propofol. Hypotension is a frequent side effect, especially with bolus administration of the drug. A 25% to 40% decrease in blood pressure may be seen. This is a dose-dependent phenomenon and is usually transient. It can often be avoided by careful patient selection and adequate volume repletion.

Of more concern clinically than this easily managed hypotension is the propofol infusion syndrome, which was first described in 1992 in children and has since been reported in adults. The syndrome is usually associated with high-dose infusions of propofol, and it has been hypothesized that concomitant steroid or catecholamine use, sepsis, systemic inflammatory response syndrome (SIRS), and brain injury may contribute to its occurrence. Abnormalities in the mitochondrial and fatty acid metabolism are thought to be part of the pathogenesis of this syndrome. The clinical aspects of the syndrome include metabolic acidosis, hypertriglyceridemia, rhabdomyolysis, hypotension, brady-cardia, and eventually asystole and death. Although a causal relation-ship between this syndrome and propofol infusion has not been firmly established, vigilance for this spectrum of clinical findings is advised when using propofol, since cardiac impairment and death often occur without warning and the mortality rate is high. If suspected, propofol should be immediately discontinued and supportive measures insti-tuted. Therapies such as continuous hemofiltration or hemodialysis might improve outcomes.

In addition, it is important to remember that propofol is emul-sified in a soybean-based lipid formulation, which provides about 1.1 kCal/mL as fat calories. When infused at high doses it can be a significant source of calories for the patient, which should be taken into account when calculating the patient's nutritional require-ments. As a significant calorie source, it may increase CO_2 produc-tion and necessitate a greater minute ventilation to maintain acid–base balance.

Another concern with propofol infusions is the association with increased levels of triglycerides of up to 500 to 600 mg/dL in some studies, which may predispose patients to acute pancreatitis. If propo-fol is used at high dosages or for prolonged periods, triglyceride levels should be monitored. The lipid carrier may also predispose to throm-bosis by interfering with prothrombin times, but information about this complication is limited.

There have been reported cases of blood-stream infections secondary to the infusion of contaminated propofol. Propofol preparations are now available with a choice of preservatives like ethylenediaminetetraacetic acid (EDTA) and metabisulfite. Current recommendations state that propofol should not be used for more than 6 hours after it has been removed from its packaging and that infusion bottles and tubing should be changed frequently to decrease the risk of infection.

Finally, propofol infusions can irritate peripheral veins and can be very painful during administration. Lidocaine injection prior to or with the propofol may be helpful but is not always effective in ameliorating the pain.

SUGGESTED READINGS

Angelini G, Ketzler JT, Coursin DB. Use of propofol and other nonbenzodiazepine sedatives in the intensive care unit. Crit Care Clin 2001;17(4):863–880.

Riker R, Fraser GL. Adverse effects associated with sedatives, analgesics, and other drugs that provide patient comfort in the intensive care unit. Pharmacotherapy 2005;25:8S–18S.

BE ALERT FOR DRUG-RELATED PANCREATITIS IN HIV/AIDS PATIENTS AND CONSIDER A PERIOD OF PROXIMAL BOWEL REST

LAWERENCE OSEI, MD

Acute pancreatitis is an inflammatory condition of the pancreas, which is manifested clinically as abdominal pain with elevated pancreatic enzymes—amylase and lipase. It is potentially life threatening. Pancreatitis is caused by a variety of insults to the pancreas. It is estimated that in the United States, gallstones and chronic alcoholism account for approximately 75% of acute pancreatitis cases. The incidence of pancreatitis in non–human immunodeficiency virus (HIV) patients is relatively low and ranges from 17 to 30 cases per 100,000 population. However, it is considerably higher in the U.S. HIV population. One study of prevalence in the HIV population found incidence rates as high as 14 cases per 100 patients over a 1-year period. This is thought to be due to comorbid conditions like ethanol use, medications frequently used in HIV patients (e.g., didanosine, stavudine, corticosteroids, sulfonamides, isoniazid, ketoconazole, metronidazole), and opportunistic infections like cryptosporidiosis, mycobacteria, and cytomegalovirus (CMV) disease.

HIV-positive patients are frequently admitted to the intensive care unit (ICU). In addition to pancreatitis, some of the leading indications for ICU admissions are pneumococcal pneumonia or meningitis, cryptococcal meningitis, toxoplasmosis, liver failure from co-infection with hepatitis B or C, or shock from either infections or drugs (abacavir hypersensitivity). The critically ill patient with pancreatitis on antiretroviral drugs is a challenge and ICU physicians typically base treatment decisions on physician experience rather than data from controlled studies (that largely do not exist). Clearly, if the presenting condition is pancreatitis related to the HIV therapy, the drugs should be stopped and a regimen of proximal bowel rest should be undertaken. However, it is often difficult to substitute with alternative regimes because of overlapping toxicities, previous drug resistance, or difficulties in administering the drug. In addition, in patients who are nil per os (NPO), abruptly stopping antiretroviral therapy may cause a sudden fall in CD4(+) cell count and a rise in viral load. Some patients may even develop an acute seroconversion illness.

Complicating matters for the HIV patients with pancreatitis is that most antiretroviral drugs can only be administered to patients with a normally functioning gastrointestinal tract (GI) who can be fed orally or through a nasogastric tube. There are few data on the absorption and pharmacokinetics of any of the antiretrovirals when given through a gastric or a postpancreatic jejunal feeding tube. Erratic absorption from a nonfunctioning GI tract means the possibility of patients being on a drug at subtherapeutic levels, which can promote resistance to highly active antiretroviral therapy (HAART). However, where it will adversely impact care, it might be prudent to discontinue antiretroviral therapy until the critical illness is over.

When restarting HAART after a period of ICU management for pancreatitis, care must be taken to review possible drug-drug interactions with the antiretroviral regimen, especially when enzyme inducers, such as phenytoin and rifampicin, have been started. There are still relatively few data on the interactions between many of the drugs used in the ICU and those used in HIV therapy. The protease inhibitors and the nonnucleosides can act as cytochrome P450 3A4 inhibitors and affect the metabolism of many of the drugs used in ICU, such as midazolam or opiates. Listed in *Table 46.1* are some drug interactions to check for.

TABLE 46.1	DRUG-DRUG INTERACTIONS ASSOCIATED WITH ANTIRETROVIRALS/PROTEASE INHIBITORS
DRUG	**PRECAUTIONS**
Amiodarone	Do not use with ritonavir.
Statins	Increases AUC for statins.
Simvastatin, lovastatin	Do not use.
Atorvastatin	Increase 5.8-fold.
Pravastatin	AUC increased 30%.
Rifampin	Decreases AUC of lopinavir and ritonavir 75%.
Rifabutin	Lopinavir and ritonavir raises rifabutin level 3 times.
Ergot alkaloids	Unpredictable ergot levels.
Voriconazole	Bidirectional.
Methadone	Decreases AUC for lopinavir and amprenavir (not ritonavir).
Oral contraceptives	Decrease ethinyl estradiol 42%.
Sildenafil	Ritonavir increases AUC 11 times.
Desipramine	Increase AUC.
Propylene glycol	Oral fosamprenavir has propylene glycol.

AUC, area under the curve.

SUGGESTED READINGS

Dutta SK, Ting CD, Lai LL. Study of prevalence, severity, and etiological factors associated with acute pancreatitis in patients infected with human immunodeficiency virus. Am J Gastroenterol 1997;92:2044–2048.

Soni N, Pozniak A. Continuing HIV therapy in the ICU. Crit Care 2001;5:247–248.

47

CONSIDER THE USE OF FLUCONAZOLE PROPHYLAXIS IN INTENSIVE CARE PATIENTS WITH SEVERE PANCREATITIS, ABDOMINAL SEPSIS, OR NEED FOR MULTIPLE ABDOMINAL SURGERIES

LISA MARCUCCI, MD

There is a growing awareness of the increasing role of fungal infections in morbidity and mortality of intensive care unit (ICU) patients. The use of the azoles in prophylaxis for fungal infection in immunocompromised patients is well described and has proven efficacy. In addition, there is an increasing body of work that azole prophylaxis may be of benefit in certain patient populations as well. In both patient populations, infections caused by *Candida* species are thought to develop from endogenous colonization, yet the value of fungal surveillance cultures in critically ill patients is uncertain and lacks a high positive predictive value.

Fungal infections may develop in up to 30% to 35% of patients with necrotizing pancreatitis, with *Candida albicans* being the most frequently isolated fungal species by far. Two recent studies showed a significant decrease in fungal infections in a fluconazole prophylaxis group compared with a control group. In patients with septic shock from abdominal nonpancreatic sources, use of empiric fluconazole showed a decreased incidence of candidemia and fungal-related deaths in three recent studies, although reduction in overall mortality was less certain. Some caution has been voiced concerning the prophylactic use of fluconazole in "moderately ill" immunocompetent patients because of the risk of developing drug-resistant (resistant to azole drugs) fungal strains, especially *Candida glabrata*, although Swoboda et al. have reported no shift to nonalbicans pathogens with a decreased risk of mortality using prophylaxis.

Of recent interest to critical care physicians is the emerging literature on the anti-inflammatory properties of fluconazole. It appears that, separate from its antifungal properties, use of fluconazole may improve outcomes in septic patients because of blunting of the systemic inflammatory response that typically occurs. In light of this effect and the high mortality of candidemia, it seems reasonable to institute a short (10- to 14-day) course of prophylactic oral azole therapy (initial bolus of 800 mg and then a minimum of 200 and preferably

400 mg/day of fluconazole) in patients with severe pancreatitis, abdominal perforation, or anastomotic breakdown, and other abdominal catastrophes.

SUGGESTED READINGS

De Waele JJ, Vogelaers D, Blot S, et al. Fungal infections in patients with severe acute pancreatitis and the use of prophylactic therapy. J Infect Dis 2003;37:208–213.

He YM, Lu XS, Ai ZL, et al. Prevention and therapy of fungal infection in severe acute pancreatitis: a prospective clinical study. World J Gastroenterol 2003;9:2619–2621.

Swoboda SN, Merz WG, Lipsett PA. Candidemia: the impact of antifungal prophylaxis in a surgical intensive care unit. Surg Infect 2003;4:345–354.

Sypula WT, Kale-Pradhan PB. Therapeutic dilemma of fluconazole prophylaxis in intensive care. Ann Pharmacother 2002;36:155–159.

48

HAVE A HIGH THRESHOLD FOR ADMINISTERING VITAMIN K INTRAVENOUSLY

MICHAEL J. MORITZ, MD

Anaphylactoid reactions in patients receiving intravenously (IV) administered vitamin K have been widely reported. A recent review of the literature along with the US Food and Drug Administration (FDA) adverse drug reaction database uncovered a total of 155 cases, 27 of which were fatal and with the true number no doubt being much higher. The manufacturer has sufficient concern over the safety of IV administration of vitamin K that it was voluntarily removed from the Canadian market. Anaphylactic reactions and fatalities have occurred even when IV vitamin K was given at low doses and by slow dilute infusion. Of the reported 155 cases, 21 cases with four fatalities occurred in patients who received doses smaller than 5 mg of IV vitamin K. Reactions in patients receiving vitamin K by a non-IV route do occur but are much less common.

WATCH OUT FOR

The pathogenesis of this reaction is unknown and may be due to vasodilatation related to the solubilizing vehicle or immune-mediated (i.e., allergic) processes. The solubilizing agent is polyethoxylated castor oil (Cremophor EL). Despite rumors to the contrary, there has been no change in the formulation of the solubilizing agent in the last several years that decreases the risk of IV use. Other drugs using this agent include paclitaxel, cyclosporine, and teniposide, and all three drugs, when administered by IV, have been associated with reactions including anaphylaxis. The incidence of anaphylaxis after IV vitamin K appears to be similar to that of other drugs known to cause anaphylaxis, such as penicillin or iron dextran.

Vitamin K is commonly used to treat overanticoagulation from warfarin, which can be life threatening. The American College of Chest Physicians (ACCP) guidelines provide recommendations for vitamin K use in overanticoagulated patients but only for IV (despite the previously described 155 cases) and oral administration. In addition to IV and oral administration, vitamin K can be given subcutaneously. However, subcutaneous vitamin K may have less reliable kinetics than the other routes. In addition, several reports have found that oral vitamin K has a more rapid effect on lowering the international normalized ratio (INR) than the subcutaneous route.

To re-emphasize, the use of IV vitamin K should be avoided in almost all patients with overanticoagulation and should be reserved for those with serious hemorrhage, inability to take oral vitamin K, and inability to administer fresh frozen plasma. If IV vitamin K must be given, it should be administered mixed into a minibag of 100 mL of D5W or saline and given over a 30-minute period. Irrespective of the risk of an anaphylactoid reaction, there is no recommendation to pretreat patients with steroids or antihistamines before administering IV vitamin K.

SUGGESTED READINGS

Crowther MA, Douketis JD, Schnurr T, et al. Oral vitamin K lowers the international normalized ratio more rapidly than subcutaneous vitamin K in the treatment of warfarin-associated coagulopathy. A randomized, controlled trial. Ann Intern Med 2002;137:251–254.

Fiore LD, Scola MA, Cantillon CE, et al. Anaphylactoid reactions to vitamin K. J Thromb Thrombolysis 2001;11:175–183.

Riegert-Johnson DL, Volcheck GW. The incidence of anaphylaxis following intravenous phytonadione (vitamin K1): a 5-year retrospective review. Ann Allergy Asthma Immunol 2002;89:400–406.

Wjasow C, McNamara R. Anaphylaxis after low dose intravenous vitamin K. J Emerg Med 2003;24:169–172.

49

DO NOT USE BENZOCAINE SPRAY: IT INCREASES THE RISK OF METHEMOGLOBINEMIA

KELLY GROGAN, MD

Topical anesthetics are commonly used for procedures including endotracheal intubation, endoscopy, bronchoscopy, laryngoscopy, orogastric tube placement, dental extractions, and office gynecological procedures. Topical anesthetics are also widely available in several over-the-counter medications such as teething gels and throat lozenges. However, one topical anesthetic whose use should be avoided is benzocaine spray (aka Hurricaine spray) due to the risk of methemoglobinemia. Benzocaine-induced methemoglobinemia is an uncommon occurrence in clinical practice; however, knowledge of this potentially life-threatening condition is necessary to those practitioners who perform procedures requiring local, topical anesthesia.

PHYSIOLOGY AND PATHOPHYSIOLOGY

Methemoglobinemia occurs when an imbalance due to either increased methemoglobin production or decreased methemoglobin reduction is present. Normal hemoglobin contains an iron molecule that exists in the divalent ferrous state (Fe^{2+}). Methemoglobin results from the conversion of the iron ferrous ion (Fe^{2+}) to the oxidized ferric (Fe^{3+}) state. The ferric hemes of methemoglobin are unable to bind oxygen. In addition, the oxygen affinity of any accompanying ferrous hemes in the hemoglobin tetramer is increased. This results in a "left shift" in the oxygen dissociation curve and oxygen delivery to the tissues is impaired (*Fig. 49.1*). Therefore, the patient with increased concentrations of methemoglobin has a functional anemia as the circulating methemoglobin-containing molecules are unable to carry oxygen and deliver it to the tissues.

Auto-oxidation of hemoglobin to methemoglobin occurs spontaneously at a slow rate in normal individuals, converting 0.5% to 3% of the available hemoglobin to methemoglobin per day. The only physiologically important pathway for reducing methemoglobin back to hemoglobin is the nicotinamide adenine dinucleotide (NADH) reductase–dependent reaction catalyzed by cytochrome b5 reductase. An alternative pathway is an enzyme utilizing nicotine adenine dinucleotide phosphate (NADPH) generated by glucose-6-phosphate

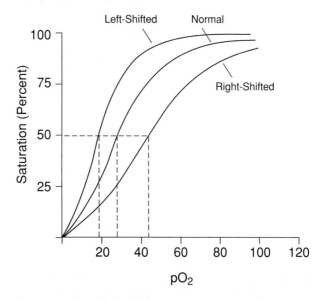

FIGURE 49.1. Oxygen Dissociation Curve

dehydrogenase (G6PD). There is normally no electron carrier present in red blood cells to interact with NADPH methemoglobin reductase, making this reaction a minor player in the conversion of methemoglobin to hemoglobin. However, its activity is markedly enhanced by electron acceptors or redox dyes, such as methylene blue.

Most cases of methemoglobinemia are acquired, resulting from increased methemoglobin formation by various exogenous agents. The mechanism involved in the formation of methemoglobin is not clear but appears to be the direct or indirect oxidation of hemoglobin to a degree that overwhelms the capacity of the reductive pathway. Local anesthetics have been implicated as a cause of methemoglobinemia for more than 50 years. Although almost all topical anesthetics have been associated, benzocaine is the most commonly implicated agent. Of the cases reported, more than half involved infants and the elderly. Cases have been reported after application to the pharyngeal mucosa, rectal mucosa, vaginal mucosa, and skin. The majority of cases of hereditary methemoglobinemia are due to a deficiency of NADPH methemoglobin reductase. This autosomal recessive disease is most common in the Inuit population and in Alaskan Native Americans. Hemoglobin M is another form of congenital methemoglobinemia characterized by an abnormal hemoglobin molecule.

CLINICAL PRESENTATION

Methemoglobinemia should be immediately suspected in any patient who has central cyanosis and a decrease in oxygen saturation that develops after the administration of benzocaine or other topical anesthetic. Clinical signs and symptoms depend on the level of methemoglobinemia. Levels greater than 15% are associated with cyanosis while headache, lethargy, tachycardia, weakness, and dizziness generally present at levels of 20% to 45%. Dyspnea, cyanosis, cardiac dysrhythmias, heart failure, seizures, and coma may occur at levels exceeding 45%. Methemoglobin levels above 70% are associated with a high mortality rate. The clinical effects may appear earlier and be more severe in patients with underlying anemia or cardiopulmonary disorders.

DIAGNOSIS

Methemoglobinemia may be clinically suspected by the presence of clinical "cyanosis" in the face of a normal arterial PO2 (PaO2) as obtained by arterial blood gases. The blood in methemoglobinemia has been variously described as dark red, chocolate, or brownish to blue in color, and, unlike deoxyhemoglobin, the color does not change with the addition of oxygen. Pulse oximetry is inaccurate in monitoring oxygen saturation in the presence of methemoglobinemia, and it cannot be used to make the diagnosis of the disorder. Pulse oximetry is based on differential light absorption of oxyhemoglobin and reduced hemoglobin at two wavelengths of light (typically 660 and 940 nm). The ratio of absorbance is used to provide an estimate of SpO2, calibrated so that a 1:1 ratio corresponds to a saturation of 85%. Methemoglobin has an absorbance pattern similar to reduced hemoglobin and exceeding that of oxyhemoglobin at 660 nm, and greater absorbance than either reduced hemoglobin or oxyhemoglobin at 940 nm. Therefore, in the presence of methemoglobin, light absorbance is greatly increased at both wavelengths and tends to drive the absorbance ratio toward unity. Based on these characteristics, SpO2 tends to be about 85% over a wide range of pathologic methemoglobin levels. Thus, oxygen saturation measurement by pulse oximetry can over- or underestimate the degree of oxygenation, depending on its severity. However, the presence of methemoglobin can be suspected when the oxygen saturation as measured by the pulse oximetry is significantly less than the oxygen saturation from arterial blood gas analysis (saturation gap).

The laboratory diagnosis of methemoglobinemia is based upon analysis of its absorption spectra, which has peak absorbance at

631 nm. A fresh specimen should always be obtained as methemoglobin will increase with storage. The standard method of assaying methemoglobin utilizes a microprocessor-controlled, fixed-wavelength co-oximeter. This instrument interprets all readings in the 630-nm range as methemoglobin; thus false positives may occur in the presence of other pigments including sulfhemoglobin and methylene blue.

TREATMENT

In acquired methemoglobinemias, the offending agents should be discontinued. In one study of 138 cases of acquired methemoglobinemia, use of dapsone accounted for 42% of all affected patients, with a mean level of methemoglobin of 7.6%. The most severe cases were seen after the use of 20% benzocaine spray for topical anesthesia (mean peak methemoglobin level 44%, range 16% to 60%).

In lesser degrees of methemoglobinemia, no therapy other than discontinuation of the offending agents may be required. In the absence of serious underlying illnesses, methemoglobin levels less than 30% usually resolve spontaneously over 15 to 20 hours. However, this condition can be life threatening when methemoglobin constitutes more than 50% of total hemoglobin. Blood transfusions or exchange transfusions may be helpful in patients who are in shock.

Methylene blue (methylthionine chloride), given intravenously in a dose of 1 to 2 mg/kg over five minutes, provides an artificial electron acceptor for the reduction of methemoglobin via the NADPH-dependent pathway, greatly increasing the enzymatic reduction of methemoglobin. Methylene blue is converted to leukomethylene blue by accepting an electron from NADPH in the presence of NADPH-methemoglobin reductase. Leukomethylene blue then donates this electron to methemoglobin, resulting in its conversion to hemoglobin. Response is usually rapid and while methylene blue may be redosed in one hour, this is frequently not necessary. It is important to note that large doses of methylene blue (>7 mg/kg) can cause dyspnea, chest pain, and hemolysis. Doses exceeding 15 mg/kg may actually cause methemoglobinemia by direct oxidation of hemoglobin. Since co-oximetry detects methylene blue as methemoglobin, this is not a useful method to determine the response of methemoglobin levels to treatment with methylene blue.

Finally, patients with G6PD deficiency who have decreased production of NADPH will not respond to methylene blue.

SUGGESTED READINGS

Anderson S, Hajduczek J, Barker S. Benzocaine-induced methemoglobinemia in an adult: accuracy of pulse oximetry with methemoglobinemia. Anesth Analg 1988;67:1099–1101.

Ash-Bernal R, Wise R, Wright S. Acquired methemoglobinemia: a retrospective series of 138 cases at 2 teaching hospitals. Medicine 2004;83:265.

Rodriguez L, Smolik L, Zbehlik A. Benzocaine-induced methemoglobinemia: report of a severe reaction and review of the literature. Ann Pharmacother 1994;28:643–649.

50

KNOW WHICH WEIGHT TO USE WHEN DOSING MEDICATIONS

EDWARD T. HORN, PHARMD

Volume of distribution (Vd) is a nebulous pharmacokinetic principle that describes the hypothetical volume of plasma into which a drug distributes. While this is not an actual physiologic parameter like cardiac output or clearance, it is an extremely useful tool that describes how widely a drug distributes throughout body fluids and tissues.

Vd is often reported in either liters or liters per kg to help normalize a particular drug's Vd to a patient's weight. As the Vd increases, so does the drug's ability to distribute into various body tissues. The body tissues that the drug distributes into will be based on drug characteristics in addition to the Vd. This is important to understand when determining the dose of a medication to administer to a patient. Dose is related to Vd by the following equation:

$$\text{peak concentration} = \frac{\text{dose (mg)}}{\text{Vd (L)}}$$

This shows that as Vd increases, the dose must increase to achieve the same concentration; the converse is also true. As a patient's weight changes through his or her stay in an intensive care unit (ICU) (early on, weight gain due to fluid resuscitation; later, weight loss due to diuresis), Vd will change as well and may affect how doses result in the therapeutic levels that are achieved. Vd can be affected by various physiologic aberrations that occur in the ICU patient because of deranged organ function. These include decreased plasma proteins (and plasma protein binding), pH differences, and fluid balance abnormalities.

These issues with Vd can be related to the weight changes and the various weight definitions that are used in critically ill patients. In drugs with a larger Vd that will distribute widely within the body, doses based on actual weight are used. To briefly review, the various weight definitions are

Actual Body Weight: The actual weight of the patient at any given time; includes fluids for resuscitation and fat.

Ideal Body Weight (IBW): Weight calculated based on height and gender.

$$\text{IBW (male)} = (\text{height in inches} > 60 \times 2.3) + 50$$

$$\text{IBW (female)} = (\text{height in inches} > 60 \times 2.3) + 45.5$$

TABLE 50.1 GUIDELINE FOR DOSING SOME COMMON ICU DRUGS

DRUG/CLASS	WEIGHT TO USE WHEN CALCULATING DOSE		NORMAL PEAK	NORMAL TROUGH
	ACTUAL BW ≤150% OF IBW	ACTUAL BW >150% OF IBW		
Aminoglycosides	Actual weight	Adjusted weight = IBW + 0.4 (Act BW − IBW)	8–10 mcg/mL	<2 mcg/mL
Heparin	Actual weight	Adjusted weight = IBW + 0.4 (Act BW − IBW)	n/a	n/a
Beta-lactams	Actual weight (use higher end of normal doses)	Actual weight (use higher end of normal doses)	Varies	Varies
Ciprofloxacin	Actual weight (use higher end of normal doses)	Actual weight (use higher end of normal doses)		
Vancomycin	Actual weight	Actual weight	n/a	15–20 mcg/mL
Amiodarone	Actual weight	Adjusted weight, but may need to give supplemental doses	n/a	n/a
Drotrecogin Alfa	Actual weight[a]	Actual weight[a]	n/a	n/a

[a] Models what was done in large randomized controlled trials.

Adjusted Body Weight: Weight calculated from the difference between ideal and actual weight.

$$\text{Adj BW} = \text{IBW} + (0.25 \text{ to } 0.40 \, [\text{Actual BW} - \text{IBW}])$$

As mentioned earlier, drug dosing is also impacted by the physiochemical properties of the drug—specifically the lipophilicity or hydrophilicity of the agent in question. For example, aminoglycosides are very hydrophilic agents. In morbidly obese patients, dosing should be based on an adjusted body weight. However, an actual weight should be used to estimate doses in a postoperative ICU patient who has large amounts of extracellular fluid on board. It should be noted that medications used as infusions should be titrated to effect, regardless of weight used.

Table 50.1 is a guide to help make dosing decisions for common ICU drugs based on weight. As a general rule, in obese patients, the actual weight should be used for drugs that distribute well into tissues (e.g., quinolones, vancomycin). An adjusted weight should be used for medications that do not distribute well into body tissues (e.g., heparin, aminoglycosides). For medications that distribute into extravascular fluid well, like aminoglycosides, any increases in weight due to fluid administration must be taken into consideration. As a general recommendation, you can add that difference in weight to the actual or adjusted weight that will be used. For example, imagine the patient weights are as follows:

> Actual: 130 kg
> Usual: 120 kg
> Ideal: 70 kg

The weight that would be used for aminoglycoside dosing for this patient would be an adjusted weight (Adj weight $= 70 + 0.4\,[120 - 70] = 90$ kg) with the addition of the extra 10 kg of fluid on board, or 100 kg total. If you wanted to add vancomycin to this regimen, then you would just use the actual weight, since vancomycin has a larger Vd and will distribute into the fat as well as the fluid on board.

SUGGESTED READINGS

Buton ME, Shaw LM, Schentag JJ, eds. Applied Pharmacokinetics and Pharmcodynamics: Principles of Therapeutic Drug Monitoring. 4th Ed. Philadelphia: Lippincott Williams & Wilkins; 2006:8–29.

Erstad BL. Dosing of medications in the morbidly obese in the intensive care unit setting. Intensive Care Med 2004;30:18–32.

51

Beware of Intensive Care Unit Medications That Can Increase Serum Potassium and Cause Hyperkalemia

Adam R. Berliner, MD
Derek M. Fine, MD

Many common medications can raise serum potassium (K^+) concentration. Although these effects are usually insignificant in healthy patients with normal renal function, the synergy between polypharmacy and the high prevalence of coexisting renal dysfunction in the intensive care unit (ICU) can make these effects very dangerous in critically ill patients. *Table 51.1* lists some frequent offenders in the ICU setting.

Diagnosis of Hyperkalemia

Electrocardiographic (ECG) changes in hyperkalemia are striking if present and include peaked T-waves, varying degrees of A-V block, QRS-interval widening, or diminutive or lost P-waves. However, the severely hyperkalemic patient (a) does not progress through these ECG changes in a predictable sequence and (b) may not have any of these changes. A benign ECG can move to ventricular fibrillation with no intervening changes. ECG changes alone are not sensitive enough to use their absence to dismiss the danger of hyperkalemia . Regardless of ECG changes, a serum K^+ of ≥ 6.0 meq/L merits prompt therapy to rapidly stabilize the myocardium to protect against arrhythmias and to rapidly lower extracellular K^+ via shifting toward intracellular stores, with an eye toward more definitive therapy thereafter. Values in the range of 5.0 to 5.9 meq/L are also cause for concern if a trend of continuing increase is expected. Otherwise, elevations to this degree (5.0 to 5.9 meq/L) may be treated with definitive therapies alone or simply minimization of offensive medications or K^+ intake.

Treatment Options

Immediate Therapy (for Cardiac Myocyte Membrane Stabilization to Prevent Arrhythmia). Generally reserved for K^+ levels ≥ 6.0 meq/L, intravenous calcium salts (most commonly 10 cc [one ampule] of 10% calcium gluconate solution) are usually given concurrently with the short-acting therapies discussed next. The effect is rapid (onset 1 to 3 min) but brief (30 to 60 min).

TABLE 51.1	COMMON MEDICATIONS THAT CAN CAUSE HYPERKALEMIA
DRUG	**MECHANISM OF HYPERKALEMIA**
Beta-2 blockers	Decreased renin release (and hence diminished aldosterone action) and impaired cellular uptake of K^+ by sodium-potassium pump.
Spironolactone, eplerenone	Aldosterone receptor inhibitor, down regulates distal nephron K^+ excretion.
Heparin (IV or SQ), ketoconazole	Impaired aldosterone metabolism leading to diminished aldosterone effect.
Angiotensin-converting enzyme inhibitors/angiotensin II receptor blockers	Suppression of aldosterone release; decreased glomerular filtration rate (GFR).
Succinylcholine	Muscle cell depolarization-induced K^+ "leak" from intra- to extracellular space.
Nonsteroidal anti-inflammatory drugs (NSAIDs)	Decreased renin release; decreased GFR.
Digoxin	Inhibition of sodium-potassium pump.
Tacrolimus, cyclosporine	Decreased renin release.
Trimethoprim, amiloride, triamterene, pentamidine	Blockade of collecting duct sodium channels, thereby reducing sodium-for-potassium exchange and hence K^+ excretion.

Short-acting Therapy (to "Shift" Potassium from Extracellular to Intracellular Sites). The foremost "shifting" therapy is intravenous insulin (usually 10 units coadministered with 1 ampule IV dextrose unless the patient is already hyperglycemic), which acts via stimulation of the cellular sodium-potassium pump. The effect begins in 10 to 20 minutes and lasts 4 to 6 hours. In persistently hyperglycemic patients an insulin drip may be required, since hyperglycemia itself can promote hyperkalemia. Nebulized beta-2 agonists, usually 10 to 20 mg albuterol (about four to eight times the dose of a common 2.5-mg nebulizer treatment), can be given as well. Lastly, the role of intravenous bicarbonate in this setting is debated. If severe acidemia is present, normalization of blood pH can help reduce hyperkalemia but otherwise bicarbonate by itself is thought to be of little intrinsic benefit in shifting K^+ intracellularly. Indeed, through the lowering of ionized calcium by increasing serum pH, the use of bicarbonate may actually be detrimental in the face of a significant hyperkalemia. In chronic dialysis patients in particular, one study showed bicarbonate to have very little potassium-lowering effect.

Definitive Therapy (to Reduce Total Body Potassium Stores). *Sodium polystyrene sulfate* (Kayexalate) is the most commonly used anion exchange resin used to treat hyperkalemia. Given orally or as a retention enema, it absorbs K^+ and other luminal cations, which are then lost in stool. It carries a finite incidence of colonic necrosis, frequently in the context of an elderly patient with widespread atherosclerotic disease who may have mesenteric hypoperfusion due to hypotension or dehydration and impaired gastrointestinal motility (usually postoperative). It should never be given to renal transplant patients.

Intravenous loop diuretics at doses sufficient to induce high urinary flow rates will clear K^+ via the urine. In the presence of severe underlying renal disease, however, this approach may be unsuccessful.

Dialysis is the most rapid method of lowering serum K^+, though since the overwhelming majority of bodily K^+ stores are intracellular, rebound hyperkalemia postdialysis can be problematic. Rebound hyperkalemia more often occurs if there is an ongoing K^+ source (e.g., ischemic tissue) or if dialysis is preceded by aggressive pharmacological shifting of K^+ to intracellular stores.

OTHER POTASSIUM FUN FACTS

- After spironolactone was shown to reduce morbidity and mortality in severe heart failure, a Canadian study showed a four- to fivefold increase in spironolactone prescriptions, a four- to fivefold increase in hospitalization for hyperkalemia, and a sixfold increase in hyperkalemia-related mortality. Extra caution is required when considering the initiation of spironolactone in hospitalized patients.
- Other causes of hyperkalemia in the ICU include severe acidemia, rhabdomyolysis, ischemic or gangrenous tissue, and hemolysis.
- Think about pseudohyperkalemia—caused by K^+ release into the already collected blood sample—in conditions when erythrocyte, leukocyte, or platelet numbers are pathologically high (e.g., leukemia, polycythemia). For an accurate assay the K^+ should be rechecked in a serum separator tube (or in a heparinized tube in the case of severe thrombocytosis).
- K^+ can hide in medication components (e.g., penicillin G potassium has 1.7 mEq potassium/million units) or dietary intake. For approximation when reading labeled food ingredients, 39 mg potassium is equal to 1 mEq (in vitro).

SUGGESTED READINGS

Blumberg A. Effect of various therapeutic approaches on plasma potassium and major regulating factors in terminal renal failure. Am J Med 1988;85:507–512.

Greenberg A. Hyperkalemia: treatment options. Semin Nephrol 1998;18:46–57.

Palmer B. Current concepts: managing hyperkalemia caused by inhibitors of the rennin-angiotensin-aldosterone system. N Engl J Med 2004;351:585–592.

Pitt B, Zannad F, Remme WJ, et al. The effect of spironolactone on morbidity and mortality in patients with severe heart failure. Randomized Aldactone Evaluation Study Investigators. N Engl J Med 1999;342:709–717.

52

ADMINISTER ACETAZOLAMIDE (DIAMOX) ON A ONE-TIME DOSE SCHEDULE ONLY

YING WEI LUM, MD

Metabolic alkalosis is usually categorized as either chloride responsive or nonchloride responsive. Common causes for chloride–responsive metabolic alkalosis in the intensive care unit (ICU) setting include diuretic therapy, vomiting (or from excessive nasogastric suctioning), and diarrhea. Nonchloride causes include alkali administration (with sodium bicarbonate or rapid infusion of more than eight units of blood that contain large quantities of citrate), mineralo-corticosteroid excess (corticosteroid administration), chronic respiratory acidosis (secondary to permissive hypercapnea from mechanical ventilation), and hypokalemia.

Therapy for metabolic alkalosis in most patients involves discontinuing the causative factor for alkalosis and undertaking volume and electrolyte repletion. Patients in an edematous state, however, follow a different principle since it may be desirable to avoid volume repletion. Treatment with acetazolamide (Diamox) may be indicated in this setting. Acetazolamide is a carbonic anhydrase inhibitor that acts by promoting the renal excretion of bicarbonate anions and hence reversing the metabolic alkalosis.

Acetazolamide is commonly administered between 250 and 500 mg every 24 hours for 3 to 4 doses; continuous dosing can cause a metabolic acidosis. A wide body of evidence to support a once-daily dosing strategy is lacking. However, there have been reports that the effect of acetazolamide lasts 24 to 72 hours after single dose administration. Marik et al. studied the effect in a population of 30 mechanically ventilated (mostly surgical) patients and noted that after the administration of a single dose of 500 mg of intravenous acetazolamide, there was a mean reduction of 6.4 mmol/L of bicarbonate at 24 hours. The onset of action was within 2 hours and peaked at a mean of 15.5 hours, although there was wide variation.

WHAT NOT TO DO

Health care providers who administer acetazolamide should be cautious about overcorrection of metabolic alkalosis, which can in turn cause a hyperchloremic acidosis. Another common precautionary measure is the monitoring of serum potassium since hypokalemia can develop as a result of increased sodium bicarbonate delivery to the collecting tubules, which in turn can enhance sodium and/or potassium channels to encourage potassium excretion. Most experienced clinicians wait for potassium to be in the high normal range before giving acetazolamide.

SUGGESTED READINGS

Marik PE, Kussman BD, Lipman J, et al. Acetazolamide in the treatment of metabolic alkalosis in critically ill patients. Heart Lung 1991;20:455–459.

Mazur JE, Devlin JW, Peters MJ, et al. Single versus multiple doses of acetazolamide for metabolic alkalosis in critically ill medical patients: a randomized, double-blind trial. Crit Care Med 1999;27:1257–1261.

53

CHECK AN ELECTROCARDIOGRAM FOR LONG QT INTERVAL BEFORE GIVING HALOPERIDOL

SHAYTONE NICHOLS, MD

Several drugs used in the intensive care unit (ICU) have the potential to prolong the QT interval. If not corrected, this can evolve into the malignant arrhythmia of *torsades de pointes*. The QT interval is the total duration of depolarization and repolarization of the ventricles; prolonged QT is due to lengthening of the repolarization phase and usually due to changes in potassium handling by sodium or potassium channels. A long QT can be inherited or acquired; the acquired form is usually induced by drugs or electrolyte abnormalities like hypokalemia and hypomagnesaemia.

Drugs commonly used in the ICU that potentiate this effect are haldol, amiodarone, metoclopramide, ibutilide, procainamide, azithromycin, clarithromycin, cisapride, erythromycin, methadone, and pentamidine. When using these drugs, an electrocardiogram (ECG) should be checked to ensure a normal QT.

WHAT TO DO

If the patient does develop a long QT interval, strong consideration should be given to stopping the medicine and correcting any electrolyte abnormalities. Experienced practitioners will give empiric magnesium in the setting of normal renal function. If the patient develops *torsades de pointes*, overdrive pacing, isoproterenol, and magnesium are the standard of care. The goal is to increase heart rate to shorten ventricular repolarization. Overdrive pacings is to a rate of 100 to 120 beats per minute either transvenously or externally. Isoproterenol may also be effective to this end.

A recent analysis of 250 people who had drug-induced long QT showed that in the majority of cases, predisposing factors can be identified. These factors included inhibition of cytochrome P450 by other concurrent medicines the patient was taking (47%); electrolyte derangements (32%); and concomitant administration of more than one QT-prolonging medicine (23%).

One important drug class that falls into the category of potentiating the long QT interval via cytochrome P450 inhibition is the azole class used to treat fungal infections. Prophylaxis for fungal infections is now standard in many ICU settings and it is important to remember that while this class has not been definitely linked to torsades, it can potentiate this effect.

SUGGESTED READING

Roden DM. Drug-induced prolongation of the QT interval. N Engl J Med 2004;350:1013–1022.

54

DO NOT USE IPRATROPIUM IN METER-DOSE INHALER FORM IN PATIENTS WITH NUT ALLERGIES

J. GREGORY HOBELMANN, MD

Ipratropium bromide is an anticholinergic agent that is commonly used in the intensive care unit (ICU) and in the treatment of asthma and chronic obstructive airways disease (COPD). Ipratropium is a competitive muscarinic acetylcholine receptor antagonist that when given intravenously is most potent at the inhibition of bronchial receptors. When given by the inhaled route, even in high dosage, the systemic effects, such as salivary, cardiac, ocular, and urinary effects, are negligible. It produces a dose-related inhibition of both substance-induced and exercised-induced bronchoconstriction. It is a potent bronchodilator in patients with COPD but is less potent in patients with asthma that is responsive to beta-2 agonists. In patients with asthma alone, the combination of ipratropium and a beta-2 agonist may be synergistic, but often beta-2 agonism may be a good solo-agent treatment. Other treatments for COPD in addition to anticholinergics and beta-2 agonists are theophylline and corticosteroids.

The onset of action of ipratropium when given by the inhaled route is slower than that of the beta-2 agonists, (around 30 to 60 minutes) and its effects last up to 4 to 6 hours with a maximal effect at 1 to 2 hours. Very little of the drug is absorbed following inhalation or ingestion so hepatic or renal impairment has little effect on its therapeutic use and there is no evidence of tolerance with prolonged use.

There are several concerns that must be considered when starting a patient on ipratropium. It should be used with caution in patients who have glaucoma, difficulty with urination, an allergy to soy or peanuts, or recreational use of betel nuts. Patients with recreational use of betel nuts are known to be more prone to allergic reactions. Patients with allergies to nuts or soy may have an allergic reaction to the metered-dose inhaler (MDI) preparation but not the nebulized form since the allergy is to a compound in the preparation of the MDI. If an allergy is present, patients may experience a constellation of symptoms consisting of chest pain; tachycardia; trouble breathing or wheezing; swelling of the face, lips, or tongue; and/or a rash or hives. The first step in therapy is to eliminate the instigating factor, namely the MDI, and then use supportive measures as for any allergic reaction, depending on severity.

SUGGESTED READINGS

Betel Nut. Wikipedia. http://en.wikipedia.org/wiki/Betel_nut

Facchini G, Antonicelli L, Cinti B, et al. Paradoxical bronchospasm and cutaneous rash after metered-dose inhaled bronchodilators. Monaldi Arch Chest Dis 1996;51:201–203.

Micromedex Healthcare Series on Ipratropium. Thomson Healthcare. http://www.thomsonhc.com/hcs/librarian

55

BE CAUTIOUS IN USING KETOROLAC IN PATIENTS WITH MARGINAL URINE OUTPUT OR RENAL FUNCTION

ANGELA D. SHOHER, MD

Ketorolac is a nonsteroidal inflammatory agent with greater systemic analgesic properties than anti-inflammatory activity. The onset and efficacy of its analgesic properties are claimed to be comparable with those of morphine. Ketorolac works by competitively inhibiting the cyclooxygenase isoenzymes (COX-1 and COX-2). These enzymes catalyze the conversion of arachidonic acid to prostaglandins. Prostaglandins E and F appear to be responsible for sensitizing pain receptors, explaining the analgesic properties of the drug. Bioavailability of the drug is 100% after oral, intravenous, or intramuscular administration. Food only decreases the rate but not the extent of absorption. Ketorolac is also 99% bound to albumin. It is metabolized by the liver to a form that is less than 1% as potent as the original form.

WHAT NOT TO DO

The dosing of ketorolac should not exceed a period of 3 days. Oral use is indicated only in combination therapy with intravenous (IV) or intramuscular (IM) forms and is rarely used in the intensive care unit (ICU). In patients who are less than 65 years of age, 30 mg can be given IV every 6 hours. Special consideration of ketorolac includes the renal effects of the drug. Prostaglandins in the kidney mediate sodium and water reabsorption. In the setting of decreased volume, prostaglandins help maintain renal blood flow. Ketorolac administration in a patient with tenuous renal function therefore may lead to decreased renal perfusion and acute renal failure. In patients with renal impairment (serum creatinine >1.9 mg/dL), the dose may need to be adjusted. These patients and those who are older than 65 years or weigh less than 50 kg should receive no more than 15 mg every 6 hours. Ketorolac can also inhibit platelet aggregation by decreasing levels of platelet thromboxane A2, which leads to an increase in bleeding time. The platelet inhibition is reversible within 24 to 48 hours. Of note, ketorolac can also cause gastrointestinal side effects including ulceration related to the COX-1 inhibition.

SUGGESTED READINGS

Katzung BG, ed. Basic and Clinical Pharmacology. 9th Ed. New York: McGraw-Hill; 2004:596–624.

Wickersham RM, Gremillion S, eds. Drug Facts and Comparisons Pocket Version. 10th Ed. St. Louis: Wolters Kluwer Health; 2005:473.

56

DO NOT CRUSH SEVELAMER HYDROCHLORIDE (RENAGEL) TO PLACE DOWN A NASOGASTRIC OR FEEDING TUBE

ASHITA GOEL, MD

Hyperphosphatemia is a common metabolic derangement seen in end-stage renal disease secondary to the inability of the kidney to excrete serum phosphate. High levels of phosphates can result in secondary hyperparathyroidism and release of calcium from bone. This loss of calcium from bone can result in osteodystrophy and ectopic calcium deposition into soft tissues including deposits in coronary or cerebral arteries.

WHAT NOT TO DO

Sevelamer (Renagel) is an aluminum- and calcium-free phosphate binder used in the treatment of hyperphosphatemia in end-stage renal disease. Sevelamer is a cationic polymer (poly[allylamine hydrochloride]) cross-linked with epichlorohydrin, which binds phosphate anions by ion exchange and hydrogen binding. Although sevelamer is hydrophilic, it is not absorbed by the gastrointestinal tract. When the polymer comes in contact with gastric or intestinal fluid, it expands through hydration; it can expand up to eight times its weight. This gelatinous form binds phosphate in the gastrointestinal tract and then is excreted in feces. This polymer cannot be crushed or broken prior to ingestion because an intact gelatinous matrix is needed for efficient phosphate binding.

Of interest to clinicians is that unlike other phosphate binders, sevelamer has the unique property to sequester bile acids in addition to phosphates. Use of this drug has been associated with lowered low-density lipoprotein (LDL) and total serum cholesterol levels. Possibly through an improved lipid profile and reductions in hypercalcemia, sevelamer has been shown to stabilize or retard coronary and aortic calcification. However, clinical correlations are unclear. Side effects of sevelamer include nausea, dyspepsia, constipation, and worsening metabolic acidosis. The metabolic acidosis is more pronounced in patients receiving an acetate-based dialysate over bicarbonate.

Currently, the most widespread method of phosphorous reduction relies on other phosphate binders. Calcium salts such as calcium acetate and calcium carbonate are currently the most broadly used agents. When compared with sevelamer, calcium salts have similar efficacy profiles in reduction of phosphate levels at significantly lower costs. However, calcium salts can result in hypercalcemia (with calcium carbonate being the most pronounced offender), adynamic bone disease, vascular calcifications, and lead toxicities. Other metallic salts can also be used in phosphate binding. Early on, aluminum salts were used as phosphate binders, but they were found to result in deposition of aluminum in soft tissue including the brain. Recently, salts of rare earth metals are under investigation for their ability to bind phosphate. Lanthanum carbonate appears to be the next promising aluminum- and calcium-free phosphate binder. Clinical trials have shown minimal gastrointestinal absorption of the metal with phosphate-binding efficacy similar to the calcium salts. These new binders do not possess any cholesterol-lowering properties.

SUGGESTED READING

Loghman-Adham M. Safety of new phosphate binders for chronic renal failure. Drug Saf 2003;26:1093–1110.

57

REMEMBER THAT MANY COMMONLY USED INTENSIVE CARE UNIT DRUGS SHOULD NOT BE USED IN PORPHYRIA

J. GREGORY HOBELMANN, MD

The porphyrias are a constellation of congenital and acquired deficiencies in the activity of enzymes involved in the biosynthesis of heme. Abnormal amounts of the heme intermediate compounds are formed, resulting in tissue accumulation and excessive excretion. All of these intermediates in the heme biosynthetic pathway can be toxic and can result in neurovisceral symptoms or photocutaneous symptoms. Some porphyrias cause life-threatening neurovisceral abnormalities and are characterized by the presence of aminolevulinic acid (ALA) or porphobilinogen in the urine. Others cause photosensitivity and skin damage with exposure to ultraviolet light with subsequent production of tissue-damaging free radicals.

WATCH OUT FOR

The diagnosis of each type of porphyria may be made by identifying the metabolite of excess in the urine, feces, or blood. The two most common types are porphyria cutanea tarda and acute intermittent porphyria. The diagnosis of porphyria cutanea tarda is strongly suggested by the presence of blistering skin lesions on areas exposed to ultraviolet light. This condition is confirmed by a high plasma porphyrin level and uroporphyrin in the urine. Liver enzymes may be elevated, but liver function is rarely affected. Risk factors for developing porphyria cutanea tarda include excessive alcohol use, hepatitis C, human immunodeficiency virus (HIV), and iron overload. Treatment consists of phlebotomy and low-dose chloroquine, which are almost always effective. Other than potential cutaneous scars, there are no long-term sequelae of the disease. Care must be taken to pad the skin during hospital care to avoid further damage.

Acute intermittent porphyria is characterized by neurologic dysfunction affecting the peripheral, autonomic, or central nervous system. There are many symptoms of an acute exacerbation including abdominal pain, nausea, vomiting, constipation, diarrhea, ileus, urinary retention, incontinence, dysuria, tachycardia, hypertension, sweating, tremor, and psychosis. Multiple factors may precipitate an attack including reduced caloric intake, stress (including surgery and illness),

TABLE 57.1	PARTIAL LIST OF DRUGS CONSIDERED UNSAFE IN PORPHYRIA	
Amitriptyline	Etomidate	Oxcarbazepine
Barbiturates	Furosemide	Phenytoin
Carbamazepine	Halothane	Pyrazinamide
Chloramphenicol	Hydralazine	Rifampin
Chlordiazepoxide	Hydrochlorothiazide	Spironolactone
Co-trimoxazole	Hydroxyzine	Sulfamethoxazole
Dapsone	Ketoconazole	Sulfonylureas
Dihydralazine	Lidocaine	Theophylline
Enalapril	Lisinopril	Valproic acid
Erythromycin	Metoclopramide	Verapamil
Ethanol	Nifedipine	

smoking, hepatocellular carcinoma, and many drugs and chemicals (*Table 57.1*). Initial treatment consists of supportive care, withdrawal of any potentially offending agents, and appropriate caloric intake. If this is not effective, the administration of intravenous (IV) heme preparations such as hematin or heme arginate to suppress non-specific delta-amino-levulinate synthase (ALAS-N) activity or administration of cimetidine may be indicated. Usually attacks last from a few weeks to several months, but lower motor lesions may be permanent, leading to bulbar paralysis.

SUGGESTED READINGS

American Porphyria Foundation. http://www.porphyriafoundation.com/about_por/drugs/drugs02.html.

Braunwald E, Fauci AS, Kasper DL, et al., eds. Harrison's Principles of Internal Medicine. 15th Ed. New York: McGraw-Hill; 2001:2264.

Miller RD. Miller's Anesthesia. 6th Rd. New York: Elsevier; 2005:1096–1097.

58

DO NOT INSERT, CHANGE, OR REMOVE A CENTRAL LINE WITH THE PATIENT SITTING UP

AARON BRANSKY, MD
HEIDI FRANKEL, MD

The insertion of central venous catheters is an extremely common procedure in the United States, accounting for more than 5 million procedures annually. There are many different complications that have been described. One of the more underrecognized and feared complications is a venous air embolism. Clinically, air embolism may present with acute chest pain, hypoxia, dyspnea, hypotension, visual changes, or convulsions.

The two most common times for air embolism to develop are upon placement or removal of a central venous catheter, including instances of intentional or inadvertent removal by the patient. Upon placement of a central venous catheter, proper care should be taken to prevent each lumen of the catheter from connecting with atmospheric air without a column of fluid within it. Furthermore, to increase central venous pressure, the catheter should be placed with the patient in a Trendelenburg position. Removal of a catheter should also be done with caution, particularly in a cachectic patient or if the catheter has been in place for a sustained time and a fibrous sheath has developed. The patient should be placed in a Trendelenburg position with his or her breath held. Upon removal of the catheter, an occlusive dressing should be placed immediately. The risk of death is related to both the volume of the air embolus and the rate at which it enters. In humans, the minimum injection rate and volume are 100 mL/sec and 300 to 500 mL, respectively.

The actual physiological mechanism that causes the hemodynamic instability from an air embolus is a right ventricular outlet obstruction caused by the slurry of churned air embolus with blood. Because gases rise, the patient should be placed in a position where the gas will exit the ventricle or prevent it from entering the ventricle. This is best accomplished by the reverse Trendelenburg position with the left side down. This places the right atrium in the least dependent position, causing air to ascend to this position. Once the patient is in this position, if the central venous catheter remains in place, an attempt can be made to aspirate the air, although this is rarely successful. Other proposed therapies include hyperbaric oxygen that addresses the neurological disturbances that occur as a result of a patent foramen ovale (present in up to 30% of the population) or a shunt. Hyperbaric oxygen is successful if utilized early after recognition of neurological symptoms.

SUGGESTED READINGS

Orebaugh SL. Venous air embolism: clinical and experimental considerations. Crit Care Med 1992;20:1169–1177.

Pronovost PJ, Wu AW, Sexton JB. Acute decompensation after removing a central line: practical approaches to increasing safety in the intensive care unit. Ann Intern Med 2004;140:1025–1033.

AVOID PLACEMENT OF CENTRAL ACCESS IN THE RIGHT INTERNAL JUGULAR IN CARDIAC TRANSPLANT PATIENTS IF POSSIBLE

BENJAMIN S. BROOKE, MD

The outcome of cardiac transplantation has improved dramatically over the past several decades, in large part because of improvements in immunosuppression and postoperative management. During the first 2 to 3 weeks after transplantation, patients are closely monitored for evidence of rejection. This includes a percutaneous transvenous endomyocardial biopsy to assess for histological signs of organ rejection and to adjust immunosuppressive medications if necessary. The first cardiac biopsy is usually performed 2 weeks posttransplant, unless earlier signs of rejection occur. The preferred site for vascular access to perform this procedure is through the right internal jugular vein, as the transvenous biotome used to take the biopsies does not need a guiding catheter or sheath when inserted through this approach. Moreover, right-sided cardiac biopsies are associated with fewer complications.

In order to preserve the right internal jugular site for cardiac biopsy in heart transplant patients, caregivers should give consideration to placing central venous catheters elsewhere in cardiac transplant patients. Catheter-related venous thrombosis may occur in up to 22% of catheterized patients and the risk of clot formation is higher with internal jugular insertion as compared with subclavian vein insertion. The preferred site for central venous access in these patients is the subclavian vein or the left internal jugular vein. The femoral vein may also be used for vascular access if necessary, but it is associated with the highest risk of overall infectious complications.

SUGGESTED READINGS

Cotts WG, Johnson MR. The challenge of rejection and cardiac allograft vasculopathy. Heart Fail Rev 2001;6:227–240.

McGee DC, Gould MK. Preventing complications of central venous catheterization. N Engl J Med 2003;348:1123–1133.

PLACE THE TIP OF A CENTRAL VENOUS CATHETER AT THE JUNCTION OF THE SUPERIOR VENA CAVA AND ATRIUM

JAYME E. LOCKE, MD

Central venous access is often necessary in order to adequately resuscitate a patient with large volumes of fluid or blood products, monitor intravascular volume, perform hemodialysis, administer parenteral nutrition, and administer antibiotics. Internal jugular and subclavian veins are most commonly used. When access is obtained via the internal jugular (IJ) vein, placement of the catheter on the patient's right side is best (except in cardiac transplant patients; see Chapter 59) secondary to the vein's superficial position and larger size in that location. Overall, the IJ vein is the preferred site for dialysis access, allows for easier control of arterial puncture, and is less likely to cause central stenosis. The subclavian vein is associated with the lowest risk for infection, but it does come with a higher risk for pneumothorax and central stenosis. Femoral venous access should be avoided unless no other access is available or it is an emergency situation. Placement of central access in the groin has the highest risk of infection and deep venous thrombosis.

Central venous catheters can be categorized as either nontunneled or tunneled. Nontunneled catheters can be placed and removed at the patient's bedside, can be easily exchanged over a guidewire, and are inexpensive. Examples of nontunneled catheters include single-, double-, and triple-lumen catheters, and Cordis, Hohn, and Shiley catheters. Some nontunneled catheters such as the Hohn can be used for up to 6 months. Hohn central lines have a silver-impregnated gelatin cuff that lies just beneath the skin surface at the puncture site, which serves as a barrier to infection.

In contrast, tunneled catheters tend to be for long-term use. These catheters are generally tunneled from the chest wall to the subclavian or internal jugular vein. They are double cuffed and designed to induce scar formation, allowing them to remain in place indefinitely. Examples include Hickman, Broviac (a small catheter used in children), and Groshong catheters (does not require heparin flushes; ideal for patients with allergies to heparin). Specialized tunneled catheters, called implanted venous ports, are best used when chronic therapy is necessary and only intermittent access is needed. The ports have reservoirs that are located infraclavicular in a subcutaneous pocket. Accessing ports requires the special noncoring Huber needle. Mediport, Infusaport, and Port-a-Cath are examples of specific implanted venous ports.

WHAT TO DO

Regardless of the type of central venous access, proper positioning is imperative. Central catheters placed in either the subclavian or internal jugular veins should be positioned with the tip at the cavoatrial junction. The cavoatrial junction is located approximately 5 cm below the tracheobronchial angle, a reliable fluoroscopic landmark. This distance is reproducible in all patients independent of gender and body habitus. Most central venous catheters are manufactured with marks denoting the length of the catheter. In general to reach the cavoatrial junction, catheters should be placed at the following lengths: RIJ ~ 12 cm, LIJ ~ 15 cm, RSC ~ 15 cm, LSC ~ 18 cm. Proper placement of catheters in both the internal jugular and subclavian veins can be confirmed using a chest x-ray or with fluoroscopy. Central catheters placed in the femoral vein should have the tip located at the confluence of the left and right iliac veins. The third lumbar vertebral body approximates this location, which can be confirmed on pelvic x-ray. Improperly placed tips of catheters can create significant morbidity and in some cases mortality. Specifically, catheter tips located in the right atrium or right ventricle can cause arrhythmias or perforate the heart, leading to tamponade and death. Catheter tips placed too proximally, in the subclavian vein or brachiocephalic vein, are associated with higher rates of thrombus formation and central stenosis.

SUGGESTED READING

Klingensmith ME, ed. The Washington Manual of Surgery. 4th ed. Philadelphia: Lippincott Williams & Wilkins; 2005:133–139.

61

Do not remove the intravenous catheter used for plasmapheresis immediately after the last treatment

Kelly Olino, MD

Plasmapheresis is performed through either centrifugation or membrane plasma separation. Centrifugation technique is the same technology used by blood banks to process blood and can be done with either intermittent or continuous flow. Blood components are separated out according to density, and plasma or cells can be removed. Intermittent flow requires only one venipuncture site but can be associated with more hypotension since larger volume shifts are needed. Continuous flow requires two venous access sites or a double-lumen catheter capable of handling high flow states. Membrane filtration technique can be used with hemodialysis equipment and uses a special filter that allows only plasma to pass through pores. Different filters or hemadsorption columns can be used depending on the indication.

A plasmapheresis treatment session usually removes 1 to 1.5 plasma volumes. Autoantibodies, immune complexes, toxins or substances bound to proteins, immunoglobulins, thrombotic factors, coagulation factors, lipoproteins, and other immunologic factors are removed during plasmapheresis for a number of different immunologic, hematologic, neurologic, renal, rheumatologic, and metabolic disorders. Replacement fluid usually consists of 60% to 80% albumin with the rest of the solution being normal saline. However, fresh frozen plasma can be used as the replacement solution when there is a concern for bleeding or in the treatment of certain conditions such as thrombotic thrombocytopenic purpura or hemolytic uremic syndrome. Anticoagulation is required for these treatments with citrate used for centrifugation, while unfractionated heparin is used for membrane filtration.

There is varying evidence for the clinical use of plasmapheresis, but according to the American Association of Blood Banks hemapheresis committee, it is standard or supportive therapy for the following: antiglomerular basement membrane disease, rapidly progressive glomerulonephritis, familial hypercholesterolemia, ABO-incompatible bone marrow transplant, thrombotic thrombocytopenic purpura-hemolytic uremic syndrome, posttransfusion purpura, acute or chronic inflammatory demyelinating polyneuropathy, Guillain-Barré, myasthenia gravis, cold agglutin disease, cryoglobinemia, rheumatoid arthritis, myeloma kidney, Lambert-Eaton syndrome, Sydenham chorea, and pediatric autoimmune disorders associated with strep (PANDAS).

WHAT NOT TO DO

The vascular access catheter used for plasmapheresis should not be removed immediately after plasmapheresis has ended, especially in cases where albumin or colloid are used as replacement fluids because of the depletion of coagulation factors. The shortest half-life of the factors is VII, which is between 1.5 to 6 hours. Factors VIII and V have a half-life of around 12 hours; IX, about 24 hours; X, 36 hours; XII, 2 days; and XI, prothrombin, and fibrinogen, 3 or more days. The prothrombin and activated partial thromboplastin times increase after a single plasmapheresis exchange and return to normal after 4 hours. However, the time to return to normal levels is dependent on how many plasma volumes are cycled and how many treatments the patient has undergone. It is best to wait 1 to 2 days before removing the catheter used for plasmapheresis whenever possible and to hold pressure up to 30 to 40 minutes, especially in cases when a catheter needs to be removed more promptly.

SUGGESTED READINGS

Clark WF, Rock GA, Buskard N, et al. Therapeutic plasma exchange: an update from the Canadian Pheresis group. Ann Int Med 1999;131:453.

Hoffman R, ed. Hematology Basic Principles and Practice. 4th Ed. New York: Churchill Livingstone; 2004:2481–2485.

Kaplan AA, Joy Fridey. Complications of therapeutic plasma exchange. Prescription and techniques of therapeutic plasma exchange. Plasmapheresis with hemodialysis equipment. Indications for therapeutic plasma exchange. UpToDate; October 2005. http://www.uptodate.com/

Smith JW, Weinstein R. The AABB Hemapheresis Committee KL. Therapeutic apheresis: a summary of current indication categories endorsed by the AABB and the American Society for Apheresis. Transfusion 2003;43:820.

62

NEVER THREAD A TRIPLE-LUMEN THROUGH A CORDIS

BRADFORD D. WINTERS, MD, PhD

Introducer catheters (i.e., Cordis catheters) are used for the placement of devices, such as pulmonary artery catheters (PACs) and certain cardiac pacing devices as well as when extremely large volume resuscitations are needed or anticipated. Since PACs and pacers may need frequent manipulation of their position, they are placed through the hemostatic valve of the Cordis, which holds them in position and prevents back leakage of blood. Different devices require and are matched to different sizes of Cordis catheters and it is imperative that the device is appropriately matched to the Cordis diameter. Occasionally, practitioners will place a standard central line catheter through the Cordis when one of the aforementioned functions is not applicable. Despite it seeming reasonable to do so, standard single-, double-, and triple-lumen central venous access catheters should not be placed through a Cordis for several reasons.

WATCH OUT FOR

First, standard single-, double-, and triple-lumen central venous access catheters are not designed to fit the cordis and so there is the risk of back leakage of blood. There is also the risk of air leakage around the hemostatic seal, leading to air emboli. Additionally, pulmonary artery catheters and pacers have sheaths that are designed to cover them so that when their position is manipulated, the catheter remains sterile so as not to introduce microorganisms into the bloodstream. Central line catheters are not designed for use with these sheaths. The port in the cordis needs to be kept covered and sterile with the sheath or an appropriate locking cap. Central line catheters are not configured in this manner and should not be jerry-rigged with one. Placing a standard central line catheter with any number of lumens through a Cordis creates an infection risk.

Thirdly, central line catheters are designed for securing to the skin with sutures using a hub and/or clamp. Placing them through the Cordis defeats this and leaves the central line catheter at risk for accidental dislodgment. This may leave the patient in a situation where he or she is not receiving a crucial medication such as an inotrope or vasopressor and the hemostatic valve port is left exposed to the environment, risking infection.

Lastly, a Cordis should not be left in any longer than necessary. They are thrombogenic and lead to central venous clotting, obstruction, and emboli. The longer it is in and the larger the diameter, the greater the risk of thrombosis. Once the Cordis is no longer needed, it should be rewired to a standard central line or removed entirely.

If it is desirable to leave the Cordis in after the PAC or pacer has been discontinued, or you anticipate short-term future need for the Cordis, one of two things must be done. It should either be capped with the appropriate locking cap, or if a second intravenous access point in addition to the sideport of the Cordis is needed, there are specially designed single-lumen intravenous catheters (SLICs) that go through and lock on the Cordis. These are the only kind of central catheters other than pulmonary artery catheters or pacing devices that are acceptable to place through a Cordis. When considering the use of an SLIC, one must recognize that a Cordis is felt to be more thrombogenic than a regular central line when the decision is made to maintain the Cordis for an extended period of time.

SUGGESTED READING

Hall JB, Schmidt GA, Wood LDH, eds. Principles of Critical Care. 2nd Ed. New York: McGraw-Hill; 1998:308–322.

63

BE METICULOUS IN TECHNIQUE WHEN INSERTING AND CARING FOR CENTRAL VENOUS ACCESS CATHETERS IN THE INTENSIVE CARE UNIT TO LOWER THE INCIDENCE OF INFECTION

LISA MARCUCCI, MD

Central venous catheters are associated with a significant rate of bloodstream infections and an estimated 10% mortality in intensive care patients. Several strategies have been shown to be effective in reducing these infections and are summarized here.

USE FULL-BARRIER PROTECTION WHEN INSERTING CENTRAL VENOUS CATHETERS

This is the most bothersome protocol for most clinicians but should be employed except in the most emergent situations. Full-barrier protection consists of the surgeon and all assistants being fully gowned (with the ties fastened as in the operating room), masked, and gloved with sterile gloves and the patient fully draped with sterile drapes. If the procedure is a change of catheter over a wire, the surgeon should change gloves between removing the old catheter and inserting the new catheter.

USE CHLORHEXIDINE FOR SKIN PREP

Chlorhexidine has a decided advantage over aqueous iodine-based preps in reducing infection, and its use should be adopted routinely with extreme care to avoid contact with the eyes and the external ear canal. The prep should be applied via a concentrically larger circular motion for at least 20 seconds and should be allowed to dry without blotting or fanning. Alcohol-based iodine preps are felt to be less effective.

USE A STERILE DRESSING ON THE INSERTION SITE

Immediately after catheter insertion, the site should be protected with a transparent sterile dressing while the insertion site is still sterile. The sterile bandage should not be placed if the site is still oozing, and a sterile gauze should be used to remove blood (the ideal culture medium) before the sterile dressing is placed. Topical antibiotic ointment has not been shown to reduce infections and should not be used. Antiseptic impregnated dressings and disks are promising adjuncts to exit-site care.

USE THE CATHETER WITH THE FEWEST NUMBER OF LUMENS POSSIBLE AND CONSIDER TREATED CATHETERS

The question of whether triple-lumen catheters have higher infection rates compared with single-lumen catheters is still somewhat uncertain, with the majority of studies showing higher infection rates for triple-lumen catheters. Contradicting this are a few studies and one recent meta-analysis that found there is no strong evidence for an increase in infections in triple-lumen catheters. This may be because the patient population studied in the literature is heterogeneous in the following variables—patient location (intensive care unit [ICU], inpatient, mixed), pulmonary artery catheters allowed, blood drawing allowed through catheters, types of catheters (antibiotic impregnated, number of lumens), sites of catheters (peripherally inserted, centrally inserted), ports included or not, tunneled and/or cuffed catheters included or not, and so on.

In addition, catheters coated with a sterilant (e.g., silver) or an antibiotic (e.g., rifampin) are also effective at decreasing infections; cost-effectiveness will vary with an institution's infection rate.

DO NOT USE STOPCOCKS ON THE LUMEN PORTS

Use of stopcocks functionally increases the number of portals in a central venous catheter, with an attendant increase in contamination, and therefore should be avoided. Catheter hubs that incorporate an antiseptic barrier should be used whenever possible.

SUGGESTED READINGS

Chaiyakunapruk N, Veenstra DL, Lipsky BA, et al. Vascular site care: the clinical and economic benefits of chlorhexidine gluconate compared with povidone iodine. Clin Infect Dis 2003;37:764–771.

Dezfulian C, Lavelle J, Nallamothu BK, et al. Rates of infection for single-lumen versus multilumen central venous catheters: a meta-analysis. Crit Care Med 2003;31:2385–2390.

O'Grady NP, Alexander M, Dellinger EP, et al. Guidelines for the prevention of intravascular catheter-related infections. Pediatrics 2002;110:e51.

Raad II, Flohn DC, Gilbreath BJ, et al. Prevention of central venous catheter-related infections by using maximal sterile barrier precautions during insertion.Infect Control
Hosp Epidemiol 1994; 231–238.

Sitges-Serra A, Hernandez R, Maestro S, et al. Prevention of catheter sepsis: the hub.
Nutrition 1997;13:30S–35S.

64

IN A PATIENT WITH A PREVIOUSLY PLACED VENA CAVA FILTER, DO NOT USE THE J-TIP ON THE GUIDEWIRE WHEN USING THE SELDINGER TECHNIQUE TO PLACE A CENTRAL VENOUS CATHETER

LISA MARCUCCI, MD
AWORI J. HAYANGA

Vena cava filters are placed for treatment of deep vein thrombosis and/or pulmonary embolism. Complications arising from the placement of these filters include migration, dislodgment, vena cava penetration, and vena cava thrombosis. One additional complication that has been increasing in frequency but is completely preventable is the ensnarement of the filter by guidewires being used to insert central venous catheters from the subclavian, jugular, and femoral approaches.

There are a variety of vena cava filters available in the United States. Some of the more commonly used filters include the Greenfield (both titanium and stainless steel models), Simon Nitinol, Bird's Nest, Vena Tech LGM, Vena Tech TrapEase, and Gunther Tulip filters. Despite design differences, they are all similar in that they allow venous flow through the filter while capturing emboli via the radiating struts of the filter.

There are various guidewires that are used during the Seldinger technique, including straight guidewires and the more commonly encountered 1.5-, 3-, and 15-mm J-tip guidewires packaged in central venous catheter insertion kits (the number describes the radius of the curve of the J-tip). In vitro studies and case reports show that ensnarement of the guidewire in the filter struts is possible with all diameters of the J-tip guidewire used in placing central venous catheters and does not occur with straight guidewires. The filters with the highest likelihood of ensnaring the J-tip guidewires are the Greenfield and Vena Tech filters with only the Gunther Tulip reported as not entrapping the J-tip guidewire.

Ensnarement of an inferior vena cava (IVC) filter occurs when the curved end of a J-tip guidewire (*see Fig. 64.1*) is pushed through a strut opening with subsequent hooking of the wire onto the strut when the catheter is pulled back. This is noted clinically as the wire becoming "stuck" during wire withdrawal. If even slight resistance to removing the wire is noted, further attempts to remove the wire must be halted immediately. Attempting to free the guidewire with force can cause

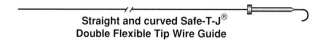

Straight and curved Safe-T-J®
Double Flexible Tip Wire Guide

FIGURE 64.1. Straight and curved J-tip double flexible tip wire guide.

shearing of the guidewire or dislodgment of the filter with potentially catastrophic complications including filter caval disruption, perforation, arrhythmias, cardiac tamponade, and death. Although some clinicians advocate attempts to free the wire at bedside by pushing the wire caudally and applying torque to rotate the J-tip away from the strut, a more cautious approach demands urgent consultation with interventional radiology. Techniques used to remove ensnared guidewires include using fluoroscopic visualization and placement of a vascular sheath and snares to work the guidewire free.

WHAT TO DO

To help prevent ensnarement of a guidewire, all patients or patient families should be queried about the presence of a cava filter before elective insertion of a central venous catheter. With an increasing proportion of filters placed percutaneously, filter placement may not be elicited as part of a "past surgical history." In the event of an elective procedure in a patient where the history cannot be obtained, a plain radiograph will show the presence of this device. Because patients usually do not know what model of vena cava filter they have received, they should be specifically asked about the placement of a "Greenfield, filter, or birdcage in the vena cava." If they answer in the affirmative, a straight guidewire (or the straight end of the J-tip guidewire) should be used to place the central venous catheter. Similarly, in emergent central venous catheter insertions, a straight guidewire should be considered to prevent ensnarement.

SUGGESTED READINGS

Dardik A, Campbell KA, Yeo CJ, et al. Vena cava filter ensnarement and delayed migration: an unusual series of cases. J Vasc Surg 1997;26:869–874.

Munir MA, Chien SQ. An in situ technique to retrieve an entrapped J-tip guidewire from an inferior vena cava filter. Anesth Analg 2002;95:308–309.

Stavropoulus SW, Itkin M, Trerotola SO. In vitro study of guide wire entrapment in currently available inferior vena cava filters. J Vasc Interv Radiol 2003;14:905–910.

65

DO NOT "WHIP THE TIP" WHEN TESTING A PULMONARY CATHETER BEFORE INSERTION

RACHEL BLUEBOND-LANGNER, MD

Prior to placement of a pulmonary artery (PA) catheter, the balloon should be tested, all ports should be flushed, the system should be primed with saline, and the equipment calibrated or zeroed with the system open to air. Flushing and priming the tubing removes air bubbles that can dampen the waveform. Leveling should be done with the patient lying flat and with the catheter held at the level of the of the patient's atrium. The distal port should be connected to the pressure transducer, which produces the characteristic placement waveform on the monitor (*Fig. 65.1*). Prior to floating the catheter, the transducer connections should be checked by placing a finger over the distal tip of the catheter. This should cause a rise in pressure of the PA waveform only. Some people shake the tip to elicit a waveform, but this is to be avoided. "Whipping the tip" will cause all pressures, including the central venous pressure (CVP), to rise and will not provide specific information about transducer connections. There is also the theoretical risk of damage to the sensing mechanism and contamination of the catheter tip.

Alternatively, the practitioner may check the PA catheter before insertion by holding the catheter still with one hand positioned at the 30-cm mark (CVP port). If the tip is slowly raised, the PA pressure waveform only should change if the system has been assembled correctly.

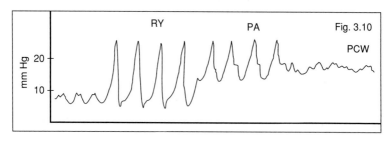

FIGURE 65.1. Pulmonary artery tracing. (Reused with permission from Chen H, Sonnenday CJ, Lillemoe KD, eds. Manual of Common Bedside Surgical Procedures. 2nd Ed. Philadelphia: Lippincott Williams & Wilkins; 2000:100.)

Selected Readings

Pulmonary Artery Catheter Education Project. http:// www.pacep.org
Summerhill EM, Baram M. Principles of pulmonary artery catheterization in the critically ill. Lung 2005;183:209–219.

66

REMOVE KINKED OR COILED PULMONARY ARTERY CATHETERS

HARI NATHAN, MD

A postplacement chest radiograph should always be obtained after placement of a pulmonary artery catheter (PAC) (*Fig. 66.1*). The post-placement radiograph serves several purposes. It checks for complications of introducer catheter placement such as pneumothorax or hemothorax. It confirms that the PAC has not been advanced too far into the periphery of the pulmonary arterial system and it also rules out kinking or coiling of the PAC.

The risk of kinking the PAC can be lessened by halting advancement of the catheter if any resistance is felt upon insertion. It should be noted that appropriate waveform changes, such as from right atrial to right ventricular or from right ventricular to pulmonary artery, should occur every 15 cm as the PAC is advanced (see Figure 65.1). If these changes are not readily observed, the PAC should be withdrawn. Minimizing insertion time and using a slow but steady insertion rate can take advantage of flow-directed positioning of the PAC (i.e., a "float" as opposed to a "push") and reduce the likelihood of the catheter kinking or coiling.

Although a kinked or coiled PAC may give good pressure and wedge tracings and allow cardiac output measurements, it should nevertheless be removed because of the risk of thrombosis and, in extreme cases, pulmonary infarction. The PAC should never be withdrawn with the balloon inflated to avoid valvular damage. Any resistance during PAC withdrawal mandates that the operator halt the procedure and obtain a chest radiograph to ensure that the catheter has not knotted. If a kink has developed, interventional radiologists should be consulted to remove the PAC under fluoroscopic guidance.

One final note is that in cardiac surgery patients, a "stuck" PAC must cause concern that the catheter was inadvertently sutured in place during surgery.

SUGGESTED READINGS

PACEP Collaborative. Pulmonary Artery Catheter Education Project. 2006. Available at http://www.pacep.org. Accessed March 9, 2006.

Voyce SJ, McCaffree DR. Pulmonary artery catheters. In: Irwin RS, Rippe JM, eds. Irwin and Rippe's Intensive Care Medicine. 5th Ed. Philadelphia: Lippincott Williams & Wilkins; 2003:45–67.

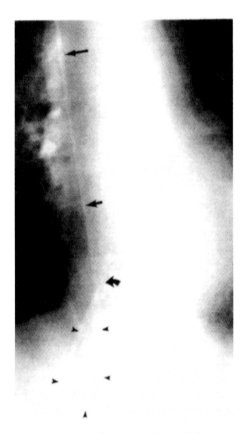

FIGURE 66.1. Swan-Ganz catheter looped in inferior vena cava and re-entering right atrium. Anteroposterior close-up view shows the Swan-Ganz catheter through the superior vena cava (*long arrow*) and right atrium (*short arrow*), looping in the inferior vena cava (*arrowheads*) and re-entering the right atrium (*curved arrow*). (Reused with permission from Umali CB. Chest radiographic examination. In: Irwin RS, Rippe JM, eds. Irwin and Rippe's Intensive Care Medicine. 5th Ed. Philadelphia: Lippincott Williams & Wilkins; 2003:707.)

67

REMOVE A PULMONARY ARTERY CATHETER IN PATIENTS WITH NEW-ONSET VENTRICULAR ARRHYTHMIA AND IN MOST ATRIAL ARRHYTHMIAS

WILLIAM R. BURNS, MD

Arrhythmias are common in the critically ill patient and can result from a wide variety of physiologic disturbances. As the potential etiologies are many (intrinsic heart disease, myocardial ischemia, electrolyte abnormalities, hypoxemia, acidosis, volume alterations, endocrine irregularities, and others), it is difficult to pinpoint the underlying pathology in most cases. However, one should certainly not overlook the role that vascular catheters play in new-onset arrhythmias. In particular, pulmonary artery catheters have a high risk of inciting both atrial and ventricular arrhythmias, and removal of the line should be strongly considered.

The incidence of arrhythmias related to pulmonary artery catheterization is best described during initial catheter insertion. Premature atrial and ventricular contractions are frequent while advancing the catheter and have been reported in 13% to 87% of patients. More concerning disturbances, such as nonsustained ventricular tachycardia and right bundle branch blocks, are also common; however, these arrhythmias are usually well tolerated. Ventricular tachycardia, ventricular fibrillation, and complete heart block, on the other hand, require emergent intervention. Fortunately, these unstable arrhythmias occur in less than 1% of all catheterizations.

WATCH OUT FOR Catheter-induced arrhythmias are initiated by direct physical contact between the catheter and the endomyocardial cells. This mechanical stimulation can be sufficient to trigger ectopic beats, as well as life-threatening arrhythmias. It should be noted that patients with a left bundle branch block are at increased risk of developing complete heart block during pulmonary artery catheterization. Newer catheters (which are often thinner and more flexible) may be less likely to trigger these rhythm disturbances.

While arrhythmias are most often noted during catheter advancement, the simple presence of a foreign body can be sufficient to initiate rhythm disturbances. Therefore, the contribution of pulmonary artery catheters to new-onset arrhythmias should always be considered, even in the absence of recent catheter manipulation. Acute myocardial ischemia, recent myocardial infarction, severe hypoxemia, acidosis, and electrolyte abnormalities are key risk factors for arrhythmias and also seem to lower the threshold for catheter-related arrhythmias. In these situations, removal of the catheter should be strongly considered.

SUGGESTED READINGS

Ermakov S, Hoyt JW. Pulmonary artery catheterization. Crit Care Clin 1992;8:773–806.

Marino PL. The ICU Book. 2nd Ed. Baltimore: Williams & Wilkins; 1997:158–159.

Roizen MF, Berger DL, Gabel RA, et al. Practice guidelines for pulmonary artery catheterization: an updated report by the American Society of Anesthesiologists Task Force on Pulmonary Artery Catheterization. Anesthesiology 2003;99: 988–1014.

68

REMEMBER THAT IN NORMAL PHYSIOLOGY THE WEDGE PRESSURE IS LESS THAN THE PULMONARY ARTERY DIASTOLIC PRESSURE

JOSE M. RODRIGUEZ-PAZ, MD

The pulmonary artery catheter (PAC) is a commonly used device in the critically ill or anesthetized patient. It allows the continuous monitoring of cardiac performance under several clinical conditions. Unfortunately, during the last few years several reports have shown its potential limitations, including the erroneous interpretation of the hemodynamic data (*Fig. 68.1*). The correct use of the PAC requires a thorough understanding of heart physiology and what the catheter is measuring.

The PAC is a flow-directed catheter. Dr. Swan conceived the idea (by looking at a sailboat in 1967) of taking advantage of the flow generated by the blood going through the heart to guide a catheter. Essentially the PAC uses the air-filled cuff as a sail to guide the catheter through the different chambers of the heart. The main objective of the PAC is to measure the pressures of the right heart and "get the closest we can to the left heart." This guided "tour" of the heart provides valuable information that includes some measured values and a variety of calculated parameters.

It is basic in the understanding of the healthy heart that the pulmonary vasculature works, under normal conditions, as a low-pressure system. This is important, since blood flows due to a pressure gradient (ΔP) between the sides of the heart, as a result of the pressures generated by the right ventricle. This can be expressed by the equation $CO = \Delta P/PVR$, where the flow (CO, cardiac output) depends on the difference between pulmonary artery pressure (PAP) and pulmonary artery wedge pressure (PAWP), and it is inversely proportional to the pulmonary vascular resistance (PVR).

WATCH OUT FOR

When placing a PAC, several different pressures are observed through their pressure tracings seen on the monitor. After the catheter is introduced into the superior vena cava (SVC), the typical tracing of the right atrium (including the a, c, and v waves) is seen. When the catheter passes through the tricuspid valve, there is a substantial change of pressures due to the higher pressure system generated by the contraction of the

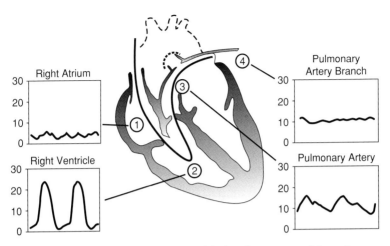

FIGURE 68.1. Hemodynamic changes with the advancement of the pulmonary artery catheter. (Reused with permission from Marino PL. The pulmonary artery catheter. In: Marino PL, ed. The ICU Book. 2nd Ed. Baltimore: Williams & Wilkins; 1998:157.)

right ventricle (RV), as seen in *Figure 68.1.* It is also apparent that the RV diastolic pressure is the same as the right atrium (RA) pressure, since at end diastole the chambers reach equilibrium. As the catheter is advanced, eventually the blood flow will guide the tip of the PAC through the pulmonary valve. That can be easily recognized by the effect that the closure of the pulmonary valve has on the tracing. At the pulmonary artery diastolic pressure (PAD), the pulmonary valve closes causing the PAD to be higher than the right ventricular diastolic pressure. That is the distinctive feature of advancing the catheter into the PA vasculature. Also, the PA pressure tracing shows a characteristic dicrotic notch (as would be expected from the closure of the pulmonary valve). The PA pressure is equivalent to the systemic pressures, in that PAS represents the pressure generated by the RV and the PAD by the recoiling of the PA vasculature until the pulmonic valve closes.

Once in the PA vasculature, the flow will guide the catheter until it reaches a vessel that is smaller in diameter than the catheter with the balloon inflated. At that point the tracing will appear dampened and look similar to the tracing obtained in the RA (atrial pressures). That value of pressure is known as the PA wedge pressure (PAWP) or PA occlusion pressure (PAOP). That pressure represents the interruption of flow generated by the RV as a result of the inflated balloon obstructing the capillary bed of the PA vasculature and corresponds

TABLE 68.1	CARDIAC PRESSURE VALUES	
CARDIAC CHAMBER	PRESSURE SYSTOLIC/ DIASTOLIC (MM HG)	MEAN PRESSURE (MM HG)
Right atrium	0–6	3
Right ventricle	S: 17–30	
	D: 0–6	
Pulmonary artery	S: 15–30	10–18
	D: 5–13	
Pulmonary artery wedge		2–12

to the pressure transmitted by the column of fluid created by the left atrium (LA) and transmitted by the pulmonary veins. Since PAOP is to the left side of the heart as the CVP is to the right side of the heart, one could make inferences of the status of the filling of the left ventricle by assuming the correlation between left ventricular end–diastolic pressure (LVEDP) and left ventricular end–diastolic volume (LVEDV). Regrettably, this correlation is difficult to make because the PAC and PAOP do not give us information on the LV compliance (volume/pressure) and contractility (the slope of that relationship).

Another important principle in the use of the PAC is that if it is correctly positioned, PAOP is always less than the PAS and PAD pressures. This occurs only if there is a patent column of fluid connecting the tip of the catheter with the pulmonary veins/LA. Also this occurs only if the tip of the PAC lies in West zone III (PA >pulmonary venous pressure >alveolar pressure), radiologically located below the LA. When the catheter is located in either of the other West zones, the pressures may be different. An easy way to visualize this is by using Dr. Swan's sailboat example. As a sailor, the goal is to bring the boat to the area of maximal wind (blood flow) and not to an area of minimal wind, which will make the boat stay still or go backward, if the wind is actually against the sail (PAOP ≥PAD).

SUGGESTED READINGS

Marino PL. The pulmonary artery catheter. In: Marino PL, ed. The ICU Book. 2rd Ed. Baltimore: Williams & Wilkins; 1998:154–165.

Summerhill EM, Baram M. Principles of pulmonary artery catheterization in the critically ill. Lung 2005;183:209–219.

Voyce SJ, McCaffree DR. Pulmonary artery catheters. In: Irwin RS, Rippe JM, eds. Irwin and Rippe's Intensive Care Medicine. Philadelphia: Lippincott Williams & Wilkins; 2003:45–66.

69

DO NOT USE PULMONARY ARTERY CATHETER MEASUREMENTS IN TRICUSPID REGURGITATION

DIMITRIS STEFANIDIS, MD, PhD
RONALD F. SING, DO

Most of the parameters obtained from pulmonary artery (PA) catheters are calculated rather than directly measured; only right atrial and pulmonary artery pressures can be directly measured. Many PA catheters use the method of thermodilution to calculate cardiac output (CO) indirectly. This method, however, is subject to a number of pitfalls that can occur during daily interpretation of PA catheter readings and invalidate measurements. Tricuspid valve regurgitation, low flow states, patient temperature, presence of intracardiac shunts, and volume of injected bolus can all interfere with accurate measurements.

WATCH OUT FOR

Thermodilution is a method of measuring blood flow. A cold electrolyte solution is injected through the proximal port of the PA catheter into the right atrium. The cold fluid mixes with blood in the right heart chambers and the cooled blood is ejected into the pulmonary artery, where it flows past a thermistor located at the distal end of the PA catheter. The changes in blood temperature over time recorded by the thermistor are used to create a temperature-time curve; the area under this curve is equivalent to the average cardiac output in the absence of intracardiac shunts. In the case of tricuspid regurgitation, the cold fluid is delayed in the right heart because of back-and-forth movement across the incompetent valve, thus leading to a prolonged thermodilution curve. This produces a falsely low cardiac output.

A study that compared cardiac output measurements by thermodilution with continuous Doppler measurements by transesophageal echocardiography (TEE) in patients with variable degrees of tricuspid regurgitation found that the thermodilution method was associated with underestimation of cardiac output. In particular, they found that the higher the degree of tricuspid valve regurgitation, the lower the CO measurements; in patients with third-degree tricuspid valve regurgitation, thermodilution produced CO measurements that were a mean of 2 L/min lower compared with those of TEE. Moreover, some degree of tricuspid valve regurgitation may be common in ventilated patients because of high right-sided cardiac pressures created by positive-pressure ventilations and may thus be a common source of CO measure error when thermodilution is used. In addition, another study has implied that just the presence of the PA catheter may lead to a low degree of tricuspid valve regurgitation.

Thus, in patients with tricuspid valve regurgitation, especially when it is severe, pulmonary artery catheter measurements that are based on the thermodilution method should be interpreted very carefully, if not avoided completely. In these cases, continuous cardiac output measurements or Doppler measurements by TEE should replace thermodilution-based measurements.

SUGGESTED READINGS

Balik M, Pachl J, Hendl J. Effect of the degree of tricuspid regurgitation on cardiac output measurements. Intens Care Med 2002;28:1117–1121.

Marino PL. The ICU Book. 2nd Ed. Baltimore: Williams & Wilkins; 1998:182.

Sherman SV, Wall MH, Kennedy DJ, et al. Do pulmonary artery catheters cause or increase tricuspid or pulmonic valvular regurgitation? Anesth Analg 2001;92:1117–1122.

70

ALWAYS TURN ON A PACING PULMONARY ARTERY CATHETER PRIOR TO FLOATING THE DEVICE

BRADFORD D. WINTERS, MD, PHD

There are several temporary transvenous pacing devices available for use in the intensive care unit (ICU). They include pacing wires, pacing catheters, paceport pulmonary artery catheters (PACs), and pacing PACs. Pacing wires are devices that use essentially bare wires, which are placed through an introducer sheath into the central circulation and advanced into the heart until pacing is captured. Pacing catheters usually have an inflatable balloon at their tip much like a PAC that allows blood flow to help guide the catheter forward as it is advanced through the introducer sheath. Since it depends on blood flow for effective placement, it is not useful in emergent episodes of asystole and may be difficult to place in the case of extreme bradycardia. Paceport and pacing PACs have similar potential problems since they are flow directed for their placement. Ideally, pharmacological treatment with atropine, epinephrine, or isoproteronol and/or transcutaneous pacing with Zoll pads will create a situation that provides time and adequate cardiac output such that a transvenous system can be placed when asystole or extreme bradycardia occurs.

Paceport and pacing PACs differ in that the paceport PAC, in addition to the normal lumens for measuring cardiac output, pulmonary artery pressures, and so on, has a special lumen through which a special wire matched to the catheter can be introduced. The wire exits through an orifice so as to come in contact with the right ventricular wall and effect capture. The pacing PAC does not have this port nor a special wire but rather has electrodes built into the wall of the catheter such that when it is in normal position for doing cardiac output measurements, the electrodes are positioned for affecting pacing capture. They are in a fixed position on the device, which can make capture difficult if the catheter is not oriented in optimal position. While the orifice on the paceport catheter is also in a fixed position, the wire exits to move somewhat independently so as to contact the ventricular wall.

Placement of either one of the pacing-capable PACs starts with central venous cannulation, preferably in the right internal jugular or left subclavian position. The reason for this is that PACs have a curve molded into them that is most amenable to placement from these two positions. The left internal jugular or right subclavian approach may be used but it is often more technically challenging to "float" the catheter from either of these two sites. Femoral placement is also an option but tends to have similar difficulties. Even brachial placement has been performed, though passing an introducer sheath into one of the arm veins is often very difficult. Once the introducer sheath is placed and secured, the PAC is flushed, covered with the sterile cover sheath, connected to the monitors, and then placed through the hemostatic valve of the introducer. Once it is advanced to the 20-cm mark on the catheter, the balloon is inflated. The distal electrode should be connected to lead V on the electrocardiogram (ECG), which should be properly grounded since any current leakage to ground above 10 μA can result in ventricular fibrillation. For the pacing PAC, the pacer pulse generator is connected and turned on to 20 mA. It is important to use this higher current for placement so as to be sure capture occurs. The electrocardiogram monitor as well as the distal port tracing should be watched as the catheter is advanced. As the catheter enters the atrium a large and possibly down-going P-wave will occur. Whether this P-wave is up or down going or biphasic will depend on the position in the atrium and the relationship of the electrode to the direction of atrial depolarization. Ideally, you should have capture when you achieve a pulmonary artery tracing that also wedges the catheter. Capture will be identified by a sudden change in the axis of the ECG and widening of the QRS. Premature ventricular contractions (PVCs) that may occur during the passage of the PAC through the ventricle should not be mistaken as capture. The PVCs are random while capture should be regular at the set rate (usually 80). Once you achieve capture, the current is turned down until capture is lost and then turned back up until capture is attained again. Clinicians usually place the final setting a couple of milliamps above the capture point for a safe margin. The catheter may need frequent adjustments to achieve capture at the lowest possible current while at the same time to allow for wedging of the catheter for hemodynamic assessments.

The paceport PAC is placed as with other PACs until a wedge position is obtained. Once this is done the wire is advanced through the pacing port with the current set on 20 mA until similar changes are seen on the ECG as described previously. Once this has occurred the current is reduced until capture is lost, raised again until capture is obtained again, and then usually set a couple of milliamperes above this for safe margin.

On average, most clinicians find paceport PACs are easier to use for maintaining capture as well as proper position for hemodynamic measurement, though others favor the pacing catheter. In general, these devices are best chosen when it is imperative to have hemodynamic measurements in addition to pacing capability. If only pacing is needed, pacing wires alone or pacing catheters that are not pulmonary artery catheters are preferred for transvenous pacing. There are a myriad of products and configurations for these devices and one should become familiar with the type available at his or her hospital so as to reduce confusion when placement is emergently required.

SUGGESTED READINGS

Bump TE, Soble JS. Cardiac pacing. In: Hall JB, Schmidt GA, Wood LDH, eds. Principles of Critical Care. 3rd Ed. New York: McGraw-Hill; 2005:423–433.
Gammadge MD. Temporary cardiac pacing. Heart 2000;83:715–720.

71

MAKE SURE ANY CORDIS IN PLACE IS THE CORRECT SIZE WHEN EMERGENTLY FLOATING A TRANSVENOUS PACING WIRE

CHRISTINA L. CAFEO, RN MSN
DAVID G. HUNT, RN, BSN
PETER J. PRONOVOST, MD, PhD

One of the most difficult and frustrating situations to occur when caring for a critically ill patient is not having all of the required supplies available, especially during a crisis situation. This situation particularly seems to occur when certain emergency procedures arise only sporadically. As a result, staff may be unsure of both the supplies and the equipment required to treat such emergencies in a timely and efficient manner.

WHAT NOT TO DO

Many clinicians have faced the misadventures associated with placing a transvenous pacing wire. Temporary transvenous cardiac pacing is a potentially lifesaving intervention used primarily to correct profound bradycardia. A transvenous pacing wire is typically placed through a 6 French Cordis catheter. If the patient does not have a Cordis catheter in place, the temptation is to break open the closest kit that contains a Cordis and proceed to gain central access. However, this is usually a mistake; usually, the closest kit that contains a Cordis is one for inserting pulmonary artery catheters. Invariably these have Cordis catheters that are 7.5F—that is, catheters that are too big to insert a transvenous pacing wire through. Similarly, if the patient already has a Cordis in place, it is almost always a 7.5F catheter.

The placement of a transvenous wire has a considerable complication rate, with a high risk-to-benefit ratio because of insertion difficulties and pacemaker malfunction. Clinically identified complications include local trauma, pneumothorax, hemothorax, arrhythmias, and cardiac perforation. In addition, blood loss, air emboli, and infection are risks that occur when Cordis catheter is used that is too large and that allows for bleeding or an air embolus around the pacer wire, which is generally 6 French.

Recommendations to reduce the risk of not having the correct-size Cordis available include identification and packaging of all appropriate supplies for an adult pacer wire insertion kit (bundle) together. Components for this bundle should include an adapter for the pacemaker, an introducer percutaneous sheath 6F combo kit, and bipolar transvenous pacing wire. This is problematic as many hospitals purchase these components from different suppliers.

WHAT TO DO

There are two potential solutions to this problem. One is to have immediately available a sheath adapter that can be used with most of the currently clinically available 4F to 8F cordis catheters (e.g., Arrow Sheath Adapter with Cath-Gard). A second solution is to store the pacer wire insertion supplies in a dedicated area and away from the routinely used cordis, central line, and pulmonary artery catheter supplies.

One final note is that the designation of a unit of French refers to the size of the external diameter of a catheter. One unit is equal to .033 mm; so a 6F catheter has an external diameter of approximately 0.198 mm and a 7.5F catheter has an external diameter of 0.2475 mm.

SUGGESTED READINGS

Fitzpatrick A, Sutton R. A guide to temporary pacing. BMJ 1992;304:365–369.
Gammage MD. Temporary cardiac pacing. Heart 2000;83:715–720.

72

TRY PLACING A SKIN LEAD TO ACT AS A GROUND WIRE IF PACING WIRES ARE NOT FUNCTIONING CORRECTLY POSTOPERATIVELY

TAMMY M. SLATER, CRNP

Temporary epicardial wires are routinely implanted in patients during cardiac surgery. Historically, four wires are placed with the distal ends of these wires being held in place on the epicardium by a suture or staple. The proximal ends are brought outside the chest wall through subcutaneous tissue. Two atrial wires are placed on the right atrium with the proximal ends of those wires being brought out through the chest wall to the right of the subcostal area. Two ventricular wires are implanted on the anterior surface of the right ventricle with the proximal ends exiting the chest wall to the left of the subcostal area. The location of the atrial wires on the right side of the chest and ventricle wires on the left side is universal. Additionally, skin (or ground wires) may be placed. These wires are the longest of the wires and usually exit on the side of the atrial wires (i.e., the right side). If a skin wire has not been placed, then one of the other wires acts as a ground wire (positive pole).

The wires that are implanted in the operating room will dictate the type of pacing that can be performed. For example, if both atrial and ventricular wires are present, then a patient can be atrially (A) paced, ventricularly (V) paced, or AV paced. More recently, in uncomplicated cardiac surgery cases, it has become routine for only two ventricular wires to be placed. Secondary to the atrial wall being thinner, there is a potential increased risk of bleeding when pulling the atrial wires. If this is the situation, and there is difficulty with capture during pacing, an extra skin or ground lead can be placed at the bedside to optimize pacing. All skin or ground wires are placed in the positive pole of the external pacer.

This procedure should be performed aseptically. Temporary pacing leads are in sterile packaging and should be available in cardiac surgical intensive care units (ICUs) or in the cardiac surgery operating rooms. The following steps can be used:

- Wash hands thoroughly.
- Cleanse the skin with ChloraPrep.
- Use sterile gloves.

- Notice the temporary pacing lead has a curved needle at one end and a long straight needle at the other end. Use the long straight needle to puncture the skin.
- Pull the needle until the wire has gone through to the protective coating.
- Take the wire with the protective coating and tie a knot. This will secure it to the skin.
- Then break the straight needle off. You will be left with a straight long stainless steel shaft in place into the temporary pacemaker.
- At this time, the curved needle can be removed (this curved needle is used in the operating room when these wires are initially placed in the epicardium).

SELECTED READINGS

Baumgartner WA, Owen, SG, Cameron DE, et al., eds. The Johns Hopkins Manual of Cardiac Surgical Care. Baltimore: Mosby; 1994:208–211.

Clochesy JM, Breu C, Cardin S, et al., eds. Critical Care Nursing. 2rd Ed. Philadelphia: W.B. Saunders; 1996:182–185.

73

KNOW THE BACKUP MECHANISM OF ACTION AND REQUIREMENTS FOR ELECTRICAL CARDIOVERSION AND ANTICOAGULATION FOR VENTRICULAR ASSIST DEVICES

ELIZABETH A. MARTINEZ, MD, MHS

More than 2 million Americans have congestive heart failure and of these, approximately 60,000 meet criteria for some type of cardiac support or transplant. Despite expansion of criteria in the donor pool, there remains a limited number of donors. This number has essentially plateaued over the last decade between 2,000 and 3,000 annually. Because heart transplantation is not a viable option for many patients, there has been significant effort and research in the development of alternative medical and mechanical therapies. Mechanical ventricular assist devices (VADs) are currently used as a temporizing measure in the setting of acute heart failure, a bridge to transplantation, or as destination therapy. These devices are reported to improve the quality of life in these patients who are otherwise crippled by their heart failure despite maximal medical therapy.

VADs can be categorized in many ways: short term or long term; pulsatile or nonpulsatile; internal or external (i.e., intra- or extracorporeal). Short-term devices include cardiopulmonary bypass, extracorporeal membrane oxygenation (ECMO), and the Abiomed BVS. Long-term devices include the Novacor, the HeartMate I and II, Thoratec, and the newer Abiomed AB5000 Ventricle. The nonpulsatile devices are cardiopulmonary bypass and ECMO in addition to the HeartMate II. The permanent devices have an internal chamber. No device has a totally implantable energy source.

All VADs except the HeartMate II, which generates nonpulsatile flow using a rotarylike motor, generate pulsatile flow because of their design with unidirectional flow valves. They operate in a fill-to-empty cycle, similar to the action of the native ventricle (i.e., diastole and systole). The determinants of the stroke volume are the pre-ejection chamber volume (preload) and the outflow resistance, either pulmonary or systemic, depending which side is mechanically supported. Emptying is initiated when the control unit senses that the chamber is nearly full. The rate of the ejection is volume, or preload, dependent. It is important to note that the rate of output is independent of the native cardiac rhythm. The goal is to maintain unloading

TABLE 73.1 CLINICAL CHARACTERISTICS OF COMMONLY USED VENTRICULAR ASSIST DEVICES

DEVICE	ABIOMED (AB5000)	THORATEC	NOVACOR	HEARTMATE I	HEARTMATE II
Arterial tracing	Pulsatile	Pulsatile	Pulsatile	Pulsatile	Nonpulsatile
Valves	Angioflex polyurethane	Mechanical	Bioprosthetic	Porcine	n/a
Implantation	Paracorporeal	Para- or intracorporeal	Intracorporeal	Intracorporeal	Intracorporeal
Control unit	Not portable, large device	Portable, not wearable	Portable, worn as "belt"	Portable, worn as "belt" (electrical model)	Portable, worn as "belt"
Anticoagulation	Coumadin	Coumadin	Coumadin	Aspirin	Coumadin
Maximum stroke volume	100 mL	65 mL	70 mL	85 mL	n/a
Backup mechanism	Backup pump (also has pneumatic hand pump)	Pneumatic handheld pump	Backup controller needed; no manual mechanism	Pneumatic handheld pump	Backup controller needed; no manual mechanism
Maximum flow rate	4–6 L/min	7 L/min	10 L/min	10 L/min	10 L/min
Electrical cardioversion	No issue[a]	No issue	No issue	Need to turn electrical device off (electrical model)[b]	External paddle cardioversion: no issue; internal paddle cardioversion: must remove controller[b]
Cautery	No issue	No issue	No issue	May produce erratic pump output	No issue
Precautions	Acetone can crack the housing device	Acetone can crack the housing device		Controller and filter port must remain free of liquids	Controller must remain free of liquids

[a] May perform external or internal cardioversion with the device functioning.
[b] Specific instructions should accompany the device. It includes multiple steps that need to be performed in a specific sequence.

of the ventricle, especially in those patients who have had this placed with planned removal after recovery of the myocardium. This typically is limited to the postcardiac surgery patient in which a temporary device is placed.

Among the commonly used VADs (*Table 73.1*) there are unique characteristics and specific clinical information that are important to recognize. These include whether they require anticoagulation, the maximum stroke volume, the requirements for cardioversion and concerns with electrocautery, and the backup mode in case of emergency. In addition to these important management issues, the key to the management of the hemodynamics of these patients is understanding that the pumps are *volume dependent* (as discussed previously) and that many of these patients have concomitant right ventricular (RV) dysfunction or failure and pulmonary hypertension, which may further compromise RV function. RV dysfunction is very difficult to manage and key hemodynamic goals include those that optimize RV function and prevention of pulmonary hypertension, which will result in improved VAD filling and emptying. These include prevention of hypoxia and hypercarbia; optimal RV coronary perfusion pressure; and maintenance of a normal intrinsic cardiac rhythm. Although the filling and emptying of the LVAD is not in synchrony with the native cardiac cycle (rate), maintenance of sinus or other stable rhythm will potentially improve RV ejection and thus LV filling.

A key aspect in the management of such devices is the need for anticoagulation, except in the case of the HeartMate I. There are clinical situations that may require discontinuation of anticoagulation (e.g., need for emergent surgery, acute hemorrhagic stroke, and central line placement). Anticoagulation may be held for brief periods of time, but it must be reinitiated as soon as it is deemed safe. These devices are thrombogenic and patients are at high risk of clotting, which is generally and universally catastrophic. Even with adequate anticoagulation, there is an estimated 30% risk of thrombus formation. Thrombosis may occur in the device itself or at a native valve (e.g., aortic). Changing out the pumps because of thrombosis is possible only with the Abiomed BVS system and the paracorporeal Thoratec. There are some reports of changing out the prosthetic valvular devices in the literature as well.

SUGGESTED READINGS

Deng MC, Naka Y. Mechanical circulatory support devices—state of the art. Heart Fail Monit 2002;2:120–128.

Mancini D, Burkhoff D. Mechanical device-based methods of managing and treating heart failure. Circulation 2005;112:438–448.

74

PLACE THE DEFIBRILLATOR IN SYNCHRONOUS MODE WHEN CARDIOVERTING

ANGELA D. SHOHER, MD

Electrical cardioversion is used to manage patients with cardiac arrhythmias that involve re-entrant circuits, such as ventricular tachycardia or atrial fibrillation. In an emergent setting any patient with a ventricular rate greater than 150 who is unstable (i.e., chest pain, hypotension, unresponsive) should be treated with synchronized cardioversion. Cardioversion may also be performed on stable patients who have an arrhythmia that is refractory to pharmacologic intervention.

Cardioversion theoretically stops the arrhythmia by depolarizing the re-entrant circuit and making it refractory to propagation. Cardioversion delivers energy that is synchronous with the early part of the QRS complex. If the energy is delivered in an asynchronous manner, it can induce ventricular fibrillation. This occurs when the energy is delivered during the early phase of repolarization. When the cardioverter is placed in synchronous mode, it automatically discharges a current that coincides with a large R or S wave, thereby avoiding the period of repolarization when ventricular fibrillation can occur. In synchronous mode there is always a delay in energy delivery while the cardioverter searches for the R or S wave. It is important to switch the mode to asynchronous delivery if the patient develops ventricular fibrillation.

WHAT TO DO

When cardioverting, there are two possible placement options of the pads on the chest wall. In the anteroposterior position, one pad is placed to the right of the sternum anteriorly and the second is placed between the spine and the tip of the left scapula posteriorly. The second option is to place the paddles in the anterolateral position with one paddle in the fourth or fifth intercostal space in the left midaxillary line. The second paddle is then placed to the right of the sternum on the second or third intercostal space. The anterior-posterior approach is optimal in patients with implantable devices to avoid diverting current to the device. Pacemakers should be 10 cm from direct contact with the paddles. The paddles should be placed firmly against the skin to prevent arcing and skin burns. Conductive gel should be used to ensure good contact with the skin.

The amount of energy used to cardiovert is controversial. Prompt cardioversion prevents prolonged ischemia and multiple shocks. Excessive energy, however, can lead to myocardial damage. The optimal amount of energy also depends on the patient's arrhythmia. For a patient who is relatively hemodynamically stable, atrial fibrillation with rapid ventricular rate (RVR) that is refractory to pharmacologic therapy, for example, 50 joules may be adequate. For ventrical tachycardias, however, advanced cardiac life support guidelines now recommend starting with 360 joules (unlike the increasing amount of joules recommended in past guidelines). This number also depends on the type of defibrillator. If it is monophasic (i.e., current travels in one direction between the paddles) more energy will be required. If the machine delivers biphasic current, consideration should be given to starting at 25 joules for a trial fibrillation and 150 joules for ventricular tachycardias.

SUGGESTED READINGS

Morgan GH, Mikhail MS, Murray MJ, et al., eds. Clinical Anesthesiology. 3rd Ed. New York: McGraw-Hill; 2002:472–473.

Podrid PJ. Basic Principles and Techniques of Cardioversion and Defibrillation. UpToDate. http://www.uptodate.com

75

TURN OFF THE SYNCHRONIZATION MODE ON THE DEFIBRILLATOR IF THERE IS NO RECOGNIZED R WAVE

NIRAV G. SHAH, MD

The difference between cardioversion and defibrillation is based on whether the synchronization mode on the cardioverter-defibrillator is turned on or off. In cardioversion, the electrical shock is delivered in synchronization ("turned on") with the QRS complex and can result in the termination of a variety of arrhythmias. Atrial fibrillation is one of the most frequently cardioverted rhythms and usually requires at least 300 J of energy on traditional defibrillators and between 75 J and 200 J on the newer biphasic defibrillators. Urgent cardioversion is undertaken in patients with hemodynamic compromise and in stable patients after anticoagulation unless the arrhythmia has lasted less than 48 hours. Direct-current cardioversion is also used for atrial flutter and most practitioners initially try 50 to 100 J with a good rate of success. Supraventricular tachycardias and ventricular tachycardias may also be cardioverted but this is done far less frequently secondary to success of intravenous antiarrhythmics and unrecognizable R waves.

Defibrillation, as opposed to cardioversion, delivers a shock at any time during a cardiac cycle and is used primarily when there is no recognized R wave, such as in ventricular fibrillation, polymorphic ventricular tachycardia, or rapid ventricular tachycardia. The energy requirement is now recommended to be 360 J for successful conversion to sinus rhythm. With prompt defibrillation the success of this procedure is usually high. In patients with ventricular tachycardia there is a chance of conversion to ventricular fibrillation requiring additional shocks for restoration of sinus rhythm.

For either cardioversion or defibrillation several considerations are important. First, adequate sedation should be provided if the patient is awake and alert. The pain associated with electrical shock is significant and ideally the patient should have adequate analgesia and amnesia for the procedure. Second, complications from the procedure include myocardial necrosis, myocardial dysfunction, pulmonary or systemic embolization, skin burns, and deterioration to a less stable rhythm. Finally, it is possible that the patient may progress to cardiopulmonary arrest and the care team should be prepared for the need to treat this should it occur.

SUGGESTED READINGS

Falk RH. Atrial fibrillation. N Engl J Med 2001;344:1067–1078.

Tracy CM, Akhtar M, DiMarco JP, et al. American College of Cardiology/American Heart Association clinical competence statement on invasive electrophysiology studies, catheter ablation, and cardioversion: a report of the American College of Cardiology/American Heart Association/American College of Physicians-American Society of Internal Medicine task force on clinical competence. Circulation 2000;102:2309.

76

DO NOT RULE OUT THE PRESENCE OF
A MYOCARDIAL INFARCTION BY
A NORMAL ELECTROCARDIOGRAM

JOSE M. RODRIGUEZ-PAZ, MD

One of the most challenging clinical scenarios that we encounter in clinical practice and specifically in the intensive care unit (ICU) environment is the diagnosis of myocardial ischemia/infarction (MI) or acute coronary syndrome (ACS). The diagnosis is made by consideration of certain risk factors for coronary artery disease, the characterization of clinical symptoms (especially pain), and the results of diagnostic studies (invasive and noninvasive). Moreover, making the diagnosis in a timely fashion is paramount in order to reduce the morbidity and mortality associated with this disease, since those patients with ST-elevation MI or new left bundle branch block require urgent reperfusion therapy.

SIGNS AND SYMPTOMS

One common clinical finding in patients presenting with MI is chest pain (located in the precordium and described as tightness or pressure radiating to left arm, jaw, or neck). Commonly these patients also present with dyspnea, anxiety, lightheadedness and syncope, nausea and vomiting, and diaphoresis. There are also many patients who present with no specific symptoms. It is accepted that one in six patients with chest pain actually have an MI, especially in elderly patients. It is important to obtain a good description of the patient's symptoms. In general, the likelihood of having an MI with chest pain increases if the patient has had other episodes of chest pain for more than 1 year, if the pain is constant and described as pressure and radiates to the arms, and if it is associated with diaphoresis, nausea, and vomiting. In some patients (e.g., diabetics) this characteristic pain may be absent. Other clinical findings that have an increased likelihood of being associated with MI include hypotension, presence of a third heart sound, and the presence of pulmonary crackles. Although these symptoms cannot rule it out, symptoms that lower the likelihood of ischemia include reproducibility of pain with palpations and positional changes, stabbing pain, and other atypical presentations. Nevertheless, the evidence published does not support the sole use of clinical signs and symptoms without the support of electrocardiography (ECG), cardiac enzymes, or other diagnostic tools to diagnose ACS or MI, as these have low sensitivity.

ECG continues to be one of the most important diagnostic tools for ACS. The current classification of ACS has moved toward dividing MI into ST-elevation MI (STEMI) and non—ST-elevation MI (NSTEMI). In the presence of characteristic symptoms, the presence of ST-segment elevation has high specificity for MI, especially for transmural MI (Q-wave infarct). In general, perioperative ischemia or MI generally is associated with ST depression rather than ST elevation. Unfortunately, ECGs can be normal in half of the patients with ACS. This is probably even more frequent in patients admitted to the ICU for other causes or in the case of intraoperative MI, in which the lack of typical symptoms or atypical ECEs changes may make the diagnosis of MI very difficult. It is important to note that ECG waveforms are determined by not only the pathophysiology of the patient but also by technical factors, thus determining the output ECG. The electrical changes registered by the ECG are related to the mass of myocardium damaged and thus the bigger the area, the more evident that the changes and the territory are affected by the MI, although this not always true. For example, in the case of concomitant right ventricular (ST elevation in V1 and V2) and posterior MI (ST depression in V1—V3), both in the territory of the right coronary artery, the electrical forces that result after MI neutralize each other and ST changes may not be seen. This is very important because the pathophysiology and treatment of the right ventricle MI is very different than the MI in the left heart, requiring volume loading and early use of inotropes to maintain preload to the left ventricle.

TABLE 76.1	RELATIONSHIP OF CORONARY ANATOMY AND ECG LEAD FINDINGS	
REGION	**ECG LEADS**	**CORONARY ARTERY**
Inferior wall	II, III, aVF	RCA
Posterior wall	Large R wave (R/S ratio >1) in V1, V2, or V3 with ST depression, T-wave changes in V1	RCA
Lateral wall	I, aVL, V4–V6	Circumflex
Anterolateral	I, aVL, V1–V6	LAD
Anteroseptal	V1–V3	LAD
Anterior	V1–V4	LAD
Right ventricle	V3R–V5R (transient changes), V4R the highest specificity and sensitivity	RCA

LAD, left anterior descending; RCA, right coronary artery; V3R, right precordial lead.

The ECG findings that characteristically are found in MI are the presence of Q waves, ST-segment elevation (≥ 1 mm) or depression, new conduction defects and T-wave depression in specific leads, depending upon the territory affected (*Table 76.1*). The change with the highest probability of being found in MI is the ST-segment elevation, especially in the presence of reciprocal changes. At the same time, and despite the number of cases of MI with normal ECG, the presence of a normal ECG decreases the probability of MI but this does not rule it out.

SUGGESTED READINGS

Birnbaum Y, Drew BJ. The electrocardiogram in ST elevation acute myocardial infarction; correlation with coronary artery anatomy and prognosis. Postgrad Med J 2003;79:490–504.

Hurford WE. Critical Care Handbook of the Massachusetts General Hospital. Philadelphia: Lippincott Williams & Wilkins; 2000:273–292.

Panju AA, Hemmelgarn BR, Guyattt GH, et al. The rational clinical examination: is this patient having a myocardial infarction. JAMA 1998;280:1256–1263.

77

DO NOT USE THE 3 OR 5 LEAD ECG MONITOR AS A 12-LEAD ELECTROCARDIOGRAM

TUHIN K. ROY, MD, PHD

Continuous electrocardiogram (ECG) monitoring is a standard monitor utilized for the detection of arrhythmias and ischemia. Many common monitoring systems utilize 3 or 5 leads instead of the 12 leads captured by the standard ECG. Even though both systems can potentially be used for detection of arrhythmias as well as ischemia, the limitations of the 3- or 5-lead system monitors should be understood so that the care of the patient may be optimized by obtaining further studies as necessary. The standard 12-lead ECG provides a 10-second snapshot of three bipolar leads (I, II, III), three augmented unipolar leads (aVR, aVL, aVF), and six precordial leads (V1 to V6); the standard 5-lead system allows the monitoring of seven different leads (I, II, III; aVR, aVL, aVF; and V5). It is important to remember that the ECG reflects only electrical activity and not heart function (e.g., pulseless electrical activity) and can be altered by physiologic factors, pathophysiological factors (e.g., electrolyte imbalances, pacemakers, pericarditis, hypothermia, subarachnoid hemorrhage), and technical factors (e.g., calibration, lead position, and body position).

ARRHYTHMIA DETECTION

Accurate detection and identification of arrhythmias is crucial since inadequate or inappropriate treatment can be harmful or fatal. Although lead II is commonly used for the detection of cardiac dysrhythmias since its direction parallels atrial depolarization and results in the maximum P-wave amplitude, lead V1 is more useful for diagnosing bundle branch blocks and discriminating between ventricular tachycardia (VT) and supraventricular tachycardia (SVT) with aberrant conduction. Both of these leads should be monitored if possible so that the relationship between atrial and ventricular depolarizations can be determined.

Premature atrial contractions typically result in abnormal P waves from an ectopic atrial focus with a variable PR interval and no compensatory pause. If part of the ventricular conduction system is refractory, the resulting aberrant conduction leads to an abnormal QRS complex and can be confused with a premature ventricular contraction. Look for a preceding (likely abnormal) P wave, a QRS complex suggestive of a right bundle branch block, an rSR' in V1, and concordance of the initial deflection with the preceding beat to distinguish these from premature ventricular contractions.

Paroxysmal SVT results from transient activity of an ectopic atrial pacemaker and is seen as a rapid regular rhythm with abnormal P waves and normal QRS complexes. SVT with aberrant conduction (as mentioned earlier) can be confused with ventricular tachycardia. Atrial flutter is characterized by sawtooth flutter (F) waves best seen in leads II and V1 with normal QRS complexes typically conducted at 2:1, 3:1, or 4:1. In atrial fibrillation, P waves cannot be identified and the QRS complexes are narrow with irregular interval.

Junctional rhythms such as atrioventricular (AV) nodal re-entry tachycardia can result from ectopic activity near the AV node that is conducted retrograde as well as anterograde, leading to inverted P waves in leads II, III, and aVF and positive P waves in aVR. High nodal rhythms produce shortened PR intervals, whereas low nodal rhythms produce P waves that follow a normal QRS. If the rhythm is midnodal, the P wave can distort the QRS complex, causing a pseudo S wave in the inferior leads and a pseudo R wave in V1.

AV re-entrant tachycardias are due to accessory conduction pathways that permit ventricular pre-excitation. Wolff-Parkinson-White syndrome (WPW) generates a regular rhythm with a delta wave and a slurred QRS complex resulting from early ventricular depolarization. Type A WPW is characterized by an upright delta wave and QRS complex in the precordial leads with an upright dominant R wave in V1; this can be confused with a right bundle branch block (RBBB). Type B WPW has a downward delta wave and QRS complex in leads V1 and V2 with upward deflections in the other precordial leads similar to a left bundle branch block (LBBB). The majority of tachycardias in WPW are classified as orthodromic and result from antegrade conduction of impulses through the AV node that return to the atria via the accessory pathway; P waves follow the normal-width QRS complexes and no delta waves are seen. Antidromic AV re-entrant tachycardia results from antegrade conduction via the accessory pathway (causing wide QRS complexes) with retrograde conduction via the AV node. Atrial fibrillation in WPW results in an irregular wide complex tachycardia.

Premature ventricular contractions result in a prolonged abnormal QRS complex since the ectopic ventricular pacemaker impulses are conducted via ventricular muscle rather than the Purkinje fibers; typically, the QRS voltage is increased and the T wave appears inverted. Retrograde or blocked atrial depolarization may lead to the presence of P waves on the tracing. A compensatory pause occurs since a subsequent depolarization from the sinoatrial (S-A) node is blocked. An R-on-T phenomenon may happen if this occurs near the vulnerable period of the preceding depolarization, leading to ventricular fibrillation. The QRS complex may be of the RBBB variant with a prominent R wave in V1 or may be of the LBBB variant with notching of the S wave with less acute downsloping.

Ventricular tachycardia appears as multiple, rapid, regular premature ventricular contractions. The QRS complexes are wide and must be distinguished from SVT with aberrancy. If the QRS complexes appear to be positive in lead V1, a ventricular origin is suggested by positive deflections in all precordial leads, a duration >0.14 seconds, and characteristic R-wave morphologies in lead V1. If the QRS complexes are negative in lead V1, a ventricular origin is suggested by negative deflections in all precordial leads and a duration >0.16 seconds . Axis deviation >40 degrees, a QS or negative complex in lead V6, and negative P waves in aVR are also suggestive of a ventricular origin. This rhythm is characterized by fusion/capture beats as well as AV dissociation. Ventricular fibrillation appears as an irregular wavy line. *Torsades de pointes*, associated with altered repolarization and QT prolongation, may have a similar appearance to polymorphic VT or ventricular fibrillation (VF).

Other causes of QRS prolongation include left ventricular hypertrophy (LVH).

CONDUCTION DEFECTS

Conduction defects include SA node block (no atrial excitation and no P wave), atrioventricular block (with altered conduction of the atrial impulse through the AV node), and intraventricular defects including RBBB and LBBB.

Although the QRS complexes are narrow in first-degree atrioventricular block (PR interval >0.21 seconds) and Type I (Wenckebach) second-degree block, the duration of the QRS complex in Type II second-degree block depends on its location within the conduction system. Complete atrioventricular dissociation (third-degree block) can result in narrow or wide QRS complexes depending on the location of the ectopic pacemaker causing ventricular depolarization. If it is near the AV node, the complexes appear normal with a ventricular rate of 40 to 60 per minute; if it is infranodal, the rate is usually <40 per minute and the complexes appear wide.

Leads I, V1, and V6 are especially important for diagnosing intraventricular conduction defects. In complete LBBB, all impulses are conducted via the right bundle, causing a widened QRS with a negative rS complex in V1 and a wide notched R wave in leads I, aVL, and V6. The QRS complex is not widened in left anterior or posterior hemiblock. Left anterior hemiblock leads to left-axis deviation with a small Q in I and aVL and a small R in II, III, and aVF; left posterior hemiblock leads to right-axis deviation with a small R in I and aVL and a small Q in II, III, and aVF. RBBB causes a wide QRS and can generate rSR' complexes in V1 to V3 with wide S waves in leads I and V6.

In summary, widening of the QRS complex can be associated with right and left bundle branch blocks as well as ectopy arising from the right and left ventricles, which may not be detected if lead II is monitored exclusively. This highlights the importance of lead V1 to assist with the accurate detection and diagnosis of conduction defects and arrhythmias during monitoring. Obtaining a hard-copy 12-lead ECG should be strongly considered when aberrant conduction or conduction defects are suspected.

ISCHEMIA DETECTION

The optimal leads for detection of ischemia are different from the optimal leads for detection of arrhythmias. Common indicators of ischemia are ST-segment changes, T-wave inversions, or the development of Q waves in leads corresponding to different areas of myocardium (*Table 77.1*); note, however, that ischemia may be present even in the absence of ECG changes.

ST-segment changes are typically measured relative to the PQ baseline. A generally accepted definition of ischemia is horizontal or

TABLE 77.1	RELATIONSHIP OF CORONARY DISTRIBUTION TO POSSIBLE ECG CHANGES	
LEADS	CORONARY DISTRIBUTION	MYOCARDIUM
II, III, aVF	RCA	Inferior LV wall RA, RV, interatrial septum SA node, AV node
I, aVL	LCX	Lateral LV wall SA node, AV node
V3–V6	LAD	Anterolateral LV wall

LAD, left anterior descending coronary artery; LCX, left circumflex artery; RCA, right coronary artery.

downsloping ST-segment depression >1 mm from baseline or ST-segment elevation >1 mm in any lead 60 or 80 milliseconds after the J point. Leads II and V5 (reflecting the inferior and anterolateral distributions) have traditionally been used for ischemia detection. A study by London et al. assessed the utility of various leads in detecting ischemia in patients with known coronary disease undergoing surgery. Lead V5 was found to be the most sensitive (75%); adding lead II (often used for arrhythmia detection) improved this to 80%, but adding leads II and V4 improved this further to 96%. A more recent study by Landesberg et al. in patients undergoing vascular surgery found that V4 was the most sensitive for ischemia among patients who had a myocardial infarction (83%) and that using 2 to 3 precordial leads detects more than 92% of all ischemia that would be picked up by using all 12 leads. Note that simultaneous recording of multiple precordial leads may not be available on all monitors.

Although the 5-lead ECG may a useful tool for detection of ischemia, as with a 12-lead, the waveforms obtained are sensitive to lead placement, especially with regard to the precordial electrodes. Often during surgical procedures or in patients with dressings in place, the placement of the leads is not ideal. Accurate ischemia detection also relies on adequate skin contact of the leads. To reduce electrical and cautery interference, monitors rely on filters that reduce artifact and drift but that may prevent accurate ST-segment analysis. Monitors should be switched to diagnostic mode to allow the appropriate bandwidth for detection of ischemia.

Continuous ST-segment tracking is available to monitor changes but is subject to limitations and requires vigilance with regard to drifting set points that need to be checked and adjusted on a regular basis. Also, ischemia may be transient and not reflected on serial ECGs, providing the rationale for continuous 12-lead ECG monitoring with simplified lead systems that have recently become available. Finally, intraoperative ECG monitoring may not detect a substantial fraction of intraoperative ischemic events as compared with the use of echocardiography to detect regional wall motion abnormalities. If ischemia is suspected based on a 3- or 5-lead ECG, a 12-lead ECG should be obtained, if possible. In addition, the use of other modalities including echocardiography should also be considered if ischemia is suspected in the absence of ECG changes.

SUGGESTED READINGS

Edhouse J, Morris F. Broad complex tachycardia: part I. BMJ 2002;324:719–722.
Edhouse J, Morris F. Broad complex tachycardia: part II. BMJ 2002;324:776–779.

Landesberg G, Mosseri M, Wolf Y, et al. Perioperative myocardial ischemia and infarction. Anesthesiology 2002;96:264–270.

London MJ, Hollenberg M, Wong MG. Intraoperative myocardial ischemia: localization by continuous 12-lead electrocardiography. Anesthesiology 1988;69:232–241.

Miller RD, ed. Anesthesia. 5th Ed. New York: Churchill Livingstone; 2000:1231–1254.

78

PUT A BOARD UNDER THE PATIENT WHEN DOING CHEST COMPRESSIONS

ELIZABETH A. HUNT, MD, MPH
CAMERON DEZFULIAN, MD

Chest compressions have long been considered one of the critical elements of basic and advanced life support, as they provide vital substrate to the brain and myocardium during cardiac arrest. The quality of compressions delivered during cardiac arrest affects the success of the patient's outcome.

WHAT TO DO

However, it has become increasingly clear that health care providers do not always perform high-quality cardiopulmonary resuscitation (CPR). To address this issue, the 2005 American Heart Association Guidelines for CPR and Emergency Cardiovascular Care provides a number of evidence-based recommendations detailing how to deliver effective chest compressions. For example, these guidelines and the evidence stress the importance of providing chest compressions as early as possible after cardiovascular collapse, minimizing interruptions to compressions, and permitting chest-wall recoil. The guidelines also give specific recommendations on how to perform chest compressions on adults, including a rate of 100 compressions per minute, a compression to ventilation ratio of 30:2 for the unintubated patient, and a compression depth of 1.5 to 2 in (4 to 5 cm).

In addition to these recommendations, the guidelines also specifically state, "to maximize the effectiveness of compressions, the victim should lie supine on a hard surface (e.g., backboard or floor)." In addition, the guidelines state, "'CPR-friendly' deflatable mattresses have been studied, and they do not provide an adequate surface on which to perform chest compressions." In animal and mannequin studies, compressions delivered on a soft surface (e.g., foam mattress or fully inflated or deflated air mattress) resulted in significant dissipation of the downward force of compression and inadequate depth of compression when compared with placement of the mannequin on the floor. Furthermore, resuscitators felt their compressions were more unstable and less effective when performed on any of the mattresses when compared with the floor.

The aforementioned studies also showed that the force of compressions decreased with the increasing height of the bed. It is possible that the floor is such an effective surface for chest compressions because of the interaction between the hard surface and the position of the rescuer over the patient's chest. With this in mind, if a patient suffers a cardiac arrest while in a hospital bed, in addition to using a backboard, rescuers should also lower the bed and/or use a stool on which to stand in an effort to ensure the patient's chest (and not just the mattress) is compressed to the suggested depth of 4 to 5 cm.

SUGGESTED READINGS

2005 American Heart Association guidelines for cardiopulmonary resuscitation and emergency cardiovascular care, part 4: adult basic life support. Circulation 2005;112:19–34.

Perkins GD, Benny R, Giles S, et al. Do different mattresses affect the quality of cardiopulmonary resuscitation? Intensive Care Med 2003;29:2330–2335.

Boe JM, Babbs CF. Mechanics of cardiopulmonary resuscitation performed with the patient on a soft bed vs a hard surface. Acad Emerg Med 1999:6:754–757.

79

KNOW THE PACEMAKER ALPHABET SOUP

ELIZABETH A. MARTINEZ, MD, MHS

Critically ill patients may require urgent or emergent pacing at any time during their hospital course. This may occur more frequently in medical or surgical cardiac intensive care units (ICU), but a working knowledge of the standard nomenclature is important for all ICU caregivers.

Many will care for patients with implanted pacemakers for long-standing conditions. An increasing number of patients will have a pacemaker plus an Automatic Implantable Cardioverter Defibrillator (AICD) or biventricular pacing wires, as this becomes more widespread in the management of patients with heart failure. Many of these implanted pacemakers have sophisticated settings. This is in contrast to the much more simplified scenario used in an urgent situation requiring transvenous pacing or epicardial pacing in post–cardiac surgery patients. However, despite being more simplified, the nomenclature is the same in both implanted and temporary pacing.

WATCH OUT FOR

The standard nomenclature for pacing is a five-letter designation for the mode of pacing and sensing of intrinsic electrical (cardiac) activity. In the setting of urgent or emergent pacing, only the first three letters of the Inter-Society Commission for Heart Disease Resources (ICHD) are typically used (*Table 79.1*). The first letter refers to the cardiac chamber paced, the second letter represents the chamber sensed, and the third letter represents the mode, or what happens in response to the sensing. The latter two-letter designations are generally used in internal pacemakers and reflect more sophisticated programming that is beyond the scope of this chapter.

The method used to pace patients depends on the wires that are used (i.e., whether there is capability to pace the atria, ventricles, or both) and the mode designated on the pacer box. The capability to pace one or both chambers depends on the type (or number) of wires placed or the type of transvenous device that has been placed. In the setting of post–cardiac surgery patients, the ground wire is placed in the positive pole of the pacer box. By convention, the ground wire is the longer of the two ventricular wires or a newly placed skin lead. For atrial epicardial wires, either can be used as the grounding wire. In the

TABLE 79.1	PACING NOMENCLATURE AND MODES			
ICHD DESIGNATION[a]	CARDIAC CHAMBER PACED (FIRST LETTER DESIGNATION)	CARDIAC CHAMBER SENSED (SECOND LETTER DESIGNATION)	RESPONSE TO SENSED EVENTS (THIRD LETTER DESIGNATION)	RESULTANT PACING MODE
AAI	Atrial	Atrial	Inhibited	Synchronous (demand)
AOO	Atrial	None	n/a (no inhibition)	Asynchronous (fixed rate)
VVI	Ventricular	Ventricular	Inhibited	Synchronous
VOO	Ventricular	None	n/a (no inhibition)	Asynchronous
DVI	Dual[b]	Ventricular	V pacing inhibited by V sensing	Synchronous
DDI	Dual[b]	Dual[b]	Inhibited	Synchronous
DOO	Dual[b]	None	n/a (no inhibition)	Asynchronous

[a] Inter–Society Commission for Heart Disease Resources code.
[b] Dual is both atrial and ventricular chambers.

setting of transvenous pacing, the positive lead on the wire is placed in the positive pole of the pacer box.

There are two general modes of pacing, asynchronous and synchronous. Asynchronous pacing will result in electrical output to the myocardium at a fixed or set rate, regardless of what the underlying rate and rhythm are. There is no feedback from the myocardium to the external pacing device. This mode is typically used for atrial pacing because the atria are difficult to sense since these chambers have less mass. Asynchronous pacing is generally not used for ventricular pacing because it increases the risk of the R-on-T phenomenon. If this occurs and the ventricle is triggered when it is in a vulnerable phase of the cardiac cycle, ventricular fibrillation can result.

Synchronous or demand pacing is used to describe modes that are responsive to the native rhythm. That is, the native rhythm is sensed by the pacing wires and give feedback to the pacer box such that it will fire an electrical current only if the native rate is below the predetermined rate (or rate set on the pacer box).

SUGGESTED READINGS

Artusio JF, Yao F-SF. Anesthesiology: Problem-oriented Patient Management. 3rd Ed. Philadelphia: Lippincott Williams & Wilkins; 1993:199–213.

Baumgartner WA. The Johns Hopkins Manual of Cardiac Surgical Care. St. Louis: Mosby; 1994:208–212.

Fuster V, Alexander RW, Schlant RC. Hurst's the Heart, Arteries and Veins. 9th Ed. New York: McGraw-Hill; 1998:1023–1052.

80

Do not use cooling blankets to cool

Iosifina Giannakikou, MD

A patient that "needs to be cooled" is not an infrequent occurrence in the intensive care unit (ICU). In order to effectively lower a patient's core body temperature, an understanding of temperature physiology is required.

The human body can be roughly divided into two thermal compartments: a core compartment, consisting of the trunk and head, excluding the skin, and a peripheral compartment, consisting of the skin and extremities. The core temperature is regulated by limiting or increasing heat transfer to the periphery through vasoconstriction and vasodilatation, respectively. Heat loss from the peripheral compartment is regulated through changes in skin perfusion (again through vasodilatation or vasoconstriction) and by increasing or decreasing the production of sweat.

When cooling blankets are placed over or under a patient, they increase sympathetic tone (with concomitant increase in systemic vascular resistance index) and induce vasoconstriction in the skin. This actually prevents heat dissipation and causes an increase in core body temperature, not a decrease. This physiological response complicates attempts to induce therapeutic hypothermia or normothermia by other means of external cooling. In addition, heat production will be increased through the shivering response and, in later phases, through the increased metabolism of fats, carbohydrates, and proteins. As a result there can be an increase (not a decrease) in body temperature.

There are more effective ways to cool the core body temperature that use the well-described four mechanisms of heat transfer: convection, conduction, evaporation, and radiation. Some of the more common ways are summarized in *Tables 80.1* and *80.2.*

TABLE 80.1 METHODS OF PERIPHERAL COOLING		
METHOD	**HEAT TRANSFER**	**COMMENTS**
Fans	Convection	Increased infection risk
Ice packs	Conduction	Neck, axilla, groin
Cold-water sponge bath	Evaporation	—

TABLE 80.2	METHODS OF CORE BODY COOLING	
METHOD	**HEAT TRANSFER**	**COMMENTS**
Antipyretic agents	—	Acetaminophen, dantrolene
Cooled intravenous fluids	Conduction	Neck, axilla, groin
Cold–water lavage	Conduction	Gastric, bladder, peritoneal
Antishivering maneuvers	Conduction, radiation	Paralysis

SUGGESTED READINGS

Creechan T, Vollman K, Kravutske ME. Cooling by convection vs cooling by conduction for treatment of fever in critically ill adults. Am J Crit Care 2001;10:52–59.

Henker R, Rogers S, Kramer DJ, et al. Comparison of fever treatments in the critically ill: a pilot study. Am J Crit Care 2001;10:276–280.

O'Donnell J, Axelrod P, Fisher C, et al. Use and effectiveness of hypothermia blankets for febrile patients in the intensive care unit. Clin Infect Dis 1997;24:1208–1213.

81

DO NOT PLACE FEMORAL ARTERIAL LINES OR VENOUS CATHETERS ABOVE THE INGUINAL LIGAMENT OR BELOW THE THIGH CREASE

SUSANNA L. MATSEN, MD

The majority of intensive care patients require arterial and central venous lines for purposes of continuous blood pressure monitoring, blood gas sampling, and the administration of large volumes of fluid and vasoactive substances. The femoral areas provide an access location for rapid arterial or venous cannulation in an emergency situation, or alternatively when other locations are not available. Despite the relative accessibility and superficial nature of these vessels, their cannulation can present risks of which the prudent clinician should be aware.

WATCH OUT FOR

Puncture sites for femoral lines should lie between the groin crease and the inguinal ligament; punctures outside of these zones risk complications. The inguinal ligament stretches from the anterior superior iliac spine down to the pubic symphysis and marks the inferior border of the peritoneum. Hence, punctures above this point will likely enter the peritoneal cavity, with potential visceral injury and bacterial seeding. Aspiration of enteric contents or ascitic fluid should immediately alert the operator of this eventuality, and a general surgical team should be alerted.

Conversely, attempting cannulation too inferiorly (below the groin crease) risks laceration of branch vessels. The common femoral artery branches into the superficial femoral and deep femoral arteries at this point. Similarly, in the venous system, the greater saphenous vein joins the deep femoral vein roughly 3 cm inferior to the inguinal ligament, forming the femoral vein. Although the operator may obtain a "flash" of blood into the syringe at a distal site, there may be difficulty threading the wire through the junction of the superficial to the common femoral artery. More significantly, the needle may lacerate the femoral artery "through and through" and also injure the vein, eventually leading to an arteriovenous fistula (usually >2 days after the injury). A patient with diminished distal pulses, a groin bruit, pulsatile mass, and potentially a drop in blood pressure after attempts at femoral cannulation should be suspected of an arteriovenous (AV) fistula, and a high-quality vascular duplex study should be ordered. Evidence of flow between the artery and vein should prompt an immediate vascular surgery consult.

Other iatrogenic etiologies of pulsatile masses in the groin include femoral artery pseudoaneurysms. These result from dissection of the arterial wall by the needle or wire during line placement, leading to weakening of the wall and aneurysmal dilatation. Given the risk of growth of the pseudoaneurysm and potential rupture, these should also be referred to vascular surgery.

Undetected bleeds from the femoral artery after attempts at cannulation may lead to retroperitoneal hematomas. Such a bleeding source should always remain in the back of the mind of an intensive care team with a patient who drops his hematocrit without any apparent bleeding source. The blood remains extraperitoneal, dissecting the potential space between the peritoneal sac and the retroperitoneum. Patients may present with leg paresis (secondary to irritation of the nerves coursing through this area), abdominal or groin pain, or simply a flank bruise. Although the blood usually courses posteriorly, it may dissect anteriorly into the space of Retzius. A continuous drop in hematocrit or a symptomatic bleed with a computed tomography (CT) scan demonstrating retroperitoneal blood should prompt surgical repair of the vessel.

One final note is that the operator must be familiar with the medial-lateral anatomy of the femoral vessels, commonly recalled by the mnemonic NAVEL when moving lateral to medial. NAVEL stands for *n*erve most laterally, then *a*rtery next most medial, then *v*ein, *e*mpty space, and *l*ymphatics most medially.

SELECTED READINGS

Marino PL. The ICU Book. 2nd Ed. Baltimore: Williams & Wilkins; 1998:53–75.
Moore KL, Dalley AF. Clinically Oriented Anatomy. 4th Ed. Philadelphia: Lippincott Williams & Wilkins; 1999:541–549.

82

CONSIDER RESPIRATORY VARIATION ON THE ARTERIAL-LINE MONITOR TRACING AS A SIGN OF HYPOVOLEMIA

JAMES F. WELLER, MD

During the inspiratory phase of spontaneous ventilation, negative intrathoracic pressure leads to augmentation of right ventricular (RV) filling. This leads to a leftward shift in the interventricular septum, decreasing the size and compliance of the left ventricle. In addition, the augmented right ventricular stroke volume pools in the pulmonary circulation, causing a further decrease in left ventricular (LV) filling volume. Decreased LV volume is associated with a decrease in LV stroke volume and systemic blood pressure. With exhalation, blood pooled in the right ventricle and pulmonary circulation returns to the left ventricle; stroke volume and systemic blood pressure increase. Under normal conditions, the inspiratory decrease in arterial blood pressure does not exceed 5 to 10 mm Hg.

A reversed pulsus paradoxus, or systolic pressure variation, has been described during mechanical ventilation. The positive intrathoracic pressure of mechanical inspiration decreases venous return to the right heart and increases RV afterload. In addition, increased alveolar pressure "squeezes" blood from the pulmonary circulation into the left ventricle. The result is an inspiratory decrease in RV stroke volume and an inspiratory increase in LV stroke volume and systemic arterial blood pressure. Given static arterial compliance, systemic arterial pulse pressure (the difference between systolic and diastolic blood pressure) is directly proportional to stroke volume. Thus, any changes in venous return or pulmonary blood flow that lead to an increase in LV stroke volume will also lead to an increase in pulse pressure.

Under hypovolemic conditions, mechanical respiratory effects on venous return, stroke volume, and arterial blood pressure are accentuated for at least four reasons: (i) the vena cava is more collapsible; (ii) an underfilled right atrium is more compliant and, therefore, more susceptible to changes in pleural pressure; (iii) more of the lung is in West zone I ($P_{alveolar} > P_{arterial} > P_{venous}$), where respiratory effects on pulmonary blood flow are most pronounced; and (iv) both ventricles are more sensitive to changes in preload when operating on the steep portion of the Frank-Starling curve. All four of these mechanisms accentuate the mechanical inspiratory decrease in RV stroke volume, suggesting that it is the subsequent expiratory decrease in LV output that is mostly responsible for the profound respiratory variation in blood pressure encountered in the setting of hypovolemia. If the difference is greater than 10 mm Hg, hypovolemia must be considered as the most common cause.

SUGGESTED READINGS

Michard F. Changes in arterial pressure during mechanical ventilation. Anesthesiology 2005;103:419–428.

Thomas S, Kramer J, eds. Manual of Cardiac Anesthesia. 2nd Ed. New York: Churchill Livingstone; 1993:134–135.

83

DO NOT USE LOW-MOLECULAR-WEIGHT HEPARIN IN PATIENTS WITH EPIDURALS

AWORI J. HAYANGA, MD
ELLIOTT R. HAUT, MD

Neuraxial anesthesia and analgesia (either by perioperative spinal or postoperative epidural catheter) has been shown to significantly improve pain control and other outcomes after major surgery as well as for trauma patients with multiple rib fractures. Simultaneously, data have shown lower rates of venous thromboembolic events in patients receiving chemical venous thromboembolic event prophylaxis with some form of anticoagulant (i.e., unfractionated or low-molecular-weight heparin [LMWH]). However, the concomitant use of anticoagulants and spinal or epidural anesthesia can result in the rare, but potentially devastating, spinal hematoma.

Patients with significant uncorrected bleeding disorders and those receiving anticoagulation are at significantly elevated risk of developing spinal hematoma in the setting of neuraxial anesthesia. The diagnosis of spinal hematoma is complicated by the concealed nature of the bleeding. A high index of suspicion must be maintained. Patients who have neurologic findings (e.g., weakness, decreased sensation, or incontinence) after undergoing a lumbar puncture or receiving spinal or epidural analgesia require emergent evaluation for possible spinal hematoma. Back pain is a common finding but is not present in all cases. Detailed physical examination should also include a rectal exam to evaluate tone. These physical examination findings should not be simply attributed to the epidural anesthetic. A computed tomography (CT) scan can often be obtained rapidly and may yield the diagnosis. However, magnetic resonance imaging (MRI) or myelography may be necessary for definitive diagnosis.

The treatment for a symptomatic patient is urgent surgical intervention, usually a laminectomy, and evacuation of the blood. Expedient decompression of the spinal hematoma (within 8 to 12 hours of onset of symptoms) is essential to avoid permanent loss of neurologic function.

Current guidelines from the Second American Society of Regional Anesthesia (ASRA) Consensus Conference on Neuraxial Anesthesia and Anticoagulation include the following suggestions related to the use of LMWH:

1) In patients receiving preoperative prophylactic LMWH, insertion of the spinal needle should be delayed for at least 10 to 12 hours after the most recent LMWH prophylaxis dose. For patients on treatment-dose LMWH, the delay should be 24 hours from the last dose.

2) Single-dose anesthetic is preferable to continuous epidural anesthesia.

3) LMWH dosing should be delayed for at least 2 hours after spinal needle placement. If a hemorrhagic aspirate occurs during the initial spinal needle placement, LMWH should not be given for 24 hours.

4) Single-daily LMWH dosing may be safely used with indwelling catheter-based continuous epidural anesthesia as long as the first postoperative dose is given at least 6 to 8 hours after surgery. The second dose should be at least 24 hours later. Catheter removal should be a minimum of 10 to 12 hours after the last dose.

5) Twice-daily LMWH dosing should not be used in patients with indwelling catheters because of the potential association with increased risk of spinal hematoma.

Any decision to implement LMWH prophylaxis in the presence of an indwelling catheter must be made with extreme care, and extreme vigilance of the patient's neurologic status is warranted.

SUGGESTED READINGS

Douketis JD, Kinnon K, Crowther MA. Anticoagulant effect at the time of epidural catheter removal in patients receiving twice-daily or once-daily low-molecular-weight heparin and continuous epidural analgesia after orthopedic surgery. Thromb Haemost 2002;88:37–40.

Horlocker TT, Wedel DJ, Benzon H, et al. Regional anesthesia in the anticoagulated patient: defining the risks (the Second ASRA Consensus Conference on Neuraxial Anesthesia and Anticoagulation). Reg Anesth Pain Med 2003;28:172–197.

84

ADMINISTER EPIDURAL TEST DOSES

RAHUL G. BAIJAL, MD

The spinal canal contains the spinal cord and its coverings (or meninges), fatty tissue, and the venous plexus. It extends from the foramen magnum to the sacral hiatus. The meninges are composed of three layers: the pia mater, the arachnoid mater, and the dura mater. The pia mater is adherent to the spinal cord, whereas the arachnoid mater is adherent to the tough, fibroelastic dura mater. The subarachnoid space, located between the pia mater and the arachnoid mater, contains cerebrospinal fluid. The epidural space is a potential space, containing fat, alveolar tissue, nerve roots, and a network of arteries and venous plexus. No fluid is present in the epidural space. The epidural space extends cephalad from the foramen magnum and caudad to the sacral hiatus. The space is bound anteriorly by the posterior longitudinal ligament, laterally by the interverterbral foramen, and posteriorly by the ligamentum flavum. The spinal cord extends from the foramen magnum to L1 in adults and L3 in children. The anterior and posterior nerve roots at each spinal level exit the intervertebral foramina forming spinal nerves from C1 to S5.

Epidural anesthesia is produced by injection of a local anesthetic solution into the epidural space. Continuous epidural anesthesia is achieved by placement of a catheter into the epidural space. The epidural space is identified by the "loss of resistance" technique, reflecting passage from an area of high resistance in the ligamentum flavum to an area of low resistance in the epidural space. After the epidural needle is positioned in the ligamentum flavum, a glass syringe with a freely movable plunger is attached to the needle and continuous pressure is applied to the plunger. If the needle is positioned correctly in the ligamentum flavum, the plunger should not inject when pressure is applied. When the needle passes into the epidural space, a loss of resistance is achieved, and the plunger will easily inject.

WATCH OUT FOR

Following successful placement of the needle in the epidural space, a catheter is placed through the needle and advanced 3 to 5 cm into the epidural space to allow repeated and incremental injections of local anesthetic solution. The shorter distance the catheter is advanced, the more likely the catheter may become dislodged. Conversely, the farther the catheter is advanced, the more likely the catheter may enter an epidural vein, puncture the dura mater and enter the subarachnoid space, exit the intervertebral foramen, or enclose a nerve root. Even a catheter successfully placed is subject to migration. Movement of a patient with an epidural catheter may dislodge the catheter from its initial appropriate position.

Epidural analgesia has the potential to produce local anesthetic-induced systemic toxicity through unintentional administration into an epidural vein. Additionally, unintentional administration of an epidural dose of local anesthetic in the subarachnoid space will produce a rapid spinal, or subarachnoid, analgesia. A test dose following placement of the epidural catheter is designed to detect both subarachnoid and intravascular injection. The classic test dose combines 3 mL of local anesthetic solution and epinephrine, typically 3 mL of 1.5% lidocaine (secondary to rapid onset) with 1:200,000 epinephrine. The lidocaine, if injected into the subarachnoid space, will produce a rapid spinal analgesia that may be manifest as analgesia to the saddle area and cardiopulmonary depression secondary to sympathetic blockade. The lidocaine, if injected intravascularly, will affect primarily the central nervous and cardiovascular systems, with the central nervous system affected at lower levels. Four to seven times the dose of local anesthetic necessary to produce convulsions is required to produce cardiovascular depression. The epinephrine, if injected intravascularly, will produce a 20% or more rise in heart rate. Reapplication of the test dose through the catheter is paramount to detect unintentional injection intravascularly or in the subarachnoid space.

Suggested Readings

Miller RD, ed. Miller's Anesthesia. 6th Ed. Philadelphia: Elsevier; 2005:1677–1678.

Morgan EG, Maged SM, eds. Clinical Anesthesiology. New York: McGraw-Hill; 2002:270–271.

Stoelting RK, Miller RD, eds. Basics of Anesthesia. Philadelphia: Elsevier; 2002:179–181.

85

CONSIDER AN INTRAVENOUS NALOXONE DRIP FOR TREATMENT OF PRURITUS ASSOCIATED WITH EPIDURAL ANALGESIA

J. GREGORY HOBELMANN, MD

Continuous epidural analgesia can be beneficial for postoperative pain control. Perioperatively, it may attenuate the physiologic response to surgery. This potentially decreases morbidity and mortality when compared with systemic opioids by improving gastrointestinal function, decreasing pulmonary complications, decreasing myocardial infarctions, improving mental status, and decreasing thrombotic events. It is indicated for patients undergoing almost all surgeries extending from the thorax to the lower extremities. There are few contraindications; these include patient refusal, coagulopathy, and local infection at the insertion site. Although continuous epidural analgesia is quite effective when properly managed, care must be taken to balance the beneficial effects with the many possible side effects.

There are several choices of medications and medication combinations that can be used for epidural infusion. Local anesthetics can produce an excellent sensory block but may also cause a motor block, hypotension, and/or bradycardia. Opioids produce good analgesia but may be associated with nausea, vomiting, urinary retention, and pruritus. Therefore, for postoperative pain control, the combination of a local anesthetic and an opioid is often the best choice. There are many different local anesthetics and opioids that are available and the choice of what to use should be tailored to the patient and situation. Adjuvant medications include clonidine and epinephrine, but their utility has not been proven to be effective.

SIGNS AND SYMPTOMS

The most frequent side effect of epidural opioid use is pruritus. The prevalence in the literature has been reported to be 0% to 100%, but experienced providers anecdotally report its occurrence in about 60% of patients. The cause is unknown, but it is not related to histamine release. There may be central activation of an itch center in the lower medulla involving the trigeminal nucleus. Pruritus may occur at any dose, but severity seems to be dose-related.

Pruritus is an undesired effect of continuous epidural opioid use but is not dangerous to the patient and should not prevent the use of perioperative epidurals. It can be controlled with an intravenous infusion of an opioid antagonist such as naloxone (Narcan). The difficulty in this strategy is finding the dose that decreases the pruritus without compromising the analgesia. A good starting dose is 1 to 5 μg/kg/hr, which can often accomplish this goal. There is also some evidence that using an opioid agonist-antagonist (e.g., nalbuphine, butorphanol) may control pruritus with better analgesia preservation. An additional benefit of these medications is that they may decrease the incidence of respiratory depression associated with epidural opioids that can be fatal if unnoticed.

SUGGESTED READINGS

Caldwell M, Wu C. Effect of post-operative analgesia on patient morbidity. Best Pract Res Clin Anesthesiol 2002;16:549–563.
Miller RD, ed. Miller's Anesthesia. 6th Ed. Philadelphia: Elsevier; 2000:2737–2744.
Raj PP, ed. Practical Management of Pain. 3rd Ed. New York: Mosby; 2000:689–707.
Richman J, Wu C. Epidural analgesia for postoperative pain. Anesthesiol Clin North America 2005;23:125–140.

86

BE METICULOUS WHEN DOSING BUPIVACAINE IN PATIENTS WITH BOTH EPIDURAL AND PLEURAL CATHETERS

PATRICIA M. VELOSO, MD

Many patients being admitted to the intensive care unit (ICU) after thoracic surgery will have both epidural and pleural catheters for postoperative pain control. The epidural catheter will usually be attached to a patient-controlled analgesia (PCA) device with both a continuous and a demand dose; pain medication administered via a pleural catheter is usually given as a continuous infusion.

This can be an area of potential confusion for ICU staff because epidural and pleural catheters often look identical; a pleural catheter is usually a catheter taken from an epidural kit and inserted into the pleural space. In addition to the identical appearance, the epidural and pleural catheters may be positioned next to each other and covered with dressings, making it extremely easy for the nursing staff to mistake one catheter for the other. To avoid this confusion, the epidural and pleural catheters should be clearly marked near the site of injection.

Given the mistakes that have occurred with epidural and intravenous (IV) catheters, such as inadvertent IV administration of bupivacaine intended for an epidural catheter or the epidural administration of potassium or lipid emulsion, it is mandatory that meticulous care should also be used when dosing epidural and pleural catheters. One drug that is particularly problematic if it is administered in the wrong catheter in the wrong dose is bupivacaine, which is a local anesthetic used in both epidural and pleural catheters for postoperative pain control. Bupivacaine works by binding to the sodium channel of a nerve cell and preventing propagation of the nerve impulse along the cell membrane. It then dissociates very slowly from the sodium channel.

The usual scenario where bupivacaine causes trouble is when the epidural dose is injected into the pleural catheter. This can cause a severe toxicity. Systemic absorption of bupivacaine from a pleural catheter (virtually 100%) is greater than from an epidural catheter because of the increased vascularity of the pleural space as compared with the epidural space. Signs of toxicity are usually manifested by the central nervous system (CNS) before the cardiovascular system. CNS manifestations include lightheadedness, tinnitus, perioral numbness, disorientation, muscle twitching, tonic-clonic seizures, unconsciousness, and respiratory arrest. Cardiovascular manifestations include hypotension, sinus bradycardia, sinus node arrest, ventricular arrhythmias, and circulatory arrest. Because of bupivicaine's slow dissociation from the sodium channel, resuscitation after cardiovascular collapse due to bupivacaine toxicity can be difficult, at times requiring cardiopulmonary bypass until bupivacaine dissociates from cardiac sodium channels.

One final note is that bupivacaine toxicity can follow inadvertent intravascular injection or systemic absorption from the epidural site with migration of the catheter.

SUGGESTED READINGS

Miller R, ed. Miller's Anesthesia. 6th Ed. Philadelphia: Churchill Livingstone; 2005:1648.

Sculz–Stubner S. Regional analgesia in the critically ill. Crit Care Med 2005;33:1400–1407.

87

Do not dismiss rib fractures as trivial and consider an epidural catheter for pain control in multiple rib fractures

BRYAN A. COTTON, MD

Rib fractures are the most common injury associated with blunt chest trauma, with a reported incidence of at least 10% to 25%. Multiple rib fractures are associated with high-energy mechanisms such as motor vehicle crashes and pedestrians struck by automobiles. In the elderly, however, they may be associated with mechanisms such as low-level falls. These injuries are frequently, and inappropriately, dismissed as trivial with inadequate attention given to the control of pain in these patients. Rib fractures are likely to be associated with concomitant injuries such as pulmonary contusions and hemo-pneumothoraces (frequently requiring tube thoracostomy). In addition, rib fractures may also serve as a marker for significant solid-organ injury. Left-sided rib fractures are associated with a 15% to 20% risk of spleen injuries, while right-sided rib fractures are associated with a 10% to 15% risk of hepatic injury.

WATCH OUT FOR

Multiple rib fractures usually cause significant pain and limited chest-wall excursion and thus restrict the patient's ability to cough and breathe deeply. This results in poor clearance of secretions, atelectasis, and decreased functional residual capacity with the clinical correlates of this being hypoxia, ventilation-perfusion mismatches, and respiratory failure. In the elderly in particular, this results in increased length of ventilator days, intensive care unit (ICU) length of stay, and pneumonia rates. As few as three rib fractures have been associated with an approximate 20% mortality and a 30% risk of developing pneumonia in those more than 65 years of age. In fact, the risk of mortality increases to almost 35% and the pneumonia rate to greater than 50% when these patients sustain six or more rib fractures. However, patients age 45 and older with more than four rib fractures are also at a dramatically increased risk of pulmonary complications and death. Therefore, aggressive pulmonary toilet and adequate pain control (as evidenced by the ability to cough, breathe deeply, and reproducibly perform large inspiratory volumes on spirometry) should not be limited to the elderly trauma patient with rib fractures.

Several options exist to achieve adequate pain control in these patients, including the use of intravenous opiates with or without nonsteroidal anti-inflammatory drug (NSAID) supplementation, intercostal blocks, paravertebral blocks or infusion catheters, and epidural analgesia. Compared with other forms of analgesia, numerous studies have noted superior pain control when patients with rib fractures receive timely placement of an epidural catheter. Even when compared to patients with lower chest-injury scores and no epidural catheter, patients with higher injury scores receiving an epidural have significantly lower morbidity and mortality. Specifically, the use of epidural analgesia for pain control is associated with a decreased risk of nosocomial pneumonia and shorter duration of mechanical ventilation. The greatest impact of epidural analgesia (as compared with intravenous opiates) appears to be among those with five or more fractures and in the elderly population. Despite the overwhelming evidence supporting the use of epidural analgesia, a recent evaluation of the National Trauma Data Bank (NTDB) noted this modality is significantly underutilized. In some centers, the lack of available experienced (or committed) anesthesia personnel is the single greatest limiting factor to obtaining an epidural for pain control.

Epidural catheter placement and analgesia are associated with the risk of hypotension, dural puncture, spinal cord injury, and urinary retention. The ability to utilize epidural analgesia is often limited by concomitant injuries and pre-existing illnesses. These include acute spine fracture, previous spine deformity, impaired mental status, hemodynamic instability, coagulopathy, and chest-wall infection and/or soft-tissue injury. Enoxaparin and other low-molecular-weight heparins should be held 24 hours prior to placement of any form of neuraxial anesthesia (epidural) and not restarted until 24 hours after removal. During this interval, subcutaneous heparin (5,000 units every eight hours) should be utilized.

In addition to conventional intravenous opiates or patient-controlled analgesia (PCA), other analgesia methods such as intercostal nerve (rib) blocks, continuous paravertebral blocks, and intrapleural blocks exist and are quite feasible. Intercostal nerve blocks are usually performed with a local anesthetic such as bupivacaine, as either a bolus dose that may be repeated or a continuous infusion via catheter. Pain control with bolus injection is usually effective for 8 to 24 hours with each injection. Studies have demonstrated that this approach, whether administered as a single injection or via continuous catheter, provide sufficient pain control in patients with multiple rib fractures. This approach carries a small risk of pneumothorax and is not suitable for posterior rib fractures. Thoracic paravertebral infusions have been shown to be an effective method of providing pain control in patients with both unilateral, as well as bilateral, multiple rib fractures. This is supported by the observation of a sustained improvement in pulmonary function testing and oxygenation. Paravertebral blocks are safer and easier to perform than thoracic epidurals and are not associated with hemodynamic instability or urinary retention. This approach also carries a small risk of pneumothorax. Pleural-based anesthetic administration lacks the potential for central nervous system depression as well as the need for repeated injections. This method, however, has decreased efficacy in the presence of hemothoraces or pleural effusions and requires interruption of chest-tube drainage.

One final note is that regardless of the modality used, adjuncts such as intermittent positive pressure breathing (IPPB) or intrapulmonary percussive ventilation (IPV) should be utilized early in the care of these patients.

SUGGESTED READINGS

Bulger EM, Arneson MA, Mock CN, et al. Rib fractures in the elderly. J Trauma 2000;48:1040–1046.

Flagel BT, Luchette FA, Reed RL, et al. Half-a-dozen ribs: the breakpoint for mortality. Surgery 2005;138:717–723.

Holcomb JB, McMullin NR, Kozar RA, et al. Morbidity from rib fractures increases after age 45. J Am Coll Surg 2003;196:549–555.

Karmakar MK, Ho AM. Acute pain management of patients with multiple fractured ribs. J Trauma 2003;54:615–625.

Pain management in blunt thoracic trauma: an evidence-based outcome evaluation. Eastern Association for the Surgery of Trauma; 2004. Available at http://east.org/tpg/painchest.pdf

88

USE A TWO-STEP TECHNIQUE WITH RADIOGRAPHIC CONFIRMATION WHEN PLACING A FEEDING TUBE

JULIUS CUONG PHAM, MD

Placement of a feeding tube is not without peril to the patient and requires a high level of concern on the part of the practitioner, as illustrated in the following scenario.

CASE

Mr. JCP was a 68-year-old male who was postoperative day four from an aortic-valve replacement complicated by a stroke. Despite having no previous history of pulmonary disease, his airway pressures on the ventilator were persistently high, as noted on morning rounds. The nurse from the night shift noted a significant amount of residual from his feeding tube. She was instructed to continue the feeds because the stomach "makes a lot of secretions." On radiology rounds, a significant left-sided pneumothorax was noted with the feeding tube positioned in the left pleural space.

DISCUSSION

Feeding tubes are commonly placed in the intensive care unit (ICU) for enteral feeding in the patient who is not able to orally take nutrition. Many types of tubes are available to accomplish this. One type of tube that is commonly used is the flexible small bore/stylet-guided tube (e.g., Dobhoff). These tubes have the advantage of being small and comfortable. They are more suitable for medium–term feeding. Because these tubes are small and flexible, they require a metal stylet to give them enough rigidity for placement. Unfortunately, this rigidity and small size make them ideal for inadvertent bronchial placement. This occurs in about 4.4% of feeding-tube placements. A correctly positioned endotracheal tube with the cuff inflated does *not* preclude placement into the main-stem bronchus. It has been postulated that the endotracheal tube may act as a guide for the feeding tube to follow. Both recognized and unrecognized, the results can be devastating and complications include pneumothorax, "isocalothorax," pneumonia, empyema, sepsis, and death.

WHAT TO DO

To minimize these potentially fatal complications, a two-step radiographic method is commonly used to detect bronchial-tube placement. The two-step technique involves taking two radiographs, one after partial insertion of the tube and the other after full insertion of the tube. The purpose of this process is to confirm that the feeding tube is in the esophagus before fully advancing it to avoid puncturing lung tissue and causing a pneumothorax. In the first step, the feeding tube is advanced to a point past the carina, but before entering the bronchials, and a radiograph is taken. If the feeding tube is in the bronchus, it will be "angled" toward one of the main-stem bronchi. If it is in the esophagus, it will be midline. After the feeding tube is confirmed to be midline and below the carina, a second radiograph is taken to confirm that it is in the stomach (as opposed to curled back into the esophagus). Implementation of this protocol significantly reduces risk of pneumothorax (0.38% vs. 0.09%).

To summarize:

1) Prior to placement, the tube should be measured to be just below the carina (typically 30 cm).
2) A radiograph is obtained at the measured length (estimated carina) to confirm that the styleted tube is in the midline position and below the carina (i.e. in the esophagus and not the airway).
3) When there is uncertainty concerning the tube position, radiology consultation should be obtained.
4) The tube can then be advanced with the stylet until in appropriate position.
5) A second x-ray should be performed to confirm that the styleted tube is in the stomach/duodenum.
6) Once in appropriate position, the stylet should be removed and cannot be reinserted for any reason.
7) Feedings can be started if the tube is in the stomach/duodenum at the discretion of the ordering physician and attending.

SUGGESTED READINGS

Mardenstein EL, Simmons RL, Ochoa JB. Patient safety: effect of institutional protocols on adverse events relating to feeding tube placement in the critically ill. J Am Coll Surg 2004;199:39–47.

Roubenoff R, Ravich WJ. Pneumothorax due to nasogastric feeding tubes. Report of four cases, review of the literature, and recommendations for prevention. Arch Intern Med 1989; 149:184–188.

Torrington KG, Bowman MA. Fatal hydrothorax and empyema complicating a malpositioned nasogastric tube. Chest 1981;79:240–242.

89

PERFORM DOPPLER ULTRASOUND BEFORE PLACING SEQUENTIAL COMPRESSION DEVICES

BRADFORD D. WINTERS, MD, PHD

Deep vein thromboses (DVTs) are extremely common in many groups of hospitalized patients and contribute to patient morbidity and mortality by their propensity to embolize to the lung, where they can lead to severe hypoxemia, increased dead space, respiratory insufficiency, and right-sided heart failure with progression to cardiorespiratory arrest. Many DVTs develop in the deep pelvic veins though a substantial number originate in the deep veins of the thigh. DVTs of the lower leg below the knee are common also but rarely embolize.

Several factors promote the tendency to develop DVTs. Ill patients tend to be hypercoagulable, especially those with certain diseases such as cancer and pancreatitis. This combined with immobility and venous stasis greatly enhances the likelihood of developing clot. Development of clot is a surprisingly rapid event. Patients undergoing surgery have been shown to develop DVTs on the operating table shortly after induction of anesthesia.

Prevention of DVTs or pulmonary embolisms (PEs) is a major concern for hospitalized patients. There are several modalities that are used to prevent this complication; recent evidence suggests that the ones chosen for an individual patient should be based on risk-stratification profiles. These modalities include subcutaneously injected heparin, heparinoids such as enoxaparin, thromboembolic deterrent (TED) stockings, and sequential compression devices (SCDs). While heparin and heparinlike compounds work pharmacologically, TED stockings and SCDs work mechanically by compressing the venous structures in the extremities. The primary mechanism of action for reducing the risk of clot formation is the release of tissue-type plasminogen activator (tPA) from the endothelium in response to the mechanical compression of the veins. The formation of plasmin is enhanced, which presumably promotes the lysis of any clot that is initiated. This is why studies have shown that placing TED stockings or SCDs on the arms of a patient is just as effective as placing them on the legs. Secondarily, the compression of the veins helps to prevent stasis, which is thought to promote clotting.

<table>
<tr><td>WATCH OUT FOR</td></tr>
</table>

WATCH OUT FOR

This mechanical effect of compressing and propelling blood by TEDs/SCDs may have deleterious effects as well. If the patient already has a clot burden in the legs, the main concern is that the mechanical compression of the deep vein by placement of the TEDs/SCDs may dislodge the clot leading to a PE. For this reason, the package insert on the most commonly used brands of SCDs direct the clinician to remove the device from the extremity where there is a known DVT. Also, it is important to assess whether any clot burden already exists prior to placing the compression devices. For ambulatory patients entering the hospital, this is usually not an issue; ideally, the SCDs would have been placed and maintained from the outset of admission. However, this may not always happen and when they are taken off for procedures or tests, it is not unusual for their replacement to be forgotten. During this unprotected time period, clot burden may already have started to develop.

WHAT TO DO

Thus when initial placement of TEDs or SCDs was not performed, they have not been replaced within approximately 6 hours after their removal, or a patient is received in transfer with an uncertain history of clot burden, many experienced clinicians will obtain a venous Doppler study to rule out the presence of DVT prior to application or reapplication of the devices. As none of the modalities for preventing DVTs are 100% effective, it would seem prudent to also perform Doppler studies on patients receiving pharmacological DVT prophylaxis when mechanical devices are to be added to the prophylactic regimen as well as after a period of immobility or in patients judged to be at high risk of DVT.

SUGGESTED READINGS

Caprini JA. Thrombosis risk assessment as a guide to quality patient care. Dis Mon 2005;51:70–78.

Goldhaber SZ, Turpie AG. Prevention of venous thromboembolism among hospitalized medical patients. Circ 2005;111:e1-e3.

Turpie AG, Chin BS, Lip GY. Venous thromboembolism: pathophysiology, clinical features and prevention. BMJ 2002;325:887–890.

90

CONSIDER CHANGING THE FOLEY CATHETER WHEN PATIENT HAS A URINARY TRACT INFECTION

MELISSA S. CAMP, MD

Urinary tract infections (UTIs) are one of the most common nosocomial infections in intensive care unit (ICU) patients. They almost always occur in the setting of a Foley catheter and the risk of developing a UTI increases with the length of time the Foley catheter is left in place. The risk of UTI is approximately 5% per day with a Foley catheter.

The diagnosis of a urinary tract infection is made based on urinalysis and urine culture. Findings on the urinalysis that are suggestive of a UTI include pyuria and bacteriuria. A urine culture with greater than 10^5 bacteria per mL is consistent with a diagnosis of a UTI. The most common organism responsible for UTIs is *Escherichia coli*. Other common organisms include *Proteus, Klebsiella, Pseudomonas, Enterococcus, Staphylococcus epidermidis, Staphylococcus aureus*, and *Candida*. Antibiotic treatment for a UTI should be based on the sensitivities from culture results, and recommended duration of therapy is 7 to 14 days depending on the severity of the infection. Urosepsis, for example, should be aggressively treated with a 14–day course of antibiotics.

WHAT TO DO

To reduce the risk of developing urinary tract infections, Foley catheters should be removed as soon as possible. Foley catheters become coated with a bacterial biofilm that encourages adherence of bacteria. The biofilm protects bacteria from the host immune response as well as from eradication with appropriate antibiotic therapy. This can make it difficult to clear the source of infection without removing or changing the Foley catheter. If a Foley catheter is still clinically indicated and a patient develops a UTI, the Foley should be changed in addition to instituting antibiotics. Contraindications to changing the Foley catheter include severe scrotal edema and recent urologic or bladder surgery, which may make it technically difficult or potentially harmful to remove and reinsert the Foley.

Candiduria may be due to asymptomatic colonization or a UTI. If a UTI is suspected, the Foley catheter should be removed or changed and antifungal therapy should be considered. Treatment of candiduria should be instituted in transplant patients and critically ill patients with multiple sites of fungal colonization as they are at high risk for disseminated fungal infection.

It should be remembered that patients with chronic indwelling Foley catheters will often have chronic bacterial colonization. Antibiotic treatment and/or changing the Foley catheter in these situations is not indicated unless the patient develops other symptoms consistent with systemic infection such as fever, hypotension, or changes in mental status.

SUGGESTED READINGS

Ferri F, ed. The Care of the Medical Patient. St. Louis: Mosby; 2001:549–554.
Lanken P, ed. The Intensive Care Unit Manual. Philadelphia: Saunders; 2001:137–139.
Nicolle L. Catheter related urinary tract infection. Drugs Aging 2005;22:627–639.

DO NOT FLUSH URETERAL STENTS IF A UROLOGICAL CONSULTATION IS AVAILABLE

JENNIFER MILES-THOMAS, MD

Postoperative urology, gynecology, and other abdominal surgical patients often come to the intensive care unit (ICU) with externally draining ureteral stents; some of these patients may have undergone reimplantation of the ureters during urinary diversion. Invariably, in the middle of the night the likely bloody urine output will decrease and the house officer may be presented with the opportunity or request to flush these stents. However, before doing so there are several important factors to consider.

The prime consideration is whether there exists any other reason the patient may have decreased urine output through the stents. The astute clinician will evaluate the postoperative fluid resuscitation, cardiac status, and infectious status of the patient. An exam should be performed to make sure the patient does not have any other catheters in place draining the bladder or kidneys. An assessment must include the amount of fluid draining around the stents in a capillary-type manner. Immediately postoperatively, ureteral edema may cause ureteral obstruction, and therefore the majority of urine output typically comes from the stents in the early postoperative period. As edema decreases, the ureters may drain urine around the stents, decreasing the output from the stents but maintaining good overall urine output.

If all other causes of decreased urine output are ruled out and the ureteral stents appear to be clogged, a urologist should be called to assess the stents. It is recommended that you do not manipulate the stent as the stent may become dislodged or penetrate the renal parenchyma, pelvis, ureter, or anastomosis. If a consultation is not possible, you should draw back on the stent with a 3- to 5-cm^3 syringe. If there is no return, you may gently flush the stent with 3 to 5 cm^3 of normal saline over 5 to 10 seconds. The stent should then be returned to straight drain. The slow introduction of a small volume helps prevent the abrupt rise of renal pelvic pressure, which can cause pyelovenous backflow of urine into the blood stream and forniceal rupture.

SUGGESTED READINGS

Walsh PC, ed. Campbell's Urology. 8th Ed. Philadelphia: WB Saunders; 2002:3745–3784.

MAKE SURE THE CUFF (PILOT BALLOON) IS COMPLETELY DEFLATED ON A CUFFED TRACHEOSTOMY TUBE BEFORE A PASSY-MUIR SPEAKING VALVE IS PLACED

MOLLY B. CAMPION, MS

A speaking valve is a one-way valve that is used with tracheostomy patients to redirect airflow, allowing them to use their voice and speak. Some speaking valves have also been shown to assist in reducing aspiration risk in the tracheostomy patient. The Passy-Muir valve is one type of speaking valve commonly used and marketed for its "no-leak" closed system design.

One-way speaking valves allow airflow into the tracheostomy tube on inhalation but close on exhalation, thus forcing air to pass between the tracheostomy tube and the walls of the trachea and ultimately through the vocal cords and upper airway (*Fig. 92.1*). This helps to establish a more "normal" airflow pattern for the patient in addition to restoring verbal communication.

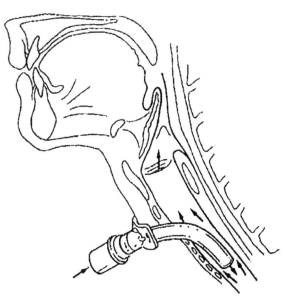

FIGURE 92.1. Uncuffed Tracheostomy Tube with Passy-Muir Closed-position "No-leak" Speaking Valve.

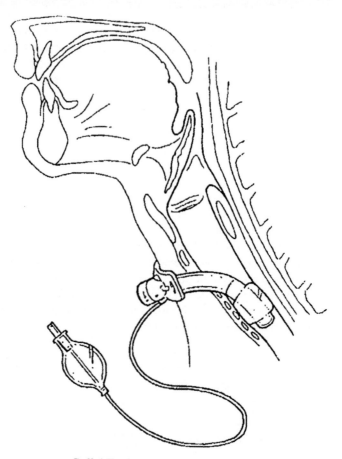

FIGURE 92.2. Cuffed Tracheostomy Tube.

In a patient with a cuffed tracheostomy tube, the cuff (pilot balloon) must be completely deflated prior to placement of the speaking valve in order for the exhaled air to move around the tracheostomy tube and airway walls. If the cuff remains inflated and a speaking valve is placed, the cuff will obstruct exhaled airflow and the patient will be unable to exhale or breathe (*Fig. 92.2*). This scenario can quickly lead to a respiratory arrest.

SUGGESTED READINGS

Suiter DM, McCullough GH, Powel PW. Effects of cuff deflation and one-way tracheostomy speaking valve placement on swallow physiology. Dysphagia 2003; 18:284–292.

93

KNOW THE CLINICALLY IMPORTANT ISSUES WITH USING AN INTRA-AORTIC BALLOON PUMP

ELIZABETH A. MARTINEZ, MD, MHS

Low cardiac output syndrome is defined as inadequate perfusion as a result of impaired pumping function and a cardiac index of <2.2 L/min/m^2. Clinical manifestations of hypoperfusion are listed in *Table 93.1*. Management of low cardiac output is characterized by optimization of hemodynamic parameters, which include heart rate, rhythm, preload, afterload, and contractility. All of these parameters play a significant role in the balance of oxygen supply and demand of the myocardium. Mechanical circulatory support must be considered to optimize these parameters, especially when there is ongoing ischemia.

The intra-aortic balloon pump (IABP) is a device that can support these hemodynamic goals. It is designed to augment coronary blood flow and can reduce the vascular impedance seen by ejecting myocardium during systole. In its capacity to optimize myocardial oxygen supply and demand and to improve cardiac output, distal perfusion generally improves as well.

The indications for placement of an IABP include complications of a myocardial infarction (including mitral regurgitation); ongoing ischemia or chest pain despite maximal medical therapy for myocardial ischemia; prophylactic support in patients scheduled for cardiac surgery with a high-grade left main coronary artery stenosis; and post–cardiac surgery in a low cardiac output state. The contraindications include aortic insufficiency, aortoiliac disease, and irreversible myocardial disease. The first, aortic insufficiency, is an absolute contraindication because inflation of the balloon during diastole will cause an increase in regurgitant flow, adding significantly to preload and increasing myocardial oxygen demand and risk of injury to the aortic valve. The other contraindications are relative. Many patients have some degree of aortoiliac disease and if the patient is suffering an acute decompensation that is reversible, then there may be a role for the IABP, even if he or she is not a candidate for revascularization, ventricular assist placement, or transplant.

The catheter part of the IABP is made up of a nonthrombogenic balloon that inflates and deflates in synchrony with the cardiac cycle. The IABP produces its desired effect through counterpulsation; the

TABLE 93.1	CLINICAL MANIFESTATIONS OF SYSTEMIC HYPOPERFUSION

Tachycardia
Hypotension
Oliguria
Dry mucous membranes
Confusion
Tachypnea
Cold and clammy or mottled extremities
Pulmonary edema
Low cardiac index
Increased calculated systemic vascular resistance
Progressive acidosis

balloon inflates during diastole and deflates during systole, or counter to what the intra-aortic blood volume and pressures are. The inflation during diastole increases the intra-aortic pressure during the portion of the cardiac cycle in which the coronary arteries are perfused, thus augmenting flow, especially through ischemic vessels that may have lost their autoregulation. The IABP deflates prior to opening of the aortic valve to decrease afterload and optimize ejection.

IABPs are often placed in cardiac catheterization labs by cardiologists under fluoroscopy or in the cardiac surgery operating rooms either with or without visualization on transesophageal echo (TEE). The correct placement of the IABP is extremely important because malposition can lead to serious complications including occlusion of the renal or mesenteric vessels and ischemia of these end organs. If it is too cephalad, it can obstruct left ventricular outflow by obstructing the valve or even perforating the aorta and flow to the proximal major vessels. The most common site for placement is a femoral artery, but it may also be placed directly into the aorta in the chest at the time of surgery if access distally is not feasible. Because of the potential complications, the position of all IABPs should be confirmed radiographically upon admission to the ICU after placement, regardless of how it was placed (fluoroscopy, TEE). The optimal placement is with the tip in the thoracic aorta, just distal to the left subclavian artery. The IABP device has a radiopaque tip that can be used to confirm appropriate positioning of the IABP and must be visualized (*Table 93.1*). If it is not visualized, the chest radiograph should be repeated either more cephalad or more caudally. If the IABP needs to be repositioned, the IABP must be paused and the catheter either advanced or withdrawn within the sterile sheath.

In order for the IABP to be properly synchronized with the cardiac cycle, the inflation of the balloon can be triggered by the electrocardiogram (ECG) tracing, the arterial tracing, detection of pacing, or an internal trigger. In the current generation of IABP devices, the ECG is the default mode. In the presence of arrhythmias, strong consideration should be given to using the arterial tracing to obtain more consistent triggering. The pacing modality is commonly used for individuals who are being paced but is not required with the newer generation of the devices. The internal trigger is reserved for nonpulsatile flow, for example, while on bypass. When evaluating for appropriate timing, the IABP should inflate at the dicrotic notch on the arterial tracing, reflecting inflation after the aortic valve has closed.

Weaning of the IABP can be accomplished by decreasing the frequency of inflation to deflation in relation to the cardiac cycle, that is, from a 1:1 ratio with every heartbeat to a 1:3 ratio with every heartbeat. The degree of balloon fill is less often adjusted. When evaluating tolerance of weaning, one should monitor the ECG and distal perfusion. A common weaning strategy is to wean from 1:1 to 1:2 to 1:3 with interval ECG and cardiac output evaluations, if available. The goal should be to remove the IABP as soon as clinically appropriate to decrease the risk of complications, which include infection, bleeding, thrombosis and compromise of distal perfusion, and visceral ischemia. Aortic dissection is also a potential complication, but it generally occurs at the time of placement.

SUGGESTED READINGS

Baskett RJ, Ghali WA, Maitland A, et al. The intraaortic balloon pump in cardiac surgery. Ann Thorac Surg 2002;74:1276–1287.

Hanlon-Pena PM, Ziegler JC, Stewart R. Management of the intraaortic balloon pump patient: pharmacologic considerations. Crit Care Nurs Clin North Am 1996;8:389–408.

Papaioannou TG, Stefanadis C. Basic principles of the intraaortic balloon pump and mechanisms affecting its performance. ASAIO J 2005;51:296–300.

94

REMEMBER THAT RIGHT HEART FAILURE IS A COMMON AND IMPORTANT COMPLICATION/ MANAGEMENT CHALLENGE FOLLOWING PLACEMENT OF A LEFT VENTRICULAR ASSIST DEVICE

ANDREW L. ROSENBERG, MD

Left ventricular assist devices (LVADs) including intra-aortic balloon pumps, percutaneous Tandem Heart devices, extracorporeal, and implanted ventricular assist devices have significantly improved the management and outcome for patients with the most severe forms of heart failure. Acute or chronic right ventricular failure, however, remains one of the most serious and difficult conditions to manage for patients with heart failure, especially following LVAD placement.

WATCH OUT FOR Causes of right ventricular dysfunction include pre-existing myocardial disease, increased preload and/or right ventricular dilatation, ischemia, arrhythmias, increased intrathoracic pressures from mechanical ventilation, and especially acute or chronic forms of pulmonary hypertension. Frequently a positive feedback cycle exists, initiated by something that causes right ventricular pressure overload, interventricular septum displacement, increased wall tension with or without reduced right ventricular perfusion of decreased right ventricular cardiac output. Experienced implant programs evaluate ventricular device candidates for the presence of severe right ventricular dysfunction *prior* to LVAD/RVAD placement using some combination of echocardiography and measures of right ventricular function including central venous pressures and the presence of upstream organ failure due to right ventricular dysfunction including renal insufficiency and hepatic synthetic failure with elevated prothrombin times, aminotransferase levels, and hyperbilirubinemia.

In addition to the older modalities, newer measures of right ventricular dysfunction include right ventricular stroke work index: (mean pulmonary artery pressure – right atrial pressure [or central venous pressure] / (cardiac index × heart rate) $RVSWI = [(PAP_m - RAP) \times CI]/HR = (mm\ Hg \cdot mL)/_m 2$. Several studies have suggested that RVSWI values less than 300 $(mm\ Hg \cdot mL)/_m 2$ are independent predictors of the need for an RVAD. A more recent measure of right ventricular failure is the tricuspid annular plane systolic excursion (TAPSE) of the lateral edge of the tricuspid annulus on a standard four-chamber echo view of the heart. A normal TAPSE is 20 to 25 mm and is usually easy to obtain. Significant decreases in the TAPSE suggest the presence of severe right ventricular dysfunction. In most cases, patients with pre-existing biventricular dysfunction will also have an RVAD inserted at the time of LVAD placement. For those patients who do not, recognizing and treating new right ventricular dysfunction is among the most important perioperative management challenges in the intensive care unit (ICU).

SIGNS AND SYMPTOMS

Right ventricular dysfunction usually manifests as some combination of low cardiac output, hypotension, and in the presence of an LVAD, decreased flows from the device. Usually, a central venous pressure measurement is available and is often elevated as the right ventricle is dilated, poorly compliant, or volume overloaded. An emergent echocardiogram is crucial to obtain and usually confirms the diagnosis especially if pre-existing echocardiography did not show right ventricular failure prior to LVAD placement. Other conditions such as tamponade, obstructions to LVAD inflow, excessive LVAD flows, excessive systemic vasopressor use, and increases in pulmonary vascular resistance can mimic, cause, or worsen right ventricular dysfunction. Rising central venous pressures with constant or decreasing LVAD flows is probably the most common presentation of RV dysfunction.

WHAT TO DO

Treatment for right ventricular dysfunction focuses on correcting the underlying cause (i.e., draining blood in tamponade, optimizing device timing and rates). Probably the most common treatment is to relieve right ventricular afterload by avoiding or treating any cause of respiratory or metabolic acidosis and hypoxemia, as well as using direct pulmonary vasodilators such as nitric oxide, inhaled prostacyclines, or, rarely, other nitric oxide donors such as nitroglycerine. If nitric oxide is not already in use, starting doses of 80 ppm down to 20 ppm is commonly used. Right ventricular dysfunction frequently manifests more slowly in patients with biventricular failure when nitric oxide is being weaned, especially at 5 ppm or less, and is often the reason nitric oxide may need very slow weaning. Inotropes are also commonly used to avoid or treat right ventricular failure. Phosphodiesterase III inhibitors such as milrinone (0.375 to 0.5 μg/kg/min) are most often used because they may have some effect on reducing pulmonary vascular tone. Dobutamine, isoproterinol, and epinephrine may also improve right ventricular dysfunction but may also cause more arrhythmias. A newer class of inotropes that act by increasing myocardial troponin sensitization to intracellular Ca^+ may soon be used. Even if hypotension is present, very careful diuresis or fluid removal with continuous renal replacement devices may also improve right ventricular function in the setting of severe volume overload with elevated central venous pressures. Finally, placement of a temporary RVAD (Abiomed or Thoratec), cardiac extracorporeal membrane oxygenation (ECMO), or emergent heart transplant may be required for worsening or refractory right ventricular failure.

SUGGESTED READINGS

Furukawa K, Motomura T, Nose Y. Right ventricular failure after left ventricular assist device implantation: the need for an implantable right ventricular assist device. Artif Organs 2004;29:369–377.

Ghio S, Recusani F, Klersy C, et al. Prognostic usefulness of the tricuspid annular plane systolic excursion in patients with congestive heart failure secondary to idiopathic or ischemic dilated cardiomyopathy. Am J Cardiol 2000;85:837–842.

Kavarana MN, Pessin-Minsley MS, Urtecho J, et al. Right ventricular dysfunction and organ failure in left ventricular assist device recipients: a continuing problem. Ann Thorac Surg 2002;73:745–750.

Ochiai Y, McCarthy PM, Smedira NG, et al. Predictors of severe right ventricular failure after implantable left ventricular assist device insertion: analysis of 245 patients. Circulation 2002;106:198–202.

95

KNOW THE COMMON PROBLEMS ASSOCIATED WITH CARDIOPULMONARY SUPPORT USING EXTRACORPOREAL MEMBRANE OXYGENATION

ANDREW L. ROSENBERG, MD

Venoarterial extracorporeal life support (VA ECMO) is among the more advanced methods to temporarily support patients with either cardiac or cardiac and pulmonary failure until patient recovery, assist device implantation, or transplant. The indications and contraindications for this type of support are listed in *Table 95.1*. Managing these patients is challenging, and sophisticated teams of perfusionists, intensivists, and surgeons are required. The advantages of using ECMO instead of a ventricular assist device include

- the ability to cannulate patients at a bedside
- immediate biventricular support
- both cardiac and pulmonary support
- ability to assess patients off ECMO prior to decannulation
- ability to change to venovenous cannulation if hemodynamic failure improves while pulmonary support is still required

The disadvantages include

- more bleeding, especially after cardiotomy or heart or lung transplantation
- increased left ventricular afterload
- limb ischemia
- thromboembolic injury to lung and/or brain

TABLE 95.1	INDICATIONS AND CONTRAINDICATIONS OF ADULT ECMO	
INDICATIONS	**CONTRAINDICATIONS**
Cardiogenic shock	Unwitnessed cardiac arrest
Cardiac trauma	Aortic insufficiency
Respiratory insufficiency	Aortic dissection
Status asthmaticus	Cardiac arrest >30 minutes
Smoke inhalation	No correctable anatomic defect
Massive pulmonary embolism	Terminal illness
Donor heart preservation	Severe diabetes mellitus
	Severe peripheral vascular disease
	Recent cerebrovascular accident

- incomplete left ventricular decompression with pulmonary edema
- uneven oxygenation to upper and lower body
- hemolysis
- increased infections
- significant expense and resource needs

Experienced ECMO providers have developed management strategies for some of these problems.

POSTOPERATIVE BLEEDING

Bleeding is the most common complication of VA ECMO. Typically, ECMO programs have protocols for treating bleeding with appropriate blood product replacement. Methods to reduce systemic anticoagulation involve some combination of decreasing doses of heparin to allow the kaolin-activated clotting time to approach very low levels such as 160 to 180 seconds for several hours or in extremely rare situations for several days, though this is a very risky procedure and requires extremely close communication among the ECMO team members. In any bleeding situation and especially when a low-dose or no-heparin condition exists, it is mandatory to have a redundant ECMO circuit primed and ready at the bedside in case the active circuit develops significant clot. Other strategies to reduce bleeding while on ECMO include aprotinin infusions; using heparin-bonded circuit tubing; increasing flow rates to reduce stagnation; and frequent surgical explorations to remove clot (surgical wounds are usually left open other than a sterile occlusive patch and electrocautery is generously applied to any bleeding points).

LOW FLOW STATES

Low flow states are usually due to reduced intravascular volume but can also be due to compression of venous inflow cannula from body position or lower-extremity edema. Increasing the intravascular volume and/or repositioning the patient frequently improves this problem. Other causes of blood-flow impedance around the heart include tamponade, tension pneumothorax, and clot in the circuit. If periodic pulsation is not detected by arterial line, echocardiography is used to determine if an atrial septostomy is needed in order to vent a noncontracting chamber, dilated a left ventricle, as well as look for the presence of left ventricular clot.

REGIONAL ISCHEMIA

Because most VA ECMO is performed using the femoral vein and artery, perfusion to the ipsilateral leg is often impaired. The usual method to reduce or treat this is to insert a small, 14-gauge perfusion cannula in the posterior tibial artery and to infuse 100 to 200 mL/min of flow through this line. Another complication of perfusing oxygenated blood into the arterial system using the femoral artery is inadequate oxygenation of the upper extremities and head. This situation manifests itself by the lower half of the body looking pink while the upper half is cyanotic. The usual treatment is to insert and perfuse oxygenated blood through a venous jugular line; this creates, in effect, a VA-V ECMO circuit.

HYPOTENSION

Blood pressure frequently requires some combination of vasopressor and inotrope support (especially when weaning patients). Norepinephrine 0.08 to 0.2 μg/kg/min and milrinone 0.375 to 0.5 μg/kg/min or dobutamine 10 to 20 μg/kg/min are often used for these purposes.

NEUROLOGICAL INJURY

Periodic sedation holidays are important to detect new onset or presence of serious neurologic morbidity in these patients.

SELECTED READINGS

Meurs KV, Lally KP, Peek G, et al., eds. Extracorporeal Cardiopulmonary Support in Critical Care. 3rd Ed. Ann Arbor, MI: ECLS Organization; 2005.

Mielck F, Quintel MI. Extracorporeal membrane oxygenation. Curr Opin Crit Care 2005;11:87–93.

96

TREAT "WRINKLING" IN THE ABIOMED DIAPHRAGM AS A POSSIBLE SIGN OF HYPOVOLEMIA

FRANK ROSEMEIER, MD

Ventricular assist devices (VADs) are indicated for patients with ventricular failure on maximum pharmacological support in the post–cardiopulmonary bypass period, following an acute myocardial infarction, as bridge to transplantation, or destination therapy for permanent use. Most of these devices, which can be used in either an intracorporeal or extracorporeal position, are displacement pumps and assist the left ventricle. In a left VAD (LVAD) configuration, a device inflow cannula connects the left atrium or left ventricular apical region to the pump chamber. Blood returns to the ascending aorta via a device outflow cannula. For a right-sided VAD (RVAD), the inflow cannula is situated in the right atrium or right ventricle with the outflow cannula connected to the main pulmonary artery. These tubular cannulae are typically radiolucent and are not easily identifiable on a plain radiograph.

The Abiomed assist device is most frequently used in an emergency for its ease of implantation, robustness of operation, and versatility as it can be configured as an LVAD, an RVAD, or BiVAD. It is simple to operate, inexpensive, and robust for transport purposes. It has the added advantage in that the pump section can be changed at the bedside in 1 minute. Drawbacks include a high re-exploration rate for hemorrhage. A clear plastic housing device that is placed below the level of the heart contains a pulsatile dual-chamber assembly in series. Filling of the upper chamber is via passive gravity drainage from the ventricle or atrium. Adjusting the height of the device relative to the patient's heart level will control preload conditions. As the device is lowered, the flow into the upper chamber will increase, shortening diastolic filling time and increasing device output. The lower chamber performs the pumping action at a constant stroke volume of around 88 mL with an output limitation of 4 to 5 L/min. High systemic vascular resistance may increase the duration of the emptying of the lower chamber, prolonging systole with a possible decrease in output.

WATCH OUT FOR	For the Abiomed device, it is important to recognize that a reduced rate of pump cycles may serve as a clinical indicator of inadequate preload

or excessive afterload. Typically, in hypovolemia the chambers might cycle slowly, causing wrinkling in the diaphragm, which may be the first sign of a problem. Volume loading will help restore device output, as can the Trendelenburg position. In addition, manipulation of the external housing device may help temporize the clinical hypovolemia. This is accomplished by increasing the height differential by lowering the device, which may improve the pressure gradient and therefore flow to the upper chamber temporarily. In addition, this maneuver may be helpful as a diagnostic procedure. Caution is advised when raising the head of the patient in an effort to increase the pressure differential as venous return to the patient's right heart may further diminish.

Although filling and output occur independently of the native cardiac rhythm, patients with assist devices generally do not tolerate ventricular fibrillation, tachycardia, or asystole well. The filling of the chamber requires a pressure gradient all the way from the right ventricle (RV) through the pulmonary vasculature bed to the left atrium/ventricle. Loss of RV output can result in a decrease of LVAD preload. Low output of an LVAD can also be related to a failing right heart, increased pulmonary resistance, or flow obstruction from tube kinking or clot formation. A careful inspection of the tubing and chambers is mandatory when unexpected clinical hypovolemia or low LVAD output is observed.

SUGGESTED READINGS

Goldstein DJ, Oz MC, Rose EA. Implantable left ventricular assist devices. N Engl J Med 1998;339:1522–1533.
Hensley FA, Martin DE, Gravlee GP, eds. A Practical Approach to Cardiac Anesthesia. 3rd Ed. Philadelphia: Lippincott Williams & Wilkins; 2003:557–573.

97

ADMINISTER ANTIBIOTICS BEFORE PLACING A CHEST TUBE IN TRAUMA PATIENTS

PETER G. THOMAS, DO
PATRICK K. KIM, MD

The role of antibiotics during the placement of tube thoracostomy for hemothorax or pneumothorax in the trauma patient remains controversial. Every year, more than 100,000 chest tubes are placed in trauma patients for hemopneumothorax. Multiple studies have been performed over the last four decades to determine whether or not antibiotics decrease the rate of infection after chest-tube insertion.

In 2000, the Eastern Association for the Surgery of Trauma (EAST) Practice Management Guidelines Work Group reviewed all of the prospective articles and two meta-analyses on the topic published between 1977 and 1997. The group identified class I (prospective randomized controlled trials) and class II (clinical studies in which the data were collected prospectively, and retrospective analyses that were based on clearly reliable data) studies upon which to base their recommendations. The authors concluded that there is sufficient data to make a level III recommendation for prophylactic antibiotic use in patients undergoing tube thoracostomy for trauma. There is no apparent effect on empyema rate, but antibiotics may reduce the incidence of pneumonia. The guidelines suggest that antibiotics should not be given for more than 24 hours. The authors were able to make only level III recommendations (defined as "supported by available data but adequate scientific evidence is lacking") because the studies had markedly different study designs and treatment criteria, and as such, consensus conclusions could not be made based by combining the data.

Wilson and Nichols reviewed the same data and published an editorial to the EAST guidelines in 2000. Their interpretation of the data re-emphasized the correlation between the use of antibiotics during chest-tube placement and the decrease in the rate of pneumonia. When the three reviewed studies that had Centers for Disease Control and Prevention (CDC)–conforming criteria for pneumonia were combined, there was a 9.4% incidence of pneumonia for the placebo group and a 0.8% ($p = 0.003$) incidence for the antibiotic group. When the eight papers that compared antibiotics versus no antibiotics were combined, the pneumonia rate was 14.8% for the placebo group and 4.1% ($p = 0.001$) for the antibiotic group.

The literature published after the EAST guidelines still fails to end this controversy. A randomized, prospective study from 1998 showed similar benefits for patients receiving antibiotics. Seventy-one patients treated with antibiotics were compared with 68 that received placebo. The treated group had no infections while the placebo group had four ($p = 0.05$).

The most recent study was a well-designed prospective, randomized, double-blind multicenter trial. It compared three groups of patients: those who received antibiotics for the entire length of chest-tube placement; 24 hours of antibiotics; and placebo. The authors concluded that there was a slight decrease in the reported empyema rate, although it was not statistically significant. They also found no decrease in the rate of pneumonia. The limitation of this study was that it was severely underpowered with an accrual rate of less than 20% of the predicted needed number of patients to prove statistical significance.

WHAT TO DO

Although it is apparent that there is no definitive answer to the question of prophylactic antibiotics when placing chest tubes for trauma, some recommendations can be made based on the existing literature. First, antibiotics do appear to decrease the rate of pneumonia in patients who undergo chest-tube placement. Second, the antibiotic used should primarily cover *Staphylococcus aureus* and *Staphylococcus epidermidis*, as these are the most common organisms recovered. Third, it appears that a single preprocedure dose of antibiotics is as efficacious as 24 hours of antibiotics. Judicious use of antibiotics should be practiced in order to limit antibiotic-resistant strains of bacteria.

SUGGESTED READINGS

Gonzalez RP, Holevar MR. Role of prophylactic antibiotics for tube thoracostomy in chest trauma. Am Surg 1998;64:617–620; discussion 620–621.

Luchette FA, Barrie PS, Oswanski MF, et al. Practice management guidelines for prophylactic antibiotic use in tube thoracostomy for traumatic hemopneumothorax: the EAST Practice Management Guidelines Work Group. Eastern Association for Trauma. J Trauma 2000;48:753–757. Also available at http://www.east.org/tpg.html

Maxwell RA, Campbell DJ, Fabian TC, et al. Use of presumptive antibiotics following tube thoracostomy for traumatic hemopneumothorax in the prevention of empyema and pneumonia: a multi-center trial. J Trauma 2004;57:742–749.

Wilson RF, Nichols RL. The EAST practice management guidelines for prophylactic antibiotic use in tube thoracostomy for traumatic hemopneumothorax: a commentary. J Trauma 2000;48:758–759.

98

BE SUSPICIOUS OF A LARGE PERSISTENT AIR LEAK IN A CHEST TUBE

DAVID T. EFRON, MD

To understand how to troubleshoot a persistent air leak from a chest tube, one must thoroughly understand the entire algorithm describing the creation and subsequent evacuation and treatment of a pneumothorax.

The chest cavity is a rigid structure made so by the bony scaffold of the rib cage, sternum, and thoracic vertebrae. The left and right hemithoraces are usually anatomically distinct cavities under normal circumstances. However, physiologically they are interdependent due to a soft, relatively compliant mediastinum. Normally, each hemithorax is composed of a rigid outer shell (musculoskeletal) lined on the inside with the parietal pleura. The lung is an aerated organ, soft and compliant, the outside of which is lined with the visceral pleura. The space between the pleurae is maintained at a pressure of negative 5cm H_2O. This pressure, in addition to intra-alveolar lubrication and surfactant, allows the lung to remain open and aerated and prevents collapse on itself. Thus, the movement of the diaphragm in a cephalad-caudad direction aided by much smaller, but not insignificant movement of the intercostals muscle brings air into and out of the lungs via the tracheobronchial tree. It is a system that is open to the outside environment but closed to the chest cavity. Violation of any of the barriers of the closed chest cavity results in release of the negative pressure in the pleural space and collapse of the lung. Ongoing leakage of air into the pleural space results in tension pneumothorax when that air is not able to escape. A chest tube that is placed to alleviate this will demonstrate an ongoing air leak in the water-seal chamber.

Air leaks result from disruption of any one part of the sealed chest cavity. Diagnosis of the source of an air leak is simple in the majority of cases and vital to undertaking appropriate action. The best way to think of a chest-tube circuit is to consider everything from the tube to the water seal (the second chamber) an extension of the pleural cavity. A persistent air leak can be caused only by one of three basic mechanisms: patient pathology; tube pathology; or Pleuravac pathology.

PATIENT PATHOLOGY

- Tracheobronchial disruption
- Parenchymal injury or tear
- Esophageal perforation
- Unsealed chest-wall disruption (i.e., open pneumothorax or "sucking chest wound")

TUBE PATHOLOGY

- Leak at insertion site (i.e., hole in chest wall too big, poor seal around hole)
- Proximal hole in tube outside of chest wall
- Perforation of chest tube
- Poor seal at connection of tube to Pleuravac tube

PLEURAVAC PATHOLOGY

- Improperly prepared apparatus
- Broken apparatus

The following is a suggested algorithm of how to diagnose the source and potentially fix the air leak:

1) Inspect the pleuravac for obvious defects in setup or components. Correct any faulty setups or, if damaged, replace the entire system.
2) Inspect all connections within the circuit and between the tubes and Pleuravacs. Remove all tape that obscures your view of these joints. Ensure that these connections are snug and airtight.
3) Inspect the chest-tube insertion site. The dressing must be taken down completely to do this properly. You need to ensure that the chest tube itself is intact and no side holes are visible outside the chest wall. A chest radiograph is also useful in obese patients where the chest wall is too thick to assess the relationship of the last hole to the chest cavity. If no obvious cause is found, it is best to replace an occlusive dressing at this site before proceeding.
4) Serial clamping of the tubes in the drainage system is then performed. Starting just above the Pleuravac, the tube is clamped and the leak assessed while the pleuravac remains on suction. If a leak persists at the Pleuravac when a clamp is applied to the tube, this means there must be a leak in the circuit distal to the clamp and a search should be directed to this area. The clamp is then serially

moved up the tubing toward the patient. If the leak disappears when the tube is clamped, then the leak is proximal (i.e., on the patient side) to the clamp.

One final note is that experienced clinicians usually report that the most frequent source of persistent air leak (and the easiest to fix) is the chest-tube circuit.

SUGGESTED READINGS

Baumann MH. What size chest tube? What drainage system is ideal? And other chest tube management questions. Curr Opin Pulm Med 2003;9:276–281.

Cerfolio RJ. Recent advances in the treatment of air leaks. Curr Opin Pulm Med 2005;11:319–323.

99

TREAT ANY MILKY FLUID COMING FROM THE CHEST OR ABDOMEN AS CHYLOUS UNTIL PROVEN OTHERWISE

D. JOSHUA MANCINI, MD
RAJAN GUPTA, MD

The anatomy of the thoracic duct can be variable; however, it usually originates at the confluence of the cisterna chili on the right side of the aorta at the L1-L2 level. It courses cephalad through the aortic hiatus and crosses the midline behind the aortic arch at the level of T4-T5. The duct then travels along the left side of the esophagus into the neck to drain into the venous system at the confluence of the left subclavian and jugular veins. The thoracic duct transports up to 4 L/day of chyle, depending on diet, drug intake, and intestinal function. Chyle is primarily lymphatic fluid from the gastrointestinal tract, with a smaller contribution from lymphatic drainage of the chest. Since 60% to 75% of absorbed dietary fat passes through this system mainly as chylomicrons, chyle is primarily composed of triglycerides, cholesterol, and fat-soluble vitamins. These components give chyle its characteristic milky white appearance. The thoracic duct is also the main conduit for the return of extravasated proteins to the circulation. The cellular component is predominantly lymphocytes.

Chyle leaks are most commonly secondary to trauma or malignancy (e.g., lymphoma, chronic lymphocytic leukemia, metastatic disease); however, they can also be congenital or secondary to sarcoidosis or infectious etiologies (e.g., histoplasmosis, tuberculosis). Traumatic chyle leaks are often iatrogenic, usually as a complication of thoracic procedures. Esophagectomy and surgical correction of congenital heart disease are surgical procedures with particularly high risk. Abdominal procedures such as open aortic aneurysm repair, retroperitoneal lymph node dissection, Nissen fundoplication, liver transplantation, and peritoneal dialysis catheter placement have also been implicated in chylous ascites. Approximately 20% of traumatic chyle leaks are secondary to penetrating or blunt trauma.

Although chyle is often milky white in appearance, it may also be clear, especially if enteral nutrition has not been recently administered. Thus, a chyle leak should not necessarily be excluded when clear pleural or peritoneal fluid is drained. Conversely, a chronic pleural effusion can have a milky character due to lysis of red blood cells and neutrophils in the fluid. These types of effusions are often secondary to tuberculosis or rheumatoid disease. Purulent ascites due to bacterial peritonitis can also have a similar appearance. Therefore, if a chyle leak is suspected or a milky or clear fluid of unknown etiology occurs, the fluid should be analyzed for triglyceride concentration and lymphocyte levels. If the triglyceride concentration is above 110 mg/dL, the fluid is chyle in 99% of the cases. If the triglyceride concentration is below 50 mg/dL, the fluid is chyle in only 5% of cases. Alternatively, Sudan III stain can be used to determine the presence of fat globules. Often, the diagnosis can be made clinically by administering cream orally and examining the change in appearance of the fluid.

WHAT TO DO

The approach to management of a chylothorax depends on the etiology. Generally, a graded approach should be considered, starting with the least invasive management strategy. A regimen of percutaneous drainage of the fluid, parenteral nutrition with volume replacement, and a fat-free diet supplemented with medium-chain triglycerides will enable 80% of nontraumatic cases to resolve within 2 to 3 weeks. Somatostatin is an additional adjunct that may be utilized. Chyle leaks secondary to malignancy usually require treatment of the malignancy itself, such as radiation for a lymphoma. Persistent chylous drainage beyond 2 weeks can begin to compromise natural immune response and more invasive procedures should be considered at this time. In addition, a chyle leak secondary to surgical or traumatic disruption is less likely to heal with conservative measures and will often require more invasive intervention. Percutaneous transabdominal catheter embolization or needle disruption of retroperitoneal lymphatic vessels has been effective in managing these leaks in 70% of cases. The advent of minimally invasive techniques such as video-assisted thoracic surgery (VATS) has led to earlier intervention in select cases. Surgical options for chylothorax include ligation of the duct, pleurodesis, and pleuroperitoneal and pleurovenous shunting.

SUGGESTED READINGS

Cope C, Kaiser LR. Management of unremitting chylothorax by percutaneous embolization and blockage of retroperitoneal lymphatic vessels in 42 patients. J Vasc Interv Radiol 2002;13:1139–1148.

Merrigan BA, Winter DC, O'Sullivan GC. Chylothorax. Br J Surg 1997:84:15–20.

100

KNOW THE CONDITIONS THAT CAUSE AN INACCURATE PULSE OXIMETRY READING

ELIAHU S. FEEN, MD
JOSE I. SUAREZ, MD

BASIC PRINCIPLES

Pulse oximetry is the technique of measuring arterial blood oxygenation through identification of pulsatile blood. The fundamental physiological principle that the technique uses is spectrophotometry, or the measurement of the absorption of light by blood and tissues. One simple way to understand the basic principle is to imagine a test tube filled with some substance and shining light of a certain wavelength upon it (incident light). Some of the light is transmitted ("transient" light) through the substance and some is absorbed. The amount of light transmitted depends upon the absorptive (and reflective) nature of the particular substance. The Beer-Lambert law relates this mathematically:

$$C = (1/d \times \alpha) \log_e (I_i / I_t)$$

where C is the concentration of the particular substance in the test tube, d is the path length of the light through the test tube, α is an absorption coefficient for the substance in question at a particular wavelength of light, I_i is the intensity of the incident light, and I_t is the intensity of the transmitted light. When this principle is applied to blood oxygenation, then the question becomes one of determining the absorption of light by hemoglobin.

In adults, there are four forms of hemoglobin, oxyhemoglobin (HbO_2), methemoglobin (metHb), carboxyhemoglobin (HbCO), and "reduced" hemoglobin (Hb). Each form of hemoglobin absorbs a different amount of light at a given wavelength. Using four different wavelengths of light, the Beer-Lambert law can be solved for each of the four forms of hemoglobin to give a concentration in a sample of blood. With these concentrations, the fractional hemoglobin saturation (percentage of oxyhemoglobin in blood) can be calculated as follows:

$$HbO_2\% = \frac{HbO_2}{(HbO_2 + Hb + metHb + HbCO)}$$

Except in pathological states, the concentrations of metHb and HbCO are low. These forms of hemoglobin do not contribute importantly to tissue oxygen delivery. Physiologically, what is important is oxygen delivery. A functional oxygen saturation has been defined as follows:

$$SaO_2 = \frac{HbO_2}{(HbO_2 + Hb)}$$

This equation requires only two wavelengths of light in order to solve for concentration through the Beer-Lambert law.

In most clinical settings, the two wavelengths are a red light wavelength and an infrared wavelength. Thus, we have oximetry through the measurement of light absorption by blood. The problem then becomes determining the light absorption of arterial blood as opposed to venous and capillary blood and tissue absorption of light. *Pulse* oximetry solves this problem by measuring the difference in total absorption of light at the greatest distance and the least distance over a fixed span of tissue containing arterioles. The least distance is the distance of tissue plus venous and capillary blood plus a distance of arteriolar blood at diastole. The greatest distance is the least distance plus the distance created by the extra volume of blood contained in the arterioles at systole (the "pulse"). The difference between these distances is created by arterial blood alone, so light absorption differences represent arterial blood. This figures into the path length of the Beer-Lambert law (*d* in the equation above). Ultimately, using this information, the oxygen saturation of arterial blood can be computed.

INACCURATE READINGS

Based upon these principles, the reasons for spurious pulse oximeter readings can be understood. Any process that limits the arteriolar blood flow into peripheral sites where pulse oximeter readings are performed will either falsely lower the readings or preclude the ability to get readings. The simple example of placing a pulse oximeter probe on a finger of an arm compressed by a sphygmomanometer will demonstrate this idea. When the cuff pressure exceeds systolic blood pressure, arterial blood flow tapers off, and the pulse oximeter reading drops off as well. Similarly, peripheral vasoconstriction due to any cause (e.g., shock) will cause falsely altered readings. Additionally, any ambient interference in light transmission (or absorption) will alter the readings. Examples include nail polish on the fingers upon which the pulse oximeter probe is placed and fluorescent light in the room. Many manufacturers develop signal-processing techniques to account for ambient light around the patient. Some intravenous dyes (e.g., methylene blue) can alter the light absorption within blood and thereby spuriously alter the pulse oximetry result. As mentioned before, in some pathophysiologic states, there is increased concentration of methemoglobin and carboxyhemoglobin, which were not figured into the functional oxygen saturation equation. In such states (e.g., carbon monoxide poisoning) the pulse oximeter reading can be false. Carboxyhemoglobin is interpreted as oxyhemoglobin by standard pulse oximeters, so a falsely elevated reading will result. Methemoglobin (which has the visual appearance of a chocolate brown color) will falsely lower the pulse oximeter reading. Other metabolic states have been reported to cause changes. Hyperbilirubinemia, on the other hand, does not alter the actual pulse oximeter reading because of this condition itself. However, many icteric patients will have elevated serum levels of carboxyhemoglobin because of the catabolism of hemoglobin, and *this* may influence the real oxygen saturation.

SUGGESTED READINGS

Barker SJ, Tremper KK, Hyatt J. Effects of methemoglobinemia on pulse oximetry and mixed venous oximetry. Anesthesiology 1989;70:112–117.

Miller RD, ed. Anesthesia. 5th Ed. Philadelphia: Churchill Livingstone; 2000.

Tremper KK, Barker SJ. Pulse oximetry. Anesthesiology 1989;70:98–108.

Veyckermans F, Baele P, Guillaume JE, et al. Hyperbilirubinemia does not interfere with hemoglobin saturation measured by pulse oximetry. Anesthesiology 1989;70:118–122.

101

REMEMBER THAT PULSE OXIMETRY IS INACCURATE AT LOWER SATURATION LEVELS

NIRAV G. SHAH, MD

Pulse oximetry is a noninvasive method to measure arterial hemoglobin saturation. The probe for the pulse oximeter consists of two light-emitting probes and a photodetector. Pulse oximeters are able to distinguish between oxygenated and deoxygenated hemoglobin on the basis of their differential absorption of two wavelengths of light. The photodiodes turn on and off several hundred times per second, allowing the absorption of light by oxyhemoglobin and deoxyhemoglobin to be continuously recorded. It is the absorption during pulsatile flow that is a measure of arterial hemoglobin saturation, while the absorption during nonpulsatile flow is a function of the surrounding tissue and venous blood.

WATCH OUT FOR

Although pulse oximetry is universally used in the intensive care unit (ICU), the experienced practitioner will understand the limitations and inaccuracies inherent in using it. First, microprocessors in pulse oximeters are calibrated using reference tables compiled by exposing healthy volunteers to decreasing FIO_2 (fraction of inspired oxygen) to produce SaO_2 (oxygen saturation) ranging from 75% to 100% by co-oximetry. Thus, any reading below 75% is a calculated value extrapolated from healthy volunteers. At 75% to 83% the bias on pulse oximetry is 8% from co-oximetry and this value does not reach an acceptable 3% bias until the saturation is >83% on pulse oximetry.

A second limitation of pulse oximetry is the insensitivity of the measured values to changes in the partial pressure of oxygen because of the flat shape of the oxyhemoglobin dissociation curve at the upper end of the spectrum. For example, in a patient receiving supplemental oxygen therapy, a fall in PaO_2 (partial pressure of oxygen in arterial blood) of 140 to 65 mm Hg would be required before a significant decrease in oxygen saturation is picked up by the pulse oximeter.

A third limitation is the inability of the photodetector to pick up adequate signals to generate a value. This can occur with poor tissue perfusion (e.g., peripheral vasoconstriction, pressor administration where the probe can cause tissue injury, or shock), excessive patient movement (e.g., seizures or shivering), excessive ambient light, severe anemia, and hypothermia.

One final note is that it is well known that the pulse oximeter cannot differentiate between oxyhemoglobin and methemoglobin or carboxyhemoglobin, and the presence of either of the latter two in the vascular system will provide an inaccurate assessment of the amount of oxygenated hemoglobin.

SUGGESTED READINGS

Schnapp LM, Cohen NH. Pulse oximetry: uses and abuses. Chest 1990;98:1244.
Weinberger SE. Recent advances in pulmonary medicine. N Engl J Med 1993;328:1389–1397.

102

CONSIDER PLACING AN INTRACRANIAL PRESSURE MONITOR IN PATIENTS WITH GLASGOW COMA SCALE ≤8

JOSE I. SUAREZ, MD

Neuronal injury is usually classified as primary or secondary. Primary injury refers to the intracranial processes themselves (i.e., ischemic or hemorrhagic strokes, trauma, neoplasms) whereas secondary injury refers to systemic conditions that may worsen the primary injury. Common processes that lead to secondary injury include fever, seizure, hypotension, and elevated intracranial pressure (ICP). Uncontrolled elevated ICP will lead to cerebral ischemia and most experienced clinicians initiate treatment at an upper threshold of 20 to 25 mmHg. Such threshold is based on prospective analysis of patients with traumatic brain injury (TBI) and outcome related to ICP elevations. The optimal predictive value of outcome was 20 mmHg although data are lacking from randomized, controlled trials investigating various ICP treatment thresholds.

ICP MONITORING

The best way to determine ICP is through continuous monitoring. The neurological examination may not reliably correlate with ICP elevations, especially in patients in coma. Most of the data available regarding selection of patients for ICP monitoring come from TBI patients and most practitioners have extrapolated such criteria for patients with various intracranial abnormalities. Current recommendations indicate that ICP monitoring is appropriate in patients with severe TBI (Glasgow Coma Scale [GCS] of 3 to 8 after cardiopulmonary resuscitation) with an abnormal admission head computed tomography (CT) scan. An abnormal head CT scan is defined as one that demonstrates hematomas, contusions, edema, or compressed basal cisterns. ICP monitoring is also appropriate in patients with severe TBI with a normal head CT scan but who present with two or more of the following: age >40 years, unilateral or bilateral motor posturing, and systolic blood pressure <90 mm Hg. Essentially, any patient with GCS ≤8 should be considered for ICP monitoring regardless of the underlying intracranial or systemic condition.

Several types of ICP-monitoring devices are commercially available today. These include intraventricular catheters (IVCs), parenchymal catheters, subarachnoid bolts, epidural catheters, and lumbar drains (to measure the cerebrospinal fluid [CSF] pressure in the lumbar spinal space). When IVCs are inserted, a pressure transducer can be connected to measure the fluid pressure of the CSF that drains. IVCs are considered the gold standard of direct ICP monitoring, because fluid conveys a pressure wave reliably. They also have the added benefit of treating ICP elevations by draining CSF. IVCs are associated with infections that may range from 5% to 20% and are more common after day five of insertion. Accordingly, some practitioners have recommended replacing catheters that are more than 5 days old. Other clinicians believe changing the catheter should be done only if there is evidence of an infection that has not been localized to a source other than the central nervous system (CNS). Other devices include parenchymal catheters, such as the Camino and Codman MicroSensor catheters, which are inserted through a burr hole in the skull with the catheters being inserted through the dura into brain parenchyma (or the ventricles, if so desired). Hemorrhagic and infectious complications appear to be about the same as with an IVC. Subarachnoid bolts and epidural catheters are less commonly used.

THE GLASGOW COMA SCALE

The best way to determine level of consciousness in the intensive care unit (ICU) is by calculating the GCS, which is a reproducible 15-point scale in which the maximum score is 15 and the minimum score is 3. The scale describes eye opening, verbal behavior, and motor responsiveness. The scale has a high interobserver reliability among physicians of multiple disciplines and nursing staff. The scale has a good sensitivity and reliability (intraclass correlation coefficient 0.8 to 1 for trained users). GCS scores between 3 and 8 correspond to unresponsive patients. Although the calculation of the GCS sum score in critically ill subjects has multifaceted applications, the presence of untestable components of the GCS limits its usefulness. The most common untestable feature of the GCS is the verbal score, which is usually due to the presence of endotracheal intubation. A predicted verbal score for subjects who are intubated has been described and validated (*Table 102.1*), with the total maximum score of the GCS in intubated patients still 15. The accuracy of this model was confirmed by comparing the predicted verbal score with the actual verbal score in the test data set ($n = 736$, $r = 0.92$, $R^2 = 0.85$, $p = 0.0001$). The derivation of the verbal score based on the eye and motor components

TABLE 102.1	CALCULATED PREDICTED GCS VERBAL SCORE FROM EYE AND MOTOR SCORES USING LINEAR REGRESSION			
	GCS EYE SCORE			
GCS MOTOR SCORE	**1**	**2**	**3**	**4**
1	1	1	1	2
2	1	2	2	2
3	2	2	3	3
4	2	3	3	4
5	3	3	4	4
6	3	4	4	5

Reused with permission from Rutledge R, Lentz CW, Fakhry S, et al. Appropriate use of the Glasgow Coma Scale in intubated patients: a linear regression prediction of the Glasgow verbal score from the Glasgow eye and motor scores. J Trauma 1996;41:514–522.

was further validated in a larger data set ($n = 24,085$, $r = 0.97$, $p = 0.0001$).

SUGGESTED READINGS

Meredith W, Rutledge R, Fakhry SM, et al. The conundrum of the Glasgow Coma Scale in intubated patients: a linear regression prediction of the Glasgow verbal score from the Glasgow eye and motor scores. J Trauma 1998;44:839–844.

Rutledge R, Lentz CW, Fakhry S, et al. Appropriate use of the Glasgow Coma Scale in intubated patients: a linear regression prediction of the Glasgow verbal score from the Glasgow eye and motor scores. J Trauma 1996;41:514–522.

Teasdale G, Jennett B. Assessment of coma and impaired consciousness: a practical scale. Lancet 1977;2:81–84.

Teasdale G, Knill-Jones R, van der Sande J. Observer variability in assessing impaired consciousness and coma. J Neurol Neurosurg Psychiatry 1978;41:603–610.

The Brain Trauma Foundation. The American Association of Neurological Surgeons. The Joint Section on Neurotrauma and Critical Care. Indications for Intracranial Pressure Monitoring. J Neurotrauma 2000;17:479–491.

The Brain Trauma Foundation. The American Association of Neurological Surgeons. The Joint Section on Neurotrauma and Critical Care. Intracranial Pressure Treatment Threshold. J Neurotrauma 2000;17:493–495.

103

KNOW HOW TO USE THE LICOX SYSTEM TO MEASURE BRAIN TISSUE OXYGENATION

AARON BRANSKY, MD
HEIDI L. FRANKEL, MD

Traumatic brain injury is a leading cause of death and disability in young people. In an attempt to direct therapy, intracranial pressure (ICP) monitoring and calculated cerebral perfusion pressure (CPP) have been used to make bedside management decisions. However, several studies have shown that cerebral infarction can occur even with normal ICP and CPP.

Given this information, brain tissue oxygen monitoring has been investigated to give an earlier marker of brain ischemia. One new technology has been the use of a Clark-type catheter to measure partial oxygenation of brain tissue (PbO_2). These probes can be placed in the brain cortex during craniotomy or in the intensive care unit (ICU) by placing a burr hole. There are differing opinions as to whether the probe should be placed in healthy brain tissue or the penumbra of injury.

However, it is generally agreed that PbO_2 levels should be maintained greater than 15 to 20 mm Hg. If an acute decrease is discovered, it may represent an earlier sign of brain ischemia than either elevated ICP or CPP. Contradictory to therapy for elevated ICP, if a patient develops low PbO_2, the physician should lower the head of the bed and consider permissive hypercapnia for cerebral vasodilatation. Additionally, raising global oxygen delivery by means such as increasing FIO_2 (fraction of inspired oxygen) and transfusing packed red blood cells, or raising cardiac output has shown some success in raising PbO_2. The manufacturer (Licox) recommends use for up to 5 to 7 days.

SUGGESTED READINGS

Stiefel MF, Spiotta A, Gracias VH, et al. Reduced mortality rate in patients with severe traumatic brain injury treated with brain tissue oxygen monitoring. J Neurosurg 2005;103:805–811.

Valadka AB, Gopinath SP, Contant CF, et al. Relationship of brain tissue PO_2 to outcome after severe head injury. Crit Care Med 1998;26:1576–1581.

van den Brink WA, van Santbrink H, Steyerberg EW, et al. Brain oxygen tension in severe head injury. Neurosurgery 2000;46:868–876; discussion 876–878.

VENTILATORS/AIRWAY/ INTUBATION/EXTUBATION

104

PREOXYGENATE PATIENTS BEFORE INTUBATION

RAHUL G. BAIJAL, MD

The purpose of preoxygenating a patient before induction of general anesthesia and paralysis is to provide maximum time that a patient can tolerate apnea. Maximum preoxygenation is achieved when the alveolar, arterial, tissue, and venous compartments are filled with oxygen. Patients in whom oxygen extraction is increased (e.g., hyperthermia, acidosis, hypercarbia) or oxygen loading is decreased (e.g., decreased functional residual capacity, hemoglobin concentration, alveolar ventilation, cardiac output) desaturate faster during apnea than a healthy patient and consequently require maximum preoxygenation. Various factors may necessitate preoxygenation when mask ventilation is not possible, including difficulty maintaining airway patency; a full stomach where pressure of the upper abdomen may induce regurgitation; anticipated difficult airway requiring increased apneic time; morbid obesity where high pressures are required to ventilate the lung; and pregnancy where increased abdominal pressure may also induce regurgitation.

WHAT TO DO

Functional residual capacity (FRC) is the volume remaining in the lungs at exhalation following normal tidal volume breathing. FRC is approximately 2,500 mL in a healthy adult and is reduced as a patient is moved from an upright to a supine or prone position. FRC is additionally reduced by 15% to 20% following induction of anesthesia. During preoxygenation, the patient inspires 100% oxygen via a face mask before induction, replacing nitrogen with oxygen in the patient's FRC. Normal oxygen consumption in a healthy adult is approximately 250 mL/min. Oxygen desaturation may occur as rapidly as 30 to 60 seconds in a healthy adult with an FRC of 21% oxygen following induction of anesthesia and subsequent apnea, despite normal initial oxygen saturation. Denitrogenation during spontaneous breathing is 95% complete within 3 minutes when a patient is breathing a normal tidal volume of 100% oxygen. This increases the margin of safety to approximately 4 to 6 times during periods of apnea following induction of anesthesia. Preoxygenation with eight maximum deep breaths over 60 seconds results in arterial oxygenation that is not different from tidal volume breathing for 3 minutes. This technique increases minute ventilation above

FRC and minimizes nitrogen rebreathing, ensuring washout of FRC; additionally, taking eight deep breaths may open collapsed airways, increasing FRC oxygen store. Four maximum breaths over 30 seconds also increases arterial oxygenation, but the time for hemoglobin desaturation is shortened compared with patients breathing normal tidal volume for 3 minutes or taking eight maximum breaths over 60 seconds.

Preventable reasons that maximum preoxygenation may not be achieved include a leak under the mask, allowing inspiratory entrainment of room air, and insufficient preoxygenation time. Avoiding a leak between the mask and the face is an important factor that cannot be compensated for by increased duration of preoxygenation.

SUGGESTED READINGS

Baraka AS, et al. Preoxygenation: comparison of maximal breathing and tidal volume breathing techniques. Anesthesiology 1999;91:612–616.

Miller RD. Miller's Anesthesia. 6th Ed. Philadelphia: Elsevier; 2005:617–719.

Eastwood WD. A study of dinitrogenation with some inhalation and anesthetic systems. Anesthesiology 1955;16:861–867.

105

USE CRICOID PRESSURE WHEN PERFORMING RAPID SEQUENCE INTUBATION OR BAG-MASK VENTILATION

RAHUL G. BAIJAL, MD

Cricoid pressure, first described by Sellick in 1961, is used to occlude the upper esophagus to reduce the aspiration of gastric contents during rapid-sequence intubation. Pulmonary aspiration of gastric contents occurs in three stages. First, gastric contents reflux into the esophagus when the lower esophageal sphincter relaxes. Esophageal contents then reflux into the pharynx when the upper esophageal sphincter relaxes. Finally, pulmonary aspiration of pharyngeal contents occurs after loss of laryngeal reflexes.

To briefly review, the cricoid cartilage is the only upper airway cartilaginous structure that is a complete ring. The esophagus begins at the lower border of the cricoid cartilage. Cricoid pressure replaces the function of the upper esophageal sphincter by compressing the lumen of the upper esophagus between lamina of the cricoid cartilage and the body of the sixth cervical vertebrae, preventing regurgitation of esophageal contents into the pharynx (the second phase of aspiration). The upper esophageal sphincter is formed anteriorly by the lamina of the cricoid cartilage and posteriorly by the cricopharyngeus muscle, which is attached to the lateral aspects of the cricoid cartilage. Upper esophageal sphincter tone is 40 mm Hg in awake patients and decreases to less than 10 mm Hg during induction of anesthesia. Regurgitation of esophageal contents into the pharynx occurs when the upper esophageal sphincter pressure is less than 25 mm Hg. Therefore, induction of anesthesia can decrease upper esophageal sphincter pressure sufficiently to allow regurgitation of esophageal contents into the pharynx. Cricoid pressure counteracts this reduction in upper esophageal pressure. It is important to note that other cartilaginous structures in the upper airway are u-shaped; mistakenly exerting pressure on these structures will be ineffective and possibly lead to airway damage or distortion during intubation.

To avoid this, the cricoid cartilage should first be identified and palpated *before* induction of anesthesia. With single-handed cricoid pressure, the thumb and middle finger can be placed on either side of the cricoid cartilage with the index finger caudal. The thumb and middle finger prevent lateral movement of the cricoid cartilage and the index finger provides anterior-posterior pressure. The disadvantage of this technique is that the extended neck will tend to collapse the arch and reduce the glottic view. Another single-handed technique is to place the palm of the hand on the sternum and apply pressure to the cricoid cartilage with only the index and middle fingers. In the two-handed, or bimanual, technique, cricoid pressure is performed as with the single-handed technique except that the assistant's other hand provides counterpressure beneath the cervical vertebrae, supporting the neck.

Cricoid pressure can withstand esophageal pressures of 50 cm H_2O (1 cm H_2O = 0.73 mm Hg). Cricoid pressure can overcome gastric pressures associated with fasting (<18 cm H_2O), delayed gastric emptying (<50 cm H_2O), eructation (<20 cm H_2O), pregnant supine patients (<35 cm H_2O), or fasiculations associated with succinylcholine administration (<40 cm H_2O). However, vomiting, which creates esophageal pressures >60 cm H_2O, can overcome cricoid pressure, leading to regurgitation and pulmonary aspiration. Cricoid pressure should begin before the patient is fully asleep, with 10 N of pressure, increasing to 30 N of pressure when loss of consciousness is established. Recommended cricoid pressure to prevent pulmonary aspiration is between 30 and 40 N (10 N ~ 1 kg), but pressure >20 N can cause pain and retching in awake patients, and pressure >40 N can distort the trachea, making intubation difficult. Retching causes a reflex relaxation of the lower esophageal sphincter and rapid distention of the esophagus, relaxing the upper esophageal sphincter and allowing expulsion of vomit. Cricoid pressure maintained during retching allows esophageal pressure to rise, increasing the risk of esophageal rupture. Cricoid pressure is additionally contraindicated in patients with cricotracheal injury, active emesis, or unstable cervical spine injuries.

Finally, bag-mask ventilation provides positive pressure ventilation with delivery of high fraction of inspired oxygen, opening atelectic alveoli and improving ventilation-perfusion mismatch. However, bag-mask ventilation may rapidly distend the stomach, increasing gastric pressure up to 30 cm H_2O. Cricoid pressure may overcome this increased gastric pressure as noted previously but may be uncomfortable in an awake patient.

SUGGESTED READINGS

Allman K. The effect of cricoid pressure application on airway patency. J Clin Anesth 1995;7:195–199.

Asai T. Cricoid pressure applied after placement of the laryngeal mask prevents gastric insufflation but inhibits ventilation. Br J Anaesth 1996;76:772–776.

Landsman I. Cricoid pressure: indications and complications. Pediatr Anesth 2004; 14:43–47.

Vanner RG. Mechanism of regurgitation and its prevention with cricoid pressure. Int J Obstet Anesth 1993;2:207–215.

Vanner RG, Hartsilver EL. Airway obstruction with cricoid pressure. Anesthesia 2000;55:208–211.

106

DO NOT USE THE PRESENCE OF END-TIDAL CO$_2$ TO RULE OUT ESOPHAGEAL INTUBATION

PATRICIA M. VELOSO, MD

SCENARIO

You are called to emergently intubate an obese woman for increasing respiratory distress who is four hours postoperative from an uneventful nephrectomy. She was successfully extubated in the operating room and initially on admission to the intensive care unit (ICU) looked like she would be a straightforward one-night ICU stay. On your arrival to the bedside, the medical student is attempting to mask-ventilate her. You ready your laryngoscope and the endotracheal tube and proceed to secure the airway. You are confident that you intubated the trachea although her body habitus made the intubation challenging. The respiratory therapist hooks up the portable end-tidal CO$_2$ monitor, gives the patient a breath, and tells you "good job" because the portable end-tidal CO$_2$ monitor detects the presence of CO$_2$. The nurse also tells you he hears bilateral breath sounds. Are you satisfied with this assessment and ready to have the respiratory therapist tape the endotracheal tube?

EXPLANATION

No! You should not be satisfied with this assessment of the placement of the endotracheal tube. Detection of CO$_2$ in one breath by the CO$_2$ monitor is not sufficient to ensure that the endotracheal tube is indeed in the trachea.

Portable CO$_2$ monitors contain litmus paper that quickly changes color (i.e., from purple to yellow) in response to exhaled CO$_2$. It is important to note that some air is always forced into the stomach when mask-ventilating a patient before intubation. During a difficult mask ventilation (as in the previous scenario with an inexperienced medical student and an obese patient), a significant amount of air can be introduced into the stomach. If the esophagus is intubated, the CO$_2$ detector will change color because it is detecting CO$_2$ from the stomach. It is only after at least 4 to 5 breaths with a continued color change on the CO$_2$ monitor that you can be confident that the trachea has been intubated.

In addition, auscultating for bilateral breath sounds is not sufficient to confirm endotracheal intubation. Sounds from air moving through the esophagus and stomach can be mistaken for bilateral breath sounds. Therefore, it is imperative to also include auscultation over the gastric region to ensure the absence of breath sounds with the more obvious auscultation of the bilateral lung fields for the presence of breath sounds.

One final note concerns the use of portable CO_2 monitors in cardiac arrest. During cardiac arrest (in the absence of adequate cardiopulmonary resuscitation [CPR]), there is no blood flow to the lungs; therefore, CO_2 is not being delivered to the lungs. The CO_2 detector will not change color even if the endotracheal tube is correctly positioned. During the resuscitation, the CO_2 detector may change color if effective chest compressions are being done and blood flow is partially restored to the lungs.

SUGGESTED READINGS

Hogg K, Teece S. Best evidence topic report: colourmetric CO_2 detector compared with capnography for confirming ET tube placement. Emerg Med J 2003;20:265–266.

Miller R, ed. Miller's Anesthesia. 6th Ed. Philadelphia: Churchill Livingstone; 2005:1648.

Nellcor Puritan Bennett, Inc. CO_2 Detection: intubation and cardiopulmonary resuscitation. Clinical Monographs. June 1, 2003. http://www.nellcor.com

107

HAVE A LOW THRESHOLD FOR CONTACTING THE MOST EXPERIENCED AVAILABLE AIRWAY PROFESSIONAL IN PATIENTS WITH DISEASES ASSOCIATED WITH DIFFICULT AIRWAYS

LAUREN C. BERKOW, MD

Patients in the intensive care unit (ICU) may require airway management for a variety of reasons, but the most common is respiratory distress or failure. Patients may also require intubation for an invasive procedure. Although the majority of patients can be safely intubated by ICU personnel trained in airway management, certain patients may require the assistance of an anesthesiologist. Anesthesiologists are trained to manage the difficult airway and can provide additional resources and skills not routinely found in the ICU setting.

WATCH OUT FOR A patient previously identified as a difficult intubation in the past may not easily be intubated by direct laryngoscopy, and enlisting the help of an anesthesiologist if the patient requires airway management may prevent complications. It is also important to keep in mind that a patient who requires reintubation postoperatively may have developed airway edema or laryngospasm that may complicate intubation. Reintubation may also be difficult if the patient has undergone surgery involving or close to the airway (cervical fusion, thyroidectomy, carotid endarterectomy) or has received large volumes of intravenous fluids or blood products that could lead to airway edema.

ICU patients in respiratory distress or failure often have decreased respiratory reserve and may be hypoxic. These patients desaturate much more quickly during airway management, so preoxygenation is critical, and the amount of time to safely secure the airway might be diminished. This is especially common in patients with obstructive sleep apnea or patients requiring continuous positive airway pressure (CPAP) or bilevel positive airway pressure (BiPAP) to maintain oxygenation. In these patients, if difficulty with mask ventilation or intubation is suspected, contacting your airway professional for assistance prior to intervention may be prudent. It may also be safer to secure the airway early, and in a controlled fashion, prior to the development of acute respiratory distress or failure.

Access to the patient for airway management in the ICU is often more difficult than in the operating room because of the smaller size of the room. Many cables and plugs are connected to an ICU bed and additional monitors or intravenous pumps may limit access to the head of the bed for airway manipulation; space for additional airway equipment may be limited. It may also be difficult for additional personnel to access the patient, for instance, if a cricothyroidotomy or tracheostomy needs to be performed. This can increase the challenge of difficult airway management.

Patients with specific diseases may have an increased likelihood of difficult intubation (*Table 107.1*). Some of these patients may be previously identified as a difficult intubation, but many may not. In addition, these patients may have undergone procedures that may further complicate mask ventilation or intubation, such as cervical fusion or uvulopalatoplasty. These patients may also be more likely to require intensive care management postoperatively after a major procedure because of either their underlying disease state or their difficult airway status.

The ICU setting should contain equipment for both the routine and nonroutine intubation in an easily accessible location, and staff members should be familiar with the location and the equipment. Specialized airway equipment such as a fiberoptic scope, intubation stylets (Eschmann, gum elastic bougie), laryngeal mask airways, cricothyrotomy set, and so on can be assembled into a cart for quick access. Emergency contact numbers for anesthesiology and trauma or ear, nose, and throat (ENT) surgery should also be clearly posted in the ICU.

So, in a patient with a known or suspected difficult airway, who should perform the intubation? It is recommended that the most skilled

TABLE 107.1	DISEASE STATES ASSOCIATED WITH DIFFICULT AIRWAY MANAGEMENT
CONGENITAL	**ACQUIRED**
Pierre Robin syndrome	Morbid obesity
Treacher Collins syndrome	Acromegaly
Goldenhar syndrome	Infections involving the airways
Mucopolysaccharidoses	(Ludwig angina)
Achondroplasia	Rheumatoid arthritis
Micrognathia	Obstructive sleep apnea
Down syndrome	Ankylosing spondylitis
	Tumors involving the airway
	Trauma (airways, cervical spine)

Adapted from Barash PG, Cullen BF, Stoelting RK, eds. Clinical Anesthesia. Philadelphia: Lippincott Williams & Wilkins; 2001; and Benumof JL, ed. Airway Management: Principles and Practice. St. Louis: Mosby; 1996.

professional should perform the procedure. Depending on resources available and the urgency of the intubation, this may be an ICU professional, an anesthesiologist (preferable), or a trauma or ENT surgeon. Having a variety of airway equipment available at all times in the ICU setting is crucial, especially if additional resources are not quickly available. In case of emergency, especially if supraglottic pathology is a possibility, there should be a physician available who is able to perform a cricothyroidotomy if needed.

SUGGESTED READINGS

Benumof J. Airway Management: Principles and Practice. St. Louis: Mosby;1996:129–130.

Practice guidelines for management of the difficult airway. An updated report by the American Society of Anesthesiologists Task Force on Management of the Difficult Airway. Anesthesiology 2003;98:1269–1277.

Stoetling RK, Barash PG, Cullen BF. Clinical Anesthesia. Philadelphia: Lippincott Raven, 1997.

108

ALWAYS USE A VERTICAL INCISION WHEN PERFORMING A CRICOTHYROIDOTOMY

BRANDON R. BRUNS MD
HEIDI L. FRANKEL, MD

No situation in medicine is as stressful as the management of a patient with an unstable airway after multiple failed attempts at endotracheal intubation. Cricothyroidotomy can save the day if performed correctly. The indication for cricothyroidotomy is simple: the inability to obtain an airway by any other means. The maneuver is theoretically simple to perform. However, the stressful situation surrounding a compromised airway requires full understanding of the technique of cricothyroidotomy and a steady hand.

If a prepackaged cricothyroidotomy kit is available, the operator may request it. Otherwise, an antiseptic, a scalpel, and an airway device are all that will be required. Chlorhexidine is a better antiseptic than is an iodine-based solution, but this is of secondary concern. The airway device may either be a small-caliber tracheostomy tube or an endotracheal tube. The anatomical landmarks used to identify the cricothyroid membrane are the thyroid cartilage (Adam's apple) above and the cricoid ring below. The thyroid cartilage is grasped in the operator's nondominant hand while the other hand is used to make a generous *vertical* incision through the skin and subcutaneous tissue. A vertical incision avoids the anterior jugular veins to minimize bleeding. Making a generous incision will allow the necessary exposure. Once the cricoid membrane is located, it is perforated with the tip of the scalpel, which can be moved caudally to expose the airway opening and allow for easy placement of the tube. Once the tube has been placed in the airway, the operator or assistant should maintain control of the airway by keeping at least one hand on it to secure it in place. Tube placement should be confirmed by verifying breath sounds and checking end-tidal carbon dioxide. It should now be easy to oxygenate and ventilate the patient. It is controversial whether a cricothyroidotomy must be converted to a tracheostomy if needed long term.

Experienced practitioners will report that the most difficult aspect of performing a cricothyroidotomy is making the decision to put one in. Although avoiding the anterior jugular veins is highly desirable, speed is of the essence and should take consideration over cosmesis and an inexact entry into the trachea.

SUGGESTED READINGS

Boyd AD, Romita MC, Conlan AA, et al. A clinical evaluation of cricothyroidotomy. Surg Gynecol Obstet 1979;149:365–368.

Francois B, Clavel M, Desachy A, et al. Complications of tracheostomy performed in the ICU: subthyroid tracheostomy versus surgical cricothyroidotomy. Chest 2003;123:151–158.

109

USE BRONCHOSCOPIC GUIDANCE FOR BEDSIDE PERCUTANEOUS DILATATIONAL TRACHEOSTOMY (PDT)

SUSANNA L. MATSEN, MD
ELLIOTT R. HAUT, MD

Percutaneous dilatational tracheostomy (PDT) has quickly become the standard method for conversion from short-term endotracheal intubation to tracheosotomy for longer-term mechanical ventilation. The procedure can be safely performed in the ICU, avoiding transport of critically ill patients to the operating room. The performance of a bedside PDT is contingent upon safety-minded advanced planning and a coordinated team effort. Given the inherent risks to the procedure, thoughtful preparation is essential. In the best case, a bedside tracheostomy proceeds smoothly; in the worst case it can end in tragedy.

Although some providers perform bedside PDT without direct visualization, most have now adopted the protocol of using direct bronchoscopic visualization. Before starting this procedure, adequate personnel must be assembled. One person is designated to manipulate the flexible bronchoscope and stands at the head of the bed. A second person is chosen to maintain control of the airway during manipulation of the endotracheal tube. Another person should be in charge of sedation, anesthesia, and monitoring. One or two people are dedicated to performing the tracheostomy itself.

There is no one best surgical technique for performing bedside percutaneous tracheostomy. A commonly used technique is the sequential dilation technique (i.e., Blue Rhino by Cook). The following steps are used by many surgeons experienced at this technique:

- Position the patient by placing a rolled sheet beneath the shoulders to extend the neck and expose its anterior structures.
- Place a bedside table above the patient's torso and prep and drape the patient.
- Test the tracheostomy balloon and lay out each instrument in the order in which they will be used.
- After infiltrating local anesthetic, use the scalpel to make a vertical incision through the skin into the subcutaneous tissue (about 2 cm superior to the sternal notch).

- Use a blunt clamp to dissect the midline connective tissues off the anterior wall of the trachea (use of a blunt technique minimizes bleeding potential).
- The bronchoscope operator advances the endoscope to transilluminate the site of the entry into the trachea (when positioned correctly the surgeons will see a glow through the trachea).
- Advance a finder needle and then a larger bore needle carefully through the trachea between the first and second or second and third tracheal rings under direct visualization with the broncohoscope.
- Pass the wire through the needle and remove the needle (Seldinger technique).
- Visualize the wire placement into the trachea and direction of passage with bronchoscopic visualization.
- Begin the sequential dilations over the wire (Seldinger technique) and eventually place the tracheostomy tube.
- Confirm tube placement by visualization of the carina when the bronchoscope is placed down the new tracheostomy tube and return of end-tidal CO_2 when ventilated.

There are a number of techniques that should keep the operator out of surgical bleeding. First and foremost, the surgeon should know the anatomy of the neck and stay between the parallel anterior jugular veins. These run on either side of the trachea between the midline and sternocleidomastoid, coursing from the region of the hyoid inferiorly to drain to the external jugular vein or subclavian vein. By staying squarely in the midline and using a vertical incision, the surgeon can avoid these structures, which may bleed profusely if entered and completely obscure the operative field. If these veins are visualized and are likely to interfere with the procedure, they may be suture ligated. Another potential source of bleeding includes the divided thyroid isthmus which can usually be controlled with direct pressure. The most serious (but thankfully rare) source of bleeding is the innominate artery, which may necessitate median sternotomy for exposure and control. The team should make every effort to remain calm in the event of profuse bleeding. Of utmost importance in this situation is to maintain the airway and protect the endotracheal tube. Provided this is done, the team can then decide on the appropriate next step, which may be a move to the operating room while maintaining direct pressure on any sources of bleeding. Often this venous bleeding will stop from tamponade once the tracheostomy is in place.

One tool that should never be used to control bleeding during tracheostomy is electrocautery. The combination of the electric current with sparks and high-flow oxygen from the endotracheal tube comprise the two ingredients for combustion, risking serious burns to the patient and staff. Although surgeons have become accustomed to using electrocautery for hemostasis, this is a case where it is contraindicated.

SUGGESTED READINGS

Bojar RM, Warner KG, eds. Manual of Perioperative Care in Cardiac Surgery. 3rd Ed. Blackwell: Malden; 1999:459–461.

Zollinger RM Jr, Zollinger RM Sr, eds. Zollinger's Atlas of Surgical Operations. 8th Ed. New York: McGraw-Hill; 2003:374–375.

http://www.cookgroup.com/cook_critical_care/features/blue_rhino.html

Delaney A, Bagshaw SM, Nalos M. Percutaneous dilatational tracheostomy versus surgical tracheostomy in critically ill patients: a systematic review and meta-analysis. Crit Care. 2006;10(2):R55. at http://ccforum.com/content/10/2/R55

Freeman BD, Isabella K, Lin N, Buchman TG. A meta-analysis of prospective trials comparing percutaneous and surgical tracheostomy in critically ill patients. Chest. 2000;118(5):1412-1418.

110

CONSIDER EARLY TRACHEOSTOMY IN SELECT PATIENTS

KONSTANTINOS SPANIOLAS, MD
GEORGE C. VELMAHOS, MD, PhD

The timing of tracheostomy presents an ongoing debate. Studies are inconsistent on what is considered early or late. Studied populations are relatively small and meta-analysis is flawed as the criteria of tracheostomy timing vary from paper to paper. The risk of the surgical procedure is not insignificant. Direct procedural complications (such as bleeding), long-term complications (such as tracheal stenosis), and indirect complications (such as risks of transporting critically ill patients to the operating room for open tracheostomy) should be balanced against the benefits of better oral and pulmonary toilet, easier weaning, and reduction of airway resistance. The risks of transportation from the intensive care unit (ICU) to the operating room include tube and line dislodgment, suboptimal monitoring during transport, and inability to manage critical events. Bedside tracheostomy by the percutaneous dilatational technique has emerged as a safe alternative to open tracheostomy. All would agree that if a tracheostomy is eventually needed, it would better be done earlier than later. The problem lies in our inadequacy to predict accurately the duration of mechanical ventilation. For patients who would need prolonged mechanical ventilation (usually defined as longer than 2 weeks), most surgeons agree that an early tracheostomy is beneficial.

The existing prospective randomized trials have failed to show a survival advantage of early tracheostomy. However, according to five randomized control trials, the length of mechanical ventilation is significantly reduced by a tracheostomy performed within 6 days of hospital admission compared with a tracheostomy performed after 14 days.

SUGGESTED READINGS

Griffiths J, Barber VS, Morgan L, et al. Systematic review and meta-analysis of studies of the timing of tracheostomy in adult patients undergoing artificial ventilation. BMJ 2005;330:1243–1247.

Moller MG, Slaikeu JD, Bonelli P, et al. Early tracheostomy versus late tracheostomy in the surgical intensive care unit. Am J Surg 2005;189:293–296.

Velmahos GC, Belzberg H, Chan L, et al. Factors predicting prolonged mechanical ventilation in critically injured patients: introducing a simplified quantitative risk score. Am Surg 1997;63:811–817.

Velmahos GC, Gomez H, Boicey CM, et al. Bedside percutaneous tracheostomy: prospective evaluation of a modification of the current technique in 100 patients. World J Surg 2000;24:1109–1115.

111

POSITION THE TIP OF THE ENDOTRACHEAL TUBE 4 CENTIMETERS ABOVE THE CARINA

LEO HSIAO, DO

Establishment of the airway is an integral part of any resuscitative algorithm. In the acute setting it is often necessary to intubate a patient in order to secure a means of providing ventilation. To this end, the position of the endotracheal tube is paramount to its success. A malpositioned endotracheal tube can be detrimental and potentially life threatening (*Fig. 111.1*).

To briefly review, the upper airway begins at the nose and mouth and ends at the carina where the trachea divides into the left and right main-stem bronchi. The nose and mouth form a common passage posteriorly called the pharynx, which is divided into three parts: nasopharynx, oropharynx, and laryngopharynx. The pharynx leads to the trachea anteriorly and the esophagus posteriorly. The glottis is the inlet to the trachea. It is bordered by the vocal cords laterally and epiglottis superiorly. The trachea, which corresponds to the C6 vertebra posteriorly, is a tubular conduit supported by semicircular cartilaginous rings leading down to the carina, the branching point for the main-stem bronchi.

WHAT TO DO

In determining the proper placement of an endotracheal tube, the length of the segments through which the tube must pass should be considered. The distance from the teeth to the vocal cords is approximately 10 to 15 cm. Once through the glottic aperture, the trachea measures another 12 to 15 cm to its end at the carina. Because the tip of the endotracheal tube is optimally positioned at 4 cm above the carina, some authors advocate empiric insertion of the endotracheal tube to a depth of 23 cm and 21 cm, measured at the lips, for men and women, respectively. Auscultation of the bilateral lung fields and stomach should follow intubation. The presence of sustained end-tidal CO_2 is confirmatory of tracheal placement. A chest radiograph then confirms the position of the tube and the need for subsequent repositioning. An improperly positioned endotracheal tube can be dangerous if left unchecked. Esophageal intubation is diagnosed by nonsustained or absent end-tidal CO_2 and epigastric gurgling on ventilation. Ventilation should be terminated immediately to avert insufflation of the stomach, which can increase gastric pressures and the risk for aspiration.

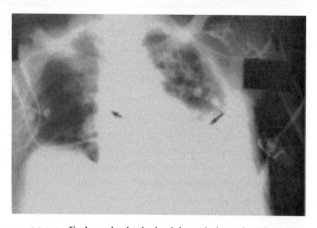

FIGURE 111.1. Endotracheal tube in right main bronchus. Portable examination, anteroposterior view, shows bilateral pulmonary edema and a dense left lower lobe (*long arrow*). The endotracheal tube is in the bronchus intermedius (*short arrow*), obstructing the left main bronchus and causing left lower lobe atelectasis. (Reused with permission from Umali CB. Chest radiographic examination. In: Irwin RS, Rippe JM, eds. Irwin and Rippe's Intensive Care Medicine. 5th Ed. Philadelphia: Lippincott Williams & Wilkins; 2003:705.)

Even when tracheal intubation is achieved, the position of the tube can be hazardous depending on its position within the trachea. If the endotracheal tube is too cephalad in position the danger of inadvertent extubation and vocal-cord injury becomes problematic. On the other hand, if the endotracheal tube is advanced too deeply, the risk of main-stem intubation is of concern. Because the right main-stem bronchus forms a more obtuse angle with the trachea than the left main-stem bronchus, it is more commonly intubated on deep advancement. Endobronchial intubation, regardless of side, is diagnosed by unequal or unilateral breath sounds, high peak airway pressures, and hypoxemia. If left unchecked there is a potential for bronchospasms, contralateral atelectasis, and ipsilateral tension pneumothorax.

Once the decision is made to reposition the endotracheal tube, the most accurate manner of determining proper positioning is with a fiberoptic bronchoscope. However, this is often impractical and typically the tube is retracted or advanced, with the cuff down, by 1-cm increments, taking care to reassess by auscultation over the bilateral lung fields. Alternatively, if there is a chest radiograph available, the degree of retraction or advancement can be estimated on film.

SUGGESTED READINGS

Miller RD, ed. Miller's Anesthesia. 6th Ed. Philadelphia: Churchill Livingstone; 2004:1617–1618,1633–1635,1648–1649.

Morgan E, Mikhail M, Murray M, et al., eds. Clinical Anesthesiology. 3rd Ed. New York: McGraw-Hill; 2002:72–74, 79–80.

REMEMBER THAT EVEN A FULLY INFLATED CUFF ON THE ENDOTRACHEAL TUBE IS NOT ADEQUATE PROTECTION AGAINST ASPIRATION

ASHITA GOEL, MD

CASE

A 45-year-old obese male presented as an emergency to the operating room (OR) for gunshot wound to the abdomen. The patient's records indicated a history of severe sleep apnea. In addition, the patient had eaten a large meal prior to his injury. On physical exam, the patient had signs of a difficult airway. Necessary precautions were taken to decrease the risk of aspiration by employing an awake fiberoptic technique for intubation. During the case, the patient's saturation declined with copious particulate secretions rising from the endotracheal tube. A diagnosis of intraoperative aspiration was made.

DISCUSSION

Aspiration can be a fatal complication of intubated patients. Although a cuffed endotracheal tube can decrease the risk, it does not eliminate the risk of aspiration. The exact incidence of clinically relevant aspiration is unknown. However, it is estimated that up to 1 of 3,000 operations is complicated by intraoperative aspiration pneumonitis. Multiple factors account for the inexactness, including subclinical microaspiration, misdiagnosis, and variations in the patient population under study. The risk of aspiration increases in patients with altered airway reflexes (e.g., drugs, general anesthesia, stroke, neuromuscular disease, encephalopathy) and in patients with altered anatomy (e.g., hiatal hernia, pregnancy, obesity, poor lower esophageal sphincter tone, full stomach). Additional patient-related risk factors include extremes of age, acuity of surgery, and abdominal surgery.

The modern cuffed endotracheal tubes come in two major types: high pressure, low volume and low pressure, high volume. The low-pressure cuff is more commonly used because it provides a greater contact area between the cuff and the tracheal mucosa. As a result, the low-pressure system decreases the risk of ischemic mucosal damage when compared with the high-pressure system. The low-pressure cuff, however, increases the risk of sore throat, aspiration, spontaneous extubation, and difficult insertion. Classically, in the low-pressure system, the endotracheal cuff is inflated to approximately 20 to 25 mm Hg, which provides reasonable protection from aspiration and limits ischemic injury to the trachea. Tracheal perfusion pressure ranges from 25 to 35 mm Hg.

It is important to note if there is evidence of aspiration, it does not necessarily mean a patient will develop aspiration pneumonitis. The risk of pneumonitis is based on gastric volume (>25 mL or >0.3 mL/kg) and acidity of gastric fluid (pH <2.5). However, gastric contents can also damage lung tissue if it contains food particulates or bacteria. Patients on H2-blockers or proton pump inhibitors are thought to be at increased risk for gastric colonization by bacteria secondary to a more neutral pH environment.

SIGNS AND SYMPTOMS

Aspiration pneumonitis results in damage to the tracheobronchial tree and the lung parenchyma. The initial reaction is the result of damage to tissue from caustic gastric secretions. Secondary damage occurs from the body's inflammatory response, mediated by neutrophils and cytokine release. Aspiration can present as dyspnea, cyanosis, coughing, wheezing, pulmonary edema, hypotension, and hypoxia. Patients can rapidly progress to respiratory distress and even death. It is estimated that 10% to 30% of anesthetic deaths are a result of aspiration pneumonitis. However, the majority of patients with aspiration are clinically asymptomatic. Radiographically, patients may show evidence of atelectasis, alveolar edema, and interstitial edema.

If aspiration is suspected, the patient's upper airway should be suctioned. In intubated patients, the lower airway should be suctioned through the endotracheal tube. Intubation should be considered for nonintubated patients that have aspirated to decrease the risk of further aspiration and to assist with ventilatory support. Generally, prophylactic antibiotics are not recommended because prophylactic treatment may result in selection of more resistant organisms. However, empiric treatment with antibiotics is recommended for patients with known aspiration and gastric dysmotility or gastric colonization (e.g., small bowel obstruction, gastric paresis, proton pump inhibitors). Also, empirical therapy is recommended for patients whose aspiration pneumonitis symptoms fail to resolve after 48 hours. Corticosteroids have been used in the past in the management of aspiration pneumonitis.

However, there is limited data on the role of these agents as therapy for aspiration pneumonitis.

SUGGESTED READINGS

Blunt MC, Young PJ, Patil A, et al. Gel lubrication of the tracheal tube cuff reduces pulmonary aspiration. Anesthesiology 2001;95:377–381.

Marik P. Aspiration pneumonitis and aspiration pneumonia. N Engl J Med 2001; 344:665–671.

Miller RD, ed. Miller's Anesthesia. 6th Ed. Philadelphia: Elsevier/Churchill Livingstone; 2005:1634–1636.

113

DO NOT OVERINFLATE THE ENDOTRACHEAL CUFF

GREGORY DALENCOURT, MD
ELIZABETH A. MARTINEZ, MD, MHS

A large percentage of patients who are cared for in the intensive care unit (ICU) are intubated with an endotracheal tube. Regardless of the reason for requiring intubation, key factors must be understood when caring for such patients. The endotracheal tube (ETT) is typically placed orally using a laryngoscope and is advanced just past the vocal cords until the cuff disappears (to the view of the operator). The cuff is then inflated. The distension of the pilot balloon, next to the injection port, reflects inflation of the ETT cuff. The appropriate position of the ETT cuff is distal to the cords with the tip 4 cm above the carina. Confirmation of ETT placement in the trachea is best accomplished with the use of end-tidal carbon dioxide confirmation. Auscultation of bilateral breath sounds may confirm placement in the trachea and is useful in evaluating whether the ETT is too deep, resulting in endobronchial intubation. This is clinically indicated by loss of breath sounds in one of the lung fields, typically the left because of the straight path to the right main-stem bronchus compared with the sharp angle to the left. The ETT is then secured with tape or other ETT-securing devices.

WATCH OUT FOR

The purpose of the ETT cuff is to facilitate positive-pressure ventilation and prevent aspiration of secretions by forming a seal within the trachea. The current practice is use of a low-pressure, high-volume cuff. The risk of high-pressure cuffs is that the pressure transmitted to the underlying tracheal mucosa can cause ischemia when the cuff pressure exceeds the capillary arteriolar pressure (approximately 32 mm Hg). The low-pressure cuffs are preferred to limit this risk of ischemia and the recommended maximum pressure of the cuff is 25 mm HG. Low-pressure, high-volume cuffs inflate more symmetrically than high-pressure cuffs, which may also decrease the risk of tracheal dilatation, and they can inflate to the shape of the patient's trachea, optimizing the seal.

The fact that cuffs are "low pressure" does not mean that one cannot overinflate them and increase the pressure such that there is risk of ischemia. Any type of cuff can become a high-pressure cuff if enough

air is injected or if inadvertent overinflation occurs, as with the diffusion of nitrous oxide into the cuff over time. In addition, the pressure
estimated by palpating the pilot balloon frequently underestimates the
actual cuff pressure, so either cuff pressure should be measured and
documented on a regular basis or the cuff should be inflated only to
the point of eliminating the leak during positive-pressure ventilation.

Commonly, a cuff leak is noted when air leaks around the cuff
during positive-pressure ventilation. When this occurs, the first maneuver is to add additional air into the cuff. This procedure not only
increases the risk of cuff overinflation and mucosal ischemia but can
also lead to unidentified herniation of the cuff above the cords. When
there is a new leak around the cuff, the position of the ETT should be
determined. On average, insertion of an ETT to 20 to 22 cm beyond
the lips in an average adult places the ETT tip in the midtrachea.
However, in patients who have had prolonged intubation, the ETT
may soften and bulge into the posterior pharynx, and thus the depth
marker may become less reliable.

When investigating and correcting a cuff leak, observe the following steps:

- Review the most recent chest x-ray.
- Obtain a repeat x-ray if time permits.
- Suction the posterior pharynx.
- Deflate the balloon to confirm how much air has been inflated.
- Reinflate the pilot balloon with the minimum volume of air required
  to prevent a leak (typically, 3 to 6 mL is sufficient with a maximum
  of 10 mL of air volume required to obtain a seal).
- If >10 mL is aspirated, one must be suspicious that the balloon
  has been hyperinflated and is either bridging the cords or migrating
  supraglottic (above the cords) and putting the patient at risk for
  inadvertent extubation.
- Consider direct visualization with laryngoscopy or a fiberoptic scope
  and advancement or repositioning of the ETT.

SUGGESTED READINGS

Braz JR, Navarro LH, Takata IH, et al. Endotracheal tube cuff pressure: need for precise
measurement. Sao Paulo Med J 1999;117:243–247.
Schmidt GA, Hall JB, Wood LDH. Principles of Critical Care. New York: McGraw-
Hill, Health Professions Division; 1992:594–595.
Stoelting RK, Miller RD. Basics of Anesthesia. 2nd ed. New York: Churchill Living-
stone; 1989:163–166.

114

CHECK FOR A CUFF LEAK IN PATIENTS WHO MIGHT HAVE TRACHEAL EDEMA BEFORE EXTUBATION

E. DAVID BRAVOS, MD

Critically ill patients often require intubation and mechanical ventilation. Along with the morbidities of intubation, problems following extubation can occur. Airway obstruction from laryngeal or tracheal edema is a significant risk and can result in respiratory distress that may require emergent reintubation. Risk factors for airway edema include traumatic or difficult intubation, duration of intubation, high balloon cuff pressure or large endotracheal tube size, inhalational injuries including burns or caustic substances, and recent self-extubation.

WHAT TO DO

The gold standard for detection of airway edema is direct visualization. However, the presence of an endotracheal tube obscures the view, making this sometimes difficult. Indirect methods of determining airway edema such as the cuff-leak test are commonly used. This test measures whether air is able to pass around the outside of the endotracheal tube through the patient's airway when the cuff of the tube is deflated and the patient exhales. This can be assessed qualitatively and quantitatively. Qualitatively, cooperative patients should breathe when the cuff is deflated with assessment for the presence of stridor. This is more commonly done in pediatric patients with croup. More recently, quantitative measurements are done by comparing the returned tidal volume of patients on volume-control ventilation when the cuff is inflated as well as deflated. The difference in the two values is the cuff leak. In practice, several tidal volumes are recorded (usually five to six) with the cuff deflated and the values averaged. Additionally, the size of the cuff leak has been hypothesized to be inversely proportional to the amount of edema and potential obstruction.

Sensitivity and specificity of the cuff-leak test have been variable in reported studies but have been as high as 100% and 99%, respectively. Additionally, positive and negative predictive values have been reported to be as high as 69% and 98%, respectively. Variability in reported values may reflect variable patient populations studied. Therefore, when deciding to extubate a patient, one should use the cuff-leak test as a guide for patients who may be at risk for postextubation airway obstruction rather than an absolute criteria for extubation.

Additionally, it may also suggest which patients may need closer monitoring after extubation and might benefit from treatment for stridor with bronchodilators, helium-oxygen mixtures, or corticosteroids.

SUGGESTED READINGS

De Backer D. The cuff-leak test: what are we measuring? Crit Care 2005;9:31–33.

Jaber S, Chanques G, Matecki S, et al. Post-extubation stridor in intensive care unit patients. Risk factors: evaluation and importance of the cuff-leak test. Intens Care Med 2003;29:69–74.

Miller RL, Cole RP. Association between reduced cuff leak volume and postextubation stridor. Chest 1996;110:1035–1040.

115

KNOW HOW TO MEASURE PLATEAU PRESSURE WHEN USING PRESSURE-REGULATED VOLUME CONTROL VENTILATION MODE AND KNOW WHAT TO DO WITH THE VALUE ONCE IT IS OBTAINED

DAVID N. HAGER, MD

Mechanical ventilation has been shown to cause ventilation-induced lung injury by at least two mechanisms. First, using a low lung volume allows the repeated opening and closing of small airways and alveoli. This is associated with high shear forces on the lung interstitium and alveolar surfactant depletion, both of which result in ventilation-induced lung injury. To reduce this low-volume injury, the use of positive end-expiratory pressure (PEEP) is advocated, though the ideal amount of PEEP continues to be the topic of intense study. Second, the use of too much PEEP and/or the use of supraphysiologic tidal volumes have been shown to cause ventilation-induced lung injury by overdistention of alveoli. Historically, alveolar overdistention has been a concern when plateau pressure (Pplat) is >30 cm H_2O. Although much attention is often given to high peak airway pressure, it is Pplat that reflects alveolar pressure, value most associated with ventilation-induced lung injury. Two approaches to limiting alveolar overdistention are (a) to reduce tidal volume until plateau pressure ≤ 30 cm H_2O during assist volume control (AC) ventilation or (b) to limit inspiratory airway pressure to ≤ 30 cm H_2O during pressure-regulated volume control (PRVC) ventilation. The astute clinician will be able to understand (a) the differences between AC and PRVC ventilation modes, (b) that alveolar pressures ≤ 30 cm H_2O might not be uniformly safe, and (c) the appropriate strategy that limits both low volume and overdistention lung injury.

CONTROLLED MODES OF VENTILATION

AC and PRVC are both "controlled" modes of mechanical ventilation. For each, the clinician sets a minimum respiratory rate, which ensures a set number of breaths even if the patient is apneic or paralyzed. A nonparalyzed/nonapneic patient who triggers the ventilator in excess of this set rate will receive full ventilator support for each additional breath. However, the modes differ in how the magnitude of tidal volumes are determined. During assist control ventilation, the clinician sets a tidal volume, inspiratory flow rate, inspiratory time, and inspiratory flow waveform. Irrespective of lung compliance, airway resistance, or simultaneous attempts at active exhalation by the patient, the set tidal volume will be delivered. For this reason, even in the apneic patient, a minimum minute ventilation (respiratory rate times tidal volume) is guaranteed, though there is the potential for high peak airway pressures. Plateau pressure is measured at end inspiration by occluding the expiratory valve of the ventilator circuit. This allows airway pressure to equilibrate throughout the lungs.

By contrast, the magnitudes of tidal volume during PRVC ventilation are dependent on the level of the inspiratory airway pressure, lung compliance, airway resistance, and even patient effort. The ventilator automatically adjusts inspiratory flow and flow waveform as it attempts to maintain a constant inspiratory pressure. Though the respiratory rate and inspiratory pressures are chosen to achieve adequate minute ventilation, tidal-volume size may vary from breath to breath. Despite this variability, some argue that PRVC is attractive because airway pressures will never exceed the prescribed level. If, for example, the inspiratory pressure is set at 29 cm H_2O, the "dangerous" threshold of 30 cm H_2O is theoretically never reached. Plateau pressures will always be *less than or equal to* the prescribed inspiratory pressure. On some ventilators, obtaining the plateau pressure value cannot be done in the PRVC mode and a brief transition to AC is required to measure plateau pressure.

AIRWAY PRESSURES

As mentioned earlier, clinicians have historically tried to avoid plateau pressures >30 cm H_2O. The focus on this threshold pressure is likely based on three observations. However, when each observation is reviewed carefully, the concept of a "safe" plateau pressure threshold appears to be misguided. First, though early animal studies did show ventilation-induced lung injury to occur predominantly in animals ventilated at airway pressures >30 cm H_2O, these studies were only a few hours long at most. When similar studies were conducted over a period of days, significant lung injury was observed even in animals ventilated at the reportedly safe inspiratory pressure of 30 cm H_2O. Second, the normal transpulmonary pressure in humans at total lung capacity is approximately 30 to 35 cm H_2O. It has been reasoned that if a person can generate these pressures spontaneously, such pressures are unlikely to cause lung injury. However, exposure to pressures of this magnitude during a solitary maneuver to achieve total lung capacity is very different than being exposed to such pressures several thousand times per day, as may occur during mechanical ventilation. Third, in the context of randomized controlled trials of low (6 mL/kg) versus traditional (12 mL/kg) tidal volumes in patients with acute lung injury and the acute respiratory distress syndrome (ARDS), only those studies in which mean plateau pressures were ≥ 32 cm H_2O among the traditional tidal-volume group was a mortality benefit associated with low tidal volumes. Some have therefore reasoned that if plateau pressure is <32 cm H_2O, there is no benefit in tidal-volume reduction. However, close inspection of the data from the largest and most rigorously conducted of these studies shows a steady decline in mortality as plateau pressure decreases well below 30 cm H_2O, irrespective of randomization group. In other words, patients randomized to the low-tidal-volume group did better even when compared with patients randomized to the traditional-tidal-volume group in whom plateau pressure was <30 cm H_2O. For these reasons, it seems inappropriate to assume that an airway pressure of 30 cm H_2O is safe, be it plateau pressure generated during AC ventilation, or the set inspiratory pressure during PRVC.

STRATEGY

Because ventilation at low lung volumes and overdistention of alveoli are the two leading causes of ventilation-induced lung injury, mechanical ventilation strategies should be tailored to limit these two types of injury. It is known that PEEP decreases low-volume injury, although how one determines the ideal PEEP is a continued topic of study. A good general guideline is to start all patients with PEEP = 5 cm H_2O and titrate upward according to oxygenation requirement as per the Acute Respiratory Distress Syndrome (ARDS) Network low-tidal-volume strategy. Like PEEP, recommendations for determining the appropriate tidal volume are in evolution. It is generally agreed that tidal volumes >10 mL/kg are excessive even in uninjured lungs. However, the best evidence to date shows that among patients with acute lung injury or ARDS, tidal volume should be set to 6 mL/kg predicted body weight, even when plateau pressures are not >30 cm H_2O. This is easily done in the AC mode by dialing in the desired tidal volume. However, during PRVC ventilation, tidal volume is set by adjusting the inspiratory pressure. Though this too is easily accomplished, it requires close follow-up and frequent adjustments because a given inspiratory pressure may ultimately deliver tidal volumes that are too small in a patient whose lung compliance is worsening or too big in a. It should not be assumed *a priori* that inspiratory airway pressures ≤ 30 cm H_2O are safe.

SUGGESTED READINGS

Dreyfuss D, Saumon G. Ventilator-induced lung injury: lessons from experimental studies. Am J Respir Crit Care Med 1998;157:294–323.

Hager DN, Krishnan JA, Hayden DL, et al. Tidal volume reduction in patients with acute lung injury when plateau pressures are not high. Am J Resp Crit 2005;172:1241–1245.

Ventilation with lower tidal volumes as compared with traditional tidal volumes for acute lung injury and the acute respiratory distress syndrome. The Acute Respiratory Distress Syndrome Network. N Engl J Med 2000;342:1301–1308.

116

USE PLATEAU OR MEAN PRESSURE AS A MORE ACCURATE ASSESSMENT OF BAROTRAUMA THAN PEAK PRESSURE

BENJAMIN KRATZERT, MD
ANUSHIRVAN MINOKADEH, MD

Monitoring lung mechanics during mechanical ventilation has become an important parameter for managing pulmonary disease and acute changes in respiratory status in patients. Additionally, this monitoring is used to adjust ventilator settings for prevention of alveolar overdistention (or barotrauma) and to attempt to improve clinical outcomes. The two most common airway-pressure parameters used are peak inspiratory pressure (PIP) and plateau pressure (Pplat).

PIP is measured at the end of inspiratory inflation (see *Fig. 116.1*) and is a function of the inflation volume, the flow resistance of the airways, and the compliance of the lungs and chest wall. Since PIP is greatly influenced by resistance in the upper airways and ventilator equipment, it represents a poor marker of alveolar pressures. The most accurate measurement of alveolar pressure is plateau pressure. This value reflects airway pressure during a 1- to 2-second inspiratory

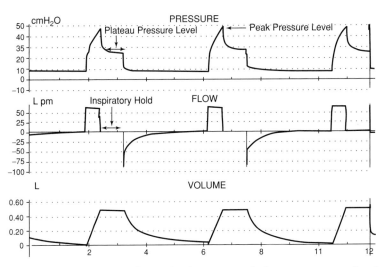

FIGURE 116.1. Pressure, flow, and volume curves during measurement of peak and plateau pressures.

pause and therefore is less influenced by ventilator equipment. The Pplat approximates small airway and alveolar pressure more closely than PIP. It is believed that control of the Pplat is important as excessive stretch of alveoli has been implicated as the cause of ventilator-induced lung injury. The recent Acute Respiratory Distress Syndrome (ARDS) Network multicenter prospective randomized trial showed that maintaining plateau pressures at ≤ 30 cm H_2O, with resultant permissive hypercapnia, resulted in a statistically significant decrease in the number of ventilator days and improved mortality.

Different ventilator strategies are useful in modifying Pplat. These strategies include lowering tidal volume, shortening inspiratory time, decreasing inspiratory flow rate, avoiding auto positive end-expiratory pressure (PEEP), permissive hypercapnia, pressure control ventilation, pressure-regulated volume control ventilation, and treating pulmonary edema.

SELECTED READINGS

ARDS Network. Ventilation with lower tidal volumes as compared with traditional tidal volumes for acute lung injury and the acute respiratory distress syndrome. N Engl J Med 2000;342:1301–1308.

Dreyfuss D, Saumon G. Ventilator-induced lung injury: lessons from experimental studies. Am J Respir Crit Care Med 1998;157:294–323.

Marino PL. The ICU Book. 2nd Ed. Baltimore: Williams & Wilkins; 1998:421–423.

Tobin MJ. Principles and Practice of Mechanical Ventilation. New York: McGraw-Hill; 1994.

117

CONSIDER AIRWAY PRESSURE RELEASE VENTILATION FOR DELIVERING AN OPEN-LUNG STRATEGY

ANTHONY D. SLONIM, MD, DRPH

Airway pressure release ventilation (APRV) is a newer mode of mechanical ventilation that alternates between two levels of continuous positive airway pressure (CPAP). The set rate for this mode of ventilation is normally 20 or fewer breaths per minute to prevent inverse ratio ventilation. The levels of CPAP are referred to as the high-pressure and low-pressure limits and also need to be set to allow adequate oxygenation. In addition, the provider needs to set two times, which allow the ventilator to cycle between the high- and low-pressure levels for 0.5 to 1.5 seconds. When the machine cycles to the lower CPAP level, exhalation occurs.

Since APRV is a newer mode of ventilation, it has not been fully evaluated in clinical trials, but early data are encouraging regarding its effectiveness. The value of APRV is derived from its ability to provide adequate oxygenation at lower pressure levels. Intrapulmonary shunt with spontaneous breathing appears to be reduced with APRV. The high-pressure limit provides for an open-lung strategy, and the low-pressure limit prevents shear stress and cyclic alveolar collapse with atelectasis, both of which contribute to ventilator-induced lung injury. As the patient's condition improves, the lung can be "deflated" by reducing the pressure limits and times to allow for normal pressure-limited mechanical ventilation. When the patient is able, the ventilator rate can be reduced to allow the patient to take on more of the work of breathing in preparation for extubation.

The major challenges occurring with APRV include the need to monitor the level of hypoventilation, hypercarbia, and respiratory acidosis. While permissive hypercapnia is a valuable technique for lung protection, patients on APRV may develop considerable hypercarbia with a resulting respiratory acidosis. In addition, the need to maintain the pressure levels to support an open-lung strategy may lead to hypotension if the patient is hemodynamically unstable or has a reduced preload. Volume loading can assist with this problem. However, on some occasions, hemodynamic compromise may not allow this mode of ventilation to be used effectively.

SUGGESTED READINGS

Goldman L, Ausiello D, eds. Cecil Textbook of Internal Medicine. 22nd Ed. Philadelphia: Saunders; 2004:410–424.

Wrigge H, Zinserling J, Neumann P, et al. Spontaneous breathing with airway pressure release ventilation favors spontaneous ventilation in dependent lung regions and counters cyclic alveolar collapse in oleic-acid-induced lung injury: a randomized controlled computed tomography trial. Crit Care Med 2005;9:780–789.

118

REMEMBER THAT STATIC COMPLIANCE OF THE RESPIRATORY SYSTEM IS NOT THE SAME THING AS DYNAMIC COMPLIANCE

NIRAV G. SHAH, MD

Compliance is a measure of lung distensibility and is measured as a change in lung volume per unit change in pressure. There are two different types of lung compliance—static and dynamic. Static lung compliance is represented by the slope of the pressure-volume curve during deflation from total lung capacity. In a patient who is being mechanically ventilated, this can be measured by dividing the exhaled tidal volume by the difference between the plateau pressure (Pplat) and the positive end-expiratory pressure (PEEP) after temporary occlusion of the expiratory limb of the ventilator circuit. The peak pressure is the most accurate reflection of static compliance.

Dynamic compliance is the ratio of the change in volume to the change in pressure over a tidal breath. Insofar as there is no abnormality in the exhaled tidal volume, a decrease in dynamic lung compliance would suggest disease or narrowing of the smaller airways. The plateau pressure most accurately reflects this measurement.

When optimizing the settings for mechanical ventilation, it is important to be able to control the tidal volumes as well as the airway pressures. There have been several large trials suggesting that a low-tidal-volume strategy improves mortality. This is thought to result from the pressure-volume curves in acute respiratory distress syndrome (ARDS) patients who show a flattened curve initially at low lung volumes, indicating that a small increase in pressure results in large changes in volume. One goal is to keep the PEEP above the point at which compliance significantly decreases. This is known as the lower inflection point.

There is great debate about the most optimal mode of ventilation chosen for patients with poor lung compliance. Pressure-control ventilation controls airway pressures but can result in large variations in tidal volume to maintain the set pressure. Volume-control ventilation controls the tidal volume but can result in increased airway pressures if faced with air trapping, decreased lung compliance, or worsening respiratory mechanics. As a patient's compliance worsens, it may be necessary to alternate modes of ventilation to achieve the needs of the patient while minimizing the effects of acute lung injury. Conversely, as compliance improves, the plateau pressures and peak pressures may decrease, indicating an improved readiness for weaning from mechanical ventilation, depending on the ventilation mode.

SUGGESTED READINGS

Byrne K, Cooper KR, Carey PD, et al. Pulmonary compliance: early assessment of evolving lung injury after onset of sepsis. J Appl Physiol 1990;69:2290–2295.

Ware LB, Matthay MA. The acute respiratory distress syndrome. N Engl J Med 2000;342:1334–1349.

119

REMEMBER THAT RECRUITMENT OF ALVEOLI USING AN INCREASED LEVEL OF POSITIVE END-EXPIRATORY PRESSURE CAN TAKE 6 TO 12 HOURS

DAVID N. HAGER, MD

There are two forms of positive end-expiratory pressure (PEEP). These are extrinsic PEEP and intrinsic-PEEP (aka, auto-PEEP). Extrinsic PEEP is the pressure applied to the airways by the ventilator at end expiration. Intrinsic PEEP is the pressure remaining in the airways in excess of extrinsic PEEP upon occluding the expiratory valve at end expiration. Extrinsic PEEP is typically used for three reasons: (a) to decrease work of breathing in patients with intrinsic PEEP, (b) to reduce or avoid atelectasis, and (c) to improve arterial oxygenation and avoid or limit low-volume lung injury. The purpose of this chapter is to review the use of PEEP in each of these situations.

WORK OF BREATHING AND PEEP

The use of extrinsic PEEP in the context of obstructive lung disease may decrease the work of breathing. At end expiration, many of these patients will have measurable intrinsic PEEP. They must therefore drop their pleural pressure far enough to (a) overcome their intrinsic PEEP and (b) trigger the ventilator. For example, if a given patient has an intrinsic PEEP of 5 cm H_2O and the ventilator trigger threshold is set at negative 2 cm H_2O, the patient has to decrease his or her pleural pressure by 7 cm H_2O before the ventilator will deliver the next assisted breath. In this situation, that application of 5 cm H_2O of extrinsic PEEP will decrease the patient's work of breathing. The patient will then need to decrease his or her pleural pressure by only 2 cm H_2O. The often cited concern that the use of *low* levels of extrinsic PEEP (5 cm H_2O) will substantially increase the hazards of hyperinflation have been overemphasized.

ATELECTASIS AND PEEP

Ventilation at low lung volumes with deep sedation predisposes patients to the development of atelectasis. Though there are no convincing data to suggest that important outcomes such as duration of mechanical ventilation, morbidity, or mortality are reduced by the empiric use of low levels of PEEP (5 cm H_2O) in healthy patients, many clinicians have adopted this practice based on physiologic measurements that show that such maneuvers reduce shunt.

LOW-VOLUME LUNG INJURY, OXYGENATION, AND PEEP

In patients with acute lung injury (ALI) and the acute respiratory distress syndrome (ARDS), higher levels of PEEP will improve oxygenation by opening (recruiting) atelectatic lung. It has also been suggested that PEEP will limit low-volume lung injury, which results from the repeated opening and closing of small airways and alveoli during tidal ventilation. This action is associated with high shear forces on the lung interstitium and surfactant depletion, both of which exacerbate ventilator-associated lung injury. Though the use of PEEP is strongly advocated in these patients based on observations in animal models, the extent to which PEEP should be raised in adults with ALI or ARDS is not clear despite a large body of literature that focuses on different approaches to the identification of "optimal" PEEP. Some investigators have suggested adjusting PEEP to a pressure slightly above the lower inflection point on a pressure-volume curve based on the belief that tidal derecruitment will not occur at this end-expiratory pressure. However, it has been clearly shown that substantial lung recruitment and derecruitment continue to occur even when PEEP exceeds the lower inflection point of the pressure-volume curve. Further, a quasistatic pressure-volume curve does not characterize the mechanical properties of the lung alone. Rather, it characterizes the combined mechanical properties of the lung and the chest wall. This is important to understand, as the extent to which the chest wall affects the pressure-volume curve is unpredictable.

The largest study to date in ALI/ARDS patients found no mortality benefit with the use of higher (average = $\sim$15 cm H_2O) versus lower (average = $\sim$9 cm H_2O) levels of PEEP. In addition, there is recent data to suggest that some patients are PEEP responders and others are PEEP nonresponders. Further investigation is clearly needed to better clarify an effective way of establishing the optimal level of PEEP for individual patients. For the time being, a reasonable approach that attempts to balance the benefits and limitations of PEEP and fraction of inspired oxygen (FIO_2) is the protocol used by the ARDS Network investigators. In this protocol, increases in FIO_2 are alternated with increases in PEEP until the goal PaO_2 of 55 to 80 mm Hg is achieved.

Lastly, it should be noted that the statement in this chapter's title can be helpful when thinking about a patient's response to the level of PEEP administered. In the context of the previous discussion, it seems prudent to apply PEEP according to the ARDS Network protocol to achieve oxygenation goals. Over time, as PEEP is increased, one may observe that PaO_2 dramatically improves. This effect may be the result of lung units opening gradually over the course of several hours or resolving inflammation.

SUGGESTED READINGS

Acute Respiratory Distress Syndrome Network Ventilation with lower tidal volumes as compared with traditional tidal volumes for acute lung injury and the acute respiratory distress syndrome. N Engl J Med. 2000;342(18):1301–1308.

Bindslev L, Hedenstierna G, Santesson J, et al. Ventilation-perfusion distribution during inhalational anaesthesia; effects of spontaneous breathing, mechanical ventilation, and positive end-expiratory pressure. Acta Anaesthesiol Scand 1981;25:360–371.

Brower RG, Lanken PN, MacIntyre N, et al. Higher versus lower positive end-expiratory pressures in patients with the acute respiratory distress syndrome. N Engl J Med 2004;351:327–336.

Dreyfuss D, Saumon G. Ventilator-induced lung injury; lesions from experimental studies. Am J Respir Crit Care Med 1998;157:294–323.

Grasso S, Fanelli V, Cafarelli A, et al. Effects of high versus low positive end-expiratory pressures in acute respiratory distress syndrome. Am J Respir Crit Care Med 2005;171:1002–1008.

Levy MM. Optimal PEEP in ARDS; changing concepts and current controversies. Crit Care Clin 2002;18:15.

Smith TC, Marini JJ. Impact of PEEP on lung mechanics and work of breathing in severe airflow obstruction. J Appl Physiol 1988;65:1488–1499.

120

HAVE A HIGH SUSPICION OF AUTO POSITIVE END-EXPIRATORY PRESSURE WHEN ATTEMPTING TO WEAN PATIENTS WITH CHRONIC OBSTRUCTIVE PULMONARY DISEASE

JOSE RODRIGUEZ-PAZ, MD

CASE

You are in the intensive care unit (ICU) and you are called to see Mrs. Smith, a woman with chronic obstructive pulmonary disease (COPD) who had been admitted for respiratory failure secondary to pneumonia. You quickly go to her bed to evaluate. You are told that she was doing well with the planned weaning from mechanical ventilation, but she became acutely unstable. Upon your arrival she is found to be tachypneic, diaphoretic, and hypotensive. Of course, today is your first day in the ICU and you have not received sign-out yet. All of a sudden the ICU fellow arrives and quickly disconnects Mrs. Smith from the ventilator and her blood pressure improves and she starts looking better. What happened?

DISCUSSION

Patients with COPD have regions of the lung with flow limitation, needing longer time constants for their alveoli to deflate (i.e., they take longer to complete expiration). In these patients, especially during mechanical ventilation, these areas that take longer to deflate may still be in expiration once the lung is making the next inspiratory effort, therefore trapping air in the alveoli. This phenomenon is called auto positive end-expiratory pressure (PEEP) or intrinsic PEEP (iPEEP). This basically means that the patient's expiratory flow gets interrupted before the alveoli are completely empty, thus creating a pressure difference between the alveoli and the proximal airway.

How do you measure if a patient has autoPEEP? The easiest method in a ventilated patient is to review the expiratory flow in the ventilator graphics. If the expiratory flow does not reach zero and continues until the onset of the following inspiratory cycle, your patient has autoPEEP (*Fig. 120.1*). There are also more sophisticated and more complicated ways to measure. Using an esophageal balloon, the intrapleural pressure can be measured and related to the onset of inspiratory flow in patients who take spontaneous breaths. If the patient is not triggering the ventilator, the static autoPEEP can be measured by

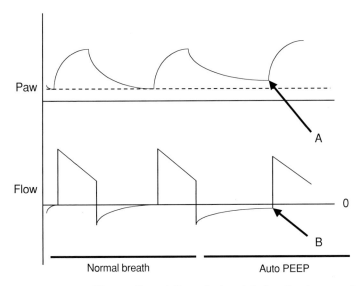

FIGURE 120.1. The ventilator delivers the breath before flow has ceased (it does not reach the baseline) **(B)**; therefore Paw (peak airway pressure) increases **(A)**.

occluding the expiratory port of the ventilator, allowing the pressure of the alveoli to equilibrate with the pressure of that port (not all ventilators allow you to do this fancy measurement). Another way to measure autoPEEP can be done by applying an end–expiratory pause for 1 to 2 seconds and measuring the pressure in excess of the PEEP set on the ventilator.

WATCH OUT FOR

There are several reasons autoPEEP is important in COPD patients. First, two–thirds of mechanically ventilated patients with COPD have autoPEEP. This is especially true in these patients who are mechanically ventilated with high minute ventilation and reduced expiratory time. Second, autoPEEP is associated with hemodynamic instability, by reducing venous return with increased intrathoracic pressure. Importantly, autoPEEP is a possible cause of pulseless electrical activity in a mechanically ventilated patient.

Third, autoPEEP can cause difficulty triggering the ventilator and increase the work of breathing, with associated failure to wean from mechanical ventilation. Because of this hyperinflation the patient needs to generate more negative intrapleural pressure (increased work of breathing) to overcome the gradient of pressure generated by autoPEEP and achieve similar levels of tidal volume. Also, autoPEEP can cause worsening of the gas exchange with lower PaO_2. In an attempt to decrease the risk of this from occurring in a mechanically ventilated patient, the expiratory time can be increased to account for the air trapping in such patients.

Several maneuvers can be implemented to optimize the ability to successfully wean patients with COPD. First, flow resistance must be decreased. This can be accomplished with bronchodilators and minimizing secretions. Second, attempts should be made to overcome the autoPEEP by applying external PEEP. This seems counterintuitive but the function of external PEEP is to open the airway to increase expiratory flow and reduce the work of breathing. It needs to be applied gently, with the objective of giving PEEP that is less than or equal to the autoPEEP. This establishes equilibrium throughout the airway and decreases the work of breathing.

Another possibility for COPD patients who are comfortable and tolerate minimal settings is to extubate to a mode of noninvasive ventilation (NIV). Of course, this approach has the risk of failure and need for reintubation, and the risk-to-benefit ratio must be evaluated for each individual patient and ICU setting depending on local resources and experience.

SUGGESTED READINGS

Irwin RS, Rippe JM, eds. Irwin's and Rippe's Intensive Care Medicine. 5th Ed. Philadelphia: Lippincott Williams & Wilkins; 2003:515–524.

Mughal MM. Auto-positive end-expiratory pressure: mechanisms and treatment. Cleve Clin J Med 2005;72:801–809.

Plant PK, Elliott MW. Chronic obstructive pulmonary disease 9: management of ventilatory COPD. Thorax 2003;58:537–542.

121

BE CAUTIOUS IN USING POSITIVE END-EXPIRATORY PRESSURE AFTER SINGLE-LUNG TRANSPLANTS

ERIC S. WEISS, MD
ASHISH S. SHAH, MD

CASE

A 63-year-old man with an extensive history of cigarette smoking and severe chronic obstructive pulmonary disease (COPD) (first expiratory volume in 1 second [FEV_1] <25% predicted and resting PaO_2 <55 mm Hg) presents to a pulmonary specialist for management. He states that he has been free of cigarettes for almost 1 year but his poor oxygenation severely limits his functional ability. He is thus deemed a suitable candidate for lung transplantation. After a relatively short period on the transplant list, the patient receives a left single lung from an otherwise healthy 24-year-old donor who died from head injuries in a motorcycle crash.

The operation progresses smoothly and the patient is transferred to the cardiac surgical intensive care unit (CSICU) postoperatively. Initial arterial blood gas measurement shows the arterial partial pressure of oxygen to be only 55 mm Hg on a fraction of inspired oxygen (FIO_2) of 100%. The resident physician orders an increase in the positive end-expiratory pressure (PEEP) on the ventilator from 5 to 10. Subsequent blood gas shows a worsening of oxygenation with a PaO_2 of 45 and $PaCO_2$ of 55. In an effort to improve the patient's respiratory status, he is disconnected from the ventilator and hand bagged. His oxygenation continues to decline and now his blood pressure drops precipitously. He becomes bradycardic and ultimately arrests.

DISCUSSION

First performed in a human by Dr. James Hardy in 1963, lung transplantation has become a lifesaving procedure for many patients with a variety of pulmonary disorders. Patients who have severe disabling pulmonary disease but who are otherwise healthy are generally considered good candidates for lung transplantation. This patient presented with chronic obstructive pulmonary disease. The indications for lung transplantation in COPD include a predicted FEV_1 of less than 30%, resting partial pressure of oxygen of less than 55 mm Hg, development of pulmonary hypertension, severe disabling symptoms, or rapid decline of function.

PEEP has an important role in the early management of all lung-transplant patients. The newly reperfused allograft is stiff and sensitive to volume and oxygen injury. As a result, PEEP helps to maintain alveolar recruitment, limit pulmonary overcirculation, and minimize the inspired oxygen. All this likely reduces the dreaded complication of primary allograft failure and may contribute to better long-term allograft function. In the specific setting of single-lung transplantation, however, ventilator management must take into consideration the nontransplanted, native lung. In this situation hyperinflation, due to excessive PEEP, insufficient expiratory time, and air trapping leads to hypoventilation and mechanical compression of the heart and lung allograft. This lethal scenario is further worsened by manual bagging. In double-lung transplant patients, unless there is an isolated airway problem, unilateral hyperinflation is unlikely. However, even double-lung transplant patients may air trap if they have insufficient expiratory time.

For most lung transplants, experienced physicians often keep PEEP at 8 cm H_2O on the first night of surgery. This not only maintains alveolar recruitment (which minimizes the oxygen requirement) but also limits pulmonary blood flow and may prevent reperfusion injury. In patients with pulmonary hypertension, a higher PEEP of 10 to 12 cm H_2O is used to further limit blood flow and alveolar fluid leak. Typically, PEEP is continued overnight until the patient is ready for extubation, at which point conventional settings are used as tolerated.

SUGGESTED READINGS

De Perrot M, Bonser RS, Dark J, et al. Report of the ISHLT Working Group on Primary Lung Graft Dysfunction part III: donor-related risk factors and markers. J Heart Lung Transpl 2005;24:1460–1467.

De Perrot M, Imai Y, Volgyesi GA, et al. Effect of ventilator-induced lung injury on the development of reperfusion injury in a rat lung transplant model. J Thorac Cardiovasc Surg 2002;74:1658–1662.

122

SELECT AN INITIAL PRESSURE SETTING THAT IS JUST SLIGHTLY HIGHER THAN THE PATIENT'S PEAK PRESSURE WHEN ATTEMPTING A PRESSURE SUPPORT WEAN

ANTHONY D. SLONIM, MD, DRPH

Pressure-support ventilation is a flow-cycled mode of ventilation. During inspiration, inspiratory flow in this mode decreases as lung volumes reach full inhalation. This mode is also patient triggered, meaning that the patient is able to initiate the inspiratory cycle. This leads to increased patient comfort by enhancing patient-ventilator synchrony. Finally, pressure-support ventilation is considered to be pressure limited, whereby the pressure-support ventilation level is determined by the provider and programmed into the machine to assist the patient. The patient controls the rate and timing of respirations.

WHAT TO DO

As a mode to assist with weaning mechanical ventilation, the pressure-support level can be adjusted so that the patient is achieving an adequate tidal volume (6 to 10 cm^3/kg) with a comfortable respiratory rate (10 to 14 breaths per minute). As a starting point, the pressure-support level can be placed 2 to 5 cm H_2O above the peak pressure limit and adjusted as necessary to accomplish the previously recommended parameters. Of course, the assessment of acid-base balance and oxygenation by either arterial blood gas measurements or end-tidal CO_2 and pulse oximetry will allow more definitive adjustments.

Pressure-support ventilation has some clear advantages as a weaning mode. It is more comfortable than other modes and often well tolerated by patients. However, it should be remembered that pressure-support ventilation is a spontaneous breathing mode and that there is no backup rate if the patient should become apneic or more heavily sedated. One sensitive method of assessing a patient's failure to wean on pressure-support ventilation is to regularly assess the respiratory rate. Minute ventilation is determined by the product of the respiratory rate and tidal volume, as depicted in the following equation:

$$\text{minute ventilation} = \text{respiratory rate} \times \text{tidal volume}$$

If the patient develops atelectasis or is insufficiently supported by the applied pressure-support ventilation, tidal volume will decrease and the minute ventilation will become compromised. This will manifest itself clinically as an elevation in the respiratory rate. If patients on pressure-support ventilation become tachypneic, consideration should be given to increasing the level of pressure support or providing a backup rate.

SUGGESTED READINGS

Brochard I, Rauss A, Benito S, et al. Comparison of three methods of gradual withdrawal from ventilatory support during weaning from mechanical ventilation. Crit Care Med 1994;150:896–903.

Fink MP, Abraham E, Vincent JL, et al. Textbook of Critical Care. 5th Ed. Philadelphia: Elsevier Saunders; 2005:120–123.

123

DO NOT REVERSE NEUROMUSCULAR BLOCKADE UNLESS THE PATIENT IS WARM

JAMES F. WELLER, MD

Neuromuscular blocking agents (*Table 123.1*) are used routinely during general anesthesia to facilitate endotracheal intubation and to provide optimal surgical conditions. These drugs block transmission at the neuromuscular junction through their effects on the postsynaptic acetylcholine receptor. Since these drugs block transmission of impulses from the nerve to the muscle, they cannot prevent muscle contraction in response to direct application of electrical stimulation (e.g., from electrocautery).

The agents used to provide muscle relaxation fall into two classes: depolarizing and nondepolarizing. The only depolarizing agent used clinically in the United States is succinylcholine. Binding of succinylcholine to the postsynaptic acetylcholine receptor causes the channel to open, leading to an initial wave of depolarization that causes the muscle to fasciculate. However, unlike acetylcholine, succinylcholine remains bound to the receptor, leading to a period of flaccid paralysis lasting several minutes. It is degraded by plasma pseudocholinesterase and cannot be reversed.

The nondepolarizing neuromuscular relaxants work by competitive inhibition of acetylcholine at the same receptor site. The choice of nondepolarizer is generally made on the basis of time of onset, duration of action, and side-effect profile. Elimination generally involves renal and/or hepatic metabolism, which may also impact drug choice in some patients. Exceptions include mivacurium, which like succinylcholine is degraded by plasma pseudocholinesterase, and atracurium and cisatracurium, which are eliminated by Hoffman degradation (a nonenzymatic phenomenon that results in breakdown of these drugs at physiologic temperature and pH).

Because their physiologic effect depends upon competitive inhibition, the nondepolarizing agents can be "reversed" by administration of acetylcholinesterase inhibitors (e.g., neostigmine, edrophonium), which lead to accumulation of acetylcholine at the neuromuscular junction and elsewhere in the body. In order to prevent undesirable cholinergic side effects outside the neuromuscular junction (e.g., bradycardia, salivation, lacrimation), an antimuscarinic agent (e.g., glycopyrrolate, atropine) is generally administered concomitantly with the cholinesterase inhibitor.

TABLE 123.1   COMPARISON OF COMMON NEUROMUSCULAR BLOCKING AGENTS

GENERIC NAME	TRADE NAME	TIME OF ONSET (MIN)	CLINICAL DURATION (MIN)	MODE OF ELIMINATION	SIDE EFFECTS
Succinylcholine	Anectine	1–1.5	5–8	Plasma cholinesterase	Fasciculations; hyperkalemia; malignant hypothermia (MH)
d-tubocurarine		4–6	80–120	Renal elimination; hepatic clearance	Hypotension; histamine release
Atracurium	Tracrium	2–4	30–60	Hoffman degradation	Histamine release
Cisatracurium	Nimbex	2–4	30–60	Hoffman degradation	
Mivacurium	Mivacron	2–4	12–18	Plasma cholinesterase	Histamine release
Rocuronium	Zemuron	1–2	30–60	Hepatic metabolism	
Vecuronium	Norcuron	2–4	60–90	Hepatic metabolism; renal clearance	
Pancuronium	Pavulon	4–6	120–180	Renal elimination	Tachycardia

Among the many deleterious effects of perioperative hypothermia is prolongation of the effects of neuromuscular relaxants. The effects of hypothermia on paralytic agents appear to be pharmacokinetic rather than pharmacodynamic. The duration of action of vecuronium is doubled at 34°C; however, there is no change in the concentration effect (i.e., pharmacodynamic) relationship at the same temperature. Furthermore, hypothermia itself is associated with muscle relaxation, even in the absence of neuromuscular blocking agents.

Because of prolongation of the duration of action of neuromuscular blockade, attempted reversal in the hypothermic patient may be unsuccessful. Despite failing to restore strength adequate for extubation, however, early reversal may unmask the innate physiologic shivering response to hypothermia. Although shivering does not increase metabolic demands by 400% as once thought, it is associated with an increase in metabolic oxygen demand. This may be undesirable in patients with limited cardiac reserve and is uncomfortable for many patients. Although all opioids reduce shivering, the most efficacious choice remains meperidine. Other pharmacologic treatments for postoperative shivering include low-dose ketamine, clonidine, and physostigmine.

In the contemporary practice of anesthesia, extensive efforts are made to monitor and maintain core body temperature in the operating room. Nonetheless, when a patient arrives to the intensive care unit hypothermic (e.g., following massive resuscitation or prolonged exposure to the environment), aggressive measures should be instituted to rewarm the patient prior to reversal of neuromuscular blockade. These include application of external forced-air devices, warming of intravenous fluids, and humidification of inhaled gases. While awaiting achievement of normothermia, the patient should be sedated appropriately.

SUGGESTED READINGS

Hardman J, Limbird L, Goodman Gilman A, eds. Goodman and Gilman's the Pharmacologic Basis of Therapeutics. 10th Ed. New York: McGraw-Hill; 2001.

Heier T, Caldwell JE, Sessler DI, et al. Mild intraoperative hypothermia increases duration of action and spontaneous recovery of vecuronium blockade during nitrous oxide-isoflurane anesthesia in humans. Anesthesiology 1991;74:815–819.

Heier T, Caldwell JE, Sharma ML, et al. Mild intraoperative hypothermia does not change the pharmacodynamics (concentration-effect relationship) of vecuronium in humans. Anesth Analg 1994;78:973–977.

124

Use glycopyrrolate before using neostigmine when reversing neuromuscular blockade

Leo Hsiao, DO

During surgery it is often necessary to achieve dense-muscle relaxation to facilitate surgical technique or to ensure patient safety. To this end, the use of neuromuscular blocking agents have become an integral part of a balanced anesthetic technique. The two main classes of neuromuscular relaxing agents are the depolarizing muscle relaxants and the nondepolarizing muscle relaxants. Depolarizing agents mimic the action of acetylcholine at the neuromuscular junction (NMJ) and prevent the normal recovery of the muscle unit from its refractory state, rendering it unexcitable. Depolarizing relaxation is terminated when the agent diffuses from the neuromuscular junction to the plasma, where it is metabolized by plasma pseudocholinesterases. In contrast, nondepolarizing agents work as competitive antagonists of acetylcholine (ACH) at the NMJ. Their effects dissipate either when the drug diffuses away from its site of action or when there is an effective surge of ACH at the neuromuscular junction that competitively displaces the agent. The latter mechanism is the principle behind reversal of nondepolarizing neuromuscular blockade.

To briefly review, during normal transmission of an action potential, influx of calcium at the nerve terminal triggers the release of storage vesicles containing acetylcholine. The membrane packages diffuse across the synaptic cleft to bind with the ACH receptors at the motor endplate. This binding results in a conformational change in the ligand-activated receptor at the motor endplate that allows the influx of ions, producing a depolarization of the motor endplate. When the membrane depolarization reaches a threshold, an action potential is produced and the muscle fiber fires. Stimulation is terminated when ACH is degraded by acetylcholinesterase located at the neuromuscular junction.

Neostigmine is a potent inhibitor of cholinesterase enzyme activity at the NMJ. The typical dose is weight based at 0.08 mg/kg with a maximum dose of 5 mg. By preventing acetylcholine degradation, neostigmine indirectly elevates the concentration of neurotransmitter at the NMJ. Acetylcholine in turn competitively displaces residual nondepolarizing drug and "reverses" the waning effects of blockade.

Unfortunately, this acetylcholine surge ubiquitously affects both muscarinic and nicotinic receptors throughout the body. This results in side effects such as bradycardia or asystole, hyperperistalsis, nausea, and vomiting, increased bronchial secretions, and urinary urge. These effects are particularly worrisome in a patient emerging from anesthesia and should be averted if possible.

WHAT TO DO Glycopyrrolate is an anticholinergic-class medication given in an intravenous formulation as an adjunct to counter the untoward effects of neostigmine during neuromuscular blockade reversal. The typical dose of glycopyrrolate for this indication is 0.2 mg per 1 mg of neostigmine. Because of its quaternary structure, glycopyrrolate is essentially devoid of central effects. It does, however, produce an impressive blockade of acetylcholine at the peripheral muscarinic receptor sites. The result is a constellation of side effects including intense drying of mucous membranes, significant rise in heart rate, diminished intestinal motility, and urinary retention.

Not surprisingly glycopyrrolate's pharmacodynamic profile negates many of the side effects produced by neostigmine. This is a model example of an advantageous drug-drug interaction whereby one drug counterbalances the side effects of another drug without negating its principle therapeutic activity. To facilitate this beneficial interaction, proponents advocate the administration of glycopyrrolate minutes in advance of neostigmine. The rationale behind this sequence of administration is to achieve a significant blockade of muscarinic receptors so as to mitigate the impending surge of acetylcholine. The result is a smooth reversal of muscle blockade. An alternative anticholinergic is atropine.

SUGGESTED READINGS
Miller RD, ed. Anesthesia. 6th Ed. Philadelphia: Churchill Livingstone; 2005:518–523.
Morgan E, Mikhail M, Murray M, et al. Clinical Anesthesiology. 3rd Ed. New York: McGraw-Hill; 2002:179–187,199–204,207–210.

125

DO NOT ATTEMPT TO REVERSE NEUROMUSCULAR BLOCKADE IF THERE ARE NO TWITCHES

E. DAVID BRAVOS, MD

Paralysis through the use of neuromuscular blockers can provide optimal conditions for many surgical procedures and can help facilitate intubation for patients requiring mechanical ventilation. These drugs can be broadly classified as being depolarizing or nondepolarizing not only by their mechanism of producing paralysis but by their response to peripheral nerve stimulation and reversal of blockade.

Neuromuscular blockers are structurally similar to acetylcholine and produce their effects by interacting with acetylcholine receptors at the neuromuscular junction. Depolarizing neuromuscular blockers such as succinylcholine bind to the acetylcholine receptor and cause a conformational change resulting in activation of the receptor. This leads to depolarization of the muscle membrane and an action potential if the threshold potential is reached. This explains the muscle fasciculation seen with use of succinylcholine. These drugs remain bound to the receptor and prevent acetylcholine from binding, thus producing paralysis. Nondepolarizing agents bind the acetylcholine receptor as well; however, they do not cause a conformational change and therefore do not cause depolarization. Similarly, acetylcholine cannot bind to any bound receptor with resultant paralysis.

WATCH OUT FOR

Once neuromuscular blockade has occurred, the depth of blockade can be measured using peripheral nerve stimulation. Different responses to nerve stimulation can be seen depending on the type of neuromuscular blocker used, as well as the pattern of stimulation used. The most common patterns of stimulation are the train of four (TOF) and tetany. With depolarizing neuromuscular blockade, TOF stimulation produces a decreased response to successive stimulation known as fade. This is thought to be due to exhaustion of acetylcholine with each successive stimulation in the TOF (and therefore there is less acetylcholine available to overcome the antagonistic block). With tetanic stimulation, fade is seen as well. Depolarizing neuromuscular blockers do not produce fade with a single TOF. However, fade may be seen with successive TOFs. Rather, a constant but diminished response may be seen if more than one twitch is present. The percent of receptor blockade can be roughly estimated by the number of twitches present. Three twitches is roughly a 75% block; two twitches, an 80% block; and one twitch, a 90% block.

When testing for twitches, the adductor pollicis and the orbicularis oculi are frequently used. Twitches in these muscles can be seen by stimulation of the ulnar and facial nerves, respectively. In general, muscles have different sensitivities to neuromuscular blockers. More centrally located muscles including the laryngeal muscles and diaphragm are quicker to respond to neuromuscular blockers than more peripheral ones. Additionally, the orbicularis oculi is relatively more resistant compared with the adductor pollicis. The best area to place the pads of the nerve stimulator is one that isolates the nerve and will not directly stimulate the muscle. For the orbicularis oculi, pads should be placed superolateral and inferolateral to the lateral canthus. For the ulnar nerve, pads should be placed just proximal and distal to the ulnar nerve as it travels through the groove between the medial epicondyle and the medial aspect of the olecranon process of the arm.

When neuromuscular blockade is no longer needed, reversal of the blockade may be warranted. Reversal is done with the use of non-depolarizing agents, but succinylcholine should never be reversed and the use of anticholinergics while succinylcholine is still present may actually prolong its effects. Before reversal is attempted, the number of twitches should be checked using the TOF to be sure at least one twitch is present. This especially holds true when using longer-acting agents such as pancuronium. When one twitch is present, spontaneous recovery is starting to occur. However, if no twitches are present then full blockade is still occurring and the effect of the neuromuscular blocker may outlast the effects of the reversal agent. Patients may have generalized weakness with possible respiratory failure if extubated.

SUGGESTED READINGS

Miller RD, ed. Miller's Anesthesia. 6th Ed. Churchill Livingstone; 2005:518–525.
Morgan GE. Clinical Anesthesiology. 3rd Ed. Lange/McGraw-Hill; 2002:120–123.

126

REMOVE CONTINUOUS POSITIVE AIRWAY PRESSURE AND BILEVEL POSITIVE AIRWAY PRESSURE MASKS PERIODICALLY

BRADFORD D. WINTERS, MD, PhD

Continuous positive airway pressure (CPAP) and bilevel positive airway pressure (BiPAP) are two noninvasive ventilatory modes that are commonly used in the intensive care unit (ICU) as well as other settings. CPAP is commonly used on an outpatient basis to alleviate sleep apnea. Although less common, BiPAP may also be used for this purpose. While both of these modes may also be used for patients in the ICU who have this diagnosis, these modes are also commonly used to assist ICU patients who are having respiratory difficulty unrelated to sleep apnea. These situations include avoiding the need for invasive mechanical ventilation (e.g., endotracheal intubation) or to help bridge patients from invasive ventilation to supplemental oxygen only. This may be done in a variety of disease settings, including cardiogenic pulmonary edema; chronic obstructive pulmonary disease exacerbations postoperatively; adult respiratory distress syndrome; and others. Variable effectiveness has been described depending on the disease state.

Regardless of the disease state being treated or whether one is attempting to avoid intubation or bridging from invasive ventilation, close attention needs to be maintained so that the clinician is able to recognize when the patient is failing this noninvasive mode. While several studies point to these modes' effectiveness in prevention of or weaning from invasive ventilation, it is clear that early recognition of the patient's failing the noninvasive strategies is crucial to preventing morbidity. In general, a patient who is getting worse after an hour or so of noninvasive ventilation, as determined by his or her blood gas values and clinically assessed work of breathing, should be considered for intubation. If the patient is not improving but is not deteriorating, the CPAP or BiPAP may be continued, perhaps with adjustments to the pressure settings.

WHAT TO DO

CPAP uses a consistent pressure setting throughout the respiratory cycle while BiPAP uses a bilevel setting with the inspiratory phase being set higher than the expiratory phase. Values for the pressures set generally range from 5 to 15 cm H_2O. Delivery of these airway pressures requires tight-fitting masks. These are usually full-face masks that cover the nose and mouth, though there are nasal masks that fit only over the nose. For these nasal masks to function well the patient must be cooperative enough to keep his or her mouth closed, or all of the pressure will escape through the mouth and ventilation might be ineffective.

The tight-fitting nature of CPAP and BiPAP masks poses the risk of pressure necrosis of the underlying tissues, particularly over the bridge of the nose where the skin is thin and bone and cartilage lie just near the surface. This is because the tightness required to overcome the flow pressures and prevent leakage of gas often will exceed tissue-perfusion pressure. It is for this reason that every few hours (4 hours is a commonly used interval) the mask should be removed to allow the tissue to receive adequate blood flow. This time period is generally less than a half hour and then the mask is reapplied unless the patient demonstrates the ability to remain off support during that time. If the patient does not tolerate being off the mask for even a short time periodically, the clinician should consider moving to intubation.

SUGGESTED READINGS

Masip J, Roque M, Sanchez B, et al. Noninvasive ventilation in acute cardiogenic pulmonary edema: systematic review and meta-analysis. JAMA 2005;294:3124–3130.

Peter JV, Moran JL, Phillips-Hughes J, et al. Effect of non-invasive positive pressure ventilation (NIPPV) on mortality in patient with acute cardiogenic pulmonary oedema: a meta-analysis. Lancet 2006;367:1155–1163.

127

EMPIRICALLY COVER THE COMMON NOSOCOMIAL MICROBES IN VENTILATOR-ASSOCIATED PNEUMONIA UNTIL THE CULTURES ARE RETURNED

ANTHONY D. SLONIM, MD, DRPH

Nosocomial pneumonia is an important hospital-acquired infection that occurs 48 hours or more after hospital admission. It is the leading cause of death from nosocomial infections. A subset of nosocomial pneumonia occurs in patients receiving mechanical ventilation. These patients have what is termed ventilator-associated pneumonia (VAP). The use of a ventilator by the patient increases the risk of developing pneumonia by a factor of 10. As a result, VAP frequently occurs in patients requiring significant mechanical ventilatory support such as patients with acute respiratory distress syndrome (ARDS), shock syndromes, and multiorgan failure.

It is important to understand that the etiology of VAP is dependent upon the fundamental relationship between the host, the microbial agent, and the environment. The host refers to the intensive care unit (ICU) patient who may be at particular risk of acquiring a nosocomial infection. Alterations in underlying host defenses like the endotracheal tube, which suppresses the normal ability of the body to eliminate respiratory pathogens by coughing; host diseases like cancers; and underlying respiratory diseases such as cystic fibrosis affect both the colonization of and predisposition to VAP. The microbial agents themselves have specific properties that increase their pathogenicity. Pili, microbial toxins, and adherence factors all play a role in the ability of particular organisms to have a propensity to cause diseases. Gram-negative bacteria are more likely than gram-positive organisms to cause VAP (60% vs. 40%). The gram-negative microbial organisms that are responsible for causing VAP include *Pseudomonas aeruginosa, Escherichia coli, Klebsiella pneumoniae,* and *Acinetobacter* species. The gram-positive spectrum primarily involves *Staphylococcus* species. In addition, the environment of the ICU, the hospital, and the region will all affect the spectrum of microbials that colonize the environment and predispose the patient to infections.

WATCH OUT FOR

Host factors that increase the likelihood of acquiring VAP include patients with ARDS, chronic obstructive airways disease (COPD), malnutrition, burns, trauma, a higher severity of illness, and the administration of specific medications and treatments. The overuse of broad-spectrum antimicrobial agents suppresses some organisms but increases the risk of the patient to other organisms that are prone to infect the respiratory tract. In addition, the use of H2-blockers reduces the gastric pH and leads to increased colonization of organisms that can cause nosocomial pneumonia.

There are strategies that can be used to reduce the risk of VAP. Aggressive postpyloric, early feeding has a beneficial effect on the patient's ability to guard against acquiring nosocomial pneumonia. Elevation of the head of the patient's bed has a beneficial effect on the rate of VAP. From an environmental perspective, appropriate hand washing is helpful in preventing all types of nosocomial infections. Health care workers are particularly poor at using this method of prevention for their patients' benefit. The respiratory equipment itself may lead to increased rates of pneumonia because of the colonization of bacteria in the tubing and condensate. Similarly, appropriate cleaning of patient rooms and multipatient equipment needs to be performed. Finally, an understanding of the common pathogens in the ICU and hospital as well as their antibiograms can be helpful in selecting appropriate empiric therapy.

WHAT TO DO For patients developing VAP, the goals of therapy include the appropriate stabilization, early diagnosis, and empiric treatment followed by specific therapy for isolated organisms. The American Thoracic Society has proposed guidelines for the diagnosis and treatment of VAP. When suspected, the early culture of blood and respiratory secretions may be beneficial in identifying an organism prior to the initiation of antimicrobial agents. These culture techniques may include direct specimen examination by use of bronchoscopy with protected specimen brush specimens or bronchoalveolar lavage. If the cultures are positive, then the initiation of antibiotics can be helpful with a fine-tuning of the antimicrobial spectrum when the sensitivity results are known. The length of antibiotic coverage for VAP should be 8 days (unless it is *Pseudomonas*, requiring a 14-day course) and should include the following antibiotic regimens:

Vancomycin plus piperacillin and tazobactam (Zosyn)
or
Vancomycin plus meropenem with or without an aminoglycoside
or
Vancomycin plus cefepime

SUGGESTED READINGS

Fink MP, Abraham E, Vincent JL, et al., eds. *Textbook of Critical Care*. 5th Ed. Philadelphia: Saunders; 2005:542–544.

Ibrahim EH, Ward S, Sherman G, et al. Experience with a clinical guideline for the treatment of ventilator associated pneumonia. Crit Care Med 2001;29:1109–1115.

128

KEEP THE HEAD OF BED ELEVATED AT LEAST 30 DEGREES FOR INTUBATED PATIENTS IF NO CONTRAINDICATIONS EXIST

DEBORAH B. HOBSON, BSN
SEAN M. BERENHOLTZ, MD, MHS

Mechanical ventilation is a common intervention in the intensive care unit (ICU). It places patients at an increased risk for death and complications, such as ventilator-associated pneumonia and gastrointestinal bleeding. Efforts to decrease the morbidity and mortality and improve the quality and safety of care for patients requiring mechanical ventilation are paramount. One simple no-cost intervention that improves outcomes in ventilated patients is to keep the head of the bed elevated ≥30 degrees. Elevating the head of bed ≥30 degrees can reduce the frequency and risk for nosocomial pneumonia compared with the supine position, decrease duration of mechanical ventilation, and decrease ICU length of stay. The evidence supporting this intervention is from a well-done randomized study of mechanically ventilated patients that found the incidence of pneumonia was reduced from 38% in the supine group to 8% in the ≥30-degrees group. Days on the ventilator and ICU length of stay were also reduced.

Other strategies, in combination with elevating the head of the bed ≥30 degrees, have been shown in the medical literature to be very effective in decreasing the morbidity, mortality, and cost of care for patients receiving mechanical ventilation. These therapies are often termed the "ventilator bundle" and include head of bed elevation ≥30 degrees; appropriate peptic ulcer disease (PUD) prophylaxis; appropriate deep venous thrombosis (DVT) prophylaxis; appropriate sedation; and daily assessment of ability to extubate. Each of these interventions is supported by medical evidence and independently decreases patient morbidity and/or mortality. A recent prospective multicenter observational trial evaluating the impact of improving compliance with the ventilator bundle found that for the 35 ICUs that consistently collected data on ventilator bundle compliance and VAP rates, an average 45% reduction of VAP was observed. In addition, three of these interventions, elevating the head of the bed ≥30 degrees, PUD prophylaxis, and DVT prophylaxis, have been selected by the Joint Commission on Accreditation of Healthcare Organizations (JCAHO) for inclusion into the initial core set of ICU quality measures.

SUGGESTED READINGS

Dodek P, Keenan S, Cook D, et al. Evidence-based clinical practice guideline for the prevention of ventilator-associated pneumonia. Ann Intern Med 2004;141:305–313.

Drakulovic MB, Torres A, Bauer TT, et al. Supine body position as a risk factor for nosocomial pneumonia in mechanically ventilated patients: a randomised trial. Lancet 1999;354:1851–1858.

Kollef MH. The prevention of ventilator-associated pneumonia. N Engl J Med 1999;340:627–634.

Resar R, Pronovost P, Haraden C, et al. Using the bundle approach to improve ventilator care processes and reduce ventilator-associated pneumonia. Jt Comm J Qual Patient Saf 2005;31:243–248.

129

TREAT VENTILATOR-ASSOCIATED PNEUMONIA FOR 8 DAYS

B. ROBERT GIBSON, MD

Ventilator-associated pneumonia (VAP) refers to a pneumonia that arises after 48 hours of mechanical ventilation. Unfortunately, it is common, costly, and life threatening. It is the most frequent intensive care unit (ICU)–acquired infection among patients receiving mechanical ventilation, and it is the second most common nosocomial infection in the United States. VAP has also been found to increase hospital stay by an average of 7 to 9 days and results in an increase in health care–related costs of $12,000 to $40,000 per case. In addition, approximately 50% of all antibiotics prescribed in the ICU are administered for respiratory tract infections. Crude ICU mortality associated with VAP ranges from 30% to 70% with an increased relative risk of mortality of approximately 2.5.

Despite the undisputed clinical importance of VAP, little consensus exists regarding its prevention, diagnosis, or treatment. Some of the risk factors for VAP are clearly known: supine body positioning; transfusion of blood products; and duration of ventilation. Duration of ventilation has been closely associated with an increased risk of pneumonia as a direct function of time. The daily risk of VAP has been estimated to start at approximately 3% per day for the first five days, followed by 2% per day for days six through ten, before finally decreasing to 1% per day for every day of mechanical ventilation thereafter.

SIGNS AND SYMPTOMS

When it comes to diagnosing ventilator-associated pneumonia, there is little consensus in the literature because of different interpretation of the clinical signs and symptoms suggestive of lung infection, variable differentiation between colonization and infection of the lower respiratory tract, and poorly specified prior antibiotic use in the ICU. As clinical signs are nonspecific and subjective, no single clinical criterion has been specifically diagnostic for VAP. Fever, tachycardia, and leukocytosis are all relatively nonspecific. Chest radiographs are most helpful when normal, as they can rule out pneumonia. Air bronchograms or alveolar opacities on a chest radiograph in patients without acute respiratory distress syndrome (ARDS) are most correlated with pneumonia and have a 68% diagnostic accuracy. When chest radiographs have been compared with subsequent autopsy findings, a localized infiltrate was 87% sensitive for VAP but only 25% specific. Furthermore, approximately 10% of the cases of pneumonia failed to have a new or worsening infiltrate at all.

The clinical pulmonary infection score (CPIS) was developed in an attempt to find more reliable criteria for the diagnosis of VAP. The CPIS combines clinical, radiographic, physiological, and microbiologic data into a single numerical result. The score is derived by awarding 0, 1, or 2 points for each of seven variables: temperature; white blood count; volume and quality of tracheal suctions; oxygenation; chest radiograph findings; and semiquantitative culture of tracheal aspirate. When the CPIS exceeds 6, good correlation with the presence of pneumonia, as defined by quantitative cultures of bronchoscopic and nonbronchoscopic lavage specimens, has been found. When compared with postmortem quantitative lung cultures as the reference standard, the CPIS has a sensitivity of 77% and a specificity of 42% for VAP.

Increased specificity at the cost of sensitivity over the CPIS may be obtained by using diagnostic criteria of a radiographic infiltrate and at least two of the three following clinical features of VAP: fever greater than 38°C; leukocytosis or leukopenia; and purulent tracheal secretions. Use of these criteria resulted in a 69% sensitivity and a 75% specificity for VAP, which represents the most accurate clinical criteria for starting empiric antibiotic therapy.

Once the diagnosis of VAP is being considered, a lower respiratory tract sample for culture to guide therapy should be collected before antibiotic administration. If cultures are obtained after initiation of antibiotics, a 40% false negative rate ensues. If there is a high pretest probability of pneumonia, or in the 10% of patients with evidence of sepsis, prompt therapy is required, regardless of whether bacteria are found on microscopic examination of lower respiratory tract samples.

The diagnosis and treatment of VAP is difficult in part because of the multiple etiologic agents associated with the disease. The causes of VAP are legion and will vary by hospital, patient population, and type of ICU, emphasizing the need for timely, local surveillance data. One of the main goals of surveillance and guiding principles of treatment of VAP is to determine whether the patient has VAP associated with antibiotic-resistant organisms or not.

VAP associated with antibiotic-resistant microorganisms can usually be predicted by the duration of ventilation of 5 days or more; the length of stay before the onset of VAP; a history of prior antibiotic treatment; or knowledge of a high frequency of antibiotic resistance in the community or hospital. Typically, antibiotic-resistant organisms associated with VAP are *Pseudomonas aeruginosa*, *Acinetobacter*, methicillin-resistant *Staphylococcus aureus* (MRSA), and multidrug-resistant gram-negative bacilli. In these patients suspected of having VAP due to antibiotic-resistant organisms, initial empiric coverage should be broad.

Those without risk factors for resistant organisms (less than 5 days of ventilation, no prior antibiotic exposure, no prior contact with the health care system) frequently have VAP due to antibiotic-sensitive bacteria such as *Haemophilus influenzae*, *Streptococcus pneumoniae*, MSSA (methicillin-sensitive *S. aureus*), or antibiotic-sensitive enteric gram-negative bacilli. These patients may be empirically started on antibiotic monotherapy. *Legionella* species, anaerobes, fungi, and even viruses should also be mentioned as potential rare causes of pneumonia in ventilated patients. This being said, it is not uncommon to isolate *Candida* species from endotracheal aspirates of ventilated patients. This distinction arises because candidal colonization of the airways is common, yet infection is rare, with a maximum of 20% of patients with positive candidal endotracheal aspirates actually having invasive candidal disease. Therefore, a positive endotracheal aspirate rarely mandates antifungal therapy.

Once the diagnosis of VAP is made, selection of an appropriate empiric antibiotic regimen is key to patient survival. In one study, inappropriate initial antibiotic therapy (pathogen resistant or not covered) for VAP was documented in as many as 33% of cases, and initial inappropriate therapy independently increased the risk of mortality by nearly sevenfold. This increased risk of mortality persisted even when the treatment was changed appropriately based upon subsequent culture data.

The previous facts drive the approach to antibiotic treatment of VAP. To reduce patient mortality, one must avoid inappropriate treatment by initiating empiric, broad-spectrum multiagent antibiotic therapy. The goal is not for redundant coverage of a pathogen, but to increase the chance that the initial antibiotic regimen is appropriate for the etiologic agent once it becomes known. There has been no documented clinical superiority of double coverage as opposed to appropriate monotherapy. Therefore, initial antibiotic therapy should be tailored to institutional patterns of antibiotic resistance and patient factors that have an influence upon the etiologic agents and antibiotic-resistance patterns for VAP in the individual.

WHAT TO DO

Given the above, antimicrobial therapy for VAP typically follows a two-stage process. The first stage involves initial broad-spectrum coverage to avoid inappropriate treatment. Once the decision to treat is made, cultures should be obtained and antibiotic therapy should be initiated. Delays in the initiation of appropriate antibiotic therapy can increase the mortality of VAP, and thus therapy should not be postponed for the purpose of performing diagnostic studies in patients who are clinically unstable. Initial empiric therapy is based upon patient risk for multidrug-resistant pathogens. When it is determined that there is a low risk for resistant organisms, then monotherapy including ceftriaxone, a fluoroquinolone, or ampicillin/sulbactam should be initiated. For patients with risk factors for multidrug-resistant pathogens, empiric coverage should be broad and initiated as follows:

> Cefepime/ceftazidime or imipenem/meropenem
> *and*
> Ciprofloxacin/levofloxacin or amikacin/gentamicin/tobramycin
> *and*
> Vancomycin/linezolid

Note that the goal of combination therapy is not to provide redundant coverage so much as to ensure initial appropriate empiric therapy.

The second stage of antimicrobial therapy focuses on maintaining appropriate coverage without overusing antibiotics. Therapy may be modified in patients with a low probability of disease based upon clinical response on days two and three. Antibiotic coverage may be switched to monotherapy or otherwise narrowed based upon culture data, and the duration of therapy may be shortened to 8 days. Antibiotic spectra should be narrowed as culture data become known. Once the results of respiratory tract and blood cultures become available, therapy can often be narrowed on the basis of the identity of specific pathogens and their susceptibility to specific antibiotics.

Once treatment for VAP is initiated, a question arises as to when it is appropriate to stop. Unfortunately, therapy cannot be guided by chest radiographs as they are of limited value for defining clinical improvement in severe pneumonia. Initial radiographic deterioration is common, especially among patients who are bacteremic or who are infected with highly virulent organisms. In addition, radiographic improvement often lags behind clinical parameters. Clinical improvement usually becomes apparent after the first 48 hours of therapy and, therefore, the selected antimicrobial regimen should not be changed during this time unless progressive deterioration is noted or initial microbiologic studies so dictate. Consequently, failure to respond to therapy is not clinically evident until treatment day three. Fortunately, this is about the time that microbiologic data become available to guide further therapy.

A recent study has shown that using the CPIS system to identifies patients with a low clinical suspicion of VAP (CPIS <6) who could be treated with 3 days of antibiotics as opposed to the conventional practice of 10 to 21 days of antibiotic therapy. Patients receiving the shorter course of antibiotics had better clinical outcomes than those receiving longer therapy and had fewer subsequent superinfections with antibiotic-resistant pathogens. In another recent trial, patients who received appropriate, initial empiric therapy for VAP for 8 days had equivalent mortality and risk of pulmonary reinfection as those of patients who received therapy for 15 days, while having significantly more antibiotic-free days. A trend to greater rates of relapse for short-duration therapy was seen if the etiologic agent was *P. aeruginosa* or an *Acinetobacter* species. Hence the recommendation for an 8-day course of antibiotics for VAP except in the case of a pseudomonal or *Acinetobacter* pneumonia, where treatment should be taken out to 14 days.

SUGGESTED READINGS

American Thoracic Society; Infectious Diseases Society of America. Guidelines for the management of adults with hospital-acquired, ventilator-associated, and healthcare-associated pneumonia. Am J Respir Crit Care Med 2005;171:388–416.

Chastre J. Conference summary: ventilator-associated pneumonia. Respir Care 2005;50:975–983.

Fink MP, Abraham E, Vincent JL, Kachanek PM, eds. Textbook of Critical Care. 5th Ed. Philadelphia: Elsevier Saunders; 2004:663–677.

DO NOT ROUTINELY EXTUBATE ON CLINICAL PICTURE ALONE

RONALD W. PAULDINE, MD

The benefits of separating patients from mechanical ventilation include decreasing the risk of ventilator-associated pneumonia and ventilator-induced lung injury, increasing patient comfort, and decreasing cost. These benefits, however, must be weighed against the complications of removing mechanical ventilation too soon, which include the potential for difficulty in re-establishing the airway and in complications related to impaired gas exchange.

Decisions to discontinue mechanical ventilation cannot be based on the clinical picture alone. "Foot of the bed" assessment is notoriously unreliable in predicting patient suitability for weaning and extubation. Studies have documented sensitivities as low as 35%, implying that often patients who may successfully wean are missed. Overall, clinical assessment is better at predicting those who will fail to wean but still has only a specificity of less than 80% at best. To this end, guidelines for ventilator weaning have been adopted by several professional organizations including the American College of Chest Physicians, the Society of Critical Care Medicine, and the American Association for Respiratory Care.

The guidelines are based on the best currently available evidence and recommend criteria to determine whom should be considered for discontinuation of ventilation, principles to guide that assessment, how to treat patients who fail their weaning assessment, as well as considerations for long-term ventilator dependence and the design and use of weaning protocols by nonphysicians. Criteria suggested prior to a formal assessment of discontinuation include evidence of some reversal of the underlying reason for the patient's respiratory failure; adequate oxygenation ($PaO_2/FIO_2 \geq 200$ mm Hg, PEEP ≤ 5–8 cm H_2O, $FIO_2 \leq 0.4$–0.5, and pH ≥ 7.25; FIO_2, fraction of inspired oxygen; PEEP, positive end-expiratory pressure); hemodynamic stability; and patient ability to generate an inspiratory effort. Spontaneous breathing trials (SBTs) may be attempted when these criteria are met. Trials may be carried out on either T-piece or with so-called "minimal" ventilator settings of 5 cm H_2O continuous positive airway pressure (CPAP) and 5 cm H_2O pressure support. The decision to use one method or the other does not seem to affect outcome. The former has the advantage of removing all supportive positive pressure from the airway but has the disadvantage of removing the patient from any apnea alarms on the ventilator. At these settings, conceptually CPAP will maintain recruitment of alveoli and pressure support will overcome the resistance to the ventilator circuit. The patient should be observed for respiratory pattern, quality of gas exchange, hemodynamic changes, and subjective comfort. Patients who pass an SBT of 30 to 120 minutes duration should be considered for separation from the ventilator. Patients successfully completing a 2-hour trial have a 90% chance of staying off mechanical ventilation at 48 hours. Patients who fail should be placed on a mode of ventilation that will provide rest and be reassessed for weaning in 24 hours. Other considerations should include the amount and quality of secretions combined with the patient's ability to protect the airway and the potential for airway edema.

WHAT TO DO

Many parameters have been proposed and used to assess patients for discontinuation of mechanical ventilation. Commonly used maneuvers to test ventilatory muscle strength include measurement of the peak inspiratory pressure or negative inspiratory force (NIF) and the vital capacity (VC). Peak inspiratory pressure is performed by measuring the pressure generated by the patient with maximal inspiratory efforts against a closed shutter over 20 seconds. Values of negative $20 - 30$ cm H_2O are thought to be predictive of success. This technique predominantly tests isometric muscle strength as opposed to endurance, and the predictive value is poor. Vital-capacity maneuvers may give some indication of reserve capacity. Vital-capacity values of greater than 1 liter or greater than two times the tidal volume suggest sufficient reserve function to attempt an SBT. The poor predictive value of individual tests like the NIF and VC has led to the development of integrative indices. The rapid shallow breathing index (RSBI; aka Tobin index) is one of the most widely used because of its ease of calculation and improved predictive value. It is useful as a screening tool to assess patients for the ability to proceed to an SBT. The RSBI is calculated by counting the number of breaths in 1 minute divided by the average tidal volume in liters. Values greater than 105 are predictive of inability to wean while values less than 80 are associated with maintained separation from the ventilator at 24 hours. Patients with values between 80 and 105 are at increased risk for reintubation.

In summary, no single test is predictive of success in discontinuation of mechanical ventilation. Patients should be assessed daily for ability to wean and proceed to an SBT if indicated. Proper implementation of protocols can aid in identifying patients who are ready to wean, thus decreasing the complications associated with both unnecessarily prolonged mechanical ventilation and premature separation from the ventilator.

SUGGESTED READINGS

Esteban A, Frutos F, Tobin MJ, et al. A comparison of four methods of weaning patients from mechanical ventilation. Spanish Lung Failure Collaborative Group. N Engl J Med 1995;332:345–350.

MacIntyre NR. Respiratory mechanics in the patient who is weaning from the ventilator. Respir Care 2005;50:275–286; discussion 284–286.

131

CONSIDER USING HELIOX IN THE MECHANICALLY VENTED ASTHMATIC PATIENT

ANTHONY D. SLONIM, MD, DrPH

Therapeutic strategies in pulmonary medicine frequently employ bronchodilators or steroids to decrease airway resistance and improve airflow. As an alternative strategy, the viscosity and density of inspired air may be manipulated to achieve this same desired effect. Air consists of 21% oxygen, with most of the remainder being nitrogen. Oxygen and nitrogen have nearly equivalent densities, and thus altering the percentage of FIO_2 (fraction of inspired oxygen) does not appreciably change the physical properties of the gas mixture. However, replacing nitrogen with the less-dense helium can dramatically decrease the overall air density. This in turn reduces airway resistance, even without anatomical changes in airway caliber.

There are no evidence-based guidelines directing the use of heliox. However, given that heliox does not have any significant side effects, therapeutic trials may be used in patients with obstructive upper-airway conditions and respiratory compromise. Low-density gas mixtures have the greatest beneficial impact in large airways with turbulent density-dependent flow, resulting in improved alveolar emptying and reduced plateau pressures. Considering this, patients with severe asthma (requiring mechanical ventilation) may be ideal candidates for heliox therapy. Indeed, in trials of intubated patients with status asthmaticus, those treated with heliox demonstrated decreased airway pressures, decreased $PaCO_2$(partial pressure of carbon dioxide, arterial), and improved acidosis. Patients with other severe upper-airway diseases such as postextubation obstruction or chronic obstructive pulmonary disease may benefit as well.

WHAT TO DO

It is recommended that heliox therapy be initiated early to reduce respiratory muscle fatigue. Commonly used mixtures contain 80:20, 70:30, or 60:40 helium-to-oxygen ratios. Clinically, the best strategy is to use the highest helium content that maintains an oxygen saturation $\geq 90\%$. Using increasing helium concentrations linearly maximizes the benefit of low-density gas inhalation. Conversely, adequate oxygen fractions are necessary to maintain alveolar oxygenation. The favorable effects of heliox therapy are often seen within minutes. Importantly, ventilators and instrumentation must be calibrated for heliox use. There are published algorithms for these calibrations.

SUGGESTED READINGS

Gluck EH, Onorato DJ, Castriotta R. Helium-oxygen mixtures in intubated patients with status asthmaticus and respiratory acidosis. Chest 1990;98:693.

Kass JE, Castriotta RJ. Heliox therapy in acute severe asthma. Chest 1995;107:757.

Rodrigo G, Rodrigo C, Pollack CV. Use of helium-oxygen mixtures in the treatment of acute asthma: a systematic review. Chest 2003;123:891–896.

INFECTIOUS DISEASE

CONSIDER PARVOVIRUS B19 INFECTION IN PATIENTS WITH ANEMIA OR PANCYTOPENIA

JAYME E. LOCKE, MD

Parvovirus B19 is a nonenveloped virus with single-stranded DNA that has a tropism for erythroid progenitor cells. The virus replicates within these cells and is cytotoxic, resulting in a pure red cell aplasia. It is a common viral disorder that is transmitted via droplets, transplacentally, and through blood transfusions. It is acquired early in life and is so common that greater than 90% of the elderly are seropositive. In general, a normal host clears the infection and at most develops a transient clinically insignificant anemia. This infection, however, becomes hematologically significant in patients with chronic hemolytic anemias, such as sickle cell, thalassemia, and congenital spherocytosis; in patients with acute malaria; and in patients with human immunodeficiency virus/acquired immunodeficiency syndrome (HIV/AIDS).

Parvovirus B19 can pose considerable risk to a critically ill patient. Any patient with pancytopenia or red cell aplasia of unknown origin should be tested for parvovirus B19 infection. The virus can be detected in a patient's blood using a dot-plot analysis and confirmed with DNA hybridization. The virus can also be detected in bone-marrow aspirates, where giant proerythroblasts with eosinophilic nuclear inclusion bodies are seen. Once diagnosed, parvovirus B19 is easily treated with administration of immunoglobulin. Treatment results in prompt reticulocytosis and resolution of the anemia.

SUGGESTED READINGS

Strickland GT, ed. Hunter's Tropical Medicine and Emerging Infectious Diseases. 8th ed. Philadelphia: WB Saunders; 2000:37.

Young NS, Abkowitz JL, Luzzatto L. New insights into pathophysiology of acquired cytopenias. Hematology (Am Soc Hematol Educ Program). 2000:18–31.

Consider Prophylactic Antibiotics When Leeches Are Applied to Free Flaps

Benjamin A. Mandel, MD

The use of leeches for medicinal purposes dates back at least 2,000 years. This practice peaked in the 18th and 19th centuries when practitioners employed the parasites to treat pathologies including gout, headaches, mental illness, obesity, and whooping cough among others. Leech therapy rapidly declined by the beginning of the 20th century when the intervention was found to have little recognizable benefit.

More recently, however, modern medicine has seen a resurgence in the application of leeches. Surgeons now commonly use the parasites to treat acute venous congestion after free-tissue transfer or replantation. This microvascular complication stems from inadequate venous drainage from the tissue in question. Quite literally, blood backs up and compromises arterial inflow, which leads to hypoxia and ultimately to surgical flap demise. Signs of acute venous congestion include dusky or bluish-purple discoloration, edema, brisk capillary refill, and relative tissue warmth.

To combat this venous congestion, medicinal leeches (*Hirudo medicinalis*) are applied to the compromised tissue, allowing the collected blood an alternative route of egress. This decongestion allows the return of arterial flow and prevents tissue ischemia and necrosis. Several leeches will consume from 5 to 15 mL of blood over approximately 25 minutes. After parasite detachment, up to another 50 mL of blood may exit from the bite wound; it is this secondary blood loss that provides the major benefit for tissue salvage. In large-volume bloodletting, transfusion may be necessary.

The leech salivary gland secretes several substances that facilitate the beneficial effects of this therapy. Leech saliva contains anticoagulants including hirudin, a selective thrombin inhibitor, which prevent thrombus formation. In addition, an anesthetic component renders the bite painless, and a histaminelike vasodilator increases blood flow to the parasite. It is generally accepted that the hirudin is largely responsible for the therapeutic postdetachment blood loss.

The leech gut contains *Aeromonas hydrophila*, a gram-negative anaerobic bacillus that aids in the digestion of consumed blood. This penicillin-resistant bacterium can be transmitted to the host via regurgitation of gut contents, leading to cellulitis, abscess formation, flap failure, and sepsis. For this reason, many experienced tissue-transfer surgeons advocate a 10- to 14-day antibiotic prophylaxis for leech therapy with trimethoprim-sulfamethoxazole, fluoroquinolones, or a third-generation cephalosporin, although there are few high-quality clinical trials supporting this practice.

SUGGESTED READINGS

Clark NM, Femino JE, Chenoweth CE. Aeromonas infection after medicinal leech therapy: case reports and review of the literature. Infect Dis Clin Pract. 2001;10(4):221–218.

Weinfeld AB, Yuksel E, Boutros S, et al. Clinical and scientific considerations in leech therapy for the management of acute venous congestion: an updated review. Ann Plast Surg. 2000;45(2):207–212.

134

TREAT METHICILLIN-RESISTANT STAPHYLOCOCCUS AUREUS WITH A MINIMUM OF 14 DAYS OF ANTIBIOTICS

IOSIFINA GIANNAKIKOU, MD

There are approximately 2 million nosocomial infections in the United States each year. About 30% of these infections are by *Staphylococcus aureus*, of which 40% are methicillin-resistant *S. aureus* (MRSA). In intensive care units (ICUs), the percentage of antibiotic-resistant Staph infections approaches 60%. The major reservoir of MRSA in institutions is colonized and infected inpatients. Nasal carriage of MRSA in ICU patients was associated with an MRSA bacteraemia rate of 38%, four times higher than methicillin-sensitive *S. aureus*. One-third of colonized patients become infected and one-half of these have pneumonia or bloodstream infection. Mortality rates for nosocomial-acquired MRSA infections may reach 50% for bloodstream infections and 33% for pneumonia.

WHAT TO DO

Vancomycin (a glycopeptide) is the standard treatment for MRSA. Vancomycin 15 mg/kg q12h, or usually 1g qd, is administered intravenously for 14 to 21 days. Recent randomized control studies have shown linezolid to be as efficacious as vancomycin and with a predictable bacteriostatic activity for suspected or proven MRSA infections. Linezolid, an oxazolidinone antibiotic, is available in an intravenous and an oral form, which is 100% bioavailable. Linezolid's dose is 600 mg intravenously or orally (IV/PO) q12h. However, vancomycin is still preferred by some authorities in order to increase longevity of linezolid's activity. In Europe, teicoplanin (also a glycopeptide) is commonly used.

In cases of vancomycin-treatment failure or allergy, other drugs used for treating MRSA bacteremia are quinupristin-dalfopristin, 7.5 mg/kg IV q12h and daptomycin, 6 mg/kg IV qd.

MRSA bacteremia should be treated with at least a 14-day course of antibiotics if there is prompt (within 72 hours) clinical response. If there is persistent bacteremia (more than 3 days), some advocate 4 weeks of treatment even with a negative echocardiogram. In the case of endocarditis, the treatment course should increase to at least

6 weeks. Recurrence or relapse rates are high if patients are treated for less than the suggested course.

SUGGESTED READINGS

Cepeda JA, Whitehouse T, Cooper B, et al. Linezolid versus teicoplanin in the treatment of Gram-positive infections in the critically ill: a randomized, double-blind, multicentre study. J Antimicrob Chemother. 2004;53(2):345–355.

Chaix C, Durand-Zaleski I, Alberti C, et al. Control of endemic methicillin-resistant *Staphylococcus aureus*: a cost-benefit analysis in an intensive care unit. JAMA.1999;282:1745–1751.

Haddadin AS, Fappiano SA, Lipsett PA. Methicillin resistant *Staphylococcus aureus* (MRSA) in the intensive care unit. Postgrad Med J. 2002;78(921):385–392.

Li JZ, Willke RJ, Rittenhouse BE, Rybak MJ. Effect of linezolid versus vancomycin on length of hospital stay in patients with complicated skin and soft tissue infections caused by known or suspected methicillin-resistant staphylococci: results from a randomized clinical trial. Surg Infect (Larchmt). 2003;4(1):57–70.

Lowy FD. *Staphylococcus aureus* infections. N Engl J Med. 1998;339:520–552.

Merrer J, Santoli F, Appere de Vecchi C, et al. "Colonization pressure" and risk of acquisition of methicillin-resistant *Staphylococcus aureus* in a medical intensive care unit. Infect Control Hosp Epidemiol. 2000;21:718–723.

Pujol M, Pena C, Pallares R, et al. Nosocomial *Staphylococcus aureus* bacteremia among nasal carriers of methicillin-resistant and methicillin-susceptible strains. Am J Med. 1996;100:509–516.

Romero-Vivas J, Rubio M, Fernandez C, et al. Mortality associated with nosocomial bacteremia due to methicillin-resistant *Staphylococcus aureus*. Clin Infect Dis. 1995;21(6):1417–1423.

Sharpe JN, Shively EH, Polk HC Jr. Clinical and economic outcomes of oral linezolid versus intravenous vancomycin in the treatment of MRSA-complicated, lower-extremity skin and soft-tissue infections caused by methicillin-resistant *Staphylococcus aureus*. Am J Surg. 2005;189(4):425–428.

Stevens DL, Herr D, Lampiris H, et al. Linezolid versus vancomycin for the treatment of methicillin-resistant *Staphylococcus aureus* infections. Clin Infect Dis. 2002;34(11):1481–1490.

Vincent JE, Bojaro DJ, Suter PM, et al. The prevalence of nosocomial infection in intensive care units in Europe. JAMA. 1995;274:639–644.

Weigelt J, Itani K, Stevens D, et al. Linezolid versus vancomycin in treatment of complicated skin and soft tissue infections. Antimicrob Agents Chemother. 2005;49(6):2260–2266.

Weigelt J, Kaafarani HM, Itani KM, et al. Linezolid eradicates MRSA better than vancomycin from surgical-site infections. Am J Surg. 2004;188(6):760–766.

135

BE ALERT FOR THROMBOCYTOPENIA AND NEUTROPENIA WITH LINEZOLID

SHAYTONE NICHOLS, MD

Linezolid is an antibiotic in the class oxazolidinones and it is effective against all Gram-positive infections. It is usually reserved for resistant Gram-positive organisms, especially vancomycin-resistant *Enterococcus* (VRE) and methicillin-resistant *Staphylococcus aureus* (MRSA). It is also sometimes considered if outpatient treatment with oral medicines is required.

Linezolid exhibits a mechanism of action that is different than any other antimicrobial class, thus making cross-resistance with other antibiotics uncommon. The drug works by inhibiting the bacterial translation process. Linezolid binds to the 23S peptidyltransferase of the 50S subunit, thus preventing the formation of a functional 70S initiation complex, an essential step in the bacterial translational process. This prevents bacteria from multiplying.

WATCH OUT FOR

The most significant side effect of linezolid is myelosuppression, causing thrombocytopenia, neutropenia, and anemia. The thrombocytopenia is reversible upon discontinuation of the drug. In phase III trials, the rate of thrombocytopenia was found to be 2.4%. However, recent prospective and retrospective studies have found rates as high as 47% in patients treated for longer than 10 days with this antibiotic. There have also been recent reports of toxic optic neuritis in patients receiving linezolid for 10 months. These symptoms also resolved with discontinuation of the antibiotic. In addition, since linezolid possesses monoamine oxidase inhibitor (MAOI) activity, it should not be administered with adrenergic and serotonergic agents such as the antidepressant selective serotonin reuptake inhibitors (SSRIs).

If linezolid must be stopped, there are several alternative antimicrobials currently available to treat resistant Gram-positive organisms. Quinupristin-dalfopristin was approved in 1999 and is a streptogramin antibiotic with activity against Gram-positive organisms. It is effective against both methicillin- and vancomycin-resistant *S. aureus* and it can be used to treat vancomycin-resistant *Enterococcus faecium* but not vancomycin-resistant *E. faecalis*. Resistance develops rapidly with its use and as a result is a less reliable antimicrobial than linezolid.

Daptomycin (the only antibiotic in this class) was recently approved in 2003 and has shown good utility. It is a cyclic lipopeptide and is effective against all Gram-positive microbes including VRE, MRSA, and VRSA. In 2005 tigecycline was approved and has extended spectrum coverage including all Gram positives and resistant Gram positives. It also has activity against anaerobes and Gram negatives, including extended-spectrum beta-lactamases.

SUGGESTED READINGS

Rao N, Ziran B, Wagener MM, et al. Similar hematologic effects of long term linezolid and vancomycin therapy in a prospective observational study of patients with orthopedic infections. Clin Infect Dis. 2004;38:1058–1064.

Senneville E, Legout L. Risk factors for anemia in patients on prolonged linezolid therapy for chronic osteomyelitis: a case-control study. J Antimicrob Chemother. 2004;54:798–802.

136

HAVE A HIGH THRESHOLD FOR USING CASPOFUNGIN AND VORICONAZOLE IN PATIENTS WITH LIVER DISEASE

LEO HSIAO, DO

Caspofungin is a member of a class of antifungals known as echinocandins. This family of antifungal exerts its effect by destabilizing the fungal cell wall through noncompetitive inhibition of β-(1,3)-D-glucan synthase. Inhibition of this enzyme prevents the synthesis of glucan, which is a key component of cell-wall stability. Not surprisingly, the relative amount of β-(1,3)-D-glucan making up the cell wall of various fungal species correlates to its susceptibility to caspofungin. Of note, caspofungin's antifungal mechanism limits its activity to branch points where there is new cell-wall synthesis.

Caspofungin is effective against a wide range of fungi including *Aspergillus* species (*fumigatus, flavus, terreus*), *Pneumocystis carinii*, and *Candida* species. Its efficacy has been evaluated in the treatment of invasive candidiasis where caspofungin demonstrated a 74% success rate versus a 62% success rate of conventional therapy with amphotericin B. Because of limitations in formulation, caspofungin's role in the treatment of oral or esophageal candidiasis should be limited either to patients who cannot tolerate azole therapy or to cases of documented failure to azole therapy. In the setting of empiric treatment of febrile neutropenia, caspofungin has been shown to be as effective as liposomal amphotericin B and with fewer side effects. Lastly, caspofungin was initially approved for salvage therapy for the management of invasive aspergillosis. Although there are some data to support its efficacy as primary therapy for invasive aspergillosis, there is concern that use of a fungistatic agent in immunocompromised patients might lead to relapse of disease.

WATCH OUT FOR

Common adverse reactions to caspofungin include fever, nausea, vomiting, and venous irritation. Caspofungin has also been shown to cause rash, bronchoconstriction, wheezing, and facial edema and flushing, denoting a probable correlation to histamine release. Alterations in liver function tests are mostly transient; however, in a patient with moderate pre-existing liver disease, defined as a Child-Pugh score of 7 to 9, dosage adjustments should be instituted. Since there are no good data available to support the safety of caspofungin in patients with Child-Pugh scores >9, it may prudent to limit the use of caspofungin in this patient population. Also, because caspofungin is metabolized by N-acetylation in the liver, its use in cirrhotic patients potentially lacking this essential metabolic pathway should be judicious.

Voriconazole is a second-generation triazole derivative of fluconazole. It exerts its antifungal activity by inhibiting the cytochrome P-450 enzyme 14-α demethylase. This inhibition prevents the conversion of lanosterol to ergosterol. Ergosterol is an important constituent of the fungal cell membrane and therefore its absence, coupled with the accumulation of toxic sterol precursors, ultimately leads to fungal demise.

The spectrum of activity and clinical efficacy of voriconazole has been well documented in both in vitro testing and clinical trials. For example, voriconazole is highly effective against most strains of *Candida* despite indications of potential cross-resistance with fluconazole among certain isolates. In the treatment of oral candidiasis, voriconazole has proven to be as efficacious as fluconazole. Moreover, there is evidence that voriconazole is effective against invasive candidiasis both as primary and salvage therapy and that its safety profile is superior to that of amphotericin B. Likewise, voriconazole can be considered an alternative to amphotericin B for the treatment of *Cryptococcus neoformans*.

Voriconazole demonstrates impressive in vitro activity against *Aspergillus* species, even against isolates resistant to itraconazole and amphotericin B. These data have been borne out in clinical trials in which voriconazole has shown to outperform amphotericin B against invasive aspergillosis. Lastly, voriconazole has shown promise against less common fungal infections including the *Scedosporium*, *Pseudallescheria*, and *Fusarium* species.

WATCH OUT FOR

Adverse reactions to voriconazole were evaluated in recent clinical trials. The most common reactions were visual disturbances (blurry vision, altered color perception, and photophobia), rash, and alterations in liver-function tests. Other reactions include hypoglycemia, pneumonitis, worsening psoriasis, and visual or auditory hallucinations. Of note, up to 20% of study participants developed elevation in liver-function tests (defined as three times the upper limit of normal). Although most of these elevations normalized after discontinuation of drug, there have been reports of hepatic failure and death associated with the use of voriconazole. It is therefore prudent to consider pre-existing liver disease as a relative contraindication to voriconazole therapy.

In addition to caspofungin other members of the echinocandin family of drugs include micafungin and anidulafungin. These drugs may be considered alternatives to caspofungin although further studies need to be done to better define their clinical role. The same can be said of voriconazole with respect to its sister second-generation azole derivatives posaconazole and ravuconazole. Lastly, combination therapy utilizing both voriconazole and caspofungin/liposomal amphotericin B has shown promise in the setting of invasive aspergillosis, giving yet another alternative to single-agent therapy.

SUGGESTED READINGS

Kofla G, Runhke M. Voriconazole: review of a broad spectrum triazole antifungal agent. Exp Opin Pharmacother. 2005;6(7):1215–1229.

Pacetti S, Gelone S. Caspofungin acetate for treatment of invasive fungal infections. Ann Pharmacother. 2003;37(1):90–98.

Zaas A, Alexander B. Echinocandins: role in antifungal therapy, 2005. Exp Opin Pharmacother. 2005;6(10):1657–1668.

137

Do not use caspofungin or voriconazole to treat yeast in the urine because a very small amount of these drugs are excreted in the urine

Harjot K. Singh, MD
Lesia K. Dropulic, MD

Candiduria, or yeast in the urine, is commonly encountered in the intensive care unit (ICU) setting. Risk factors for candiduria include increased age, female sex, urinary drainage catheters, antibiotic use, prior surgical procedures, and diabetes mellitus. Detection of the *Candida* species of yeast in the urine can represent colonization or infection and distinguishing between the two can be difficult because of the lack of appropriate diagnostic tests. Clinical findings used to diagnose bacterial infections of the lower urinary tract are not applicable to candiduria because patients are often asymptomatic and yeast colony counts and pyuria do not correlate with infection. Most of the time, candiduria is a benign process. However, caution is warranted because candiduria may represent disseminated or upper urinary tract infection in certain high-risk ICU patients.

The Infectious Diseases Society of America's guidelines for treatment of candidiasis recommend antifungal treatment of candiduria in the following circumstances: symptomatic patients; patients who will undergo urinary tract manipulation; patients with neutropenia; patients with renal allografts; and infants with low birth weight. Treatment of these select patients might reduce the risk of ascending infection and/or disseminated infection or might treat occult disseminated candidiasis. In addition, antifungal treatment should be considered for patients with candiduria who have urinary tract obstruction or an abnormal urinary tract, patients who are to have surgery to implant prosthetic devices [e.g., valves, joints, ventricular assist devices (VADs)], and critically ill patients who already have implanted VADs.

Fluconazole, dose adjusted for renal insufficiency, is the antifungal agent of choice for treatment of fluconazole-susceptible *Candida* species isolated from urine. Seven to 14 days of therapy is recommended and duration depends on the extent of symptoms and on the severity of the underlying disease. *C. albicans* is the most common isolate and is susceptible to fluconazole. *C. glabrata* isolates might exhibit dose-dependent susceptibility or may be resistant to fluconazole. *C. krusei* is intrinsically resistant to fluconazole. For such fluconazole-resistant isolates, amphotericin B deoxycholate is recommended at a range of doses and for a range of days (0.3 to 1.0 mg/kg per day for 1 to 7 days).

Caspofungin and voriconazole are not recommended for the treatment of candiduria because a very small amount of these drugs is excreted in the urine. In addition, bladder irrigation with amphotericin only transiently clears candiduria and is not recommended. Relapse of candiduria is frequent after antifungal treatment and commonly occurs with continued use of a urinary catheter or stent. Discontinuation of catheter use alone may result in eradication of candiduria in up to 40% of patients. If possible, catheters and stents should be removed concomitantly with institution of antifungal therapy.

Persistent candiduria in immunocompromised patients requires evaluation of the kidneys with ultrasound or computed tomography scan. Since candiduria can be a manifestation of disseminated infection, blood cultures should be obtained in patients with systemic signs and symptoms.

SUGGESTED READINGS

Kauffman CA. Candiduria. Clin Infect Dis. 2005;41(suppl 6):S371–S376.
Pappas PG, Rex JH, Sobel JD, et al. Guidelines for treatment of candidiasis. Clin Infect Dis. 2004;38:161–189.

138

ADMINISTER A DOSE OF ANTIBIOTIC BEFORE THE BILE SYSTEM IS INSTRUMENTED OR MANIPULATED

KELLY OLINO, MD

Bile ducts are normally sterile. However, in cases where the ducts become obstructed or instrumented, the presence of bacterobilia with some series reporting 90% with positive bile cultures. The most common organisms found are *Escherichia coli*, *Klebsiella*, *Enterobacter*, *Enterococcus*, *Pseudomonas*, *Candida* species, grampositive cocci, bacteroides, and *Clostridium*. In addition, in immunocompromised populations, one should keep in mind unusual organisms such as cryptosporidium and in patients from tropical locations, parasites such as *Ascaris*.

WHAT TO DO

When a patient is undergoing a biliary tract procedure such as percutaneous transhepatic cholangiography (PTC), endoscopic retrograde cholangiopancreatography (ERCP), or open or laparoscopic surgical operations, preprocedural antibiotic treatment is indicated. When selecting appropriate antibiotic coverage it is crucial to look at local institutional microbiological profiles as well as identifying risk factors for bacterobilia. For low-risk patients, namely those who are not severely ill, have not had previous biliary procedures, and have community-acquired illness, a one-time preprocedural treatment with 1 g of cefotetan intravenously (IV) or a fluoroquinolone IV with additional anaerobic coverage with metronidazole 500 mg IV is sufficient, with no proven benefit for postprocedural antibiotics. In patients who are severely ill, with previous instrumentation or hospital-acquired illness, broader-spectrum treatment with piperacillin/tazobactam 3.375 mg IV or a fluoroquinolone with additional anaerobic coverage is indicated. A one-time dose is sufficient, except in cases where adequate drainage is not achieved or in cases of sepsis or cholangitis, where anywhere from 5 to 14 days of treatment may be required.

To briefly review, cholangitis may present secondary to obstruction or after biliary procedures, with up to a 1% to 3% incidence after ERCP. Common etiologies leading to obstruction include gallstones, neoplasms, benign strictures, postoperative stricture, sclerosing cholangitis, papillary stenosis, and malfunction of indwelling stents. There is a broad spectrum of presenting signs and symptoms of cholangitis, ranging from around two-thirds of patients with at least two symptoms of Charcot triad (right upper quadrant pain, fever, jaundice) to 5% of patients with Reynold's pentad (Charcot's triad plus shock and change in mental status). Most patients will have an elevated white blood cell, jaundice, mild right upper quadrant pain, and abnormalities in liver-function tests. The treatment of cholangitis is centered around appropriately timed drainage of the infected bile, IV fluid hydration, and antibiotic treatment, and the mortality rate has been described to be 5%.

SUGGESTED READINGS

Cameron JL, ed. Current Surgical Therapy. 8th ed. New York: Mosby; 2004.

Lipsett PA, Pitt H. Acute cholangitis. Front Biosci. 2003; (Sept. 1):1229–1239.

The American Society for Gastrointestinal Endoscopy. Complications of ERCP. Gastrointest Endosc. 2003;57(6):633–638.

139

ADMINISTER AN ANTIBIOTIC BEFORE URINARY TRACT OBSTRUCTION IS RELIEVED

JENNIFER MILES-THOMAS, MD

Bacteriuria can become bacteremia with associated systemic complications in the setting of urinary tract obstruction. Most bacteria enter the urinary tract system through the urethra from the fecal reservoir. In addition, the kidneys can be secondarily infected by *Staphylococcus aureus* or *Candida* by hematogenous spread. *Escherichia coli* (most common), *Proteus*, *Klebsiella*, and *Enterococcus faecalis* are frequently found to cause infection in the urinary tract.

When there is an increased pressure in the upper urinary tract, pyelovenous backflow may allow infected urine to enter the bloodstream. In addition, there is a change in renal blood flow and decreased neutrophil delivery. This is the proverbial "pus under pressure." Clinical signs and symptoms of urinary tract obstruction are dependent on the time course of the obstruction, whether the obstruction is complete or unilateral, and the cause of the obstruction. Frequent symptoms include flank pain, nausea, and vomiting. Some clinical signs include rising blood urea nitrogen (BUN) or creatinine, electrolyte abnormalities, and hypertension.

WHAT TO DO

Urinary tract infection in a setting of urinary obstruction is an emergency. The patient should be hydrated and started on intravenous (IV) antibiotics as soon as possible. If the patient is septic, broad-spectrum antibiotics such as ampicillin (2 gm IV q6) and gentamicin (1.5 mg/kg q8) or a fluoroquinolone should be given as soon as blood cultures and urine culture are sent. In any patient with a suspected urinary tract obstruction, a Foley catheter should be placed to provide maximal urinary drainage. Once stabilized, the patient should undergo either ureteral stent placement or percutaneous nephrostomy tube placement. Once the obstruction is relieved, the patient should continue to be observed closely for signs of sepsis. An obstructed urinary system should not be instrumented without the protective antibiotics on board, as the bacterial load released into the bloodstream can cause acute and profound physiological derangements.

The patient should also be monitored for postobstructive diuresis, which might be manifested by polyuria with salt wasting, hypotension, or rising BUN. It is typically defined as marked polyuria after the relief of ureteral obstruction. This may be physiologic in which case, renal function quickly returns to normal and the diuresis ceases. In some cases it may be pathologic in nature with continued impairment of sodium reabsorption and impaired renal concentrating ability. The patients most likely to exhibit postobstructive diuresis are those with a history of congestive heart failure, hypertension, edema, and chronic obstruction. After the release of the obstruction, the patient should be monitored for urine output >200 cc per hour for more than 2 hours. If brisk diuresis continues, the patient should have replacement of half of the hourly urinary output with D5 $^1/_2$ normal saline with serial electrolyte checks. Typically, BUN and creatinine will return close to baseline in 24 to 48 hours.

SUGGESTED READINGS

Rubenstein JN, Schaeffer AJ. Managing complicated urinary tract infections. The urologic view. Infect Dis Clin N Am. 2003;17:333–351.
Walsh PC, ed. Campbell's Urology. 8th ed. Philadelphia: WB Saunders; 2002:452–454,515–516,3340.

140

REMEMBER THAT ENTEROCOCCUS IS A RARE INVASIVE PULMONARY TRACT INFECTION

ARUNA K. SUBRAMANIAN, MD

Enterococci rarely cause lower respiratory tract infections, though they are capable of colonizing the oropharynx. Respiratory tract infections due to enterococci are exceedingly unusual, but case reports of enterococcal pneumonia and lung abscess exist in patients with severe and debilitating diseases. These rare cases of enterococcal pneumonia have been described in the setting of broad-spectrum antimicrobial therapy, especially with cephalosporins, along with enteric feeding in severely debilitated patients. However, most experienced clinicians will not attribute a pneumonia to *Enterococcus* even if a respiratory culture returns results positive for this organism.

It is known that enterococci are not as intrinsically virulent as organisms such as *Staphylococcus aureus* and *Streptococcus pyogenes*. They do not secrete exotoxins or produce superantigens. However, studies of patients with enterococcal bacteremia have shown an attributed mortality of 31% to 37% and some studies suggest vancomycin resistance to be an independent predictor of mortality.

Although enterococci do not generally cause trouble in the respiratory tract, infection at other sites can be clinically significant. Enterococci can cause catheter-related bloodstream infections. These organisms adhere to heart valves and renal epithelial cells and thus can cause endocarditis and urinary tract infections. Enterococci are commonly found in cultures of intra-abdominal and pelvic infections. It is thought that enterococci act synergistically with other bacteria in intra-abdominal sepsis to enhance morbidity and mortality. Enterococci by themselves rarely, if ever, cause cellulitis or other soft-tissue infections. They are frequently isolated from mixed cultures in surgical wound infections, decubitus ulcers, and diabetic foot infections, but their significance is difficult to assess in these cases.

In contrast to the *Enterococcus*, *Streptococcus pneumococcus* remains the leading cause (16% to 60%) of acute community-acquired pneumonia (CAP) in most series. Classically, community-acquired pneumonia presents with a sudden onset of a chill followed by fever, pleuritic chest pain, and cough with purulent sputum. Three percent to 38% of cases of CAP are caused by *Haemophilus influenzae*, and *S. aureus* accounts for 2% to 5% of cases. Aerobic Gram-negative bacteria, mixed aerobic and anaerobic infections, and atypical organisms (*Legionella, Mycoplasma*, and *Chlamydia*) cause most of the remaining cases of acute community-acquired pneumonia.

The clinical features of nosocomial pneumonia are nonspecific and may include fever, changing chest radiographs, purulent sputum, and an elevated white blood cell count in a critically ill patient. Approximately 60% of cases of nosocomial pneumonia are caused by aerobic Gram-negative bacilli, with members of the family Enterobacteriaceae (*Klebsiella pneumoniae, Escherichia coli, Serratia marcescens*, and *Enterobacter* species) and *Pseudomonas* species accounting for the majority of these. *S. aureus* causes 13% to 40% of cases and is more common in burn units, in patients with wound infections, and in patients on a ventilator after neurosurgery or head trauma. *S. pneumoniae* causes only 3% to 20% of nosocomial pneumonias, mainly early in the hospital course. Anaerobic bacteria play a role when aspiration is likely to have occurred. Pneumonia caused by *Legionella* species may occur sporadically or as part of outbreaks, especially in immunosuppressed patients. Twenty-five percent to 46% of ventilator-associated pneumonia may be polymicrobial. Nosocomial viral infections are most commonly caused by respiratory syncytial virus, influenza, and parainfluenza, which can cause pneumonitis.

SUGGESTED READINGS

Mandell GL, Bennett JE, Dolin R, eds. Mandell, Douglas, and Bennett's Principles and Practice of Infectious Diseases. 6th ed. New York: Churchill Livingstone; 2005:831–836, 2411–2417.

141

KNOW HOW TO CALCULATE THE CLINICAL PULMONARY INFECTION SCORE

B. ROBERT GIBSON, MD

Ventilator-associated pneumonia (VAP) refers to pneumonia that occurs more than 48 hours after patients are intubated and treated with mechanical ventilation, and it is the second most common nosocomial infection in the United States. Despite this clinical frequency, VAP has been surprisingly difficult to diagnose as there is no single clinical criterion that is specific to VAP. In addition, there is variation in the literature as to what constitutes the clinical diagnosis of VAP. Depending upon the study reviewed, there have been varying interpretations of clinical signs and symptoms suggestive of lung infection, different definitions of colonization versus infection, and different use of antibiotics in the intensive care unit (ICU).

Consistent and timely diagnosis is no small matter as early and appropriate treatment of VAP has been directly linked to favorable patient outcomes. Conversely, late or inappropriate therapy has been found to increase risk of in-hospital mortality by as much as a factor of seven. Typically, pneumonia is suspected if the patient has a radiographic infiltrate that is new or progressive concurrent with clinical findings suggesting infection: new onset of fever, purulent sputum, leukocytosis, or a decline in oxygenation. Unfortunately, these clinical signs are nonspecific and subjective. At best, no single radiographic sign has greater than 68% diagnostic accuracy.

In an effort to enhance diagnostic sensitivity and specificity for VAP, and to provide some consistency within the literature, Pugin et al. developed the clinical pulmonary infection score (CPIS). This clinical scoring system establishes the likelihood of VAP based upon several clinical parameters that can be scored 0, 1, or 2 points (as adapted by Singh et al.) (*Table 141.1*).

When the total CPIS exceeds 6, there is a 93% sensitivity and a 96% specificity for the presence of pneumonia, as defined by quantitative cultures of bronchoscopic and nonbronchoscopic bronchoalveolar lavage (BAL) specimens. The sensitivity and specificity of the CPIS does vary to some degree upon the reference standard used for diagnosis of pneumonia. For instance, when compared with postmortem quantitative lung cultures as the reference standard, the CPIS has a lower sensitivity of 72% to 77% and specificity of 42% to 85%. Varying

TABLE 141.1	CLINICAL PULMONARY INFECTION SCORE (CPIS)
PARAMETER	**POINTS**
Temperature (C)	
36.5–38.4	0
38.5–38.9	1
<36.4 or >39.0	2
WBC Count	
4,000–11,000	0
<4,000 or >11,000	1
with >50% bands	+1
Tracheal Secretions	
None	0
Nonpurulent	1
Purulent	2
Oxygenation: PaO_2/FIO_2 (mm Hg)	
>240 or ARDS	0
<240 without ARDS	2
CXR	
No infiltrate	0
Diffuse/patchy infiltrate	1
Localized infiltrate	2
Infiltrate Progression	
No progression	0
Progression (in absence of CHF or ARDS)	2
ET Suction Culture	
No/light growth	0
Heavy growth	1
Same growth on Gram stain	+1
TOTAL (Range)	0–14

ARDS, acute respiratory distress syndrome; CHF, congestive heart failure; CXR, chest x-ray; ET, endotracheal; FIO_2, fraction of inspired oxygen; WBC, white blood cell.

sensitivity and specificity aside, the overall interpretation based upon these studies is that the CPIS is reasonably accurate for the clinical diagnosis of VAP. Furthermore, if the CPIS is >6 there should be suspicion of VAP and empiric antibiotics should be started.

In addition to being used for the diagnosis of VAP, the CPIS has also been used to guide the duration of antibiotic therapy. Singh et al. explored whether the CPIS could serve as a tool to limit antibiotic overuse in the ICU. Subjects who were less likely to have an infection (CPIS ≤6) were randomized to either "standard," 10- to 21-day antibiotic therapy or a 3-day course of empiric ciprofloxacin, followed by re-evaluation, with discontinuation of treatment if the CPIS remained ≤6. Outcome, measured as mortality and length of ICU stay, was the same for both the short-course group and the longer-course group receiving standard therapy. It is postulated that the shorter-course patients will have a decrease in superinfections and a decrease in antibiotic resistance. Thus, in patients with an initial CPIS ≤6 and an improving clinical course, longer antibiotic regimens of 10 to 21 days may not be necessary.

SUGGESTED READINGS

American Thoracic Society; Infectious Diseases Society of America. Guidelines for the management of adults with hospital-acquired, ventilator-associated, and healthcare-associated pneumonia Am J Respir Crit Care Med. 2005;171(4):388–416.

Pugin J, Auckenthaler R, Mili N, et al. Diagnosis of ventilator-associated pneumonia by bacteriologic analysis of bronchoscopic and non-bronchoscopic "blind" bronchoalveolar lavage fluid. Am Rev Respir Dis. 1991;143:1121–1129.

Singh N, Rogers P, Atwood CW, et al. Short-course empiric antibiotic therapy for patients with pulmonary infiltrates in the intensive care unit: a proposed solution for indiscriminate antibiotic prescription. Am J Respir Crit Care Med. 2000;162:505–511.

142

REMEMBER THAT LACK OF POSITIVE BLOOD CULTURES DOES NOT RULE OUT BACTERIAL ENDOCARDITIS

HARJOT K. SINGH, MD
ARUNA K. SUBRAMANIAN, MD

Infective endocarditis (IE) is generally defined by vegetative cardiac lesions in the setting of positive blood cultures. However, the lack of a single diagnostic test has led to several diagnostic algorithms, of which the Duke criteria are the most widely accepted. The Duke criteria have been shown to have a specificity of 99% and a negative predictive value of 92%. Despite the diagnostic difficulty, when infective endocarditis is suspected, empiric therapy is warranted because of its high morbidity and mortality.

SIGNS AND SYMPTOMS

The signs and symptoms of infective endocarditis can vary greatly and have a low sensitivity and specificity for infective endocarditis. Fevers, chills, and sweats are common. Fatigue, syncope, congestive heart failure, and embolic events can occur. On exam, patients can have fever, new or louder pre-existent murmurs, splinter hemorrhages, Janeway lesions, Osler nodes, or Roth spots. Risk factors endocarditis include presence of prosthetic valves, structural heart disease, intravenous drug use, and indwelling catheters.

Definitive diagnosis using the Duke criteria requires fulfillment of two major criteria, one major and three minor, or five minor criteria.

MAJOR CRITERIA

- Two separate positive blood cultures for a typical organism (community-acquired *Staphylococcus aureus* or enterococci without another infectious focus, *Streptococcus viridans*, *Streptococcus bovis*, or HACEK[1] group), or persistently positive blood cultures with any organism (e.g., two specimens drawn 12 hours apart, all of three separate cultures at least 1 hour apart, or most of ≥ four cultures)
- Vegetation/abscess/new prosthetic valve dehiscence on echocardiogram, or new valvular regurgitation (increase or change in pre-existing murmur is *not* sufficient)

---

[1]HACEK group: *Haemophilus* species, *Actinobacillus actinomycetemcomitans*, *Cardiobacterium hominis*, *Eikenella* species, and *Kingella kingae*.

MINOR CRITERIA

- Predisposing condition (previous endocarditis, injection drug use, prosthetic valve, structural heart disease)
- Fever >38°C
- Embolic event
- Immunologic phenomenon (e.g., Osler nodes, glomerulonephritis, positive rheumatoid factor)

Even with careful diagnostic techniques, blood cultures remain negative in approximately 5%–10% of patients with infective endocarditis. Negative cultures are especially common when HACEK group organisms,*Coxiella burnetii*, or other atypical organisms (*Chlamydia*, *Mycoplasma*, *Brucella*) are responsible because they do not grow in standard medium or require longer growth of 7 to 21 days. Most laboratories can test for these if asked. The typical organisms that cause infective endocarditis include *S. aureus*, *S. bovis*, *S. viridans*, and *Enterococcus* species. Gram-negative bacilli and fungi are less common causes of endocarditis.

WHAT TO DO

The organism, valvular location, and presence of prosthetic devices determine treatment of infective endocarditis. A long duration of parenteral antibiotics is necessary because of the high density of micro-organisms within the vegetation. Uncomplicated right-sided infective endocarditis with penicillin-sensitive streptococci can be treated either with penicillin (12 to 18 million units/day) and gentamicin (1 mg/kg intravenously q8h) for 2 weeks (most other regimens require longer therapy) or with penicillin alone for 4 weeks. *S. viridans* and *S. bovis* are treated with penicillin (18 mu/day) and gentamicin, while enterococci are treated with ampicillin (12 g/day) and gentamicin for 4 to 6 weeks. Penicillin-allergic patients either undergo desensitization or vancomycin is used.

Methicillin-sensitive *S. aureus* is best treated with nafcillin or oxacillin 2 g IV q4h for 4 to 6 weeks, with the optional addition of gentamicin 1 mg/kg IV q8h for 3 to 5 days. For MRSA or penicillin allergy, vancomycin is used at 15 mg/kg IV q12h. If prosthetic material is present, at least 6 weeks of therapy is required with nafcillin, oxacillin, or vancomycin; rifampin is added for synergy for 6 weeks and gentamicin is used for 2 weeks. Surgical intervention is usually required in addition for prosthetic valve IE. HACEK organisms are treated with ceftriaxone (2 g/day) for 4 weeks.

SUGGESTED READINGS

Bartlett JG, ed. Pocket Book of Infectious Disease Therapy, 2005–6. Philadelphia: Lippincott Williams & Wilkins; 2004:253–261.

Mandell GL, Bennett JE, Dolin R, eds. Mandell, Douglas, and Bennett's Principles and Practice of Infectious Diseases. 6th ed. New York: Churchill Livingstone; 2005:975–1002.

143

TREAT BLACK LIPS OR A BLACK SPOT ON THE ORAL MUCOSA AS A SURGICAL EMERGENCY

ARUNA K. SUBRAMANIAN, MD

Mucormycosis is the common name given to several different diseases caused by fungi of the order Mucorales. It is also called zygomycosis after the class Zygomycetes, which are molds that grow in the environment and in tissue as hyphal forms. *Rhizopus* species are the most commonly isolated agents of mucormycosis, followed by *Rhizomucor* and *Cunninghamella*.

Mucormycosis is mostly limited to people with severe immunocompromise, diabetes mellitus, or trauma. Solid-organ and hematopoietic stem-cell transplant recipients represent a growing population at risk. More than half of patients have rhinocerebral disease; approximately 10% have pulmonary, cutaneous, or disseminated disease; and 2% have kidney or gastrointestinal involvement. Three-quarters of transplant patients with mucormycosis also had diabetes or had received antirejection therapy. It is rarely seen in immunocompetent hosts.

Most commonly, the fungus gains entry to the body through the respiratory tract and is inhaled from the nasal turbinates. In the case of primary cutaneous mucormycosis, spores are introduced directly into abraded skin. They then proliferate and can invade more widely. Once the fungus begins to grow, the hyphae invade tissue and have a special affinity for blood vessels. Direct penetration and growth through the blood-vessel wall explain the propensity for thrombosis and tissue necrosis, two major hallmarks of the histopathology of mucormycosis.

Rhinocerebral mucormycosis is most often found in patients with diabetes mellitus, particularly in the presence of acidosis, and in patients with leukemia who have been neutropenic for long periods and who have been receiving broad-spectrum antibacterial drugs. Patients complain of facial pain and/or headache, and fever and orbital cellulitis occur. Invasion often involves the palate and perioral tissues, first with erythema and then the development of ulceration (where it can mimic a herpetic lesion), which may turn black, reflecting the characteristic tissue necrosis. It is important to consider the possibility of mucormycosis before the development of the necrotic ulcer. With invasion of the orbit loss of extraocular muscle function, proptosis, and marked swelling of the conjunctiva become evident. Loss of vision may result from thrombosis of the retinal artery and the development of cranial nerve dysfunction is manifested by ptosis and pupillary dilatation, which represents a serious prognostic event. Cerebral abscess, cavernous sinus, and internal carotid artery thrombosis are additional complications.

Pulmonary mucormycosis is marked by fever, dyspnea, and cough. With continued tissue necrosis, hemoptysis may develop; should a major blood vessel be eroded, fatal pulmonary hemorrhage can result.

The hallmarks of mucormycosis are vascular invasion and tissue necrosis; black eschars and discharges should be aggressively sought. The presence of a black nasal discharge should not be dismissed as merely dried blood as it may reflect tissue necrosis. Similarly, black necrotic lesions of the nasal mucosa or hard palate may reflect invasive mucormycosis. Diagnosis depends on demonstration of the organism in the tissue of a biopsy specimen. Swabs of discharge or abnormal tissue are not appropriate and often result in erroneous information. Fungal hyphae can be seen on potassium hydroxide preparations of touch slides prepared from the biopsy specimen. Fixed tissue can be stained with routine or special fungal stains to demonstrate fungal hyphae.

WHAT TO DO

In mucormycosis aggressive correction of hyperglycemia and acidemia should be pursued. If possible, doses of immunosuppressive drugs, including steroids, should be decreased or stopped. The prognosis often depends on the ability to reverse the predisposing conditions. The standard therapy for invasive mucormycosis is treatment with amphotericin B. Because the fungus is relatively refractory to medical treatment, the maximum tolerated dose of amphotericin B deoxycholate is usually recommended, typically 1.0 to 1.5 mg/kg/day. High doses are not usually tolerated before renal function deteriorates; therefore, lipid preparations such as amphotericin B lipid complex (Abelcet) and liposomal amphotericin B (AmBisome) are recommended at a dose of at least 5 mg/kg daily.

None of the currently available azoles (ketoconazole, itraconazole, fluconazole, or voriconazole) or echinocandins has a role in the treatment of mucormycosis. A new, broad-spectrum triazole, posaconazole (not yet clinically available), has been shown to be active in a murine model of mucormycosis. Successful use of posaconazole has been reported after initial therapy with amphotericin B and often surgery.

Although reports have appeared in the literature of recovery of patients with mucormycosis with antifungal therapy alone, these are clearly the exception and aggressive surgical debridement of necrotic tissue is advisable. Repeated operations may be required for satisfactory removal of continuously appearing necrotic tissue. The overall historical mortality rate has been about 50%, although higher survival rates (up to 85%) have been reported more recently.

SUGGESTED READING

Mandell GL, Bennett JE, Dolin R, eds. Mandell, Douglas, and Bennett's Principles and Practice of Infectious Diseases. 6th ed. London: Churchill Livingstone; 2005:2973–2981.

144

CHECK FOR CRYPTOSPORIDIUM IN IMMUNOSUPPRESSED PATIENTS WITH CHRONIC, SEVERE, OR REFRACTORY DIARRHEA

ALA' S. HADDADIN, MD

Diarrhea, the principal manifestation of intestinal infection among the critically ill, affects approximately one-third of all patients (reported incidence of 2% to 63%) admitted to the intensive care unit (ICU). Although many definitions exist in the literature, diarrhea is best defined as bowel movements that, because of increased frequency, abnormal consistency (the normal water content of stool is 60% to 85% of total weight), or increased volume (stool volume output >250 mL or 250 g/day), are deleterious to the well-being of the patient. Potentially deleterious consequences in these patients include perianal and sacral skin ulcers with secondary superinfections and decreased absorption of enterally administered medications. For the critically ill patient, the dehydration that accompanies severe diarrhea strains a circulatory system already limited by impaired cardiac function and septic hemodynamics, which might ultimately culminate in multisystem organ failure. Diarrhea can also precipitate metabolic derangements including electrolyte imbalances and anion gap acidosis with all their debilitating consequences.

Three main types of diarrhea include secretory, osmotic, and inflammatory diarrhea.

SECRETORY DIARRHEA

In this disorder, there is both active intestinal secretion of fluids (commonly described as "watery" diarrhea) and electrolytes as well as decreased absorption. Common causes of secretory diarrhea include enterotoxins (e.g., cholera, rotavirus, *Escherichia coli*); hormones (e.g., vasoactive intestinal peptide in the Verner-Morrison syndrome); bile salts (in the colon) following ileal resection; fatty acids (in the colon) following ileal resection; and laxatives (e.g., a docusate sodium). Secretory diarrhea occurs even when the patient is fasting because the secretory process is independent of enteral intake or the absorptive process.

OSMOTIC DIARRHEA

This type of diarrhea results from consuming nonabsorbable solutes by mouth, nasogastric tube, or nasoenteral tube. This type of diarrhea resolves once the osmotic load is eliminated (i.e., on the outset of fasting). Some medications causing this type of diarrhea include sorbitol; a solution of polyethylene glycol and electrolytes (GoLYTELY); and magnesium-containing medications. It can also be secondary to malabsorption and incomplete digestion of protein (azotorrhea), fats (steatorrhea), or carbohydrates.

INFLAMMATORY DIARRHEA (MUCOSAL DESTRUCTION)

Inflammatory diarrhea occurs secondary to damage to the intestinal mucosal cell so that there is loss of fluid and/or blood. In addition, there is defective absorption of fluids and electrolytes. Common causes are infective conditions (e.g., clostridial infections, dysentery due to *Shigella*, particularly *S. dysenteriae*, and *Cryptosporidium*) and inflammatory conditions (e.g., inflammatory bowel disease). This type of diarrhea worsens after feeding and persists after fasting. Fecal leukocytes are present.

Cryptosporidiosis is caused by *Cryptosporidium parvum*, a microscopic one-celled parasite that can live in the intestines of humans, farm animals, wild animals, and pets. The parasite is protected by an outer shell called an oocyst. This protective shell allows it to survive outside the body for an extended period. *C. parvum* is highly infectious, requiring only 10^1 to 10^3 oocysts to cause human disease (50% infectious dose, 10^2). The oocysts are infectious immediately, and the life cycle of the parasite produces forms that invade the intestine. Location of the parasite in the intestine is intracellular but extracytoplasmic, which might contribute to the marked resistance of *C. parvum* to treatment. Large numbers of oocysts are excreted and are resistant to harsh conditions, including chlorine in levels usually applied in water treatment. Cryptosporidiosis is a frequent cause of infectious diarrhea, especially in immunocompromised patients whose CD4+ lymphocyte count falls below 200 cells/μL. Cryptosporidiosis parasites are passed in the stool of infected persons and animals. People get cryptosporidiosis when they swallow the parasites. Sources of disease include parasite-containing stool, food, and water.

The mechanism by which *C. parvum* causes diarrhea is not known for certain, but it appears to be a combination of secretory and malabsorptive processes. In patients who are not immunocompromised, the infection is limited to the jejunum. In patients with acquired immunodeficiency syndrome (AIDS), the entire gastrointestinal tract and respiratory tract may be involved. After an incubation period of 7 to 10 days (range 5 to 28 days), the patient develops diarrhea and may have abdominal cramps and a low-grade fever. Patients with AIDS can have voluminous diarrhea (up to 17 L/d). Biliary infection in patients with AIDS is associated with right upper quadrant pain, nausea, and vomiting. Physical findings are nonspecific. Temperature higher than 39°C is not characteristic of cryptosporidiosis and warrants investigation for other infections.

There are many diagnostic tests ordered for patients with the possibility of *Cryptosporidium*. On stool microscopy modified acid-fast staining of stool shows red-stained round oocysts against a blue-green background. White and red blood cells should not be seen in the stool. Stool cultures are usually performed to rule out the presence of other bacterial pathogens: Elevated alkaline phosphatase and glutamyl transpeptidase without hyperbilirubinemia are typical signs of biliary infection. $CD4^+$ lymphocyte counts predict the duration of disease in patients infected with human immunodeficiency virus (HIV). When the counts are greater than 200, the diarrhea is likely to resolve spontaneously. Abdominal ultrasound will show dilated or irregular intrahepatic and extrahepatic bile ducts, along with a thickened gallbladder in biliary involvement. Identification of *Cryptosporidium* in bile on endoscopic retrograde cholangiopancreatography confirms the diagnosis of cryptosporidiosis. Papillary stenosis may be present.

Results of antibiotic treatment for cryptosporidiosis in patients with AIDS have been disappointing. Most experienced clinicians use a protocol involving atovaquone, azithromycin, and/or paromomycin. Fortunately, the incidence of cryptosporidiosis is reduced greatly where HAART (highly active antiretroviral therapy) is used widely. Symptomatic therapy includes treatment with antidiarrheal agents such as loperamide or diphenoxylate-atropine. Treatment usually is not required for cryptosporidiosis in patients who are immunocompetent and no clinical trials have convincingly demonstrated the efficacy of antimicrobials. Enteral nutrition frequently exacerbates the diarrhea.

SUGGESTED READINGS

Dionsio D. Cryptosporidiosis in HIV-infected patients. J Postgrad Med. 2002;48(3):215–216.

Hunter PR, Nichols G. Epidemiology and clinical features of cryptosporidium in immunocompromised patients. Clin Microbiol Rev. 2002;15(1):145–154.

Xiao L, Ryan UM. Cryptosporidiosis: an update in molecular epidemiology. Curr Opin Infect Dis. 2004;17(5):483–490.

145

PAY ATTENTION TO THE MORPHOLOGY REPORTED BY THE MICROBIOLOGY LAB FOR FUNGAL CULTURES

SHELLEY S. MAGILL, MD
WILLIAM G. MERZ, PhD

Fungi cause a wide variety of diseases in the critically ill patient, from mucocutaneous infections to bloodstream infection and deep-seated, tissue-invasive disease. The high mortality of invasive fungal infections and the availability of new antifungal agents with different spectra of activity make prompt, accurate, specific diagnosis critical. When an invasive fungal infection is suspected, appropriate specimens, such as blood, body fluids, and/or tissue, should be sent to the laboratory specifically for fungal microscopic examination and fungal culture. The microscopic examination involves preparing a slide of the specimen with potassium hydroxide, a Calcofluor White stain, or a Gram stain.

There are two common morphologic forms of fungi that may be seen on microscopic examination and in the culture plate or tube: yeasts and molds (or filamentous fungi). Yeasts are fungi that reproduce by budding or, in rare cases, by binary fission. If the laboratory reports yeastlike forms on a microscopic examination, the most common organisms to consider would be *Candida* species and *Cryptococcus* species, although endemic fungi such as *Histoplasma* (agent of histoplasmosis), *Blastomyces* (agent of blastomycosis), and *Paracoccidioides* (agent of paracoccidioidomycosis) would also be possible, but less likely. *Candida* species are common colonizers of sites such as the oropharynx, gastrointestinal tract, and female genitourinary tract, but they may also cause devastating invasive infection. *Cryptococcus neoformans* should always be considered a pathogen. If the laboratory reports the growth of yeast in culture, the same organisms should be considered, although *Histoplasma*, *Blastomyces*, and *Paracoccidioides* would be much less likely since they are dimorphic fungi and more often grow as molds.

WATCH OUT FOR

If the laboratory reports the detection of fungal hyphae by microscopic examination, this means that the fungus in question is a mold. It is important to distinguish hyphae that are morphologically consistent with *Aspergillus* species and related molds from those that are consistent with Zygomycetes (e.g., *Rhizopus, Cunninghamella, Mucor*), since the treatments differ. Zygomycotic hyphae are wide (up to 10 to 12 microns in diameter), have wavy/ribbony cell walls, infrequent branching at right angles, and relatively infrequent septa. The agents of hyalohyphomycosis (*Aspergillus, Pseudallescheria, Fusarium*) are narrower (up to 8 microns in diameter), have parallel cell walls, frequent branching at acute angles, and usually frequent septa.

When molds are recovered in culture, they form colonies made up of masses of hyphae from which spores are produced. The colony morphology and microscopic morphology of cultured molds allow them to be identified in the laboratory. Because molds tend to grow slowly, identification to the genus level may take several days or even longer. Many molds may be deadly pathogens in the proper clinical context, but they may also be colonizers or laboratory contaminants.

Some fungi are dimorphic, meaning that they exist in two different morphologic forms, most commonly yeastlike and mold forms. These fungi typically exist in their yeastlike state in human tissues and grow in nature (and in culture in the laboratory) as molds. Examples of well-known dimorphic fungi that fit this definition are *Histoplasma capsulatum, Blastomyces dermatiditis, Sporothrix schenckii*, and *Paracoccidioides brasiliensis. Coccidioides immitis* is also a dimorphic fungus but forms large saclike structures called spherules (not budding yeast cells) in tissue. These dimorphic fungi are always pathogens.

If there is uncertainty regarding the clinical significance of a yeast or mold appearing on a microscopic examination or growing from a culture of a patient specimen, prompt infectious disease consultation should be obtained.

SUGGESTED READINGS

Doctor Fungus. http://www.doctorfungus.org

Merz WG, Hay RJ, ed. Topley and Wilson's Microbiology and Microbial Infections: Medical Mycology. 10th ed. Washington, DC: ASM Press; 2005.

Murray PR, Baron EJ, Pfaller MA, et al., eds. Manual of Clinical Microbiology. 8th ed. Vol. 2. Washington, DC: ASM Press; 2003.

146

CONSIDER POSSIBLE FUNGAL INFECTION IN PATIENTS WITH HYPOTHERMIA AND BRADYCARDIA

SUNEEL KHETARPAL, MD
ANDREW J. KERWIN, MD

Infections in the intensive care unit (ICU) remain a major source of morbidity and mortality. Typically infections are bacterial. However, with an increasing level of patient acuity, more advanced procedures, and more aggressive therapy, fungal infections are increasingly common. Certain academic surgical ICUs now find fungal isolates as the fourth most common bloodstream infection. Furthermore, the attributable mortality for such infections remains between 20% and 60%. Contributing to this mortality is the difficulty in diagnosing this entity. Despite a better understanding of fungal infections, there remains a delay in diagnosis as there is no rapidly available microbiological markers and cultures suggestive of systemic fungal infections are positive in only 30% to 50% of cases. Often, they are not positive until late in the process.

SIGNS AND SYMPTOMS

However, despite the difficulty in diagnosis, the key to treatment of fungal infections is early recognition. Risk factors for fungal infection include ventilated patients, prolonged ICU stays, previous antibiotics, total parenteral nutrition (TPN), high APACHE (Acute Physiological and Chronic Health Evaluation) scores, and previous abdominal surgery. Because of the delay in diagnosis, any individual with an atypical presentation of sepsis should be considered to have the possibility of a systemic fungal infection. Such presentations include: hypothermia; bradycardia; ongoing elevation in temperature or white blood cell count; or ongoing sepsis despite being on the "appropriate" empiric antimicrobiological therapy. In order to increase the accuracy of diagnosis, the role of colonization has been extensively evaluated. Emerging evidence has shown that the risk of candidemia may be related to the density and extension of fungal colonization over time. The risk of death has actually been found to be similar in patients with multiple-site fungal colonization and those with confirmed invasive candidiasis. As a result the concept of early empiric therapy has emerged. This therapy recognizes the high-risk patient who begins to show evidence of *Candida* colonization by positive cultures from multiple sites. It has been suggested that such high-risk patients be started on antifungal therapy, not as prophylaxis, but as treatment. On the other hand, some experienced clinicians believe prophylactic strategies against fungal infections have proven to be ineffective at significantly reducing systemic fungal infections in an ICU. Select groups of patients such as pancreatic transplant patients may, however, benefit from such strategies.

The most common fungal infection seen in ICUs are that of *Candida* species, with 50% being *C. albicans*. An increasing number of isolates are nonalbicans species such as *C. glabrata, C. parapsilosis, C. tropicalis*, and *C. krusei*. First-line therapy remains fluconazole (400 to 800 mg/d). However, with the increasing nonalbicans species the limitation of fluconazole to treat *C. glabrata* and *C. krusei* must be recognized. Currently there is a second-generation azole (voriconazole) with improved efficiency against nonalbicans species. Another new class of antifungals are the echinocandins (caspofungin, anidulafungin), which can be used for therapy against candidiasis. It should be noted that most experienced clinicians no longer consider the use of amphotericin B to be an appropriate first- or second-line agent.

Although rare, mold infections such as *Aspergillus* species remain a problem in the ICU. High-risk patients are usually significantly immunosuppressed, such as solid-organ transplant or bone-marrow transplant patients; however, any patient whose normal immune system has been altered can be considered at risk. Once again early recognition plays a key role in successful treatment. Treatment of systemic molds has been traditionally by amphotericin; however, recent literature suggests that second-generation azole (voriconazole) or the echinocandins may have improved efficiency. Despite these recent advances, the mortality rate for Aspergillus infections remains high.

SUGGESTED READINGS

Ibanez-Nolla J, Nolla-Salas M, Leon MA, et al. Early diagnosis of candidiasis in non-neutropenic critically ill patients. J Infect. 2004;48(2):181–192.

Kullberg BJ, Sobel JD, Ruhnke M, et al. Voriconazole versus a regimen of amphotericin B followed by fluconazole for candidaemia in non-neutropenic patients: a randomised non-inferiority trial. Lancet. 2005;366(9495):1435–1442.

Vardakas KZ, Samonis G, Michalopoulos A, et al. Antifungal prophylaxis with azoles in high-risk, surgical intensive care units: a meta-analysis of randomized, placebo-controlled trials. Crit Care Med. 2006;34(4):1216.

147

GIVE SPECIAL CONSIDERATION TO THE EXTENDED-SPECTRUM BETA-LACTAMASE-PRODUCING ORGANISMS BEFORE ADMINISTERING ANTIBIOTICS

JOHN J. LEWIN III, PHARMD

Extended-spectrum beta-lactamase (ESBL)-producing organisms represent one of the largest infectious disease–related challenges in the intensive care unit (ICU) environment worldwide. The β-lactamase enzymes are capable of hydrolyzing the beta-lactam ring of penicillins and related compounds, rendering them inactive. To date, there have been hundreds of different types of β-lactamase enzymes identified. There have been many classification schemes proposed for β-lactamases. The classification initially introduced by Ambler in 1980 is based on the amino-acid sequence and recognizes four molecular classes designated A to D. This scheme is based on amino-acid similarity, with classes A, C, and D being serine-β-lactamases and class B being metallo-β-lactamases. The scheme proposed by Bush is a functional classification that defines four groups according to their substrate and inhibitor profiles.

The ESBL-producing organisms are noteworthy as they represent significant challenges in prevention, identification, and treatment. The ESBL enzyme is capable of hydrolyzing essentially all β-lactam antibiotics except carbapenems and cephamycins (cefotetan and cefoxitin). The first reports of ESBLs came in the early 1980s, after the development and widespread use of third-generation cephalosporins. Of note, ESBL enzymes are plasmid-mediated, rendering the DNA encoding the ESBL enzyme (as well as other types of resistance) easily transferable. Therefore, ESBL-producing organisms are frequently resistant to other classes of antibiotics such as fluoroquinolones, aminoglycosides, and trimethoprim/sulfamethoxazole.

WATCH OUT FOR

Identification of ESBLs can be problematic for many clinical microbiology labs. The National Committee for Clinical Laboratory Standards has developed standards to improve upon the early and reliable recognition of ESBLs. However, some studies indicate an inability for many labs to reliably identify ESBL isolates and as such, clinicians should be familiar with their microbiology laboratory's methods and abilities to detect and report ESBLs. It is not uncommon to see an initial sensitivity profile indicating susceptibility to third-generation cephalosporins (especially ceftriaxone and cefotaxime) in vitro. However, using one of these agents to actively treat an ESBL infection is likely to lead to treatment failure in vivo. As such, if an ESBL-producing organism is suspected, cephalosporins should not be utilized.

Because of the ESBLs' ability to hydrolyze most β-lactams, and their plasmid-mediated transmission of resistance to other classes of antibiotics, treatment choices are severely limited. Carbapenems are considered the drugs of choice for severe infections due to ESBL-producing organisms. Theses agents exert the most consistent activity against these organisms and are highly resistant to the hydrolytic effects of ESBLs.

Most ESBLs are effectively inhibited by β-lactamase inhibitors (clavulanic acid, sulbactam, and tazobactam) to varying degrees. However, the β-lactam/β-lactamase-inhibitor combinations are not recommended in the management of infections due to ESBL-producing organisms. Many ESBL-producing organisms may also generate non-ESBL β-lactamase resistant to the β-lactamase inhibitors or generate multiple types of ESBL, rendering the β-lactamase inhibitors inactive, and the antimicrobial agent susceptible to hydrolysis. In patients with a severe beta-lactam allergy in whom an alternative to carbapenems is desired, fluoroquinolones and aminoglycosides can be considered if the organisms are shown to be susceptible.

SUGGESTED READINGS

Ambler RP, Coulson AF, Frere JM, et al. A standard numbering scheme for the class beta-lactamases. Biochem J. 1991;276 (Pt 1):269–270.

Bush K, Jacoby GA, Medeiros AA. A functional classification scheme for beta lactamases and its correlation with molecular structure. Antimicrob Agents Chemother. 1995;39(6):1211–1233.

Paterson DL, Bonomo RA. Extended-spectrum β-Lactamases: a clinical update. Clin Microbiol Rev. 2005;18(4):657–686.

Steward CD, Wallace D, Hubert SK, et al. Ability of laboratories to detect emerging antimicrobial resistance in nosocomial pathogens: a survey of project ICARE laboratories. Diagn Microbiol Infect Dis. 2000;38(1):59–67.

148

HAVE A HIGH THRESHOLD FOR THORACENTESIS WHEN LOOKING FOR A SOURCE OF INFECTION

DEBA SARMA, MD

The onset of a new fever or presence of a new or increasing leukocytosis is a problem that is encountered frequently in any intensive care unit (ICU) and can lead to an extensive workup, which subjects patients to many tests and often produces inconclusive results. Fevers may be a generalized response to a noninfectious inflammatory state such as those related to postoperative changes, alcohol or drug withdrawal, transfusion of blood products, fever, pancreatitis, adrenal insuffiency, deep venous thrombosis, and various other etiologies. Infections, however, are a much more common cause of fever with the prevalence of nosocomial infections in ICUs ranging from 3% to 31%. The most commonly reported infections in the ICU are ventilator-associated pneumonia, bloodstream infection, and catheter-related infections. The onsent of new fever will usually result in a workup obtaining tests that are directed to the most common and likely etiologies. This will often include cultures obtained from blood, urine, and sputum and a chest radiograph to assess for the presence of atelectasis or in-filtrates. If the etiology is not obvious based on preliminary studies, further workup such computed tomography (CT) scans to rule out fluid collections will be done based on the next most likely sources. By this point noninfectious etiologies are considered, as are less common infectious causes such as central nervous system (CNS) infections and infected pleural effusion (parapneumonic effusions or empyemas).

During routine daily testing of ICU patients, the presence of a pleural effusion is often noted on chest radiograph. In a recent study of medical ICU patients, it was noted that most of the ICU patients were admitted for conditions other than pleural disease, but the presence of pleural effusions was common secondary to pleural effects of pulmonary parnenchymal disorders and dysfunction of other organ systems. In this study, pleural effusions resulted from noninfectious causes in 82% of patients found to have an effusion. Of these patients the most common cause of pleural effusions was heart failure diagnosed as either a primary condition or developing after aggressive fluid resuscitation. Only 11% of patients in this study were determined to have an infected pleural effusion. The suspicion for infection was raised when a patient remained toxic despite antiobiotic coverage. Of all the study patients with an effusion, 21% of the patients underwent a thoracentesis to rule out a malignant effusion or an infection. Only three of eight with a suspected infection had a successful thoracentesis, with others being unsuccessful secondary to small size of effusion or termination of procedure secondary to instability. The patients who did not undergo a thoracentesis had resolution of their pleural effusion after initiation or changes in antibiotics. Another study looking specifically at febrile medical ICU patients and assessing the utility of ultrasound for diagnosis of empyemas found that 62% of patients with fevers and a pleural effusion did have an infectious exudate. The prevalence of empyemas (a potentially life-threatening condition), however, was only 16%. In this particular study, the specific findings such as complex, septated patterns on ultrasound increased the likelihood that an effusion was truly an empyema that would require drainage. The remainder of pleural effusions were found to be parapneumonic effusions or transudative (noninfectious/noninflammatory collections), which have been found to resolve with appropriate antibiotic coverage and observation, respectively.

Another recent study assessing the frequency of positive culture results from pleural effusions showed that the positive yield of microbiologic cultures is low. In this study the strongest predictor of a true positive result was the presence of loculated pleural effusions. Of the remaining effusions that were free-flowing, only 1.1% were positive for a true pathogen. Even when analyzing fluid from patients expected to have the highest likelihood of having an infectious cause for their effusion, the frequency of true positive results was only 18%, suggesting that the sensitivity of pleural fluid cultures is low, thereby arguing against frequent analysis of pleural fluid.

WATCH OUT FOR

Of the few studies that have looked at the presence of infected pleural effusions in the ICU, none has looked at the the yield of thoracentesis during a fever workup in surgical ICU patients. It is known, however, that in surgical patients, especially after thoracic or cardiac procedures and even intra-abdominal surgeries, the presence of pleural effusions as seen in chest radiographs is fairly common and inconsequential. Furthermore, the postoperative resuscitation is often aggressive and results in fair amount of pulmonary congestion leading to pulmonary effusions. As is the case in the studies seen in medical ICUs, the formation of pleural effusions is very common in patients in positive fluid balance, usually resolves within days, and, as such, is not a likely source of infection in ICU patients with a fever. Furthermore, a thoracentesis is not a benign procedure, and though it can be performed in the ICU even on mechanically ventilated patients, it does run the risk of several complications. Major complications include pneumothorax, hemopneumothorax, hypotension due to vasovagal response, hemorrhage, and re-expansion pulmonary edema.

WHAT TO DO

Thus, the recommendation in various studies is to have a high clinical suspicion and possibly further workup such as ultrasound or CT before doing a thoracentesis, as the incidence of infection and the yield of thoracentesis are fairly low. Some studies generally recommend thoracentesis if other sources of fever are ruled out and if the patient has a large loculated effusion or source such as those related to possible malignancy, pancreatits, possibility of a chylothorax, or esophageal leak/rupture. These are the exudative effusions resulting from local inflammation or movement of fluid from the peritoneal space and drainage is usually required to aid in diagnosis and relieve the inflammatory process.

SUGGESTED READINGS

Barnes TW, Olson EJ, Morgenthaler TI, et al. Low yield of microbiologic studies on pleural fluid specimens. Chest. 2005;127:916–921.

Marik PE. Fever in the ICU. Chest. 2000;117:855–869.

Mattison LE, Coppage L, Alderman DF, et al. Pleural effusions in the medical ICU: prevalence, causes, and clinical implications. Chest. 1997;111:1018–1023.

Tu C, Hsu W, Hsia T, et al. Pleural effusions in febrile medical ICU patients: chest ultrasound study. Chest. 2004;125:1274–1280.

149

AIM FOR A PEAK OF TEN TIMES THE MINIMUM INHIBITORY CONCENTRATION (MIC) TO KILL PSEUDOMONAS WHEN USING AN AMINOGLYCOSIDE

EDWARD T. HORN, PHARMD

Aminoglycosides (gentamicin, tobramycin, and amikacin) are bactericidal antibiotics that are active against aerobic Gram-negative and Gram-positive organisms. Clinically these agents are utilized for serious Gram-negative infections, as well as in combination with beta-lactams for Gram-positive synergy. This chapter discusses how to dose aminoglycosides for serious Gram-negative infections.

When designing dosing regimens, one must consider the pharmacodynamics of the agent in question. For aminoglycosides, this means understanding how these agents exert their bactericidal effects. Aminoglycosides display concentration-dependent killing (*Table 149.1*), which simply means that the higher the peak concentration increases above the minimum inhibitory concentration (MIC), the better the killing effectiveness. Time-dependent agents are the opposite. Their killing effectiveness is solely dependent on the amount of time the drug concentration remains above the MIC and not the degree to which they are over the MIC. To take advantage of this, time-dependent drug doses are administered multiple times during the day to keep the serum concentrations above the MIC as much as possible.

Multiple studies have shown a dose-response relationship with aminoglycosides, both clinically and experimentally. A series of papers were published in the mid 1980s that show initial "therapeutic" peaks were important predictors of successful treatment outcomes with aminoglycosides. The last paper in this series, published by Moore et al. (1987), discussed the importance of the peak:MIC ratio. Maximum peak:MIC ratio, defined as >10, was one of two statistically significant variables shown to be a predictor of a favorable outcome (the other was a favorable underlying prognosis). These studies were done with initial doses of gentamicin 2 mg/kg, and amikacin 8 mg/kg.

Subsequent studies have utilized higher doses of aminoglycosides for the therapy of these serious infections. A study of a dose 3 mg/kg, based on either an ideal or adjusted body weight, of gentamicin or tobramycin was evaluated in critically ill surgical patients. This

TABLE 149.1	DIFFERENTIATION OF ANTIMICROBIAL AGENTS BASED ON PHARMACODYNAMIC PROFILE	
TIME-DEPENDENT AGENTS	**CONCENTRATION-DEPENDENT AGENTS**
Penicillins	Aminoglycosides
Cephalosporins	Quinolones
Carbapenems	Metronidazole
Monobactams	Daptomycin
Vancomycin	
Linezolid	
Clindamycin	

study showed that the increased dose resulted in a higher initial peak (8.1 μg/mL), but this was achieved in only 50% of patients. A dose of nearly 4 mg/kg was extrapolated from study data to achieve a peak 10 μg/mL and can be reliably used. Postinfusion levels can be obtained, and even experienced providers will consult an ICU PharmD for discussion of the next dose.

An example of how to dose one of the aminoglycosides follows, but keep in mind that doses may need to be adjusted in order to maintain the peak:MIC ratio > 10 if MICs at any particular institution are higher than 1 μg/mL. The stepwise protocol is as follows:

1) After the gentamicin dose is administered, obtain 1-hour peak concentration and 8-hour postinfusion concentration.
2) Use the following equations in this sequence to calculate when the next dose can be safely given and how much to give:

a) $$Vd = \frac{dose\ (mg)}{peak\ concentration\ (mg/L)}$$

If you give a 400-mg dose of gentamicin and the resulting peak is 8 mg/dL (8 μg/mL), then the Vd = 50 L.

b) $$K_e\ (elimination\ constant) = \frac{(\ln\ [peak/8\text{-}hour\ level])}{\Delta\ time}$$

The levels after your 400-mg dose are a peak of 8 mg/dL and an 8-hour level of 4 mg/dL. The resulting K_e would be (ln [8/4])/7 hours = 0.099 hours^{-1}.

c)
$$t_{1/2} = \frac{0.693}{k_e}$$

The half-life for this example would be $0.693/0.099 = \sim 7$ hours. It is generally safe to redose in three to four half-lives, so a q24h regimen would be appropriate if renal function remains stable.

d) Next dose

You know that you can give the next dose 24 hours after your first dose. At that time, the serum concentration is approximately 1 μg/mL. If you are targeting a peak of 10 μg/mL, the next dose is calculated by rearranging the Vd equation: Dose (mg) = Vd × goal peak. In determining the follow-up doses, realize that the serum levels are not 0 μg/mL, but usually between 1 and 2 μg/mL. The trough level must be taken into consideration when giving these follow-up doses. For this example:

$$\text{Dose (mg)} = 50 \text{ L} \times 9\mu g/mL$$

$$\text{Dose (mg)} = 450 \text{ mg (not 500 mg)}$$

SUGGESTED READINGS

Leggert JE, Ebert S, Fantin B, et al. Comparative dose effect relationships at several dosing intervals for beta-lactam, aminoglycoside, and quinolone antibiotics against Gram-negative bacilli in murine thigh infection and pneumonitis models. Scand J Infect Dis Suppl 1990;74:179–184.

Moore RD, Smith CR, Leitman PS. Association of aminoglycoside plasma levels with therapeutic outcome in Gram-negative pneumonia. Am J Med 1984;77:657–662.

Moore RD, Smith CR, Leitman PS. The association of aminoglycoside plasma levels with mortality in Gram-negative bacteremia. J Infect Dis 1984;149:443–448.

Moore RD, Leitman PS, Smith CR. Clinical response to aminoglycoside therapy: importance of the ratio of peak concentration to minimal inhibitory concentration. J Infect Dis 1987;155:93–99.

150

KNOW THE DEFINITION OF A CATHETER-RELATED BLOODSTREAM INFECTION

BRADFORD D. WINTERS, MD, PHD

Catheter-related bloodstream infections (CRBSIs) are a major cause of morbidity and mortality in critical care units with an estimated 28,000 patients dying from this complication every year in the United States alone. However, this complication is largely preventable. Recent evidence shows that a process that incorporates evidence-based guidelines from the Centers for Disease Control and Prevention (CDC), the Society of Critical Care Medicine, and others into a comprehensive safety-based program can virtually eliminate CRBSIs.

A formal definition of a CRBSI can be found through the CDC. The patient must have a central venous catheter in place at the time of the suspected infection and there must be no other identifiable source of infection present. Both the catheter and peripheral blood must grow the same organism while the catheter was in place. Proper culture of the catheter requires that the intradermal portion of the catheter be cultured, not the tip as is commonly and incorrectly done. If at all possible, the peripheral blood drawn should be at least 10 mL, drawn from two separate peripheral sites. Blood drawn through the suspect catheter is invalid unless it is done through a special protocol and the lab performs quantitative cultures. This is usually done only for certain permanent catheters such as Hohn and Hickman catheters and occasionally with special lines dedicated for hyperalimentation. Colony counts for regular central catheters that report >15 colony-forming units for the catheter are considered positive.

Prevention of CRBSIs requires a multiple-element program whose most important component is education and reinforcement. The first step is developing awareness of the magnitude and implications of the problem among the staff. Creating a central location where all necessary supplies are immediately available is essential. Ideally this would be mobile such as a cart. This helps reduce breaches of sterility by preventing the need to obtain materials once the procedure of placing a catheter has begun.

WHAT TO DO

The supplies required include full gown, sterile gloves, mask, and hair covering just as for surgery. Chlorhexidine for skin prep should be used, as it has been shown to be effective in reducing the incidence of infection. Full-body draping of the patient and bed, not just the immediate procedure site, is a must. It is thought that a major source of contamination is secondary to the wire used for the Seldinger technique contacting nonsterile equipment near the field. Widespread coverage with a full drape helps to eliminate this. All participants in the sterile portion of the procedure must wash their hands prior to gowning and gloving. Chlorhexidine soap or alcohol-based hand washes are appropriate. Strict sterility must be maintained at all times. Any time there is a breach in this sequence of steps, the procedure should be stopped and the situation rectified even if it means starting the whole procedure over. Nurses should be empowered through education and a checklist to ensure that strict adherence to practice is maintained. With the exception of dialysis or possible dialysis patients, the subclavian site selection is preferred as it is associated with the lowest risk of CRBSIs. Limiting the number of lumens to the lowest needed may also help.

A final component to best practice for reducing CRBSIs is to evaluate daily whether a particular catheter is needed and, if not, remove it as soon as possible. The risk of catheter infection and CRBSI increases with the passage of time and catheters that have been in place for greater than or equal to 7 days are especially at risk and ones present for more than 21 days are quite prone to getting infected. Catheters that are placed in a nonsterile fashion such as emergent lines or trauma lines should be removed within 24 hours and replaced, if necessary, with central lines in accordance with the guidelines described here.

SUGGESTED READINGS

Berenholtz, SM Pronovost P, Lipsett PA, et al. Eliminating catheter related bloodstream infections in an intensive care unit. Crit Care Med 2004;32:2014–2020.

Mermal LA. Prevention of intravascular catheter related infections. Ann Intern Med 2000;132:391–402.

151

STRONGLY CONSIDER STOPPING PROPHYLACTIC ANTIBIOTICS AFTER 24 HOURS IN PENETRATING ABDOMINAL TRAUMA

KONSTANTINOS SPANIOLAS, MD
GEORGE C. VELMAHOS, MD, PhD

Despite abundant evidence to the contrary, multiple and prolonged antibiotics are still used following penetrating abdominal trauma. In 515 randomized patients, Fabian et al. showed that 1 day of a second-generation cephalosporin prophylaxis was equally effective as 5 days of the same antibiotic. Cornwell et al., in a prospective randomized study of 63 high-risk patients with penetrating colon injury, found no difference in infectious morbidity between 1 and 5 days of a second-generation cephalosporin. Dellinger et al. randomized 116 patients with small or large bowel injuries to 12 hours versus 5 days of antibiotics and failed to identify any significant differences in morbidity or mortality. Velmahos et al., in a prospective study of 250 critically injured patients, found that antibiotic prophylaxis for penetrating abdominal trauma longer than 1 day did not decrease septic morbidity and was an independent risk factor for delayed resistant infection.

WHAT TO DO

Multiple studies have been performed comparing different types of antibiotics in penetrating abdominal trauma. Moxalactam, gentamicin with clindamycin, cefoxitin, cefotetan, cefotaxime, aztreonam, ampicillin/sulbactam, and piperacillin/tazobactam are some of the many prophylactic agents that have been tested. The general conclusion is that a single broad-spectrum antibiotic is as effective as multiple antibiotics. Second-generation cephalosporins have shown a decreasing efficacy in some studies, probably because of bacterial resistance from prolonged use or because of inability of enterococcal coverage. Ampicillin/sulbactam seems to be cost-effective and provides adequate coverage.

Standard dosing of prophylactic antibiotics in the majority of trauma patients with abdominal trauma is sufficient. However, the pharmacodynamics of these agents in critical illness is poorly understood. Increased volume of distribution, metabolic changes affecting drug excretion, and multiple drug interactions alter the required doses. More often than not, critically ill patients are underdosed. Although higher targets and monitoring algorithms have been established for the aminoglycosides and vancomycin, such research is lacking for most other antibiotics used for prophylaxis. Although most experienced practitioners consider a single day of a single broad-spectrum antibiotic to be adequate for prophylaxis following penetrating abdominal trauma, a low threshold should exist for increasing the dose and/or shortening the dosing interval (according to the class of antibiotic) for patients who are critically injured.

One final note is that consideration should be given to redosing antibiotics in the face of continuing blood loss (>120 to 1,500 cc) in the intensive care unit or at repeat laparotomy.

SUGGESTED READINGS

Cornwell EE III, Dougherty WR, Berne TV, et al. Duration of antibiotic prophylaxis in high-risk patients with penetrating abdominal trauma: a prospective randomized study. J Gastroint Surg. 1999;3:648–653.

Dellinger EP, Wertz MJ, Lennard ES, et al. Efficacy of a short-course antibiotic prophylaxis after penetrating intestinal injury: a prospective randomized trial. Arch Surg. 1986;121:23–30.

Eastern Association for the Surgery of Trauma (EAST) evidence-based guidelines: prophylactic antibiotics in penetrating abdominal trauma. http://www.east.org

Fabian TC, Croce MA, Payne LW, et al. Duration of antibiotic therapy for penetrating abdominal trauma: a prospective trial. Surgery. 1992;112:785–792.

Hooker KD, DiPiro JT, Wynn JJ. Aminoglycoside combinations versus beta-lactams alone for penetrating abdominal trauma: a meta-analysis. J Trauma. 1991;31:1155–1160.

Velmahos GC, Toutouzas KG, Sarkisyan G, et al. Severe trauma is not an excuse for prolonged antibiotic prophylaxis. Arch Surg. 2002;137:537–541.

Weigelt JA, Easley SM, Thal SR, et al. Abdominal surgical wound infection with improved perioperative enterococcus and bacteroides therapy. J Trauma. 1993;34:579–584.

152

Use clindamycin in necrotizing fasciitis to cover group A streptococcus

Carrie A. Sims, MD, MS
Patrick K. Kim, MD

Necrotizing fasciitis is a life-threatening surgical emergency. Immediate wide surgical incision, drainage, and debridement is the cornerstone of therapy. Broad-spectrum intravenous antibiotics should be instituted as soon as the diagnosis is suspected. At operation, tissue cultures should be obtained and antibiotic coverage should be tailored to culture growth. The most common causative agents of necrotizing fasciitis are *Staphylococcus aureus*, *Clostridium* species, group A *Streptococcus*, enterococci, and *Bacteroides* species. Many necrotizing infections are mixed aerobic/anaerobic in origin. Controversy still remains about the use of hyperbaric therapy in these cases. However, if it is utilized, hyperbaric treatment should never delay aggressive surgical treatment.

Infections caused by group A *Streptococcus* (e.g., *S. pyogenes*, aka "flesh-eating bacteria") deserve special mention. Group A *Streptococcus* is responsible for a range of skin and soft-tissue infections, including impetigo, erysipelas, cellulitis, and necrotizing fasciitis. Group A *Streptococcus* necrotizing fasciitis is commonly associated with septic shock and multiorgan failure—the streptococcal toxic shock syndrome. This is secondary to the presence of M protein, a virulence factor present on the bacterial surface that is highly antigenic and inhibits phagocytosis. In addition, streptococcal pyrogenic exotoxins cause fever and contribute to organ failure and shock by stimulating host synthesis of tumor necrosis factor α, interleukin-1 β, and interleukin-6.

WHAT TO DO

Penicillins are generally effective for the staphylococcal and streptococcal infections of erysipelas, impetigo, and cellulitis. However, penicillin monotherapy is much less effective in deep necrotizing infections. Experimentally, penicillins lose effectiveness in the presence of large numbers of organisms and when bacteria are in the stationary growth phase. In deep infections, combination penicillin and clindamycin therapy improves survival compared with penicillin monotherapy. This clinical effect is supported by several experimental findings: clindamycin suppresses synthesis of group A *Streptococcus* exotoxins; inhibits M-protein synthesis; suppresses synthesis of proteins involved in bacterial cell-wall synthesis; and might suppress host tumor necrosis factor synthesis. Its mechanism is independent of bacterial inoculum and growth stage. Finally, group A *Streptococcus* resistance to clindamycin is extremely rare.

SUGGESTED READINGS

Bisno AL, Stevens DL. Streptococcal infections of skin and soft tissues. New Engl J Med. 1996;334:240–245.

Stevens DL. The flesh-eating bacterium: what's next? J Infect Dis. 1999;179(Suppl 2): S366–S374.

Stevens DL, Bisno AL, Chambers HF, et al. Practice guidelines for the diagnosis and management of skin and soft-tissue infections. Clin Infect Dis. 2005;41(10):1373–1406.

153

BE CAUTIOUS IN USING ANTIBIOTICS FOR UNINFECTED PANCREATITIS

BENJAMIN BRASLOW, MD

The best way to think about acute pancreatitis is to equate it to an internal chemical burn. The acute resuscitation, complicated fluid and electrolyte abnormalities, and infectious complications associated with acute pancreatitis must be addressed in a similar fashion to the management of severe external burns. The pathophysiology of acute pancreatitis involves a cascade of events initiated by acinar cell injury and pancreatic duct obstruction. These processes allow the inappropriate extracellular leakage of activated digestive enzymes and the consequent autodigestion of pancreatic and extrapancreatic tissues.

A wide range of etiologies of acute pancreatitis have been identified. In the United States, more than 75% of cases are attributable to either gallstones or alcohol. Other less common causes include iatrogenic causes such as endoscopic retrograde pancreatography (ERCP), cardiopulmonary bypass, and abdominal operations. Patient-based causes include blunt or penetrating abdominal trauma, periampullary neoplasm, pancreas divisum, sphincter of Oddi spasm, hyperlipidemia, hypercalcemia, and ischemia. More than 85 medications have also been implicated in causing acute pancreatitis. The highest incidence is noted with immunosuppressive agents (azathioprine and 6-mercaptopurine) and the antiviral didanosine. Other drugs incriminated include estrogen, nonsteroidal anti-inflammatory drugs (NSAIDs) (sulfasalazine, sulindac, salicylates), some diuretics (furosemide, thiazide diuretics, ethacrynic acid), numerous other antibiotics (pentamidine, metronidazole, tetracycline, trimethoprim-sulfamethoxazole, nitrofurantoin), valproic acid, procainamide, and several angiotensin-converting enzyme (ACE) inhibitors.

Most episodes of acute pancreatitis (80%) do not require any significant intervention, since they are mild and self-limiting. However, approximately 20% of patients go on to develop a severe form of acute pancreatitis associated with multisystem organ failure and/or local complications like necrosis, abscess formation, or hemorrhage. These patients have prolonged intensive care unit (ICU) stays and hospitalizations with an in-house mortality exceeding 30% despite improvements in diagnostic and treatment modalities.

SIGNS AND SYMPTOMS

The clinical diagnosis of acute pancreatitis is considered after the typical presentation of severe epigastric pain radiating through the back. Associated nausea and vomiting are frequently seen. Low-grade fevers are common; high-grade fevers are unusual in the absence of localized or systemic infection. Depending on the causative etiology (i.e., gallstones), jaundice may be present.

Biochemical evidence of pancreatic injury helps to confirm the diagnosis of acute pancreatitis. In the unexaminable, obtunded patient, laboratory abnormalities may be the first clue of pancreatic injury. In acute pancreatitis a variety of digestive enzymes escape from acinar cells and enter the systemic circulation. Amylase and lipase are the most widely assayed to confirm the diagnosis. Amylase levels rise within several hours after the onset of symptoms and typically remain elevated for 3 to 5 days. However, because of the short serum half-life of amylase (2.5 to 3.0 hours), levels may normalize within 24 hours of disease onset. Lipase has a longer serum half-life and may be useful for diagnosing acute pancreatitis later in the course of an episode. It is important to remember that the magnitude of increases in amylase or lipase concentrations does not correlate well with the severity of pancreatitis. High levels do not predict worse disease. Other serum biomarkers such as C-reactive protein, neutrophil elastase, interleukin-6, procalcitonin, and urinary concentrations of trypsinogen-activating peptide (TAP) tend to correlate better with disease severity. However, because assays of these markers are not widely available they are of limited clinical utility to predict outcomes or triage patients for ICU admission.

Radiographic imaging is often essential to rule out other potential etiologies, confirm the diagnosis, and stage the severity of acute pancreatitis. Contrast-enhanced computed tomography (CT) is the preferred study following adequate fluid resuscitation (*Fig. 153.1*). It has 90% sensitivity for detection of pancreatic necrosis, which is a finding that is predictive of severe disease. On contrast-enhanced CT scan, pancreatic necrosis appears as focal or diffuse zones of nonenhanced parenchyma. This finding may not be evident until 48 to 72 hours after presentation and delaying the scan several days to identify local complications may be beneficial. The importance of intravenous (IV) contrast dye cannot be overemphasized. However, for patients unable to receive it, the diagnosis of acute pancreatitis can be inferred from homogeneous glandular enlargement and the presence of peripancreatic fluid collections. Magnetic resonance imaging (MRI) depicts necrosis

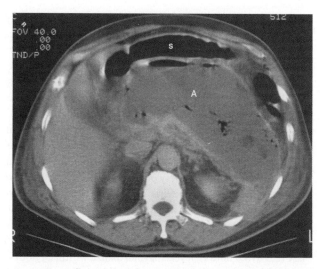

FIGURE 153.1. Contrast-enhanced computed tomographic scan at the time of transfer shows infected pancreatic necrosis with a water-density mass containing gas bubbles, completely replacing the normal pancreas. (Reused with permission from Solomkin JS, Moulton JS, Luchette FA. Diagnosis and management of intraabdominal sepsis. In: Irwin RS, Rippe JM, eds. Irwin and Rippe's Intensive Care Medicine. 5th ed. Philadelphia: Lippincott Williams & Wilkins; 2003:1670.)

vividly when present and is an excellent alternative to CT for stable patients unable to receive IV contrast dye.

WHAT TO DO

The most important component of initial management of acute pancreatitis is fluid resuscitation and electrolyte replacement. In severe cases, up to one-third of the plasma volume can be sequestered due to third space losses. Urine output must be closely monitored via placement of an indwelling urinary catheter and central venous pressure monitoring may by helpful in guiding volume replacement. Multisystem organ failure is common and early supportive management (e.g., mechanical ventilation, renal replacement therapy, vasopressors, nutrition) is imperative.

Patients with severe acute pancreatitis are severely hypercatabolic and nutritional support must start early to avoid a malnourished state. Accumulating evidence strongly supports enteral feeding over the parenteral route (total parenteral nutrition, or TPN). It is strongly recommended that enteral nutrition be initiated early after initial resuscitation via the nasojejunal route. If this is not possible, naso-gastric feeds are also acceptable. Parenteral nutrition should be implemented only when attempts at enteral nutrition have failed after a 5- to 7-day trial secondary to proximal obstruction or ileus. Enteral nutrients delivered to the jejunum appear to have minimal stimulatory effects on pancreatic exocrine secretion and convey the theoretic advantage of maintaining the integrity of the intestinal mucosal barrier. This mechanism potentially limits bacterial translocation, which is often credited with infecting sterile pancreatic necrosis. Regardless of the route of nutritional support, supplemental glutamine and tight glycemic control are associated with decreased complication rates. Clinical trials of agents that inhibit activated pancreatic enzymes (gabexate mesilate, aprotinin), inhibit pancreatic secretions (somatostatin, octreotide), or blunt inflammation (Lexipafant, anti–tumor necrosis factor α) have failed to demonstrate improved outcomes in patients with acute pancreatitis.

Infection of the necrotic pancreas develops in 30% to 50% of patients with CT-scan-documented necrosis. Although sometimes evident within a week of presentation, its incidence tends to peak in the third week of the disease and the associated multisystem organ failure and mortality escalate. Although the exact mechanism by which the necrotic pancreatic tissue becomes infected is unclear, gut bacterial translocation appears to be involved. Recent evidence suggests that patients with proven pancreatic necrosis should receive antibiotic prophylaxis with either imipenem or meropenem for a 14-day course to reduce the risk of infected necrosis. This prophylactic therapy has not been shown to increase the incidence of subsequent fungal infections as once feared.

Infection of necrotic pancreatic tissue is usually suspected in patients who develop clinical signs of sepsis. Subsequent CT scans may identify air bubbles within previous areas of sterile necrosis. Ultrasound- or CT-guided fine-needle aspiration (FNA) of pancreatic or peripancreatic tissue with Gram stain and culture should be performed once infection is suspected. If the FNA is positive for the presence of bacteria, surgical debridement (necrosectomy) and drainage is indicated. Often multiple subsequent debridements are necessary. Patients with sterile necrosis should not be surgically explored unless they display signs of overwhelming clinical deterioration. If possible, delaying operative necrosectomy and/or drainage at least 2 to 3 weeks confers lower mortality rates and fewer debridements.

SUGGESTED READINGS

Heinrich S, Schafer M, Rousson V, et al. Evidence-based treatment of acute pancreatitis: a look at established paradigms. Ann Surg. 2006;243(2):154–168.

Nathens AB, Curtis JR, Beale RJ, et al. Management of the critically ill patient with severe acute pancreatitis. Crit Care Med. 2004;32(12):2524–2536.

Uhl W, Warshaw A, Imrie C, et al. International Association of Pancreatology. IAP guidelines for the surgical management of acute pancreatitis. Pancreatology. 2002;2(6):565–573.

154

WASH YOUR HANDS

SANDRA SWOBODA, MSN

"Wash your hands!" Most health care providers have heard these simple words over and over again their entire lives—whether from their mother in childhood or at work from infection-control colleagues. Despite the fact that this simple action decreases nosocomial infection and constitutes only a fraction of a provider's day, compliance with hand hygiene is dismal. Alarmingly the intensive care unit (ICU) is associated with the lowest overall hand-hygiene compliance rates (about 50%) in the hospital, despite the fact that the need for frequent and effective hand hygiene is paramount. The consequences of poor hand hygiene are uniformly injurious and contribute to nosocomial infections that are an important source of morbidity and mortality in patients. On average, infections can complicate 8% to 10% of all hospital admissions; infection rates in the ICU occur at an even increased incidence. Studies have shown that as hand-hygiene rates improve, nosocomial infection rates go down. Reasons associated with poor compliance for proper hand hygiene include higher professional status; reluctance to experience skin irritation; poor access to supplies; "being too busy;" inattention to existing protocols; and the wearing of gloves (which is thought to "negate" the need for hand hygiene).

To briefly review, hand hygiene encompasses both hand washing with soap and water and hand rubbing with waterless alcohol-based solutions. Many health care workers falsely believe that traditional hand washing is both more efficacious and gentle on the skin. However, alcohol-based solutions are microbiologically superior, gentler on skin with less disruption to the skin's lipid layers, and more likely to be used correctly when compared with soap-and-water washing.

Some common definitions pertaining to hand hygiene are as follows:

- Hand hygiene: hand washing, antiseptic hand wash, antiseptic hand rub, surgical hand antisepsis
- Hand washing: washing hands with plain (nonantimicrobial) soap and water
- Hand antisepsis: antiseptic hand wash or antiseptic hand rub
- Antiseptic hand wash: washing hands with soap and water or detergents containing an antiseptic agent

- Antiseptic hand rub: application of waterless antiseptic agent to hands. Does not require the use of water (alcohol-based product)

The Centers for Disease Control and Prevention (CDC) guidelines for hand hygiene in the health care setting suggest the following:

- If hands are visibly dirty or contaminated or soiled with blood or other body fluids, wash hands with nonantimicrobial soap and water or an antimicrobial soap and water.
- If hands are not visibly soiled, use a waterless antiseptic agent (an alcohol-based hand rub) for routine decontamination.
- Perform hand hygiene after touching blood, body fluids, secretions, excretions, and contaminated items, whether or not gloves are worn. Perform hygiene immediately after gloves are removed, between patient contacts, and when otherwise indicated to avoid transfer of micro-organisms to other patients or environments. It may be necessary to perform hand hygiene between tasks and procedures on the same patient to prevent cross-contamination of different body sites.

Listed below are some of the "nasty bugs" that surround patients in the ICU and procedures for performing hand hygiene when providers are exposed to them.

METHICILLIN-RESISTANT STAPHYLOCOCCUS AUREUS (MRSA)

Staphylococcus aureus is a common bacterium found on the skin, and strains that are resistant to methicillin are becoming increasingly common. MRSA can be present in the nose, on the skin, or in the blood or urine and is spread through physical contact. MRSA is transferred to patients by the hands of health care workers who have been contaminated by contact with patients, surfaces in the workplace, or medical devices. This organism can survive for an hour or more on environmental surfaces such as floors, sinks, and blood-pressure cuffs. Hand hygiene with waterless antiseptic agents is recommended.

VANCOMYCIN-RESISTANT ENTEROCOCCI (VRE)

There are two common clinical isolates of enterococci that are resistant to vancomycin (*Enterococcus faecalis* and *Enterococcus faecium*). These strains can survive for 60 minutes on gloved and ungloved fingers. *E. faecalis* has been recovered on countertops for up to 5 days and *E. faecium* for 7 days. Both can survive on bedrails for up to 24 hours;

for 60 minutes on a telephone receiver; and for 30 minutes on the diaphragm of a stethoscope. VRE can be spread person to person by the hands of health care workers or in directly on contaminated environmental surfaces and patient care equipment. Hand hygiene with waterless antiseptic agents is recommended.

CLOSTRIDIUM DIFFICILE

Clostridium difficile (*C. difficile*) is a spore-forming, Gram-positive anaerobic bacillus that produces two endotoxins: endotoxin A and endotoxin B. It accounts for 15% to 25% of all episodes of antibiotic-associated diarrhea. It is shed in feces and any surface, device, or material (bedpan, toilet, thermometer, bedside commode, equipment, bedrails, etc.) that is contaminated with feces serves as a reservoir. Spores are transferred to patients by the hands of health care workers who have touched the contaminated skin of a patient, a contaminated surface, or a contaminated piece of equipment.

Alcohol-based products are *not effective* against this spore-forming bacterium; thus the use of nonantimicrobial soap and water or antimicrobial soap and water, which helps to physically remove spores from the surface of contaminated hands, is required. This is indicated especially in an outbreak situation.

BACILLUS ANTHRACIS (ANTHRAX)

Bacillus anthracis is a spore-forming bacterium. It is most commonly found in the wild in cattle, sheep, goats, camels, antelopes, and other herbivores. However, it can also occur in humans when they are exposed to infected animals or tissue from infected animals.

Alcohol-based products do not have activity against this spore so hands must be washed with either antimicrobial or nonantimicrobial soap and water.

ACINETOBACTER

Acinetobacter is a group of Gram-negative bacteria that is commonly found in soil and water. It can also be found on the skin of healthy people, especially health care workers. While there are many types or species of *Acinetobacter* and all can cause human disease, infections with *Acinetobacter* are fortunately not common. *Acinetobacter baumannii* is a waterborne organism that is sensitive to few antibiotics. This multiresistant pathogen is often cultured from patient sputum, respiratory secretions, wounds, and urine. It has also been found in irrigating solutions. Outbreaks typically occur in ICUs and this organism can be spread by person-to-person contact, contact with contaminated surfaces, or environmental exposure. It can live on the skin and survive on environmental surfaces for several days. Use of alcohol-based hand rub between and before patient and equipment contact has been shown to decrease transmission during outbreaks.

SUGGESTED READINGS

Centers for Disease Control and Prevention. Hand hygiene in healthcare settings. http://www.cdc.gov/handhygiene/

Noskin GA, Stosor V, Cooper I, et al. Recovery of vancomycin-resistant enterococci on fingertips and environmental surfaces. Infect Control Hosp Epidemiol. 1995;16(10):577–581.

Pittet D. Hand hygiene: improved standards and practice for hospital care. Curr Opin Infect Dis. 2003;16:327–335.

Shafie S, Alishaq M, Garcia M. Investigation of an outbreak of multidrug-resistant *Acinetobacter baumannii* in trauma intensive care unit. J Hosp Infect. 2004;56:101–105.

Swoboda S, Earsing K, Strauss K, et al. Electronic monitoring and voice prompts improve hand hygiene and decrease nosocomial infections in an intermediate care unit. Crit Care Med. 2004;32(2):358–363.

Swoboda S, Lipsett P. Handwashing compliance depends on professional status. Surg Infect (Larchmt). 2001;2(3):241–245.

155

CONSIDER VENTRICULOPERITONEAL SHUNT INFECTION IN PATIENTS WITH SEPSIS

JOSE I. SUAREZ, MD

Hydrocephalus is a common problem in patients with intracranial diseases. Under normal circumstances, cerebrospinal fluid (CSF) production and absorption are in dynamic equilibrium with approximate balance between them. Many intracranial processes will lead to either increased production or decreased absorption of CSF, overwhelming the balance and thus leading to hydrocephalus. Operationally, hydrocephalus can be classified as obstructive and communicating. Obstructive hydrocephalus is usually due to a mass lesion protruding into the ventricular system or arising from the ependymal lining. Communicating hydrocephalus can be seen in patients with processes in the subarachnoid space such as hemorrhage, infection, or inflammation.

Most CSF (about 50% to 80%) is produced in the choroid plexuses that line the walls of the lateral ventricles and roof of the third and fourth ventricles. The brain's ependymal lining and the brain parenchyma itself are also sources of CSF production. Once formed, CSF circulates throughout the ventricular system, exits the foramina of Magendie and Luschka in the fourth ventricle, circulates through the subarachnoid space of the brain and spinal cord, and is eventually absorbed by the arachnoid villi into the venous system.

CLINICAL PRESENTATION

In adults symptoms of hydrocephalus include headaches, diplopia, and mental status changes. Clinical signs may include papilledema and impaired upward gaze. Sudden death may occur with severe increases in intracranial pressure. In patients with chronic hydrocephalus (i.e., normal-pressure hydrocephalus among others), symptoms may include gait disturbance, urinary incontinence, and memory loss with or without any other signs or symptoms of elevated intracranial pressure as described previously.

ACUTE CSF DIVERSION

Acute hydrocephalus is best treated with insertion of an intraventricular catheter (IVC). IVCs are placed via burr holes or similar techniques into the ventricular system, usually the lateral ventricles (*Fig. 155.1*). IVCs can be used to temporarily drain CSF in the hope that

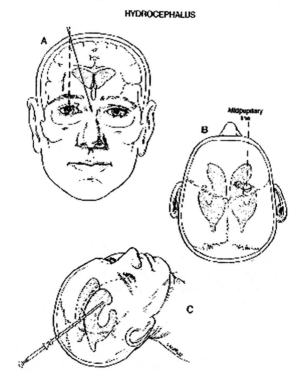

FIGURE 155.1.

normal CSF circulation is restored (e.g., in the case of intraventricular hemorrhage). The insertion site of IVCs is usually the right frontal or posterior parietal region. The right side is usually chosen, as it is rarely the dominant hemisphere. IVC placement has an overall infection rate of 4% to 10%. The optimal duration of an IVC in order to decrease infection has not been clearly established. However, many practitioners recommend inserting a new IVC by day 5 if there is still a need. The common organisms include coagulase-negative *Staphylococcus*, methicillin-resistant *Staphylococcus*, and Gram-negative bacteria such as *Escherichia Coli*, *Klebsiella*, and *Pseudomonas aeruginosa*. If a patient with an IVC becomes febrile and/or septic, CSF sampling should be obtained and appropriate antibiotic coverage should be empirically initiated. Recommended empiric antibiotics include the combination of a third-generation cephalosporin and vancomycin, or meropenem and vancomycin. Sterile technique should be used for CSF sampling and it should be obtained from the sideport of the external tubing system.

PERMANENT SHUNT PLACEMENT

Most permanent shunts in adults include ventriculoperitoneal shunts (VPSs). Other techniques include ventriculoatrial or ventriculopleural shunts. A complete description of the surgical technique is beyond the scope of this chapter. However, a summary of VPS insertion is presented in (*Figures 155.2* and *155.3.*) One important point to realize is that VPSs have a valve and a reservoir that are attached to the tubing. The valve is used to grade the pressure at which CSF is drained and current devices have programmable valves that can be easily adjusted. The IVC reservoir is usually felt near the entry burr hole. The side arm of the reservoir is attached to the proximal end of the valve and subsequently to the peritoneal tubing. There are several types of VPSs and each has its own peculiarities. However, most VPSs have a pumping mechanism, which is usually located at the valve, or a reservoir that should be used to test proper functioning. The most common complications after VPS insertion are obstruction, disconnection, and infection.

VPS INFECTION

Infection remains an important complication of VPSs. Mortality has been reported as being high (up to 40% in one series). Thus, it is very important to have a high index of suspicion to diagnose these infections. The overall infection rate after VPS insertion has been estimated to be around 7% with an acute rate of infection of about 6%. Approximately 70% of VPS infections will manifest themselves within the first 2 months after insertion. This underscores the fact that most VPS infections probably result from direct contamination at the time of surgery with few stemming from other sources such as hematogenous seeding, extension from contiguous tissue, or direct exposure of the tubing. Thus, it is not surprising that most organisms found are skin commensals such as *Staphylococcus epidermidis*. However, methicillin-resistant *S. aureus* and Gram-negative bacteria such as *E. Coli*, *Klebsiella pneumoniae*, and *P. aeruginosa* are also important organisms to consider, since they have been reported in up to 20% of cases.

The clinical presentation of VPS infections varies. Patients may experience swelling and redness over the VPS tract or have signs of peritonitis. Septicemia is also possible but is more common in patients with ventriculoatrial shunts. Patients can present acutely with headache, nausea, vomiting, fever, and decreased level of consciousness. Frank meningeal signs can also be seen.

Because the clinical signs of VPS infections can be nonspecific, practitioners should have a high index of suspicion and secure CSF

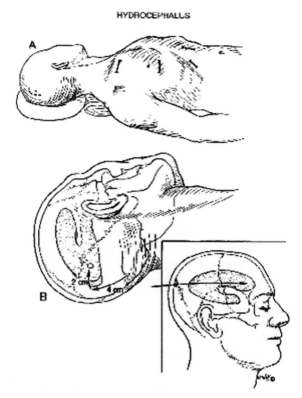

FIGURE 155.2.

sampling for culture as soon as feasible. This is even more important in patients with unexplained sepsis, unexplained fever, or shunt malfunction. A single negative CSF culture is not sufficient to rule out VPS infection; many experts recommend serial CSF sampling (although the number of cultures needed has not been determined) to increase the yield for detecting the culprit organisms. CSF sampling should be done under sterile techniques and by direct puncturing of the reservoir. CSF should be sent for aerobic and anaerobic bacteria and fungal organisms. It is equally important to send cultures from the various incision sites along the VPS tract.

Treatment of VPS infections usually involves medical and surgical management. The medical management usually consists of prompt initiation of antibiotics and supportive general care. Antibiotic therapy should include a third-generation cephalosporin (because of good CSF penetration) and vancomycin (usually at 1.5 times the usual

TECHNIQUES FOR CSF DIVERSION

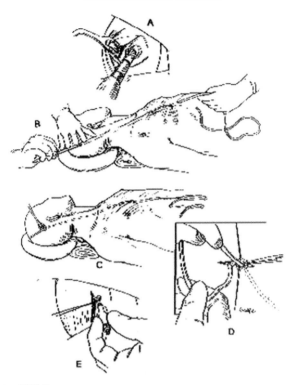

FIGURE 155.3.

dosage). Other alternatives include meropenem and vancomycin. It is common practice to add intrathecal antibiotics (usually gentamicin or vancomycin) daily. Antibiotics should be continued for at least 2 to 3 weeks after negative CSF cultures are obtained. In addition to antibiotic administration, VPS hardware should be removed and a new IVC inserted. Old VPS tips should be sent for culture. Once the cultures are negative from daily CSF sampling from the IVC, then a new VPS can be reinserted. Many neurosurgeons wait for CSF cultures to remain negative for 72 to 120 hours prior to considering VPS reinsertion.

SUGGESTED READINGS

Borgbjerg BM, Gjerris F, Albeck MJ, et al. Risk of infection after cerebrospinal fluid shunt: an analysis of 884 first-time shunts. Acta Neurochir (Wien). 1995;136:1–7.

Edwards MS, Baker CJ, Butler KM, et al. Penetration of cefuroxime into ventricular fluid in cerebrospinal fluid infections. Antimicrob Agents Chemother. 1989;33:1108–1110.

156

RECOGNIZE THAT VANCOMYCIN HAS VERY POOR CENTRAL NERVOUS SYSTEM PENETRATION

ELIAHU S. FEEN, MD
JOSE I. SUAREZ, MD

WATCH OUT FOR

Until the late 1960s, penicillin was considered optimal antibiotic therapy for meningitis secondary to *Streptococcus pneumoniae* and some staphylococcal species. Beginning with the earliest reports in the late 1960s, there has been increasing recognition of penicillin-resistant pneumococcal and staphylococcal meningitis. For many years cefotaxime and ceftriaxone, broad-spectrum cephalosporins, were adequate to treat most strains of these penicillin-resistant bacteria. However, with the advent of strains of pneumococcus that had even higher levels of penicillin resistance, alternative therapies were sought. Vancomycin is one of the most effective alternative antibiotics for penicillin- and cephalosporin-resistant pneumococcal meningitis. It has also been a mainstay of therapy for methicillin-resistant *Staphylococcus aureus*. The problem with using vancomycin to treat meningitis lies in its erratic penetration of the blood–brain barrier (BBB). Evidence from both animal models and human patients consistently demonstrates that when vancomycin is administered intravenously, only about 10% of the serum level is found in the cerebrospinal fluid (CSF). Inflammation within the meninges seems to play a role in inhibiting crossing of the BBB. The use of steroids in the acute treatment of meningitis has become more prevalent in light of recent evidence in both children and adults that steroid use acutely lessens the burden of neurologic sequelae. However, the use of steroids also seems to limit the amount of vancomycin that passes through the BBB. As an example, in animal models, the addition of dexamethasone has been found to lower the concentration of vancomycin in the CSF. Either through stabilization of the BBB by decreasing inflammation or through some other mechanism, penetration of the BBB by vancomycin is impaired.

WHAT TO DO

In order to counter this impaired penetration of the BBB, one strategy has been to use higher dosages of vancomycin. When the vancomycin dose for treating standard systemic infections is used, CSF levels are usually inadequate to achieve appropriate bactericidal activity. By increasing the dose by one-third, some researchers have shown clinical success in treating penicillin-resistant pneumococcal meningitis. However, while using higher dosages of vancomycin can increase the CSF levels, it can be difficult to maintain consistently high levels, and in addition there is increased risk of vancomycin-induced hypoacusia and other side effects. Vancomycin alone as therapy for pneumococcal and staphylococcal disease, therefore, is not recommended (some experienced intensive care unit [ICU] pharmacists feel that vancomycin should never be used alone or in conjunction with dexamethasone). By adding vancomycin to cefotaxime or ceftriaxone (or another broad-spectrum cephalosporin), a synergistic effect is achieved. This is one strategy to employ vancomycin in the treatment of beta-lactam-resistant organisms.

Some clinicians use rifampin as an alternative to vancomycin for resistant pneumococcal meningitis. Rifampin alone is inadequate, both because of the reports of rifampin resistance now extant and also because of the rapid development of bacterial resistance that can occur in certain settings. Animal and in vitro evidence supports the addition of rifampin to broad-spectrum cephalosporins. Some research has shown that the addition of rifampin to the cephalosporins has as much efficacy as adding vancomycin to the cephalosporins. In summary, when a patient has pneumococcal or staphylococcal meningitis, if there is any evidence that the causative organism carries beta-lactam resistance, vancomycin or rifampin should be added to a regimen of antibiotics including broad-spectrum cephalosporins such as cefotaxime or ceftriaxone.

SUGGESTED READINGS

Ahmed A, Jafri H, Lutsar I, et al. Pharmacodynamics of vancomycin for the treatment of experimental penicillin- and cephalosporin-resistant pneumococcal meningitis. Antimicrob Agents Chemother. 1999;43:876–881.

American Academy of Pediatrics, Committee on Infection Diseases. Therapy for children with invasive pneumococcal infections. Pediatrics. 1997;99:289–299.

Gump DW. Vancomycin for treatment of bacterial meningitis. Rev Infect Dis. 1981; 3:S289–S292.

Paris MM, Ramilo O, McCracken GH Jr. Management of meningitis caused by penicillin-resistant *Streptococcus pneumoniae*. Antimicrob Agents Chemother. 1995;39:2171–2175.

Viladrich PF, Gudiol F, Linares J, et al. Evaluation of vancomycin for therapy of adult pneumococcal meningitis. Antimicrob Agents Chemother. 1991;35:2467–2472.

157

BE ALERT FOR SEIZURES WITH IMIPENEM USE

ANTHONY D. SLONIM, MD, DrPH

Imipenem, meropenem, and ertapenem are members of the class of antibacterial agents named carbapenems. Carbapenems are one of four types of beta-lactam antibiotics. The other three are the penicillins, cephalosporins, and monobactams. Imipenem shares many of the other characteristics of these beta-lactam antibacterials: a bactericidal mechanism of action; renal excretion; and a broad spectrum of activity that covers many Gram-positive and Gram-negative aerobic organisms. In the case of imipenem and many of the penicillins, activity also includes anaerobes. Imipenem, in its commercial formulation, is complexed with cilastin to reduce its renal metabolism.

WATCH OUT FOR

Carbapenems have a number of adverse effects that can be classified by the affected system. Carbapenems can cause hypersensitivity reactions. These reactions will often present as skin rashes, urticaria, or even Stevens-Johnson syndrome in severe cases. Gastrointestinal side effects include nausea, vomiting, and abnormal liver-function tests and transaminases. From a bone-marrow perspective, marrow suppression and a positive Coombs test can result. Renal dysfunction can result from imipenem use and all beta-lactam antibacterial agents (including imipenem) require dosage adjustment in the setting of renal insufficiency and failure because of their renal excretion. Neurologically, imipenem can cause myoclonus and seizures. Seizures are a fairly common complication and result from a lowering of the seizure threshold in susceptible patients. Fortunately, this complication is not nearly as common with the use of meropenem. Seizures also occur in the setting of new-onset renal dysfunction if the carbapenem dose is not adjusted.

In patients where the risk of seizures is prohibited, other agents that can be used in place of imipenem include the broad-spectrum cephalosporins or the penicillins. It must be noted that cephalosporins will not provide the coverage of enterococcus or anaerobes that imipenem provides and penicillins, particularly the extended-spectrum penicillins, while providing adequate antimicrobial coverage might also cause seizures and twitching. Quinolones may be another alternative antibacterial, but they are also known to cause seizures.

SUGGESTED READINGS

Goldman L, Ausiello D, eds. Cecil Textbook of Internal Medicine. 22nd ed. Philadelphia: Saunders; 2004:1753–1764.

Helinger WC, Brewer NS. Carbapenems and monobactams: imipenem, meropenem, and aztreonam. Mayo Clin Proc. 1999;74:420–434.

158

REMEMBER IF THERE IS A NORMAL PLATELET COUNT IT CANNOT BE HANTAVIRUS PULMONARY SYNDROME

ANTHONY D. SLONIM, MD, DrPH

Several species of Hantavirus (family Bunyaviridae) can cause disease in humans, but in the United States, Sin Nombre virus is the most notorious and severe. Sin Nombre virus was first reported in 1993 in the Four Corners region of the southwestern United States (Arizona, Colorado, New Mexico, Utah). Physicians working for the Indian Health Service in that region noted a cluster of young healthy persons who developed severe respiratory illnesses characterized by rapidly progressive, noncardiogenic pulmonary edema, and a high case fatality rate. Though it was first clinically detected in the United States in 1993, retrospective serologic data as early as 1959 indicates that Sin Nombre virus was present decades earlier. From 1993 to 2005, 396 cases of hantavirus pulmonary syndrome (HPS) were reported in the United States, with 20 to 50 cases occurring annually.

The epidemiology of HPS in the United States usually affects healthy adults (mean age 38 years) residing in rural areas. Approximately 77% of affected patients are Caucasian and 19% American Indian. Hantaviruses are transmitted to humans by rodents via aerosolization of infected excreta. While contaminated urine is most commonly implicated, rodent droppings, saliva, and nesting materials can also aerosolize to cause illness. Rarely, hantaviruses may also be transmitted through direct mucous-membrane contact or inoculation. These viruses do not cause apparent illness in their rat reservoirs. Several murine species can transmit hantaviruses, but in the United States, deer mice (*Peromyscus maniculatus*) are the primary reservoir for Sin Nombre virus. The cotton rat, rice rat, and white-footed mouse transmit other hantavirus species in the United States. Therefore, given that there is neither an effective vaccine nor therapy, the primary strategy for combating HPS is rat control. No human-to-human cases have been reported, nor have pets or farm animals been implicated in disease transmission.

The differential diagnosis includes other infectious diseases that attack immunocompetent patients who have the environmental exposure. This includes pulmonary anthrax, plague, tularemia, histoplasmosis, coccidioidomycosis, leptospirosis, Lyme disease, ehrlichiosis, chlamydia, mycoplasma, Q fever, and Legionnaires disease.

The incubation period of HPS is approximately 3 weeks after the patient inhales the virus, during which time the patient is generally asymptomatic. The prodrome lasts for 3 to 5 days with nonspecific symptoms of fever, chills, myalgias, headache, and nausea, vomiting, and diarrhea. There may also be cough, dizziness, arthralgias, dyspnea, tachypnea, and tachycardia. Generally, rhinorrhea and sore throat are absent as are conjunctival and cutaneous symptoms.

WATCH OUT FOR

During the prodrome phase the platelet count is almost always normal but a dramatic decrease in the platelets marks the beginning of the pulmonary edema phase. In addition to thrombocytopenia, there is a leukocytosis with a marked left shift and the presence of atypical lymphocytes. There is also often hypoalbuminemia, elevated transaminases, and elevated serum lactate. Clinically, the drop in platelets corresponds with a severe and acute decompensation with a rapid progression to septic shock with a low cardiac output and an increased systemic vascular resistance. Patients may progress to sinus bradycardia and malignant ventricular arrythmias. Patients invariably require intubation and show a bilateral diffuse interstitial edema and pleural effusion.

WHAT TO DO

The treatment of HPS is largely supportive. While the antiviral compounds have been shown to inhibit hantaviruses in vitro, their clinical efficacy has not been proven. Early aggressive intensive care unit (ICU)-level care with careful monitoring of oxygenation and hemodynamic parameters is imperative, as decompensation and death can occur within hours. The patient should receive fluid resuscitation, inotropic support, and mechanical ventilation. Blood and sputum samples should be sent to a reference laboratory (e.g., Centers for Disease Control and Prevention) for detection of the Hantavirus RNA sequence by polymerase chain reaction (PCR) or detection of Hantavirus-specific IgM or a rising IgG titer. Even with excellent management, mortality still ranges from 30% to 40%. Somewhat surprisingly, HPS patients who survive the infection have a rapid recovery and are often extubated and discharged within days of the acute decompensation.

SUGGESTED READINGS

Dolin R. Principles and Practice of Infectious Diseases. Philadelphia: Elsevier; 2005.
Outbreak of acute illness—southwestern United States, 1993. Morb Mortal Wkly Rep. 1993;42:421.

159

CONSIDER EMPIRIC HELICOBACTER PYLORI TREATMENT WHEN GASTRIC OR DUODENAL ULCERS ARE FOUND

ANTHONY D. SLONIM, MD, DRPH

Peptic ulcer disease is a common condition that manifests its changes on either the gastric or duodenal mucosa and accounts for nearly half of all upper gastrointestinal bleeds admitted to the intensive care unit (ICU). The two major predisposing factors for peptic ulcer disease are infections with *Helicobacter pylori* and nonsteroidal anti-inflammatory drug (NSAID) use. The lesions caused by these two agents depend not only on the agents but on the characteristics of the gastrointestinal mucosa in the area that they affect. *H. pylori* is a Gram-negative organism that grows well in the acidic environment of the duodenal bulb. The damage caused by the bacteria in this location leads to further injury and colonization by additional bacteria, which perpetuates the inflammation. In contrast, NSAIDs inhibit cyclo-oxygenase, the enzyme that assists in prostaglandin production. Prostaglandins are an important defense mechanism for the gastric mucosa and inhibition results in a propensity for ulcer formation. Of importance for patients with NSAID-induced ulcer disease, treatment of *H. pylori* infection, even empirically, might help in achieving a cure and alleviating recurrences. Smoking and stress contribute to the occurrence of both types of peptic ulcer disease and patients should be encouraged to reduce both types of insult.

   H. pylori infection is a chronic condition. The organism can be identified by using several different diagnostic tests. Noninvasive diagnostic techniques include an enzyme-linked immunosorbent assay (ELISA) that is available for the detection of antibodies to *H. pylori*, a stool antigen test, and a urea breath test that can be used to detect the presence of organisms in gastritis or peptic ulcer disease. These tests have sensitivities and specificities that exceed 85%, but clinicians need to realize that false positive and false negative tests can still occur, particularly when patients have been pretreated with antibiotics. In addition, endoscopic specimens can be tested for the detection of *H. pylori* on histologic examination or culture, but these tests require that the patient undergo endoscopy.

WHAT TO DO

The treatment of peptic ulcer disease needs to include therapy for the hyperacidity and the underlying *H. pylori* infection. However, during acute bleeding episodes in the ICU, the focus should be on resuscitation, the restoration of hemodynamic stability, and the treatment of hyperacidity. The treatment of *H. pylori* will occur after the acute gastrointestinal bleeding subsides. This treatment should include hyperacidity treatment and treatment with two antibiotics. A number of effective regimens exist (e.g. the "prevpack") and are able to achieve cure rates of up to 90% for those patients who complete the 2-week course of therapy.

Acceptable regimens for the treatment of H pylori infection are (all for one week):

PPI bid
amoxicillin 1 gm bid
clarithromycin 500 mg bid

or

PPI bid
metronidazone 500 mg bid
clarithromycin 250 mg bid

or

PPI bid
Pepto Bismol 2 tabs qid
metronidazole 250 mg qid
tetracycline 500 mg qid

SUGGESTED READINGS

Conrad SA. Acute upper gastrointestinal bleeding in critically ill patients: causes and treatment modalities. Crit Care Med. 2002;30:S365–S368.

Huang JQ, Sridhar S, Hunt RH. Role of *Helicobacter pylori* infection and non steroidal anti-inflammatory drugs in peptic ulcer disease: a meta analysis. Lancet. 2002;35:14–22.

SHOCK/FLUIDS/ELECTROLYTES

160

ADMINISTER EMPIRIC BROAD-SPECTRUM ANTIBIOTICS WHEN A PATIENT MAY BE IN SEPTIC SHOCK

WILLIAM R. BURNS III, MD

Sepsis is a state of physiologic derangement attributed to either known or suspected infection (*Table 160.1*). When accompanied by organ dysfunction and/or hypoperfusion, the condition is termed severe sepsis. Septic shock is diagnosed if severe sepsis and hypotension persist in spite of fluid resuscitation. Despite numerous attempts to minimize the morbidity and mortality associated with these conditions, the proper administration of empiric, broad-spectrum antimicrobials is one of the few interventions to have demonstrated utility.

WHAT TO DO

Once severe sepsis or septic shock is recognized, resuscitative measures should be initiated immediately, if not already under way. Efficient delivery of broad-spectrum antimicrobial therapy is a treatment of critical importance. Potential sources of infection, common pathogens, patient risk factors, and local resistance patterns should be considered to determine the ideal drugs for first-line administration. These should almost always include broad bacterial coverage (Gram-positives, Gram-negatives, and anaerobes), may often be directed at resistant Gram-positives such as methicillin-resistant *Staphylococcus aureus* (MRSA) and/or vancomycin-resistant enterococci (VRE), and may occasionally target virulent Gram-negative bacilli and/or fungi. In patients with severe sepsis, the use of an antipseudomonal penicillin (such as piperacillin/tazobactam), a fourth-generation cephalosporin (such as cefepime), or a carbapenem (such as meropenem) is recommended; alternatively, an antipseudomonal fluoroquinolone (such as ciprofloxacin) in addition to metronidazole is suitable for those with a beta-lactam allergy. The use of vancomycin (for MRSA coverage) or linezolid (for VRE coverage), aminoglycosides (for extended Gram-negative coverage), and fluconazole (for antifungal coverage) is often indicated for patients experiencing septic shock or specific cases of severe sepsis.

While medications are being prepared (all orders for antibiotics should be written on a "stat" basis), appropriate cultures should be obtained. Typically blood from two peripheral sites, urine, and sputum

TABLE 160.1   PHYSIOLOGICAL STATES

Sepsis	Presumed or documented infection, resulting in 2 or more of the following criteria	T > 38° C or T < 36° C; HR > 90; RR > 20 or P_{CO_2} < 32; WBC > 12,000 or WBC < 4,000 or bands > 10% of neutrophils
Severe sepsis	Criteria for sepsis, plus the following	Organ dysfunction, hypoperfusion, or hypotension
Septic shock	Criteria for severe sepsis, plus the following	Hypotension despite resuscitation, perfusion abnormalities (lactic acidosis, oliguria, acute alteration in mental status), vasopressor use

T, temperature; HR, heart rate; RR, respitory rate; WBC, white blood cells.

are sampled. Furthermore, samples from vascular access and percutaneous drainage catheters may be analyzed as well. Microbial titers are highest at the time of diagnosis of severe sepsis or septic shock and the ability to isolate pathogens becomes increasingly more difficult with antibiotic treatment. As such, acquisition of cultures should occur expeditiously. This process, however, should not delay the administration of antimicrobial therapy, which should ideally be delivered within the first hour of diagnosis.

Beyond antibiotic therapy, septic patients require supportive therapy and intensive monitoring. Additional cultures must be obtained in the case of worsening physiologic derangements, and considered every 24 hours. Culture data and sensitivity information should be reviewed regularly to consider narrowing antimicrobial therapy and/or the institution of coverage for untreated organisms. If there is no evidence of MRSA and/or VRE within 48 to 72 hours, antibiotics specifically targeting these pathogens should be discontinued. Otherwise, it is often prudent to continue a short course of empiric therapy while initial and follow-up cultures are pending, keeping in mind that fungi often take 7 days to grow in culture (if they grow at all).

SELECTED READINGS

Ibrahim EH, Sherman G, Ward S, et al. The influence of inadequate antimicrobial treatment in bloodstream infections on patient outcomes in the ICU setting. Chest. 2000;118:146–155.

Leibovici L, Shraga I, Drucker M, et al. The benefit of appropriate empirical antibiotic treatment in patients with bloodstream infection. J Intern Med. 1998;244:379–386.

Souba WW, Fink MP, Jurkovich GJ, et al., eds. ACS Surgery: Principles and Practice. New York: WebMD Professional Publishing; 2006:1260–1270.

161

DO NOT ADMINISTER THE COSYNTROPIN TEST WITHIN 24 HOURS OF USING ETOMIDATE

MEGHAN C. TADEL, MD

Hypoadrenalism is a life-threatening syndrome in critically ill patients. It can be found in patients with chronic adrenal insufficiency as well as those with adrenal suppression who are simply unable to mount the expected stress response to common conditions in the intensive care unit (ICU), including infection, sepsis, trauma, and surgery. Adrenal insufficiency can manifest as a broad number of signs and symptoms including weakness, hyponatremia, hypoglycemia, disruption of acid-base status, and hypotension (specifically hypotension refractory to therapy with pressors). Patients suffering from hypoadrenalism have significantly reduced mortality when this condition is diagnosed and therapy initiated.

The widely accepted test for primary adrenal insufficiency is the cosyntropin stimulation test. Cosyntropin is a synthetic analogue of adrenocorticotropic hormone (ACTH), consisting of the first 24 amino acids of the naturally occurring ACTH. This test consists of a baseline blood sample sent for cortisol level, followed by a single intravenous (IV) dose of 250 μg of cosyntropin, with further blood samples collected at 30 and 60 minutes after administration, although the 30-minute measure may be superfluous as the cortisol levels peak at 60 minutes. There exists some controversy over what constitutes a positive and negative stimulation test, but even the more conservative proponents seem to agree that adrenal insufficiency is not present if the baseline cortisol level is >20 μg/dL and a normal response to cosyntropin stimulation is present (i.e. the cortisol level increases by greater than 9 μg/dL in response to the above test). If a patient meets these criteria, he or she does not have adrenal insufficiency and no supplementation of adrenal hormones is necessary.

One cause of adrenal insufficiency that is often seen in the ICU is the prior administration of etomidate. Etomidate is an imidazole, nonbarbiturate, sedative-hypnotic. It was formerly used as a long-term sedative infusion for ICU patients but was found to have high rates of associated hypoadrenalism with poor outcomes and such use has been mostly abandoned. However, etomidate is still frequently used, particularly in the ICU setting as an agent for induction of anesthesia, particularly for intubating unstable patients. This is because etomidate is accepted as having a more hemodynamically stable profile. More recent investigations of usage of etomidate demonstrate that even this single intubating dose of etomidate (standard dose 0.3 mg/kg) can cause adrenal suppression for anywhere from 5 to 24 hours. This is because etomidate inhibits both 11β-hydroxylase and cholesterol side chain cleavage enzyme, both of which are active in adrenal steroid synthesis. Thus, the use of etomidate within the previous 24 hours will obscure the results of a cosyntropin stimulation test.

SUGGESTED READINGS

Annane D. ICU physicians should abandon the use of etomidate! Intens Care Med. 2005;31:325–326.

Miller R, ed. Miller's Anesthesia. 6th ed. New York: Elsevier/Churchill Livingstone; 2005:350–355,1041.

162

Switch from Hydrocortisone to Dexamethasone if the Cosyntropin Stimulation Test is to be Administered

Meghan C. Tadel, MD

Patients diagnosed with adrenal insufficiency are generally treated with hydrocortisone in the range of 60 to 80 mg intravenously (IV), 3 to 4 times daily for a total dose of 200 to 300 mg per day. However, in a patient who has not had a cosyntropin stimulation test to confirm the diagnosis of adrenal insufficiency, hydrocortisone should be switched to dexamethasone 2 to 4 mg IV every 6 to 8 hours for three doses until that test can be completed. Since therapy with supraphysiologic doses of any corticosteroid for even as few as five days can result in adrenal suppression for up to 1 year following cessation of therapy, use of steroids should not be undertaken lightly and as such a stimulation test should be considered. The reason for switching from hydrocortisone to dexamethasone is that hydrocortisone directly interferes in the assay used by labs to determine cortisol levels in blood samples while dexamethasone does not.

Additionally, there may be situations where a patient's clinical picture (hypotension refractory to pressor infusion) warrants immediate therapy with glucocorticoids even before the stimulation test can be initiated. In these instances, therapy can begin immediately with dexamethasone 4 to 8 mg IV bolus with consideration given to adding a fludrocortisone (a mineralocorticoid) 50 μg (PO) per day. Once the cosyntropin test has been completed, therapy can be converted to hydrocortisone. Mineralocorticoids are equally affected by adrenal insufficiency and play an important role in volume status and electrolyte balance so they should not be overlooked in the therapy of hypoadrenalism. Dexamethasone is purely a glucocorticoid with no mineralocorticoid effects. On the other hand, at doses greater than 50 to 100 mg daily, hydrocortisone exhibits both glucocorticoid and mineralocorticoid effects. Doses in this range are recommended in the acute therapy of adrenal crisis or when a patient presents in sepsis. After that time, when hydrocortisone doses may be tapered to a standing 20 to 30 mg daily, fludrocortisone 100 μg PO should be added for mineralocorticoid therapy.

SUGGESTED READINGS

Brunton L, Lazo J, Parker K, eds. Goodman and Gilman's the Pharmacological Basis of Therapeutics. 11th ed. New York: McGraw-Hill; 2006:1599–1606.

Goldman L, Ausiello D, eds. Cecil Textbook of Medicine. 22nd ed. Philadelphia: WB Saunders; 2004:1416–1418.

Larsen P, ed. Williams Textbook of Endocrinology. 10th ed. Philadelphia: WB Saunders; 2003:528–532.

163

USE VASOPRESSORS INSTEAD OF LARGE-VOLUME RESUSCITATION IN THE TREATMENT OF SHOCK FROM MASSIVE PULMONARY EMBOLISM

ANDREW L. ROSENBERG, MD

Massive pulmonary embolism (PE) occurs when more than 50% of the pulmonary circulation is acutely obstructed by a venous embolus, usually originating in the lower extremities. In massive PE, severe hemodynamic derangements result from pulmonary artery obstruction; profound pulmonary vasoconstriction due to local mediator release; and hypoxemia-induced vasoconstriction. The resulting increased right ventricular (RV) afterload results in acute right ventricular dilatation as the normally thin-walled RV is tasked with overcoming high pulmonary vascular resistance. Other consequences of acutely increased RV pressures include tricuspid regurgitation and sometimes a significantly shifted intraventricular septum. This can lead to impaired left ventricular (LV) filling and ultimately decreased cardiac output and hypotension. In addition, decreased aortic diastolic pressures and increased RV pressure may result in RV ischemia due to poor coronary perfusion, further reducing RV work and exacerbating the shock state. This scenario may occur so rapidly that the patient immediately experiences syncope or death manifested by pulseless electrical activity.

The diagnosis of this physiological process is made by recognizing the clinical scenario of an acutely ill patient, with agitation, dyspnea, shock, and hypoxemia in an appropriate host with risk factors for deep venous thrombosis including immobility, major surgeries, bed rest, malignancy, family history, oral contraceptives use, and/or trauma. Usually, in massive PE, there is scant time for confirmatory tests; often the patient is too unstable for transport. However, a variety of modalities exist if time permits, the patient is stable, and the clinical situation is uncertain. Probably the most important noninvasive exam would be an emergent computed tomography (CT) scan to both suggest and/or rule out other mimics of PE. Other tests that can be used to suggest the presence of a PE are an echocardiogram, arterial blood gases (may reveal hypoxemia and hypocarbia due to increased minute ventilation), and a d-dimer (may be of some value in ruling out a PE if it is negative, although a positive does not confirm the diagnosis in all cases).

WHAT TO DO The usual initial treatment for suspected or confirmed massive pulmonary embolism is intravenous (IV) fluid administration. An initial bolus of 500 mL to 1,000 mL of isotonic crystalloid may be especially helpful if/when patients are intubated with resulting decrease in right ventricular preload due to increased intrathoracic pressures from positive pressure ventilation. However, intravenous fluids, especially if given too quickly or in too large a volume, may worsen RV dilatation, increase RV wall stress, decrease RV perfusion, and shift the ventricular septum leftward, resulting in decreased LV output and worsening the cycle of RV failure.

An alternative treatment is to judiciously initiate a vasoconstrictor with some inotropic effect, such as norepinephrine at 0.05 to 0.2 μg/kg/min or perhaps dopamine at 5 to 15 μg/kg/min. Several animal studies have suggested that these agents improve systemic blood pressure, cardiac output, pulmonary vascular resistance, and right ventricular pressure compared with volume resuscitation alone in models of massive PE. Ultimately, thrombolytic agents, surgical or interventional radiologic clot removal, and/or anticoagulation are the treatments of choice in the setting of massive pulmonary embolism with hypotension and/or severe hypoxemia.

SUGGESTED READINGS

Benotti JR, Dalen JE. The natural history of pulmonary embolism. Clin Chest Med. 1984:5(3):403–410.

Ghignone M, Girling L, Prewitt RM. Volume expansion versus norepinephrine in treatment of low cardiac output complicating an acute increase in right ventricular afterload in dogs. Anesthesiology. 1984;60(2):132–135.

Riedel M. Venous thromboembolic disease. Acute pulmonary embolism 1: pathophysiology, clinical presentation, and diagnosis. Heart. 2001;85:229–240.

164

CONSIDER THE DISEASES THAT MIMIC SEPTIC SHOCK IN THE DIFFERENTIAL OF THIS CONDITION

ANTHONY D. SLONIM, MD, DrPH

Septic shock is an example of a particular type of shock known as distributive or hyperdynamic shock. In this condition, the patient demonstrates a high cardiac output and vasodilatation resulting in the maldistribution of blood flow. Despite a circulatory system that is working vigorously, the cells and tissues are unable to receive the appropriate nutrients and substrate necessary for appropriate functioning. The cells begin to convert from aerobic to anaerobic metabolism and a lactic acidosis develops.

Hemodynamically, these patients may have a decreased or near-normal filling pressure (central venous pressure or pulmonary capillary wedge pressure) initially. When the vasodilatation (manifested by a reduction in the systemic vascular resistance) and maldistribution become severe enough, a relative hypovolemia occurs and the mean arterial pressure decreases. The cardiac output remains characteristically increased in this type of shock and is accompanied by increased venous oxygen saturation.

WATCH OUT FOR

A number of conditions are often associated with this hemodynamic profile. When patients present with a shocklike state that is characteristic of hyperdynamic or distributive shock, the differential diagnosis and treatment strategies need to be broad. Adrenal insufficiency, anaphylaxis, thyrotoxicosis, neurogenic shock, cirrhotic liver disease, drug intoxications, and several infectious diseases can all resemble this hemodynamic profile. Additional clues to the presence of adrenal insufficiency include the sodium and potassium levels. The administration of corticosteroids can be lifesaving in this circumstance. Thyrotoxicosis can manifest itself in patients with pre-existing thyroid disease or on thyroid medication. Neurogenic shock can accompany major trauma with neck or back injuries and spinal-cord contusion or transection. Cirrhotic liver disease patients with impending liver failure can also present with this hemodynamic profile. Finally, drug intoxications, particularly the toxidromes associated with anticholinergics, can precipitate this spectrum of findings.

In addition to the numerous medical conditions listed previously, there are a number of infectious agents that can present with a similar spectrum of disease. Malaria can be accompanied by hypotension and shock with an elevated cardiac index. This usually occurs with a high parasitemia. Rickettsial diseases that are due to intracellular bacteria like Rocky Mountain spotted fever, babesiosis, and ehrlichiosis can also present with a vasodilatory shock often accompanied by a skin rash. The last two conditions should be suspected in patients in shock with a recent or suspected Lyme disease diagnosis and it must be noted that Lyme disease is now found in all parts of the continental United States and is endemic in much of Canada and Western and Eastern Europe.

SUGGESTED READINGS

Fink MP, Abraham E, Vincent JL, et al. Textbook of Critical Care. 5th ed. Philadelphia: Elsevier Saunders; 2005:1367–1382,897–904.

165

BE ALERT FOR A LARGE SYSTEMIC INFLAMMATORY RESPONSE AFTER BACK SURGERY

ASHITA GOEL, MD

SIRS (systemic inflammatory response syndrome) is a complex immune response that is characterized by hyperdynamic cardiac function and low afterload. This syndrome is manifested by signs of inflammation including hyperthermia or hypothermia, tachycardia, tachypnea, and elevated or depressed white blood cell count. This state lies in a spectrum with septic shock with the notable exception that septic shock is associated with the presence of an infection. The multiple triggers of SIRS include trauma, surgery, medications, and transfusions. The proinflammatory reaction of SIRS correlates to the severity of tissue damage. Depending on the injury, the response can progress to a shock state including hypotension, oliguria, mental status changes, and coagulopathies.

One of the strongest surgical triggers of SIRS is spine surgery. During spine surgery, destruction of bone and soft tissue activates macrophages to release proinflammatory cytokines such as tumor necrosis factor α (TNF-α), and interleukin 1 (IL-1). These factors then induce the production of IL-6 and IL-8 from endothelial and epithelial cells, fibroblasts, and monocytes, propagating SIRS. The onset of these factors occurs immediately following the procedure and is manifested clinically as elevations of body temperature and erythrocyte sedimentation rate (ESR), leukocytosis, and an increase in C-reactive protein (CRP). In severe reactions, patients may experience hypotension, coagulopathies, and shifting of intravascular fluid to the interstitial space. Much of the proinflammatory phase peaks on postoperative day one but can continue to linger up to postoperative day four. ESR will continue to be elevated for weeks following surgery. The extent of SIRS is affected by the duration and extent of spinal surgery, the volume of blood loss, the level of postoperative pain, and the degree of instrumentation during the procedure. Instrumentation results in a dramatic increase in the inflammatory response possibly from increased tissue destruction with implant placement or a direct physiological reaction to the implant material.

Treatment during the proinflammatory phase usually involves adequate pain control and fluid resuscitation. However, in severe cases, pressor agents may be needed to control the loss of systemic vascular resistance. Also during this period, patients may experience hemorrhage secondary to coagulopathy. Management may require transfusion of blood factors or platelets. In an extensive bleed or critically located hematomas, patients may need surgical treatment for the source of bleeding.

Following the initial proinflammatory phase, a subacute phase occurs, referred to as a compensatory anti-inflammatory reaction syndrome (CARS). This reaction down regulates the SIRS response and is carried out by IL-10, IL-13, IL-14, and transforming growth factor β (TGF-β). This phase results in the reversal of SIRS manifestations including the hypotension, leukocytosis, coagulopathies, and fevers. However, it can lead to a depression of the immune system and place patients at risk for infections.

WATCH OUT FOR
In patients recovering from spinal surgery, an inflammatory response beyond postoperative day four may suggest the presence of occult or overt infection. Gram-positive bacteria such as *Staphylococcus aureus* are the common causes of infection; however, Gram-negative bacteria can result in severe infections. Many Gram-negative bacteria possess endotoxins that can result in the development of severe sepsis. CRP levels are more accurate markers of infection than ESR. ESR remains elevated for weeks following uncomplicated surgery; however, CRP should normalize by day four in uncomplicated spinal cases.

The postoperative response of spinal procedures that involve neoplastic resections have variable courses depending on the nature of the tumor and the procedure. A SIRS response is generally predicted but can be complicated in patients on chemotherapy. Also, coagulopathies can be more pronounced in this group.

SUGGESTED READINGS

Lanken P, ed. The Intensive Care Unit Manual. Philadelphia: WB Saunders: 2001:93–101.

Takahashi J, Ebara S, Kamimura M, et al. Early-phase enhanced inflammatory reaction after spinal instrumentation surgery. Spine. 2001;26(15):1698–1704.

Takahashi J, Ebara S, Kamimura M, et al. Pro-inflammatory and anti-inflammatory cytokine increases after spinal instrumentation surgery. J Spinal Disord Tech. 2002;15(4):294–300.

166

BE ALERT FOR THE DEVELOPMENT OF ABDOMINAL COMPARTMENT SYNDROME

AWORI J. HAYANGA, MD

The terms *intra-abdominal hypertension* and *abdominal compartment syndrome* have sometimes been used interchangeably. However, it is important to recognize there is a distinction between these entities. Intra-abdominal hypertension exists when intra-abdominal pressure exceeds a measured numeric parameter. This parameter has generally been set at between 20 and 25 mm Hg. Abdominal compartment syndrome exists when intra-abdominal hypertension is accompanied by manifestations of organ dysfunction, with reversal of these pathophysiologic changes upon abdominal decompression. These include the pulmonary, cardiovascular, renal, splanchnic, musculoskeletal/integumentary (abdominal wall), and central nervous system.

The exact incidence of abdominal compartment syndrome is yet to be established, but it is clearly increased in certain population groups. These include patients with the following:

- severe blunt and penetrating abdominal trauma
- ruptured abdominal aortic aneurysms
- retroperitoneal hemorrhage
- pneumoperitoneum
- neoplasm
- pancreatitis
- massive ascites
- liver transplantation
- massive fluid resuscitation
- accumulation of blood and clot
- bowel edema
- forced closure of a noncompliant abdominal wall
- circumferential abdominal burn eschars

In one prospective series of 145 patients who were identified as being at risk for development of the abdominal compartment syndrome, the reported incidence was 14%. The incidence following primary closure after repair of ruptured abdominal aortic aneurysm was reported in one series as 4%.

In the trauma population, the group that is especially at risk includes those patients undergoing abbreviated or "damage control" laparotomy, especially with intra-abdominal packing. It must be noted that having an open abdomen does not necessarily preclude the diagnosis of intra-abdominal hypertension or abdominal compartment syndrome, particularly where intra-abdominal packing has been used.

SIGNS AND SYMPTOMS

Clinical manifestations of organ dysfunction in abdominal compartment syndrome include respiratory failure that is characterized by impaired pulmonary compliance that results in elevated airway pressures with progressive hypoxia and hypercapnia. In this situation, extremely high driving pressures may be required to maintain minimally sufficient tidal volumes, often with loss of delivered tidal volume by distension of ventilatory tubing. The high airway pressures are needed to overcome high extrathoracic pressure exerted through the diaphragm and not to overcome an intrinsic lung problem. Some authors report pulmonary dysfunction and elevated peak airway pressures as the earliest manifestation of abdominal compartment syndrome. Chest radiography may show elevated hemidiaphragms with loss of lung volume.

Hemodynamic indicators consistent with abdominal compartment syndrome include elevated heart rate, hypotension, elevated pulmonary artery wedge pressure and central venous pressure, reduced cardiac output, and elevated systemic and pulmonary vascular resistance. In this situation measurement of right ventricular end-diastolic volume may be a more accurate predictor of a patient's position on the Starling curve. The pathophysiology is related to decreased venous return.

In abdominal compartment syndrome impairment in renal function is manifested by oliguria progressing to anuria with resultant azotemia. Renal insufficiency as a result of intra-abdominal hypertension is only partly reversible by fluid resuscitation. Renal failure in the absence of pulmonary dysfunction is not likely to be the result of intra-abdominal hypertension. Elevated intracranial pressure is an additional clinical manifestation of abdominal compartment syndrome.

Clinical confirmation of intra-abdominal hypertension requires bedside measurements indicative of intra-abdominal pressure. Experimental and clinical data indicate that intra-abdominal hypertension is present when intra-abdominal pressure exceeds 20 mm Hg. Contemporary measurement of intra-abdominal pressure outside of the laboratory is accomplished by a variety of means. These include direct measurement of intra-abdominal pressure by means of an intraperitoneal catheter, as is done during laparoscopy. Bedside measurement of intra-abdominal pressure has been accomplished by transduction of pressures from indwelling femoral vein, rectal, gastric, and urinary bladder catheters. Of these methods, measurement of urinary bladder and gastric pressures are the most common clinical applications. In 1984, Kron et al. reported a method to measure intra-abdominal pressure at the bedside with the use of an indwelling Foley catheter as follows:

- Sterile saline (50 to 100 cc) is injected into the empty bladder through the indwelling Foley catheter.
- The sterile tubing of the urinary drainage bag is clamped just distal to the culture aspiration port.
- The end of the drainage bag tubing is connected to the Foley catheter.
- The clamp is released just enough to allow the tubing proximal to the clamp to drain fluid from the bladder, then reapplied.
- A 16-gauge needle is then used to Y-connect a manometer or pressure transducer through the culture aspiration port of the tubing of the drainage bag.
- Finally, the top of the symphysis pubic bone is used as the zero point with the patient supine.

An alternative bedside technique has been described in which intragastric pressure measurements are taken from an indwelling nasogastric tube. This method has been validated and found to vary within 2.5 cm H_2O of urinary bladder pressures. Of these techniques, measurement of urinary bladder pressure appears to have gained widest clinical acceptance and application.

One final note is that the clinician must know if the pressure readings have been reported in cm H_2O or mmHg. To convert cm H_2O to mm Hg, multiply the reported value by 0.736.

SUGGESTED READINGS

Bailey J, Shapiro MJ. Abdominal compartment syndrome. Crit Care. 2000;4(1):23–29.
Gracias VH, Braslow B, Johnson J, et al. Abdominal compartment syndrome in the open abdomen. Arch Surg. 2002;137(11):1298–1300.
Kron IL, Hartman PK, Nolan SP. The measurement of intra-abdominal pressure as a criterion for abdominal re-exploration. Ann Surg. 1984;199:28–30.
Saggi BH, Sugerman HJ, Ivatury RR, et al. Abdominal compartment syndrome. J Trauma. 1998;45:597–609.
Sugrue M. Abdominal compartment syndrome. Curr Opin Crit Care. 2005;11(4):333–338.

167

TREAT ABDOMINAL PAIN OUT OF PROPORTION TO PHYSICAL EXAM AS MESENTERIC ISCHEMIA UNTIL PROVEN OTHERWISE

D. JOSHUA MANCINI, MD
RAJAN GUPTA, MD

Acute mesenteric ischemia is an abdominal emergency with high mortality and devastating morbidity. Perioperative mortality is 20% to 80%, depending upon the etiology of the acute process, and the overall mortality rate remains above 60%. In acute mesenteric ischemia, initial tissue injury occurs as a result of compromised end-organ perfusion. Secondary injury at the cellular level likely occurs through amplification of an inflammatory response with free-radical generation during reperfusion. Acute mesenteric ischemia is usually divided into four categories, based upon etiology. Arterial embolism is the most common type and represents 40% to 50% of all acute mesenteric ischemia cases. Emboli most commonly originate from a cardiac source and occlude the superior mesenteric artery (SMA). Acute mesenteric arterial thrombosis accounts for 25% to 30% of acute mesenteric ischemia. The proximal SMA is the most common site of thrombosis. Nonocclusive mesenteric ischemia represents approximately 20% to 30% of the acute mesenteric ischemia cases. This condition is usually a result of relative hypovolemia, low cardiac output, and splanchnic vasoconstriction. Mesenteric vein thrombosis is the least common cause of acute mesenteric ischemia, accounting for approximately 5% to 10% of the cases. These cases are often associated with a concomitant intra-abdominal process such as malignancy or inflammation, or with primary clotting disorders such as factor V Leiden mutation.

SIGNS AND SYMPTOMS

Diagnosis of acute mesenteric ischemia may be difficult because the signs and symptoms often mimic other intra-abdominal processes. This often results in significant delays in diagnosis, especially in the intensive care unit (ICU). Because these delays can adversely affect outcome, heightened clinical suspicion is paramount. The four types of acute mesenteric ischemia present with different patterns of signs and symptoms. An embolic event usually causes a sudden onset of symptoms, while acute mesenteric ischemia due to thrombosis may present suddenly or with a progressive history of postprandial pain, nausea, and weight loss. Nonocclusive mesenteric ischemia presents less acutely and often occurs in elderly patients in the ICU suffering from global hypoperfusion. Patients with mesenteric vein thrombosis classically present late with previous symptoms of nonspecific abdominal pain, anorexia, and diarrhea.

Abdominal pain out of proportion to physical exam is the hallmark of acute mesenteric ischemia. Physical exam is often not helpful in the diagnosis of acute mesenteric ischemia and can be unreliable in the ICU. In fact, early in the course of acute mesenteric ischemia, physical exam can be normal or remarkable only for distention. Peritoneal signs are late findings that develop only after infarction has occurred. Occult blood in the stool can also indicate acute mesenteric ischemia; however, bloody diarrhea is more common with colonic ischemia.

Laboratory tests in patients with acute mesenteric ischemia will commonly demonstrate an increased white blood cell count and acidosis. However, these findings are usually nonspecific and manifest too late in the disease process to be truly helpful to make a timely diagnosis. In the ICU, abdominal pain accompanied by metabolic acidosis should prompt early consideration of acute mesenteric ischemia. Findings on plain abdominal radiograph are often nonspecific (e.g., ileus) or occur late in the course (e.g., pneumoperitoneum, pneumatosis, portal venous air). Colonoscopy or sigmoidoscopy may be useful in suspected cases of colonic ischemia. Duplex ultrasonography is often limited because of bowel gas patterns. Computed tomography (CT) has become the gold standard to evaluate abdominal pain and has the advantage of being able to evaluate the entire abdomen and identify processes that may clinically mimic acute mesenteric ischemia. With the advent of multislice CT, the sensitivity of this modality using CT angiography has improved for primarily diagnosing acute mesenteric ischemia. Intravenous (IV) contrast is necessary to obtain appropriate results. Magnetic resonance imaging can be employed, especially if CT is contraindicated; however, it does not appear to have any additional value when compared with CT angiography. Selective mesenteric angiography remains the gold standard in the diagnosis of acute mesenteric ischemia. Conventional angiography has the added benefit of offering potentially therapeutic interventions such as angioplasty, stent placement, embolectomy, and the infusion of thrombolytics and vasodilators.

The treatment for acute mesenteric ischemia begins with volume resuscitation to optimize mesenteric (and global) perfusion. Broad-spectrum antibiotics should be administered and systemic anticoagulation should be considered. In patients without peritonitis, selective mesenteric angiography should be performed and appropriate therapeutic measures should be initiated based on the findings. Thrombolytic therapy is indicated for acute mesenteric occlusion secondary to embolus or thrombosis. Vasodilators (e.g., papaverine) can be used in patients with both occlusive and nonocclusive mesenteric ischemia. They are a first-line therapy in patients with nonocclusive mesenteric ischemia and can decrease occlusive vasospasm in other causes of acute mesenteric ischemia as well. For patients who fail interventional angiographic therapy for thromboembolic disease, surgical intervention is required to re-establish adequate mesenteric circulation. Surgical embolectomy is usually performed for embolic disease and bypass grafting is commonly necessary for thrombotic disease. Other than resection of nonviable intestine, there is no surgical option for nonocclusive mesenteric ischemia. Surgical intervention for mesenteric vein thrombosis (e.g., venous embolectomy for superior mesenteric vein or portal vein thrombosis) is associated with poor outcomes.

Patients who present with or develop peritonitis during the diagnostic and resuscitation phase need emergent laparotomy with resection of nonviable intestine. A planned "second look" operation 24 to 48 hours later is often required to determine the true extent of bowel necrosis. Long-term anticoagulation is indicated in patients with embolic or thrombotic causes of acute mesenteric ischemia. The use of antiplatelet agents postoperatively in cases of acute mesenteric ischemia is less well established.

SUGGESTED READINGS

Agaoglu N, Turkyilmaz S, Ovali E, et al. Prevalence of prothrombotic abnormalities in patients with acute mesenteric ischemia. World J Surg. 2005;29(9):1135–1138.

Oldenburg WA, Lau LL, Rodenberg TJ, et al. Acute mesenteric ischemia: a clinical review. Arch Intern Med. 2004;164(10):1054–1062.

Schoots IG, Levi MM, Reekers JA, et al. Thrombolytic therapy for acute superior mesenteric artery occlusion. J Vasc Interv Radiol. 2005;16(3):317–329.

DO NOT BOLUS FLUIDS THAT CONTAIN DEXTROSE

AWORI J. HAYANGA, MD

Intravenous fluids that contain dextrose have questionable utility in the intensive care unit (ICU) and should not be administered at a rate greater than maintenance fluids. Bolusing with dextrose-containing fluids causes a rapid change in extracellular osmolarity. This can occur quite rapidly and may cause convulsions and coma. At the very least, bolusing with dextrose will cause an unacceptably high serum glucose, which is detrimental in intensive care patients.

Acceptable fluids to bolus with include normal saline, hypertonic saline, and Lactated Ringer's. Lactated Ringer's is an excellent isotonic salt solution for replacing isotonic gastrointestinal losses and pre-existing volume deficits when a patient has a normal or near-normal electrolyte level. Isotonic sodium (0.9% saline) is ideal for the initial correction of depleted extracellular fluid volume associated with hyponatremia, hypochloremia, and metabolic alkalosis. One concern with normal saline is that the high chloride concentration may exceed the capacity of the kidney to excrete it and has the potential to cause dilutional acidosis.

SUGGESTED READINGS

Boldt J. Fluid choice for resuscitation of the trauma patient: a review of the physiological, pharmacological, and clinical evidence. Can J Anaesth. 2004;51(5):500–513.

Miller RD, ed. Miller's Anesthesia. 6th ed. New York: Elsevier/Churchill Livingstone; 2005:1783–1795.

REMEMBER THAT DIURESIS MAY NOT BE THE BEST TREATMENT FOR HYPERKALEMIA IN THE EARLY POST CARDIOPULMONARY BYPASS PERIOD

FRANK ROSEMEIER, MD MRCP(UK)
ELIZABETH A. MARTINEZ, MD, MHS

Hyperkalemia is a common electrolyte abnormality following cardiac surgery which can result in serious complications. Potential causes of hyperkalemia are listed in *Table 169.1*. While evaluating patients for clinical sequelae from this disturbance; these underlying causes should be carefully considered.

Decreased Clearance of Potassium. Preexisting renal insufficiency or evolving acute tubular necrosis is the most concerning cause of hyperkalemia in the postoperative period. Cardiopulmonary bypass (CPB) is characterized by altered renal blood flow because of non-pulsatile pump flow and intraoperative hypotensive episodes. Vasodilatation induced by CPB and systemic inflammatory response syndrome (SIRS) may result in diminished renal flow, pooling of blood in venous capacitance vessels, and capillary leakage with resulting hypotension. Shear forces of CPB may cause red cell destruction resulting in intravascular hemolysis, which in turn can lead to hemoglobinurea, hyperkalemia and renal failure. Management strategies include the restoration and maintenance of normovolemia, renal blood flow, and perfusion pressure to limit further insult.

ACE inhibitors are known to result in potassium retention secondary to a lowering of plasma aldosterone levels and thus a decrease in potassium clearance. This phenomenon is note to occur in individuals with other risk factors for hyperkalemia, including disruption of homeostasis or congestive heart failure. Furthermore, ACE inhibitors may also contribute to renal insult in situations where MAP falls below 50-65mmHg, hypovolemia, or inadequate cardiac output. Therefore prior to treatment of hyperkalemia with potassium wasting diuretics, you must make certain that the patient is adequately resuscitated so as not to contribute to ongoing renal insult.

Increased Intake of Potassium. Potassium is commonly repleted in post-bypass patients to a level of 4.0 to 4.5 mEq/L to decrease the risk of perioperative arrhythmias. Continuous IV insulin infusions for the management of perioperative hyperglycemiapromote cellular uptake

TABLE 169.1	POTENTIAL CAUSES OF PERIOPERATIVE HYPERKALEMIA IN CARDIAC SURGERY PATIENTS

1. ATN
2. Chronic renal failure
3. Preop ACE inhibitors
4. Exogenous potassium administration
5. NSAIDs via the aldosterone pathway
6. Preop spironolactone or potassium sparing diuretics
7. Intraoperative use of high-potassium cardioplegia
8. Heparin via an aldosterone effect
9. Epsilon-aminocaproic acid

of potassium increasing the scale of potassium repletion. As glycemic control improves, and the insulin requirements decrease, subsequent hyperkalemia may occur because of increased total body stores.

Other. Other causes of hyperkalemia include preoperative administration of spironolactone or potassium sparing diuretics, high- potassium-containing cardioplegia and large volume red cell transfusion. Rare causes of hyperkalemia are the administration of the lysine analogue epsilon-aminocaproic acid and heparin via an aldosterone like effect. Finally, both respiratory and metabolic acidemia (the latter for example caused by hypoperfusion) may cause potassium shift from intracellular to extracelluar with an increase of 0.5 mEq K+ for a pH decrease by 0.1.

Treatment. Within the setting of acute postoperative hyperkalemia it is paramount to optimize normovolemia and adequate renal perfusion pressure to prevent further renal insult. Although furosemide or other potassium wasting diuretics may support the clearance of potassium, it may, in fact, increase relative hypovolemia thus contributing to acute tubular necrosis. However, if potassium exceeds 6meq/L or there are clinical sequelae noted from hyperkalemia with peaked T-wave being the first change seen on ECG, treatment must be initiated. Temporizing measures include the intravenous administration of calcium to stabilize myocardial membranes, and sodium bicarbonate, insulin and/or beta agonist, all of which promote an intracellular shift of potassium. Further measures are those directed at decreasing the total body potassium stores. These include potassium wasting diuretics (furosemide) and hemodialysis or hemofiltration. Caution is advised to the use of oral or rectally administered Kayexalate as it can cause ischemic bowel through the osmotic load of its sorbitol component especially in the setting of hemodynamic instability and hypoperfusion.

SUGGESTED READINGS

Day JR, Chaudhry AN, Hunt I, Taylor KM. Heparin-induced hyperkalemia after cardiac surgery. Ann Thorac Surg 2002;74(5):1698-700.

Hessell EA, Hild PG. Pathophysiology of Cardiopulmonary Bypass. In: Hensley FA, Martin DE, Gravlee GP, eds. A Practical Approach to Cardiac Anesthesia. 3rd ed. Philadelphia: Lippincott Williams & Wilkins; 2003:537-54.

Weber DO, Yarnoz MD. Hyperkalemia complicating cardiopulmonary bypass: analysis of risk factors. Ann Thorac Surg 1982;34(4):439-45.

170

REMEMBER THAT MOST PATIENTS RECEIVE MANNITOL WHEN GOING ON THE PUMP SO POSTOPERATIVE URINE OUTPUT IS NOT A MARKER FOR VOLUME STATUS OR PERFUSION AFTER CARDIAC SURGERY

MUHAMMAD I. DURRANI, MD

Current techniques in cardiac surgery sometimes require the use of cardiopulmonary bypass. The essential goal of cardiopulmonary bypass is to divert blood around a nonbeating heart through an extracorporeal circuit that functionally replaces the heart and lungs. There are several steps to be performed when placing a patient on bypass. After administration of heparin and attaining adequate activated clotting time (ACT), the arterial cannula (most commonly ascending aorta) is inserted first, to allow infusion of volume in case of hemorrhage associated with venous cannulation. When the arterial cannula is inserted, the systolic blood pressure should be decreased to 90 to 100 mm Hg to reduce the risk of aortic dissection and to facilitate cannulation. Venous blood returning to the right heart is drained by gravity to the venous reservoir through either two venous cannulas separately inserted into the inferior vena cava (IVC) and superior vena cava (SVC) or, more commonly, a single cannula inserted directly into the right atrium.

The composition of pump-priming solution generally consists of electrolytes, colloids, mannitol, and heparin. Depending upon the hematocrit of the patient, blood or packed red blood cells may be added to the priming solution. The volume of priming solution ranges from 1,800 mL to 2,200 mL. After the initiation of total cardiopulmonary bypass, mild to moderate hypothermia is induced (30° C to 32° C). The aorta is cross-clamped and cardioplegic solution is infused antegrade through the aortic root and retrograde via the coronary sinus to arrest the heart.

When crystalloid solutions alone are used to prime the cardiopulmonary bypass circuit, the resultant lowering of plasma oncotic pressure results in extravascular fluid shifts and the requirement of additional fluid during the procedure. Mannitol is added to the prime to help reduce this effect. Mannitol is an osmotic diuretic and a free-radical scavenger. In the United States, the dose of mannitol in the priming solution ranges from 12.5 g to 25 g.

Within 10 minutes of administration, the majority of the administered mannitol diffuses into the interstitial fluid. Very little, if any, penetrates the cells and so the raised extracellular tonicity results in the withdrawal of fluid from the cells. In addition, it acts to prevent further cellular edema, which would otherwise have to be treated by the addition of further fluid during bypass. The plasma-volume expansion due to mannitol has been reported as being between 1 mL and 3 mL per kg of body weight per 5 g of mannitol infused. During cardiopulmonary bypass, these actions result in a greater and more stable volume of blood stored in the oxygenator.

At the same time, mannitol is entering the kidney where it is freely filtered at the glomerulus into the renal tubules. Because it cannot enter the cells of the renal tubules, it is only poorly reabsorbed and so stays within the lumen of the tubules. The increased osmotic pressure caused by the mannitol remaining in the proximal tubules reduces water reabsorption, which results in an increased diuresis.

The addition of mannitol to the pump prime may increase diuresis for about 12 hours postoperatively. Because of this, the urine output is not reliable as an indicator for volume status in patients after cardiac surgery. The central venous pressure and pulmonary capillary wedge pressures, as determined with a pulmonary artery catheter, are the preferred measurements to be used at the bedside. In addition, venous oxyhemoglobin saturation can be measured intermittently by transcatheter aspiration or continuously by fiberoptic pulmonary artery catheters. Finally, central venous (right atrial) oxygen saturations are typically measured, and resting values are usually 75%. Assuming a 100% arterial saturation, this represents unloading of one-fourth of the available oxygen. Venous desaturation usually indicates inadequate tissue perfusion whether or not the cardiac index is depressed.

SUGGESTED READINGS

Estafanous FG, ed. Cardiac Anesthesia Principles and Clinical Practice. 2nd ed. Philadelphia: Lippincott Williams & Wilkins; 2001:415–446.

Stoelting RK, ed. Pharmacology and Physiology in Anesthetic Practice. 3rd ed. Philadelphia: Lippincott Williams & Wilkins; 1999: 440–441.

171

DO NOT USE URINE OUTPUT AS A MEASURE OF VOLUME STATUS IN PATIENTS WHO ARE COLD

JUAN N. PULIDO, MD
DANIEL R. BROWN, MD, PhD

Hypothermia is a clinical entity defined as a core body temperature less than 35° C (95° F) and is classified in four stages depending on the temperature, symptomatology, and impact on specific organ physiology (*Table 171.1*).

All organs are ultimately affected by hypothermia, including the kidneys. The renal response to cold is rapid and varies with the different stages of hypothermia. Initially, peripheral vasoconstriction results in relative central hypervolemia, producing an increase in urine output. This response, termed *cold diuresis*, has been described even in patients with mild to moderate hypothermia. The etiology of this phenomenon is multifactorial and includes an initial increase in cardiac output and renal blood flow due to hypothermia-induced changes in vascular capacitance. Other important contributors are nonosmotic suppression of antidiuretic-hormone (ADH) release by the hypothalamus and subsequent decreased renal tubular reabsorption. These responses usually begin as soon as the core body temperature reaches 35° C and become more pronounced until moderate hypothermia, when decreased renal blood flow and glomerular filtration rate (reduced 50% at 27° to 30° C) may lead to renal failure.

WATCH OUT FOR

Even in the setting of a large diuresis (the urine is usually dilute with osmolarity <300 mOsm/L and specific gravity <1.003), the kidneys are unable to handle nitrogenous waste due to tubular dysfunction. Although uncommon, electrolyte disturbances including hypernatremia, hyperchloremia, and hyperkalemia can occur and are more frequent as hypothermia progresses in duration and/or severity. Cold diuresis is exacerbated by ethanol ingestion and water submersion, which may coexist with hypothermia and can potentiate inappropriate diuresis by inhibiting ADH secretion.

It is important to understand the pathophysiology of this phenomenon when making clinical decisions regarding fluid management in hypothermic patients. The cold diuresis can be massive and generally creates a hypovolemic state that worsens with rewarming because

TABLE 171.1	SEQUELAE OF HYPOTHERMIA	
STAGE	CORE TEMPERATURE $^{\circ}$C ($^{\circ}$F)	CHARACTERISTICS
Mild	32 (89.6)–35 (95)	Increased metabolic rate, hypertension, tachycardia, shivering, cold diuresis, CNS hyperexcitability, coagulopathy
Moderate	28 (82.4)–32 (89.6)	Decreased cardiac output, hypoventilation, CNS depression, atrial arrhythmias, ↓O_2 consumption (~25% to 50%)
Severe	22 (71.6)–28 (82.4)	Progressive hypotension and bradycardia, ventricular arrhythmias, VF, decreased CBF, areflexia, loss of bulbar reflexes, decreased O_2 consumption (<50% of baseline)
Profound	<22 (71.6)	Asystole, EEG burst suppression

CNS, central nervous system; VF, ventricular fibrillation; CBF, cerebral blood flow; EEG, electroencephalogram.

of the reverse changes in vascular tone as core body temperature is raised. If overlooked or underappreciated, this phenomenon can exacerbate electrolyte disturbances, contribute to hypotension, and result in prerenal stress.

Intravascular volume status should be closely monitored to avoid complications of this "physiologically inappropriate" renal response. Initially, it should be assumed that the patient is significantly dehydrated. Frequent measurements of electrolytes and hematocrit will help guide fluid therapy and electrolyte replacement and help monitor for dehydration. Central venous access should be considered to allow for safer electrolyte replacement and rapid volume administration, though electrolyte abnormalities may increase cardiac irritability and arrhythmia risk during catheter placement. Invasive arterial blood pressure monitoring should also be considered to facilitate laboratory determinations and to evaluate fluid responsiveness.

SUGGESTED READINGS

Auerbach PS. Wilderness Medicine. 4th ed. Philadelphia: Mosby; 2001:135–155.
Irwin RS, Rippe JM, eds. Irwin and Rippe's Intensive Care Medicine. 5th ed. Philadelphia: Lippincott Williams & Wilkins; 2003:751–755.
Morgan ML. Mechanism of cold diuresis in the rat. Am J Physiol. 1983;244(2):F210–F216.

172

BE CAREFUL TO NOT OVERHYDRATE POSTOPERATIVE LIVER-TRANSPLANT PATIENTS

DORRY L. SEGEV, MD
WARREN R. MALEY, MD

The resuscitation of patients immediately following a liver transplant is similar in concept to that of cirrhotic individuals who have or are experiencing a bout of variceal hemorrhage. Like the cirrhotic patient who is suffering from gastrointestinal bleeding, the transplanted patient should be repleted to euvolemia to maximize end-organ perfusion and function. Excessive hydration of the variceal bleeder will exacerbate blood loss by further elevating central venous pressure (CVP) and portal hypertension. Likewise, overaggressive volume resuscitation of the liver recipient produces elevation of the CVP, resulting in distention of the transplanted organ and diminished liver perfusion pressure.

Allocation of livers for transplantation is currently triaged according to the Model for End-stage Liver Disease (MELD) system. Under MELD, each patient is assigned a score calculated from his or her most recent blood values of creatinine, bilirubin, and prothrombin time. MELD scores range from 6 to a capped maximum of 40 and correlate directly with the risk of 3-month mortality over a wide spectrum of etiologies of cirrhosis. Those with the highest scores within their respective blood group are the next individuals to be transplanted. Inclusion of renal function (as measured by serum creatinine) in the MELD equation recognizes the significant contribution of hepatorenal syndrome to mortality, as a late manifestation of severe cirrhotic liver disease. Using this allocation algorithm results in a significant proportion of recipients undergoing transplantation with renal insufficiency or even acute renal failure secondary to changes in renal function precipitated by their advanced liver failure. Thus, urinary output, often the best measure of tissue perfusion in the trauma or postsurgical patient, may fail to accurately represent an adequate volume of resuscitation in the liver-transplant recipient. In addition, intraoperative blood loss and hypotension, as well as the elimination of massive amounts of ascites and resultant reformation, may further worsen the patient's already tenuous renal status. In liver-transplant recipients, trends in CVP, pulmonary artery diastolic or wedge pressure, and cardiac output may better represent the hydration status of the patient.

In liver-transplant recipients, interpretation of the Swan-Ganz parameters must be predicated upon knowledge of the pathophysiology of the pre-existing cirrhotic state. Prior to transplantation, patients with cirrhosis exhibit an increased plasma volume, low systemic vascular resistance, and a hyperdynamic cardiac output. This physiologic condition persists for a significant period of time following liver transplantation and can easily be misinterpreted as being consistent with sepsis. Ordinary measures of adequate stroke volume may underestimate the need for further resuscitation given the vasodilated hyperdynamic state of the chronic liver-failure patient. Blood products provide the best volume repletion and are indicated in the setting of coagulopathy, anemia, or thrombocytopenia. Otherwise, many liver-transplant surgeons prefer albumin solutions to crystalloid, especially in patients with a history of preoperative ascites and hypoalbuminemia. The rationale for this is that a liver transplant in a patient with preoperative ascites is like a large-volume parascentesis, which is one of the few situations in which albumin use has shown clinical benefit. During volume resuscitation, a transfusion requirement beyond 4 units of blood merits strong consideration of operative exploration.

Once euvolemia is ascertained by frequent serial measures of CVP and pulmonary pressures, vasopressors may be indicated in the patient who remains hypotensive. If blood products are further required to correct anemia, coagulopathy, or thrombocytopenia in a recipient who is already adequately resuscitated, diuresis may be necessary to prevent an excessive rise in CVP and the attendant worsening of hepatic congestion. Markedly elevated CVPs are associated with diminished hepatic perfusion pressure, potentially leading to graft ischemia, hepatic artery thrombosis, or even parenchymal rupture. In patients with renal insufficiency unresponsive to diuretics, consideration should be given to early continuous venovenous hemodialysis (CVVHD).

SUGGESTED READINGS

Henriksen JH, Fuglsang S, Bendtsen F, et al. Arterial hypertension in cirrhosis: arterial compliance, volume distribution, and central haemodynamics. Gut. 2006;55(3):380–387.

Kamath PS, Wiesner RH, Malinchoc M, et al. A model to predict survival in patients with end-stage liver disease. Hepatology. 2001;33(2):46–470.

173

REMEMBER THAT UREMIA ALONE RARELY CAUSES AN ANION GAP TO BE GREATER THAN 25

LAITH R. ALTAWEEL, MD

The serum anion gap (AG) is an important tool in assessing the acid-base status of a patient and narrowing the differential diagnosis of etiologies responsible for acid-base disturbance. The anion gap is a measure of serum electrical neutrality. Total serum cations always equal serum anions. Thus, sodium + potassium + calcium + magnesium = bicarbonate + chloride + phosphate + sulfate + protein + organic acid anions. To simplify the equation, potassium, calcium, and magnesium are considered unmeasured cations (UC), and phosphate, sulfate, protein, and organic acids are considered unmeasured anions (UA). Thus, UA − UC = sodium − chloride − bicarbonate = serum anion gap. The normal range of anion gap is between 3 to 11 mEq/L, with modern techniques of measuring electrolytes. A reduction of 2.5 to 3 mEq in AG should be made for every 1-gram reduction in the serum albumin below 4.

A decrease in the anion gap is seen with a reduction in unmeasured cations or with increased anions. Albumin is an anion, and thus a low albumin will decrease the AG. Lithium, hypercalcemia, and cationic immunoglobulins contribute unmeasured cations, thus also lowering the AG.

Elevations in the anion gap can be seen with a decrease in unmeasured cations, which would include magnesium, calcium, and potassium. Increases in unmeasured anions can occur from organic acids (phosphate, sulfate), inorganic acids (keto acids, lactate, uremic anions), and exogenous toxins (salicylate).

Typical causes of AG elevation are as follows:

- Ketoacidosis (diabetic and alcoholic)
- Renal failure
- Lactic acidosis
- Rhabdomyolysis
- Toxins
- Methanol
- Ethylene glycol
- Paraldehyde
- Salicylates

SUGGESTED READINGS

Haber R. A practical approach to acid-base disorders. West J Med. 1992;155:146–151.
Salem M, Mujais S. Gaps in the anion gap. Arch Intern Med. 1992;152:1625–1629.

174

DO NOT REPLETE CALCIUM IN THE SETTING OF HIGH PHOSPHORUS OR PHOSPHORUS IN THE SETTING OF HIGH CALCIUM

PRAVEEN KALRA, MD
MEHMET S. OZCAN, MD

Calciphylaxis is an unusual condition that involves an abnormality in calcium and phosphate metabolism. It is characterized by occlusion of small subcutaneous arterioles with calcium deposits leading to ischemic skin lesions as severe as dry gangrene. Secondary hyperparathyroidism caused by chronic renal failure (CRF) is the most common setting for the disorder although it is reported in patients with multiple myeloma, primary hyperparathyroidism, vitamin D intoxication, and hypercalcemia of malignancy. About 1% of all patients with CRF and 4% undergoing hemodialysis are reported to develop calciphylaxis. It carries a very high mortality rate (60% to 78%), making prevention of paramount importance.

WATCH OUT FOR

Concurrent elevation of calcium and phosphate is crucial for the development of calciphylaxis. Multiplication of serum calcium and phosphate levels (in mg/dL) with the total equal to or greater than 56 has been associated with an increased risk. In chronic renal failure, serum phosphate is generally elevated secondary to impaired excretion. Calcium levels initially fall because of decreased intestinal absorption but subsequently increase as a result of secondary hyperparathyroidism. This leads to medial calcification and intimal hyperplasia of subcutaneous arterioles. Since not all patients at risk develop calciphylaxis, presence of other factors such as local trauma and hypercoagulable states (e.g., protein C and S deficiencies) have been suggested. Other conditions that are reported to be associated with calciphylaxis include diabetes mellitus, obesity, corticosteroid use, and anticoagulation with warfarin.

Diagnosis of calciphylaxis requires clinical suspicion in the high-risk patient. Painful skin lesions with purple discoloration are the usual initial presentation, which progress to cutaneous ulcers and subsequent eschar formation. Infection of the ulcers and dry gangrene are the main causes of morbidity and mortality. Lesions have been described in various body parts with a proximal location associated with a worse prognosis than a distal location. In many patients, laboratory reveals a calcium-phosphate product greater than 56 and increased parathyroid hormone levels. Biopsy confirms the clinical diagnosis, which typically shows a medial deposition of calcium in arteries with a diameter of 40 to 100 μm.

Management of calciphylaxis includes medical and surgical options as well as hyperbaric oxygen therapy. As a preventive measure, maintaining a calcium-phosphate product less than 56 mg^2/dL^2 is recommended in CRF and other high-risk patients. A low-phosphate diet with or without phosphate binders is an important tool to achieve this goal. Surgical options include wound management with debridement as well as parathyroidectomy. Although not a universally agreed upon technique, parathyroidectomy seems to offer a better prognosis than conservative management. In addition, hyperbaric oxygen may aid in treatment by inducing angiogenesis and fibroblast proliferation. Another benefit of hyperbaric therapy may be improvement of host defenses against infections.

SUGGESTED READINGS

Beus KS, Stack BC Jr. Calciphylaxis. Otolaryngol Clin North Am. 2004;37:941–948.
Block GA. Prevalence and clinical consequences of elevated Ca × P product in hemodialysis patients. Clin Nephrol. 2000;54:318–324.
Duffy A, Schurr M, Warner T, et al. Long-term outcomes in patients with calciphylaxis from hyperparathyroidism. Ann Surg Oncol. 2006;13:96–102.

175

CHECK POSTOPERATIVE AND SERIAL SERUM LEVELS OF PHOSPHORUS AND AGGRESSIVELY REPLETE

ROBERT K. MICHAELS, MD, MPH

Phosphate (PO_4) is a trivalent anion that is most notable for the energy-rich bonds it forms in adenosine triphosphate (ATP). Phosphate is also intimately in involved red blood cell function (2,3-diphosphoglycerate), platelet function, immune function, and the central nervous system (CNS). Phosphate homeostasis is closely linked with that of calcium, which together are controlled by parathyroid hormone, calcitonin, and vitamin D.

Patients in the intensive care unit (ICU) can have either hyperphosphatemia or hypophosphatemia. Postoperative hypophosphatemia is classically linked with liver resection and living-donor hepatectomies for liver transplantation. Classic teaching on this subject highlights the utilization of total body phosphate stores for the regeneration of the liver; however, a recent study concluded the presence of hyperphosphaturia points toward a renal origin of phosphate loss. Low serum phosphate has also been reported after other surgeries, such as colorectal surgery, renal transplantation, abdominal aortic aneurysm repair, and open heart surgery. If not prevented or treated, hypophosphatemia will frequently develop after major surgery on postoperative day one and reach a nadir on postoperative day two.

Nonsurgical etiologies of hypophosphatemia can be broadly grouped into three main causes: decreased intestinal absorption; the redistribution of phosphate intracellularly; and increased renal excretion. Examples of intestinal malabsorption include vomiting, diarrhea, vitamin D deficiency, and starvation. Cellular redistribution can be observed with respiratory alkalosis (such as that seen with anxiety or sepsis), treated diabetic ketoacidosis, and with the effects of various hormones such as insulin, catecholamines, and glucocorticoids. Increased renal excretion is seen with hyperparathyroidism, hyperaldosteronism, and other renal tubular abnormalities. Iatrogenic causes are usually related to total parenteral nutrition with inadequate amounts of phosphate ordered.

Mild hypophosphatemia (PO_4 less than 2.5 mg/dL) is usually asymptomatic but has been associated with significantly higher postoperative complications (pulmonary compromise, pancreatitis, infection, ileus, etc.) after liver resection. Severe hypophosphatemia (PO_4 less than 1.0 mg/dL) is life threatening and can result in serious morbidity including muscle weakness and respiratory insufficiency, cardiomyopathy, erythrocyte dysfunction, CNS manifestations (confusion, seizures, paresthesia), rhabdomyolysis, and skeletal demineralization. Hypophosphatemia has been linked with prolonged mechanical ventilation, prolonged ICU stay, and prolonged hospitalization.

The treatment of hypophosphatemia includes treating the underlying cause while replacing electrolytes. Phosphate salts are available for oral and parenteral use. Sodium phosphate and potassium phosphate are most commonly used, with the choice based on need for repletion of the other electrolytes. As much as 45 to 60 mmol per day of phosphate preparations can be administered per 24-hour period; overaggressive infusions can lead to hypocalcemia, hypotension, and renal failure. Repletion to a phosphate level of at least 2.5 mg/dL is not supported by high-quality evidence but is probably rational given the complications reported from even mild hypophosphatemia.

SUGGESTED READINGS

Buell JF, Berger AC, Plotkin JS, et al. The clinical implications of hypophosphatemia following major hepatic resection or cryosurgery. Arch Surg. 1998;133(7):757–761.
Salem RR, Tray K. Hepatic resection-related hypophosphatemia is of renal origin as manifested by isolated hyperphosphaturia. Ann Surg. 2005;241(2):343–348.

176

CONSIDER ELECTROLYTE DISTURBANCES WHEN THERE IS A CHANGE OF MENTAL STATUS

NIRAV G. SHAH, MD

Toxic-metabolic encephalopathy results in a change of mental status and is a common diagnosis in the intensive care unit (ICU). Electrolyte disturbances need to be high on the list of differential diagnoses when evaluating the ICU patient with altered mental status. Some commonly encountered disturbances include hyponatremia, hypernatremia, hypoglycemia, hyperglycemia, hypermagnesia, acidosis, and alkalosis.

WATCH OUT FOR

Clinical manifestations of hyponatremia include dysfunction of the central nervous system and are dependent on the severity and rate of development. For instance, the acute development of hyponatremia (<24 hours) as well as extremely low sodium concentrations (<120 mEq/L) may manifest with severe symptoms including confusion, agitation, delirium, lethargy, and seizures. The most common etiologies include syndrome of inappropriate antidiuretic hormone (SIADH), treatment with thiazide diuretics, polydipsia, and inappropriate administration of hypotonic intravenous fluids. Treatment consists of free-water restriction and, in severe cases, administration of hypertonic saline to correct the hyponatremia. To prevent central pontine myelinolysis, care must be taken to prevent too rapid a rise in serum sodium. This disorder results in quadriplegia and pseudobulbar palsy and is preventable with the judicious correction of serum sodium. The goal in patients with chronic hyponatremia and in asymptomatic patients should be a gradual correction of <10 mEq/L per 24 hours.

Similarly, hypernatremia can result in altered mental status. The most common symptoms include generalized muscle weakness, lethargy, confusion, and coma. As with hyponatremia, symptoms are dependent on the degree and rate of rise of serum sodium. Etiologies contributing to this disorder include diabetes insipidus, loop diuretics, gastrointestinal losses, and hypertonic sodium. Treatment consists of treating the underlying illness and correcting the hypertonicity. The latter is achieved by administration of hypotonic saline to lower the serum sodium concentration by 1 mEq/L per hour in acute hypernatremia and 0.5 mEq/L per hour in chronic hypernatremia (goal reduction of 10 mEq/L per day in chronic cases). A relatively slow correction helps to prevent cerebral edema and seizures.

Hypo- and hyperglycemia can also cause a state of altered mental status. In cases of hypoglycemia, symptoms may include confusion, tremulousness, coma, and seizures. The cause can be inappropriate insulin or oral hypoglycemic agent administration, insulinomas, liver failure, and infection. It is treated by administration of a dextrose load (usually one ampule of D50), which should result in resolution of clinical symptoms. Hyperglycemia can result in visual changes, lethargy, coma, and seizures and most commonly occurs as part of the clinical spectrum of diabetic ketoacidosis or nonketotic hyperglycemia. Treatment requires adequate fluid resuscitation, intravenous insulin therapy, correction of electrolyte derangements (particularly potassium), and treatment of the underlying cause.

The most common side effects of hypermagnesemia are the neurologic symptoms of obtundation, loss of deep tendon reflexes, and muscle paralysis. They are most frequently seen in patients with renal failure and women on high-dose magnesium infusions for eclampsia. In patients with compromised renal function, either hemodialysis or peritoneal dialysis must be initiated. In addition, when rapid reversal is required, calcium may be given intravenously as a magnesium antagonist. For women on magnesium infusions and with normal renal function, cessation usually results in a fairly rapid return to normal serum levels.

Finally, when assessing altered mentation the differential should always include hypoxia, acidosis and alkalosis. An arterial blood gas will indicate the degree of acidosis or alkalosis and can assist with determining whether its origin is respiratory, metabolic, or a mixed etiology. In the ICU setting, the most common etiologies are sepsis, uremia, hepatic failure, and electrolyte abnormalities. Treatment consists of correcting the underlying problem while providing supportive care for the acidosis or alkalosis.

SUGGESTED READINGS

Adrogué HJ, Madias NE. Hyponatremia. N Engl J Med. 2000;342:1581–1589.

Adrogué HJ, Madias NE. Primary care: hypernatremia. N Engl J Med. 2000;342:1493–1499.

Bolton CF, Young GB, eds. Baillere's Clinical Neurology. London: Balliere Tindall; 1996:577.

177

KEEP THE SERUM POTASSIUM AT HIGH OR NORMAL LEVELS WHEN ATTEMPTING TO CORRECT A METABOLIC ALKALOSIS

ERIC S. WEISS, MD

CASE

A 45-year-old attorney travels to the Caribbean islands for vacation. While away she develops profuse vomiting and diarrhea due to an unknown gastrointestinal (GI) pathogen. She is able to fly home but becomes profoundly dehydrated, unable to keep up with her GI fluid losses. On her second day back from the trip, her husband returns home from work to find her somnolent and minimally responsive with decreased respiratory effort. He immediately calls 911 and an ambulance arrives to transport her to her local emergency department (ED).

In the ED she is clearly dehydrated with dry mucous membranes and loss of her normal skin turgor. Her heart rate is 124 and her blood pressure is measured at 100/70 mm Hg. In addition, she appears somnolent and has a severely diminished respiratory drive, requiring endotracheal intubation for her severe hypoventilation. Her initial arterial blood gas shows a pH of 7.55 (normal 7.40 to 7.44), with a partial pressure of carbon dioxide (PCO_2) of 66 mm Hg (normal 40). Her arterial partial pressure of oxygen is normal at 95 mm Hg.

With concern for dehydration, the covering ED physician places a central venous catheter and begins intravenously administering fluids to replace volume loss. After a half hour of volume administration, the patient returns to stable vital signs and again begins to produce urine. However, the nurse is concerned because despite this improvement, the patient remains weak and lethargic, unable to follow commands. In addition, the cardiac monitor shows what the nurse believes to be an abnormal rhythm. The resident orders an electrocardiogram (ECG), which shows prominent U waves. A serum electrolyte panel is ordered, which reveals a potassium level of 1.7 mg/dL (nl 3.5 to 5.0 mg/dL). After aggressive potassium repletion, the patient once again begins following commands and regains her strength, able to tolerate eventual extubation. She is discharged home on hospital day number two.

DISCUSSION

Metabolic alkalosis is the most common acid–base abnormality seen in hospital inpatients. Severe alkalosis is an extremely serious problem as mortality rates can exceed 50%. Alkalosis can lead to diffuse arterial constriction with perfusion reduction. Thus, common signs of alkalosis include decreased mental status and seizures. In addition, severe alkalosis can cause hypoventilation, leading to hypoxemia. Finally, alkalosis can lead to life-threatening hypokalemia due to cellular shifts of potassium for hydrogen ions in an attempt to correct serum pH.

Metabolic alkalosis is defined as a pathologic increase in the serum bicarbonate (HCO_3-) concentration. This occurs either as a gain in bicarbonate or a loss of acid. Compensation occurs through action of the respiratory system, with hypoventilation to lead to retained CO_2 and increased acid. Typical blood gas values show a pH value around 7.50 with P_{CO_2} values around 60 mm Hg.

There are many causes of metabolic alkalosis. First is loss of hydrogen ions, leading to bicarbonate excess. Hydrogen losses occur commonly in the gastrointestinal tract. GI losses include vomiting and nasogastric suction. A second source of alkalosis occurs as a response to hypokalemia. In this setting, potassium will shift out of cells as compensation. Hydrogen ions shift intracellularly, leading to alkalosis. Finally, a third etiology of metabolic alkalosis is due to loss of bicarbonate-poor, chloride-rich extracellular fluid as can occur with dehydration in the setting of diuretic therapy. The lower fluid levels contain a relative excess in serum bicarbonate, leading to a "contraction alkalosis."

This patient developed a metabolic alkalosis due to a combination of GI losses from vomiting and diarrhea and also had contraction due to extracellular fluid losses. Her presentation was typical in the sense that she was somnolent and hypoventilated to compensate for her alkalosis. In the case described previously, there was failure to replete a low potassium level in the setting of metabolic alkalosis. Patients with metabolic alkalosis have intracellular shifting of potassium, which allows hydrogen ions to shift extracellularly to help correct pH. For this reason, patients with metabolic alkalosis can manifest severe hypokalemia. No potassium was checked until the patient developed ECG changes. The principal clinical manifestations of hypokalemia include lethargy and muscle weakness. In addition, U waves are often seen on ECG tracings. Hypokalemia by itself is unlikely to cause life-threatening arrhythmias. However, one must always be cognizant of other electrolyte abnormalities associated with hypokalemia, such as hypomagnesemia, which is known to cause serious arrhythmias. It is, however, important to be cautious with potassium repletion, as overaggressive repletion in the setting of alkalosis can lead to life-threatening hyperkalemia. This occurs when the alkalosis is corrected and intracellularly stored potassium returns to the extracellular compartment. This can be especially problematic in the setting of acute renal failure, which can occur in dehydrated patients. Thus, vigilance with cautious potassium repletion of potassium to normal to high normal levels is of paramount importance for patients with metabolic alkalosis.

SUGGESTED READINGS

Whittier WL, Rutecki GW. Primer on clinical acid-base problem solving. Dis Mon. 2004;50(3):122–162.

178

DO NOT REPLETE CALCIUM IN RHABDOMYOLYSIS UNLESS A PATIENT IS IN TETANY

ANTHONY D. SLONIM, MD, DRPH

Rhabdomyolysis is a condition that is associated with the destruction of skeletal muscle. There are a number of causes of rhabdomyolysis. These are classified as hereditary or nonhereditary. The hereditary causes of rhabdomyolysis usually involve the deficiency of a particular muscle enzyme (e.g., carnitine), which prevents the ability to generate adenosine triphosphate (ATP) by either fatty-acid oxidation or anaerobic glycolysis during exercise. These patients often have a family history of rhabdomyolysis or experience repeated bouts of rhabdomyolysis. The nonhereditary causes of rhabdomyolysis include trauma with large amounts of tissue damage (burns, crush injuries), sepsis, medications (statins, cocaine, amphetamines, anticonvulsants, serotonin, and protease inhibitors), electrolyte abnormalities (hypokalemia, hypophosphatemia), and sepsis.

The diagnosis of rhabdomyolysis usually begins with an appropriate clinical history that often includes excessive exercise associated with muscle pain and cramping. Associated symptoms are nonspecific and include nausea, weakness, and dehydration. The laboratory analysis is important in making the diagnosis. Usually, there is a metabolic acidosis, an elevated serum creatine kinase concentration >10,000 IU/L, hyperkalemia, hyperphosphatemia, and/or hypocalcemia. These abnormalities usually result from the breakdown products of the skeletal muscle. A clue to the diagnosis includes a urinalysis that will be positive for blood but will not demonstrate erythrocytes on the microscopic examination.

The treatment of rhabdomyolysis is focused on removing the offending agent and providing supportive care. One of the major consequences of rhabdomyolysis is acute renal failure and the treatment of the syndrome is directed at preventing this complication. Aggressive intravenous hydration is indicated to improve the solubility of the by-products, improve the dehydration, and improve urine flow. Alkalinization has been used to improve the solubility of myoglobin in the renal tubules and prevent the onset of acute renal failure. Sodium bicarbonate has been used intravenously to alkalinize the urine, but it contributes to the precipitation of calcium in ectopic locations and has not been shown to improve outcomes. This ectopic precipitation of calcium is a problem in rhabdomyolysis and increases with increasing muscle degradation. Hypocalcemia, although common in this condition, is generally not treated even when symptomatic (paresthesias, cramping, mood changes) unless severe (e.g., ionized hypocalcemia, evidence of tetany, convulsions, or hyperkalemia). This is because the serum albumin is also low and artificially reduces the serum calcium and the danger of ectopic calcium deposition is a common side effect, which may lead to hypercalcemia when the rhabdomyolysis is subsiding.

SUGGESTED READING

Vanholder R, Sever MS, Erek E, et al. Rhabdomyolysis J Am Soc Nephrol. 2000;11(8): 1553–1561.

179

CONSIDER EXCESS CHLORIDE AS A CAUSE OF AN UNEXPLAINED NON-ANION-GAP METABOLIC ACIDOSIS

ANTHONY D. SLONIM, MD, DrPH

Metabolic acidosis is traditionally classified into an elevated anion-gap metabolic acidosis or a non-anion-gap (hyperchloremic) metabolic acidosis. The importance of this classification is that it provides a differential diagnosis and guidance for priorities of treatment. The anion gap is the difference in charge between the sodium and the sum of the bicarbonate and chloride ($Na - [Cl + HCO_3]$). The normal anion gap ranges from 10 to 14. When the anion gap is elevated in a metabolic acidosis, the differential diagnosis is characterized by the mnemonic MUDPILES, which stands for methanol, uremia, diabetic ketoacidosis, paraldehyde, iron/isoniazid, lactic acidosis, ethanol/ethylene glycol, and salicylates.

A non-anion-gap metabolic acidosis is usually classified in three different ways. First, a renal tubular acidosis (RTA) must be considered and ruled out when a non-anion-gap metabolic acidosis presents itself. These disorders may be associated with either hypokalemia (proximal type II RTA) or hyperkalemia (type IV RTA). Second, a hyperchloremic metabolic acidosis may occur from the loss of fluids that are low in chloride. The most common fluids to consider are excessive stool output, drainage from pancreatic or ileostomy drains, and urinary diversions. Finally, a hyperchloremic metabolic acidosis may simply occur because of excessive administration of a chloride containing salt, such as sodium chloride, potassium chloride, or ammonium chloride. When hyperchloremia develops, the kidney exchanges bicarbonate to maintain electrical neutrality and the metabolic acidosis develops.

WHAT TO DO

In the administration of total parenteral nutrition (TPN), it is common to provide different elemental salts in the form of chloride salts. For example, sodium, potassium, and calcium are usually added to TPN complexed to a chloride ion. After 3 to 4 days of therapy, the chloride ion accumulates and the patient develops a hyperchloremic metabolic acidosis. One method of preventing this occurrence is to balance the addition of ions in TPN between chloride and acetate. This approach will both maintain the electrical and chemical neutrality and prevent the occurrence of the acidosis while giving the appropriate electrolyte constituents to the patient.

SUGGESTED READINGS

Gauthier PM, Szerlip HM. Metabolic acidosis in the intensive care unit. Crit Care Clin. 2002;18:289–308.

Rodriguez Soriano J. Renal tubular acidosis: the clinical entity. J Am Soc Nephrol. 2002;13:2160–2170.

180

CONSIDER HYPERCHLOREMIC METABOLIC ACIDOSIS TO BE A RENAL TUBULAR ACIDOSIS UNTIL PROVEN OTHERWISE IF OBVIOUS SOURCES OF BICARBONATE LOSSES LIKE DIARRHEA, URINARY DIVERSIONS, AND THE ADMINISTRATION OF CHLORIDE ARE NOT PRESENT

ANTHONY D. SLONIM, MD, DRPH

It is important to consider the diagnosis of renal tubular acidosis (RTA) when a non-anion-gap metabolic acidosis has a new onset. In RTA, bicarbonate is excreted through the kidneys and chloride ion is reabsorbed, leading to the two major serum characteristics of these syndromes: metabolic acidosis and hyperchloremia. These disorders may be associated with either hypokalemia (types I and II RTA) or hyperkalemia (type IV RTA). The other causes of a hyperchloremic metabolic acidosis include bicarbonate losses through the gastrointestinal tract (e.g., diarrhea or urinary diversions) and an excess administration of chloride, which may occur from excess chloride ion administration. The latter can occur secondary to the large-volume administration of normal saline during resuscitation from trauma or with treatment of diabetic ketoacidosis. In addition, the imbalance can occur with the excess use of chloride salts rather than acetate salts for critically ill patients receiving total parenteral nutrition.

WHAT TO DO

Type I RTA is described by a hypokalemic, hyperchloremic metabolic acidosis with a high urinary pH (>5.5). The defect results from a reduced number of distal nephron ion exchangers that result from a genetic defect, the presence of certain toxins or drugs, or diseases such as multiple myeloma, cystinosis, or systemic lupus. These patients are susceptible to urinary stones. The treatment is to provide alkali in a dose of 4 mmol/kg/day, which improves the acidosis and hypokalemia. Type 2 RTA is the type of RTA that is associated with proximal tubular dysfunction and is associated with Fanconi syndrome. The presenting symptoms include a hyperchloremic, metabolic acidosis with a low urine pH. The treatment includes alkali administration and attention to growth if the patient is a child. Type IV RTA is characterized by a hyperchloremic, metabolic acidosis with hyperkalemia and a urine pH of <5.5. These patients have a reduction in their ammonia excretion and bicarbonate production. It is common for these patients to have some degree of renal insufficiency and to have hypoaldosteronism (or aldosterone resistance). These patients are usually treated with mineralocorticoid and a loop diuretic, which corrects the aldosterone resistance, hyperkalemia, and acidosis.

SUGGESTED READINGS

Gauthier PM, Szerlip HM. Metabolic acidosis in the intensive care unit. Crit Care Clin. 2002;18:289–308.

Rodriguez Soriano J. Renal tubular acidosis: the clinical entity. J Am Soc Nephrol. 2002; 13:2160–2170.

181

BE ALERT FOR NEW-ONSET CAUDA EQUINA SYNDROME IN PATIENTS WITH SACRAL OR SPINAL FRACTURES OR SURGERY AND OBTAIN EMERGENT NEUROSURGICAL CONSULTATION IF SUSPECTED

MICHAEL J. DORSI, MD

Low back pain is the fifth most common reason for all physician visits and the second most commonly reported symptom. In most cases, low back pain signals a muscular disorder that can be managed conservatively. However, physicians should have heightened vigilance for low back pain combined with bowel and/or bladder incontinence, motor and/or sensory loss in the lower extremities, and saddle anesthesia, as this may represent a neurosurgical emergency termed cauda equina syndrome.

The cauda equina (from the Latin for "horse's tail") is the descriptive name for the lumbar nerve roots emanating from the distal tip of the spinal cord. The spinal cord terminates as the conus medullaris typically at the L1–L2 level. The lower lumbar and sacral nerve roots continue caudally in the cauda equina, exit their respective neural foramina, and ultimately provide motor and sensory innervation to the muscles and skin below the waist.

Cauda equina syndrome arises from compression of the lumbosacral nerve roots. Large herniated lumbar intervertebral discs are the most common culprit. Other sources of compression include spinal or sacral fractures or surgery common in ICU trauma patients, lumbosacral neoplasms, spinal stenosis, nonneoplastic masses such as cysts, peripheral neuropathy, and infectious processes.

SIGNS AND SYMPTOMS

Cauda equina syndrome most often can be diagnosed clinically. Compression of the lumbar and S1 nerve roots results in sensory and/or motor deficits in the lower extremities. Strength and sensation should be carefully tested in a dermatomal pattern. The patellar (L3 and L4) and Achilles (S1) deep tendon reflexes should be tested and may be decreased. The sacral nerve roots supply motor innervation to the urethral and anal sphincters, sensation to the perineum, and in a "bull's-eye" pattern to the skin surrounding the anus. Thus, decreased resting and/or volitional rectal tone are a clinical sign of sacral nerve root compression, as is numbness in the perineum. Anal sphincter reflexes may be tested by stretching the phallus (bulbocavernosus reflex) or by pinprick to the skin surrounding the anus (anal wink reflex).

Emergent imaging should be obtained in all patients presenting with suspected cauda equina syndrome. Magnetic resonance imaging (MRI) has emerged as the imaging modality of choice. Computed tomography myelography is indicated for patients with a contraindication to MRI or those with spinal instrumentation. In addition, neurosurgical consultation should be sought immediately in all cases of cauda equina syndrome. Surgical intervention aims to decompress the affected lumbosacral nerve roots within 48 hours of presentation. The approach and extent of surgery depends on the nature and location of the compressing lesion. Instrumented fusion is indicated when there is evidence of spinal instability.

SUGGESTED READINGS

Greenberg MS, ed. Handbook of Neurosurgery. New York: Thieme; 2005:298–299.
Staats P, ed. Pain: Just the Facts. Philadelphia: Lippincott Williams & Wilkins; 2004:141–146.

182

KEEP PATIENTS WITH DURAL TEARS FLAT FOR 24–48 HOURS

JAYME E. LOCKE, MD

Dural tear is a known complication of spinal surgeries, such as laminectomies, spinal fusions, and disc excisions. It most commonly occurs in the lumbar region. In general, the tear is noted at the time of operation when leakage of cerebrospinal fluid (CSF) is noted by the surgeon. A tear in the dura results in decompression of the thecal sac and reduction of local pressure on the epidural veins, allowing CSF to leak in to the operative site. Dural tears that are not noted at the time of surgery often present in the postoperative period. Patients manifest severe headaches that are exacerbated by upright posture. In addition, CSF can be seen leaking from the wound, or a subcutaneous collection may be noted. Confirmation that the fluid is CSF can be gained by testing the fluid for beta-2 transferrin.

WHAT TO DO

Whether the dural tear is noted intraoperatively or stigmata of a dural tear are noted postoperatively (e.g., headache, labile vital signs postoperatively, fluid collection), repair of the dural tear must be considered. Otherwise, the patient is at risk for the development of pseudomeningocele and meningitis. Once the condition is identified, the patient should be kept flat to minimize symptoms. The goal of the repair is to achieve a watertight closure. The tear should be repaired using 4-0 or 6-0 dural suture with a tapered or reverse cutting needle. The closure can be accomplished with simple interrupted or running locking suture technique. If the tear is too large for primary repair, then a free graft or fascial graft can be used to repair the tear. The repair should be tested by placing the patient in reverse Trendelenburg position or via a Valsalva maneuver. If the leakage of CSF persists, then the repair can be augmented with fibrin glue, additional suture, gelatin sponge, or autologous fat. Once complete, the paraspinous muscles and the fascia should be closed in two layers. The fascial layer is responsible for preventing durocutaneous fistulae. A drain should not be left behind, as the negative pressure created may encourage a persistent leak. After repair, all patients should remain on bed rest in the supine position for 24 to 48 hours.

SUGGESTED READINGS

Browner B, ed. Skeletal Trauma: Basic Science, Management, and Reconstruction. 3rd ed. Philadelphia: WB Saunders; 2003:937,1026–1027.

Canale ST, ed. Campbell's Operative Orthopaedics. 10th ed. Philadelphia: Mosby; 2003:2011–2012.

183

KNOW THE STATUS OF CERVICAL, THORACIC, AND LUMBAR SPINE STABILITY ON ALL POSTOPERATIVE AND TRAUMA PATIENTS

RACHEL BLUEBOND-LANGNER, MD

When a patient returns from the operating room following spinal surgery it is important to establish with the surgical team the stability of the spine as well as the integrity of the dura. This information is critical should the patient need to be reintubated, vomit, or elevate the head of bed. There would be no greater catastrophe than for a caregiver to cause a spinal cord injury by incorrectly manipulating a patient who has an unstable spine, particularly the cervical spine (*Fig. 183.1*).

In the patient with an unstable cervical spine requiring reintubation there are three options: direct laryngoscopy with in-line immobilization; fiberoptic intubation; or an emergent surgical airway. Direct laryngoscopy with in-line stabilization (avoiding traction on the spine) is unquestionably challenging for the uninitiated but should be attempted first. Fiberoptic intubation provides a more optimal view of the airway but requires that the equipment be readily available and that the patient is relatively stable and noncombative. Emergency surgical airway should be reserved for circumstances in which oral intubation has failed. It should be stressed that a patient does not need to be intubated to be ventilated. If the bedside provider has knowledge of an unstable cervical spine and can adequately oxygenate a patient with a bag valve mask, it may be prudent to do so while obtaining the services of an experienced airway professional that may be more adept at the procedures listed earlier.

In the patient who vomits and must lie flat, most commonly due to lumbar spine instability or a dural tear, the patient should be log rolled to protect the airway. While not uniformly agreed upon, bed rest following durotomy is thought to decrease any potential cerebrospinal fluid (CSF) leak, allow the dural tears to seal, and reduce symptoms (e.g., nausea, vomiting, dizziness). It is incumbent on the ICU provider to consider this bed-rest protocol and if instituted, start appropriate thromboembolic (deep vein thrombosis/pulmonary embolism) prophylaxis measures if the query regarding the presence of a dural tear is affirmative.

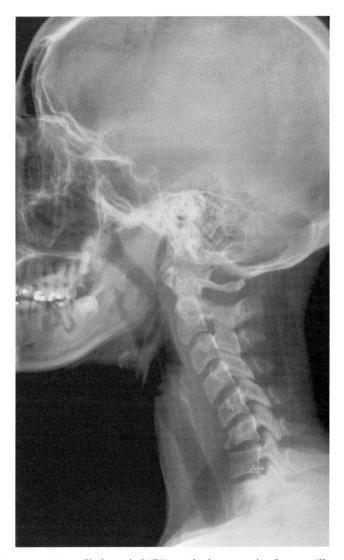

FIGURE 183.1. Sixth cervical (C6) vertebral compression fracture. (Courtesy of Robert Hendrickson, MD; reused with permission from Badawy M. Cervical vertebral compression wedge fracture. In: Greenberg MI. Greenberg's Text-Atlas of Emergency Medicine. Philadelphia: Lippincott Williams & Wilkins; 2005:629.)

SELECTED READINGS

Ghafoor AU, Martin TW, Gopalakrishnan S, et al. Caring for the patients with cervical spine injuries: what have we learned? J Clin Anesth. 2005;17:640–649.

Hodges SD, Humphreys SC, Eck JC, et al. Management of incidental durotomy without mandatory bed rest. Spine. 1999;24(19):2062–2064.

184

APPLY APPROPRIATE DEEP VEIN THROMBOSIS PROPHYLAXIS TO PATIENTS WITH SPINAL CORD INJURY

JOSE I. SUAREZ, MD

Acute spinal cord injury (SCI) is common with an estimated 8,000 to 10,000 new cases in the United States each year. The mean age of presentation is 31 years and the majority of patients are male. SCI is associated with significant long-term disability and mortality.

ETIOLOGY

SCI has traditionally been classified as traumatic and nontraumatic. Traumatic SCI is usually due to motor vehicle collisions (MVCs) (MVAs) (20% to 25%), motorcycle collisions (MCCs) (25% to 30%), or falls (20% to 25%). The most common locations for traumatic SCI are the cervical spine (50% to 55%), followed by the thoracolumbar region (15% to 20%), thoracic spine (10% to 15%), and the lumbosacral region (10%).

Nontraumatic causes of SCI are numerous. Such conditions include: various bacterial (including spinal epidural abscesses), viral, fungal, or parasitic infections; neoplastic lesions (usually extramedullary primary or metastatic tumors); vascular events (infarctions or hemorrhages from vascular malformations); demyelinating lesions such as multiple sclerosis; toxins; autoimmune disorders; and nutritional abnormalities such as vitamin B_{12} deficiency.

CLINICAL PRESENTATION

Neurologic damage and the ensuing clinical manifestations will depend on the extent and level of the SCI. Physical examination usually reveals muscle weakness and a sensory level below the level of the lesion in complete lesions. In those patients with incomplete SCI there is some preservation of motor and sensory functions below the level of compromise. Initially patients with SCI will present with atonia and arreflexia below the level of the lesion (spinal shock) and within a few days or weeks will experience spasticity and hyperreflexia.

VENOUS THROMBOEMBOLISM IN SCI

Patients with SCI who do not receive prophylactic treatment have the highest incidence of deep venous thrombosis (DVT) and pulmonary embolism (PE) among all patients. Asymptomatic DVT has been found in 60% to 100% of SCI patients and PE represents the third leading cause of death. Additional risk factors for DVT in SCI patients include age, concomitant lower limb fracture, and delayed initiation of prophylactic treatment. It has been shown that SCI patients are at greatest risk of DVT and PE during the acute care phase. However, the risk is still present during the rehabilitation period. The incidence of new DVT may be as high as 30% between 2 to 6 weeks following SCI.

THROMBOPROPHYLAXIS AFTER SCI

Six randomized studies (albeit small) have shown that the use of low-dose unfractionated heparin (LDUH) alone or sequential compression devices alone are not sufficient as thromboprophylaxis. However, adjusted-dose unfractionated heparin and low-molecular-weight heparin (LMWH) have been found to be more efficacious. This finding has also been reported in SCI patients undergoing rehabilitation (uncontrolled studies). There is also evidence that oral anticoagulants such as warfarin are also effective thromboprophylactic treatments when initiated shortly after SCI. It is important to note that thromboprophylaxis should be initiated once practitioners feel secure about having achieved effective hemostasis after SCI.

Routine insertion of inferior vena cava filters (IVCFs) in SCI patients is still controversial. There is strong evidence that when appropriate thromboprophylaxis is given IVCFs are not necessary. Even though IVCFs may theoretically reduce the incidence of PE, they are associated with complications and higher costs. Patients who have been shown to benefit from IVCF insertion include those with concomitant long bone fractures, DVT formation despite thromboprophylaxis, and those with contraindications to anticoagulation.

The current recommendations for thromboprophylaxis after SCI include the following:

1) Thromboprophylaxis for all patients with acute SCI.
2) Single prophylaxis modalities (i.e., low-dose unfractionated heparin, graduated compression stockings, or sequential compression devices alone) should be avoided.

3) Thromboprophylaxis with LMWH is the preferred treatment once primary hemostasis from the injury is obtained. Alternatives to LMWH include the combined use of sequential compression devices and either low-dose unfractionated heparin or LMWH.

4) When anticoagulation is contraindicated early in SCI, sequential compression devices and/or graduated compression stockings should be used with consideration of an IVCF.

5) During the rehabilitation phase, SCI patients should be treated with LMWH or converted to oral warfarin (international normalized ratio range 2.0 to 3.0).

6) The insertion of IVCFs as primary prophylaxis is not recommended.

SUGGESTED READINGS

Geerts WH, Pineo GF, Heit JA, et al. Prevention of thromboembolism: the seventh ACCP conference on antithrombotic and thrombolytic therapy. Chest. 2004;126:338–400.

Maxwell RA, Chavarria-Aguilar M, Cockerham WT, et al. Routine prophylactic vena cava filtration is not indicated after acute spinal cord injury. J Trauma. 2002;52:902–906.

185

BE ALERT FOR AUTONOMIC DYSREFLEXIA IN INTENSIVE CARE UNIT PATIENTS WITH A SPINAL CORD INJURY

JOSE I. SUAREZ, MD

Autonomic dysreflexia is an acute syndrome that frequently occurs in spinal cord injury (SCI) patients with a level usually above T6. It is characterized by excessive unmodulated sympathetic outflow in response to noxious stimuli below the spinal cord level. This can lead to dangerous elevations of blood pressure with disastrous clinical sequelae.

PATHOPHYSIOLOGY

In both normal and SCI patients, noxious stimulation of peripheral sensory receptors (i.e., bladder distention) will activate afferent pathways to produce a sympathetic response. The sympathetic outflow stimulates peripheral vasoconstriction, thus elevating arterial blood pressure. Arterial vessel baroreceptors are then activated and signal brain-stem inhibitory pathways that descend the spinal cord to limit the sympathetic outflow and prevent excessive arterial vasoconstriction. The brain-stem inhibitory centers increase vagal stimulation to the heart, resulting in bradycardia. In SCI patients, vagal output to the heart still occurs; however, brain-stem inhibitory descending pathways that limit sympathetic outflow are blocked in the spinal cord at the level of the spinal cord lesion. This results in excessive vasoconstriction and markedly elevated blood pressure (*Fig. 185.1*).

SIGNS AND SYMPTOMS

The main clinical signs and symptoms of autonomic dysreflexia are related to both the excessive sympathetic output below the spinal cord level and from compensatory parasympathetic output originating from above the spinal cord level. Profound hypertension occurs because of excessive peripheral vasoconstriction, and the skin will appear cool and clammy below the spinal cord level. Above the spinal cord level, parasympathetic output may result in vasodilatation of blood vessels, resulting in a pounding headache, skin flushing, sweating, and nasal congestion. Other symptoms the patient may report include visual spots, blurry vision, and anxiety. The elevated blood pressure may lead to a host of clinical sequelae, including intracranial

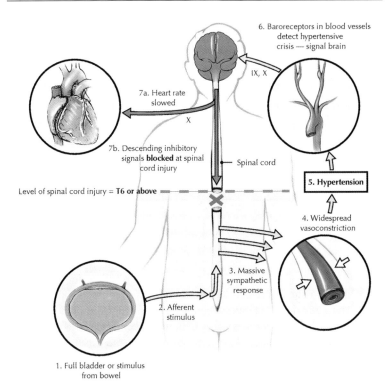

6. Baroreceptors in blood vessels
detect hypertensive
crisis — signal brain

IX, X

7a. Heart rate
slowed

X

7b. Descending inhibitory
signals **blocked** at spinal
cord injury

Spinal cord

5. Hypertension

Level of spinal cord injury = **T6 or above**

4. Widespread
vasoconstriction

3. Massive
sympathetic
response

2. Afferent
stimulus

1. Full bladder or stimulus
from bowel

FIGURE 185.1. In both normal and spinal-cord-injury patients, noxious stimulation of peripheral sensory receptors (i.e., bladder distention) will activate afferent pathways to produce a sympathetic response. From Blackmer J. Rehabilitation medicine: 1. Autonomic dysreflexia. CMAJ. 2003;169(9):931–935.

hemorrhage, seizures, hypertensive encephalopathy, cerebral edema, atrial fibrillation, pulmonary edema, renal failure, coma, and death.

PRECIPITATING FACTORS

Multiple stimuli may trigger autonomic dysreflexia. The general categories include bladder and urinary tract, gastrointestinal, dermatological, skeletal, reproductive, and hematological sources. The most common specific triggers for autonomic dysreflexia are thought to be from bladder distension and fecal impaction (*Table 185.1*).

MANAGEMENT

Immediate assessment of blood pressure should be made in patients with symptoms of autonomic dysreflexia. Normal blood pressure in

TABLE 185.1	PRECIPITATING FACTORS FOR AUTONOMIC DYSREFLEXIA
SYSTEM	**PRECIPITATING FACTORS**
Urinary tract	Bladder distention, infection, urethral distension, instrumentation, catheter traction
Gastrointestinal tract	Fecal impaction, constipation, instrumentation, infection, ulceration
Skin	Pressure sore, ingrown toenail
Skeletal	Heterotopic ossification, fracture, joint dislocation
Reproductive	Labor and delivery, menstruation, testicular torsion
Hematological	Deep vein thrombosis, pulmonary embolism
Medications	Nasal decongestants, sympathomimetics

quadriplegic patients is about 90 to 110 mm Hg systolic in the sitting position. Generally, a blood pressure above 150 mm Hg in adults warrants pharmacologic treatment. The patient should be moved to the upright position and legs lowered to allow for pooling of blood in the lower extremities, which may reduce blood pressure. Any constrictive clothing should be loosened. The blood pressure should be checked every few minutes. Pharmacologic treatment of blood pressure should be done by using rapid-onset short-acting agents. Immediate-release nifedipine 10-mg capsule is a preferred agent. This should be taken by a "bite-and-swallow" method to facilitate absorption. However, sublingual nifedipine is not advisable. Other medications that can be used include nitropaste, nitroglycerin, hydralazine, and sodium nitroprusside.

While blood pressure is being stabilized, a prompt search for the precipitating cause of autonomic dysreflexia should be made. Since bladder distension is thought to be the most common trigger, a trial of bladder catheterization should be done if no indwelling catheter is already present. A solution of 2% lidocaine jelly should be instilled into the urethra before this is done. If the patient already has an indwelling catheter, it should be checked for obstructions along the entire length. If blocked, the catheter should be irrigated with normal saline. If no problems are found with the bladder, a rectal exam and abdominal radiograph must be performed. If fecal impaction is ruled out, a systematic search for the causes listed previously must be undertaken.

SUGGESTED READINGS

Acute management of autonomic dysreflexia: individuals with spinal cord injury presenting to health-care facilities. J Spinal Cord Med. 2002;25(Suppl 1):S67–S88.
Blackmer J. Rehabilitation medicine: 1. Autonomic dysreflexia. CMAJ. 2003;169(9): 931–935.

186

CONSIDER THE USE OF STEROIDS FOR NEUROLOGICAL TRAUMA IN BLUNT SPINAL CORD INJURY ONLY

JACOB T. GUTSCHE, MD
PATRICK K. KIM, MD

Corticosteroids have been studied for decades as a treatment of traumatic central nervous system injury. The proposed mechanism of benefit is the reduction of inflammation and edema, leading to decreased ischemic injury and neuronal apoptosis. High-dose methylprednisolone was widely adopted as the standard of care for patients with blunt spinal cord injury following the publication of the National Acute Spinal Cord Injury Studies (NASCIS) II and III. These studies suggested that steroid treatment results in slight improvement in motor function at long-term follow-up. Subsequent clinical studies and critical reviews have challenged the validity of the results of the NASCIS II study. Despite its wide adoption, steroid therapy for spinal cord injury is still controversial.

Methylprednisolone (Solu-Medrol) is the steroid of choice based on NASCIS. Large doses are required, starting with a bolus intravenous infusion of 30 mg/kg of body weight over 15 minutes followed by an infusion of 5.4 mg/kg per hour. If steroid treatment begins within 3 hours of injury, the duration of the infusion is 23 hours. If steroid treatment begins between 3 and 8 hours after injury, the duration of infusion is 47 hours. If the 8-hour window is missed, steroids should not be given. The use of steroids in blunt spinal cord injury should not be extrapolated to patients with penetrating spinal cord injury (e.g., gunshot wounds, stabs). Studies have shown no improvement in neurological outcome in penetrating injury and should not be used in this patient population.

The use of steroids in acute traumatic brain injury (TBI) has also been a source of debate and has been even more extensively studied. A 1997 systematic review suggested that steroids may reduce mortality after TBI. However, the data from a 10,000-patient, multicenter, randomized, placebo-controlled trial proved the opposite. The Corticosteroid Randomisation after Significant Head Injury (CRASH) study proved a statistically significant increase in the risk of death for patients randomized to receive corticosteroids. The study was stopped early because of more deaths at 2 weeks in the steroid group. Final analysis of 6-month follow-up confirmed the higher mortality in patients treated with steroids.

It must be remembered that steroids can have severe side effects on various organ systems. These include higher rates of infection, gastrointestinal bleeding, and pancreatitis. Patients treated with steroids also have delayed wound healing and difficulty with blood sugar control. Consideration must be given to these risks, and steroids should be given only when their proven benefit outweighs these significant risks. Steroids may be considered for blunt spinal cord injury, although the data are not as persuasive as once thought. However, the data are quite convincing that steroids should *not* be used for penetrating spinal cord injury or in patients with traumatic brain injury.

SUGGESTED READINGS

Bracken MB, Shepard MJ, Collins WF, et al. A randomized, controlled trial of methylprednisolone or naloxone in the treatment of acute spinal-cord injury. Results of the Second National Acute Spinal Cord Injury Study. N Engl J Med. 1990;322(20):1405–1411.

Bracken MB, Shepard MJ, Holford TR, et al. Administration of methylprednisolone for 24 or 48 hours or tirilazad mesylate for 48 hours in the treatment of acute spinal cord injury. Results of the Third National Acute Spinal Cord Injury Randomized Controlled Trial. National Acute Spinal Cord Injury Study. JAMA. 1997;277(20):1597–1604.

Coleman WP, Benzel D, Cahill DW, et al. A critical appraisal of the reporting of the National Acute Spinal Cord Injury Studies (II and III) of methylprednisolone in acute spinal cord injury. J Spinal Disord. 2000;13(3):185–199.

Edwards P, Arango M, Balica L, et al. CRASH trial collaborators. Final results of MRC CRASH, a randomised placebo-controlled trial of intravenous corticosteroid in adults with head injury-outcomes at 6 months. Lancet. 2005;365(9475):1957–1959.

Heary RF, Vaccaro AR, Mesa JJ, et al. Steroids and gunshot wounds to the spine. Neurosurgery. 1997;41(3):576–583;discussion 583–584.

187

Start an Early Bowel Regimen in Patients After Spinal Cord Injury

Jose I. Suarez, MD

Acute spinal cord injury (SCI) is a devastating problem resulting in more than 10,000 permanently disabled patients in the United States each year. The vast majority of traumatic SCIs occur in otherwise healthy young adults between 16 and 30 years of age with a long life expectancy. Because of that SCI is associated with a significant burden on health care resources.

Gastrointestinal Consequences of SCI

SCI is associated with common gastrointestinal abnormalities including gastroesophageal reflux (GERD); delayed gastric emptying time; altered colonic motility with increased transit time; severe constipation; prolonged bowel evacuation time; abdominal distention; and hemorrhoids. Such alterations will become evident in isolation or in combination depending on the extent and level of the SCI. GERD and delayed gastric emptying time are more commonly seen in tetraplegic patients. Ileus can be seen a few days after SCI and typically in patients with complete lesions. Patients with lesions above T12 will have a spastic anal sphincter, thus retaining reflex bowel emptying. However, patients with lesions below T12 will have a flaccid anal sphincter with accompanying loss of both reflexive and voluntary reflex bowel emptying.

Management of Gastrointestinal Complications of SCI

All SCI patients should receive adequate peptic ulcer prophylaxis and a bowel care regimen from admission (*Table 187.1*). Gastrointestinal care starts with adequate fluid administration and dietary intake. Fluids are very important for stool consistency. It has been recommended that SCI patients should receive at least 2 to 3 liters of fluids daily. A diet high in fiber (at least 15 g/day) may be beneficial to increase stool bulk.

If adequate dietary management does not improve bowel function, then pharmacologic treatments should be instituted. Agents that have been used include stool softeners such as docusate; stool bulk formers such as calcium polycarbophil, methylcellulose, psyllium, or

TABLE 187.1	GASTROINTESTINAL MANIFESTATIONS AFTER SCI AND SOME TREATMENT RECOMMENDATIONS
CONDITION	RECOMMENDED MANAGEMENT
Gastroesophageal reflux	Head elevation, motility, or prokinetic agents
Peptic ulcer	Prophylaxis with H2-blockers or proton pump inhibitors
Ileus	Bowel rest, correct electrolytes (serum potassium >4 mEq/dL, consider total parenteral nutrition
Bowel obstruction	Bowel rest, correct electrolytes, decompression with nasogastric tube decompression. If medical management does not work, then consider surgery
Fecal impaction	Bowel care program, scheduled laxative

lactulose; stimulants of peristalsis and prokinetic agents such as senna; and contact irritants such as bisacodyl or glycerin suppositories. Such programs should be consistent but individualized depending upon the SCI severity, level of injury, patient's lifestyle, and plans to return to work. During the acute phase of spinal shock the rectum is usually flaccid. Therefore patients may require manual removal of stool from the rectum daily. Patients with cervical or thoracic spine lesions may retain their reflexive bowel responses. Such patients can be managed with digital stimulation of the rectum, which results in reflexive bowel emptying. Patients with incomplete SCI may not require any specific treatment beyond the dietary recommendations

SUGGESTED READINGS

Chen D, Nussbaum SB. The gastrointestinal system and bowel management following spinal cord injury. Phys Med Rehab Clin North Am. 2000;11:45–56.

Derwenskus J, Zaidat OO. Spinal cord injury and related disorders. In Suarez JI, ed. Critical Care Neurology and Neurosurgery. Totowa, NJ: Humana Press; 2004:417–432.

188

CONSIDER MODERATE HYPOTHERMIA AFTER CARDIAC ARREST

BRADFORD D. WINTERS, MD, PhD

Moderate hypothermia has been demonstrated to improve neurologic outcome and mortality in patients who remain comatose despite return of spontaneous circulation (ROSC) after ventricular fibrillation (VF) or pulseless ventricular tachycardia (VT)–induced cardiac arrest. This type of event leads to global cerebral ischemia with the potential for severe anoxic or hypoxic brain injury and progression to brain death. The patient populations studied in the original trials, which demonstrated this benefit, were those who had out-of-hospital events and as such there has been considerable debate as to whether this treatment would be useful for in-hospital cardiac arrests. In-hospital cardiac arrests are often secondary to long-developing deteriorations and are often the end result of a terminal illness. This is in contrast to out-of-hospital arrests, which are usually secondary to an acute coronary event. While the data are imperfect, there is some suggestion that inpatients with witnessed arrests from VF and VT may also benefit from this treatment.

The time between the witnessed arrest and ROSC is important. ROSC may not occur promptly and there is an outer limit that should obviate initiating hypothermia. The time limit adhered to for the out-of-hospital arrests was 60 minutes from time of collapse. Most in-hospital resuscitations do not continue this long and it is unclear what the outer limit for ROSC should be for initiating of cooling for in-hospital arrests.

The earlier the cooling is initiated after return of spontaneous circulation, the better. One of the out-of-hospital studies initiated cooling in the field. The target temperature should be between 32° and 34° Celsius core temperature (based on a bladder pressure pulmonary artery catheter or other "core" temperature measurement). It is desirable to achieve the target temperature within a 2-hour time frame. How long to maintain the hypothermia is unclear. One of the two studies maintained it for 12 hours and the other for 24 hours and both showed improved outcome. Many would advocate that unless there is a contraindication to maintaining the hypothermia for 24 hours, this would be the preferred time. After this point the patient is actively rewarmed to normothermia (37° C).

During the period of hypothermia, very close attention to a wide variety of parameters needs to be maintained. Electrolytes need to be checked frequently and volume needs to be appropriately resuscitated since hypothermia can induce diuresis and electrolyte abnormalities. Shivering must be controlled, usually with sedatives and/or paralytics, as it increases myocardial oxygen demand dramatically. Cardiac dysrhythmias may occur secondary to the hypothermia as well as a result of the original cardiac insult. Some protocols use prophylactic lidocaine infusion to control this. Coagulopathy may occur, though this is generally not a problem until well below the target temperature range. Nevertheless, the prothrombin time/partial thromboplastin time should be monitored frequently. Severe vasoconstriction occurs as a result of the hypothermia and this may place additional work on the heart in terms of increased afterload. It is prudent to place a pulmonary artery catheter to monitor cardiac performance as well as volume status during the treatment and for a period of time after rewarming.

Once the patient is rewarmed, the primary issue is neurologic assessment including frequent neurologic exams, head computed tomography scan, magnetic resonance imaging, and possibly other tests such as evoked potentials to assist in prognostication for neurologic recovery. Assessment and treatment of underlying causes of the original event also need to be performed in parallel.

SUGGESTED READINGS

Bernard SA, Gray TW, Buist MD, et al. Treatment of comatose survivors of out-of-hospital cardiac arrests with induced hypothermia. N Engl J Med. 2002;346:557–563.

The Hypothermia after Cardiac Arrest Study Group. Mild therapeutic hypothermia to improve the neurologic outcome after cardiac arrest. N Engl J Med. 2002;346:549–556.

189

BE VIGILANT FOR BLUNT CEREBROVASCULAR INJURY AFTER TRAUMA

MICHAEL D. GROSSMAN, MD

Understanding of the spectrum of blunt cerebrovascular injury has changed markedly during the past decade. In the past, these injuries were likely to be detected only after development of focal neurologic signs in patients with normal computed tomography (CT) scans of the head. Improved access to diagnostic technology and improved survival of the most severely injured trauma patients have focused attention upon earlier diagnosis and treatment of this condition.

Estimation of incidence is difficult and dependent upon specification of the population that should undergo screening, the method used to screen, sensitivity of the test, and clear agreement as to what findings constitute an injury. Published figures range between 0.1% to more than 1.0%. Incidence seems to rise as efforts at screening are intensified, suggesting the true incidence probably exceeds 1%; however, many injuries are "minimal" and their clinical consequences indeterminate.

WATCH OUT FOR

Blunt cerebrovascular injury may be caused by a variety of injury mechanisms. Relatively minor injury mechanisms may produce significant injury. Examples include hyperflexion or extension injuries of the neck producing vertebral artery occlusion and subsequent embolization into the posterior cerebral circulation. For the purposes of screening large populations of trauma patients, potential for blunt cerebrovascular injury is most often associated with severe closed head injury, cervical spine fracture (especially if the vertebral foramina are affected), skull base fractures, severe midface fractures, and presence of a "seat-belt sign" across the base of the neck. Cranial nerve findings associated with blunt force trauma to the head or neck are also suggestive of proximity to carotid and vertebral arteries.

Blunt cerebrovascular injury may affect the major trunks of the carotid or vertebral arterial systems either in the neck or skull base. Anatomic injury includes laceration or transaction with bleeding, laceration or transaction with thrombosis, development of intimal flaps, dissections, pseudoaneurysms, and arteriovenous fistulas. Occurrence of stroke or cerebrovascular accident, the most feared pathophysiologic consequences of blunt cerebrovascular injury, depends upon the presence or absence of thrombosis, embolic phenomenon, and collateral flow. Decisions regarding anticipated risks and benefits of therapy should take these factors into consideration.

WHAT TO DO The gold standard for identification of blunt cerebrovascular injury is conventional four-vessel cerebral angiography. However, because this test is invasive and resource intensive, widespread screening of populations at risk has been infrequent. Recent attention has turned to the use of magnetic resonance imaging/arteriography (MRI, MRA) and CT angiography for screening purposes. Comparison of CT angiography to angiography has been favorable in recent publications provided high-speed, multidetector devices are used ("high speed" or "light speed" scanners). CT angiography has good sensitivity and excellent specificity for carotid injuries; sensitivity for vertebral arteries may not be as good. Sixteen-slice scanners appear to provide better sensitivity for vertebral injuries. Current literature supports using CT angiography to screen for blunt cerebrovascular injury followed by angiography to establish the anatomic diagnosis.

MRI, MRA can detect vascular injury with excellent sensitivity and specificity and can identify end-organ effects of embolization or thrombosis if these have occurred. Even in the absence of identified vascular injury on CT angiography, the presence of cerebral infarction on MRI might indicate the need for treatment or at the very least more aggressive diagnostic workup using angiography. CT angiography has no utility in detection of end-organ effects of injury. MRI/A is more cumbersome to obtain than CT angiography but would seem to have greater overall utility particularly if clinical suspicion is very high.

Treatment depends upon the injury identified. While thrombosis might warrant anticoagulation, associated injuries or conditions might preclude it. There is no clear consensus on whether heparin, warfarin, or antiplatelet agents are the best therapy. Certain findings (including bleeding, pseudoaneurysm, and dissection) might warrant interventional neuroradiology procedures.

SUGGESTED READINGS

Biffl WL, Egglin T, Benedetto B, et al. Sixteen slice computed tomographic angiography is a reliable noninvasive screening test for clinically significant blunt cerebrovascular injuries. J Trauma. 2006;60(4):745–751.

Biffl WL, Ray CE, Moore EE, et al. Non-invasive diagnosis of blunt cerebrovascular injuries: a preliminary report. J Trauma. 2002;850–856.

Bub L, Hollingsworth W, Jarvik JG, et al. Screening for blunt cerebrovascular injury: evaluating the efficacy of multidetector computed tomographic angiography.
J Trauma. 2005;59:697.

Mayberry JC, Brown CV, Mullins RJ, et al. Blunt carotid artery injury: the futility of
screening and diagnosis. Arch Surg. 2004;139:609–613.

190

HAVE AN EXTREMELY HIGH THRESHOLD IN GIVING ANTIHYPERTENSIVES IN HEAD TRAUMA

M. CRAIG BARRETT, PHARMD
RONALD F. SING, DO

Blood pressure control in the intensive care unit (ICU) can result in controversial and difficult management decisions because of the paucity of data. This seems especially apparent in patients with traumatic brain injury (TBI). Hypertension can be the body's natural response to TBI in an attempt to autoregulate cerebral blood flow as the body may require an elevated blood pressure to maintain adequate cerebral blood flow. Hypertension after TBI may also be the result of a nonspecific reflex pressor response or triggers of a catecholamine response, such as pain and agitation.

Once the primary trauma to the brain has occurred, minimizing secondary insults is the primary objective to achieve maximal neurologic recovery. Avoiding hypotension (systolic blood pressure <90 mm Hg) and hypoxia (oxygen saturation <90% or PaO_2 <60 mm Hg) in TBI patients is essential to prevent cerebral ischemia, since both independently predict a worse outcome. The Brain Trauma Foundation recommends the mean arterial blood pressure (MAP) be maintained above 90 mm Hg in an attempt to maintain a cerebral perfusion pressure (CPP) greater than 70 mm Hg.

WHAT TO DO

In the event that the MAP is excessively elevated beyond that required to maintain an adequate CPP, sedation and analgesia should be optimized prior to consideration of antihypertensive administration. No antihypertensive therapy should be instituted without consultation with a senior member of the treatment team. In the very unlikely event that blood pressure reduction is warranted, the most desirable agent would have a smooth dose-response relationship providing a predictable and controllable onset. The drug would also be a short-acting, titratable infusion to allow the specific blood pressure targets to be achieved while avoiding hypotension. Additionally, the drug would have few adverse effects and would not cause intracranial pressure (ICP) elevation.

Esmolol is an acceptable choice as it is a short-acting beta-receptor antagonist administered as a constant infusion with few adverse effects. Labetalol, a beta-receptor antagonist with alpha-blocking activity, can also be used and is administered as a constant infusion or can be administered intermittently for acute elevations. Either agent is preferred in patients with baseline tachycardia. Nicardipine, a calcium-channel blocker, works exclusively as a peripheral vasodilator. Administered as a constant infusion, its smooth dose-response relationship is preferable in patients with bradycardia, heart failure, bronchospasm, or chronic obstructive pulmonary disease. These agents have no direct effect on ICP or cerebrovascular blood volume, making them acceptable treatment options.

WHAT NOT TO DO

Sodium nitroprusside should be avoided in TBI patients since it can cause ICP elevations secondary to dilatation of cerebral vasculature. Its potent effects and lack of smooth dose-response relationship can result in hypotension during infusion and rebound hypertension after discontinuation of the agent. In addition, its use puts patients at risk for its severe potential side effect of cyanide or thiocyanate toxicity with prolonged use, high doses, or in patients with liver or renal dysfunction.

SUGGESTED READINGS

Brain Trauma Foundation. Guidelines. http://www2.braintrauma.org/guidelines

Chobanian AV, Bakris GL, Black HR, et al. National Heart, Lung, and Blood Institute Joint National Committee on Prevention, Detection, Evaluation, and Treatment of High Blood Pressure; National High Blood Pressure Education Program Coordinating Committee. The seventh report of the Joint National Committee on Prevention, Detection, Evaluation, and Treatment of High Blood Pressure: the JNC 7 report. JAMA. 2003;289(19):2560–2572.

Marik PE. Management of traumatic brain injury. In Handbook of Evidence-Based Critical Care. 1st ed. New York: Springer-Verlag New York; 2001:321–330.

Rose JC, Mayer SA. Optimizing blood pressure in neurological emergencies. Neurocritical Care. 2004;1(3):287–300.

191

DO NOT GIVE MORE THAN 7 DAYS OF ANTISEIZURE MEDICATION IN HEAD TRAUMA

LAUREN PATON, MD
RONALD F. SING, DO

Among all patients with severe head trauma who receive medical attention, about 12% develop posttraumatic seizures; this rate is more than 50% for those with penetrating head injuries. Posttraumatic seizures are defined as early (occurring in the first week after injury) or late (longer than 7 days after injury) (*Table 191.1*). Seizure activity in the early posttraumatic period following head injury may cause secondary brain damage because of increased metabolic demands, raised intracranial pressure, and excess neurotransmitter release. The development of seizures complicates the acute management and rehabilitation of head-injured patients. These seizures can be physically and psychologically debilitating. However, early seizure development does not affect long-term patient outcomes.

WATCH OUT FOR

The use of antiseizure prophylaxis must be balanced against the medication's demonstrated toxicity and side effects, which may be especially disabling in this population. Valproate, phenytoin, and carbamazepine can cause a rash, hepatotoxicity, blood dyscrasias, ataxia, dizziness, and nausea. In addition, phenytoin can cause hypotension and lead to a decrease in the cerebral perfusion pressure. The impact of being on seizure medication in regard to the impact on activities of daily living should not be minimized; in some states patients on antiseizure medications are not allowed to drive a motor vehicle.

The prophylactic use of antiseizure medications (usually phenytoin or carbamazepine) after traumatic brain injury has become common, although the available data are not sufficient to support a practice standard. Class I evidence demonstrates a significantly lower rate of early posttraumatic seizures among patients treated with prophylactic antiseizure medications. Importantly, these studies had few adverse effects occurring within the first week of therapy for penetrating and nonpenetrating brain injury patients. In these patients, the benefits of seizure prophylaxis outweighed the low risk rate.

TABLE 191.1	RISK FACTORS FOR POSTTRAUMATIC SEIZURES
Glasgow Coma Scale (GCS) score less than 10	
Cortical contusion	
Depressed skull fracture	
Subdural hematoma	
Epidural hematoma	
Intracerebral hematoma	
Penetrating head wound	
Seizure within 24 hours of injury	

WHAT NOT TO DO

A common ICU error is prolonging the duration of antiseizure medication in the head-injured patient beyond 1 week. The Brain Trauma Foundation guidelines state that prophylactic use of antiseizure medications should *not* be used to prevent late posttraumatic seizures. Class I evidence exists supporting the statement that the use of phenytoin, carbamazepine, or valproate is *not* recommended in the reduction of late posttraumatic seizures. Prophylactic treatment should stop 7 days after traumatic brain injury when caring for critically ill neurotrauma patients.

One final note is that serum levels of antiseizure medications should not be tested; the half-life of these drugs is sufficiently long that steady state is not reached within 7 days.

SUGGESTED READINGS

Brain Trauma Foundation. Guidelines. http://www2.braintrauma.org/guidelines
Chang BS, Lowenstein DH; Quality Standards Subcommittee of the American Academy of Neurology. Practice parameter: antiepileptic drug prophylaxis in severe traumatic brain injury: report of the Quality Standards Subcommittee of the American Academy of Neurology. Neurology. 2003;60(1):10–16.

192

CALCULATE THE GLASGOW COMA SCALE USING THE BEST MOTOR RESPONSE

D. JOSHUA MANCINI, MD
RAJAN GUPTA, MD

The Glasgow Coma Scale (GCS) was initially developed to assess the level of brain function following injury. Recently its application has expanded to assess brain function from other neurological etiologies, especially in the critical care setting. The score is calculated by adding assigned values to different levels of function in three main categories: motor, verbal, and eye response. The GCS (*Table 192.1*) allows for a common language between health care providers during the assessment of neurologically impaired patients. Using this score to stratify the severity of brain injury assists in determining further diagnostic and therapeutic interventions. Its predictive value is limited when the score is used alone; however, when combined with other physiologic and anatomic criteria, it may be more useful in evaluating outcomes.

The severity of traumatic brain injury is often defined by the GCS. A score ≤8 is considered severe injury, 9 to 13 is moderate, and 14 to 15 is mild. The motor score may be the most reliable and accurate component and appears to correlate well with the total GCS score. The use of the motor score alone avoids problems often associated with the collection of the verbal and eye components. The eye portion of the score adds little to the overall predictive ability of the GCS score and can easily be affected by other factors. The verbal response is impossible to determine in intubated patients and has led to the adoption of annotating the GCS score with a *T* in these patients (e.g., 3T). The GCS is most reliable when used in assessing patients with isolated head injuries; however, there remains variability in calculating the score among different practitioners as well as different institutions.

TABLE 192.1 THE GLASGOW COMA SCALE		
MOTOR	**VERBAL**	**EYE OPENING**
6 Obeys commands	5 Oriented	4 Spontaneous
5 Localizes pain	4 Confused	3 To voice
4 Withdraws to pain	3 Inappropriate words	2 To pain
3 Flexion to pain (decorticate)	2 Incomprehensible sounds	1 None
2 Extension to pain (decerebrate)	1 None	
1 None		

There are several pitfalls that can often render the GCS score inaccurate and unreliable. Intoxication and substance abuse, the use of sedatives and narcotics, the need for intubation, the presence of facial injuries, hearing loss, and dementia can all be confounding factors. In addition, the motor response can be inaccurate in the setting of a spinal cord or peripheral nerve injury. However, despite its inexactness, most providers agree that patients with a GCS of <9 require emergent intubation.

SUGGESTED READINGS

Bastos PG, Sun X, Wagner DP, et al. Glasgow Coma Scale score in the evaluation of outcome in the intensive care unit: findings from the Acute Physiology and Chronic Health Evaluation III study. Crit Care Med. 1993;21(10):1459–1465.

Healey C, Osler TM, Rogers FB, et al. Improving the Glasgow Coma Scale score: motor score alone is a better predictor. J Trauma. 2003;54(4):671–680.

193

USE MAGNETIC RESONANCE IMAGING (NOT HEAD COMPUTED TOMOGRAPHY) AS THE GOLD STANDARD TEST FOR DIFFUSE AXONAL INJURY

ELIAHU S. FEEN, MD
JOSE I. SUAREZ, MD

Diffuse axonal injury develops most commonly in the setting of angular acceleration of the brain in head injury. This movement causes a shear injury between the gray and white matter with microscopic hemorrhages developing in particular areas of the brain. The shear also disrupts axons, which swell and whose severed ends eventually become the globular structures seen pathologically as the "retraction balls of Cajal." The earliest changes occur hours after injury and the pathologic changes continue for several days. The clinical manifestations of diffuse axonal injury include a period of unconsciousness (and amnesia) lasting more than 6 hours.

Prognosis for head-injury patients is difficult to predict. The severity of diffuse axonal injury can vary with the severity of head injury. Prognosis for traumatic brain injury also varies with the severity of the injury. In the most severe cases (in which patients who do not die remain in a vegetative state), about one-third of patients recover consciousness by 3 months. However, recovery continues significantly after that, with 46% of patients recovering consciousness by 6 months, and 52% by 1 year. Clinicians must therefore take extreme caution in giving a prognosis for such patients for at least 6 months. The great majority of patients in a vegetative state have diffuse axonal injury on pathological examination of their brains. Thus, when diffuse axonal injury is identified premortem (via head imaging), the same caution must be used in giving a prognosis for diffuse axonal injury.

WATCH OUT FOR

Head computed tomography (CT) in traumatic brain injury is obviously absolutely essential. Many of the various types of traumatic brain injury are easily seen on head CT and include subdural hematoma, epidural hematoma, intracranial hemorrhage, and brain contusion. Head CT is also useful in identifying acute hydrocephalus, massive cerebral edema, and midline shift or herniation. Head CT, however, is not useful in identifying diffuse axonal injury. Blood within the brain that is seen on CT imaging can be a marker for diffuse axonal injury.

However, the head CT can be normal in head-injury patients for whom diffuse axonal injury is observed on MRI. For this reason, even some patients with a normal head CT need intracranial pressure monitoring after traumatic brain injury.

The different modes of magnetic resonance imaging (MRI) sequences have better sensitivity for detecting diffuse axonal injury. Fast fluid-attenuated inversion-recovery (FLAIR), diffusion-weighted imaging (DWI), and gradient echo sequences have all been reported to have higher yield in the detection of diffuse axonal injury than regular (T2-weighted) MRI sequences. MRI can also detect microhemorrhages within the brain not visible on CT (through the use of gradient echo sequences). DWI sequences of an MRI are very sensitive for ischemia. Thus, MRI is useful in identifying diffuse axonal injury, which may not become visible until 6 to 12 days after the insult. As well, MRI is much more sensitive than CT for identifying ischemic, hypoxic, or hypotensive injuries that may be delayed or develop as secondary brain injury. Many clinicians use CT acutely and MRI in the subacute and chronic phases of traumatic brain injury for these reasons.

SUGGESTED READINGS

Adams JH, Jennett B, McLellan DR, et al. The neuropathology of the vegetative state after head injury. J Clin Path. 1999;52:804–806.

Huisman TAGM, Sorensen AG, Hergan K, et al. Diffusion-weighted imaging for the evaluation of diffuse axonal injury in closed head injury. J Comp Asst Tomography. 2003;27:5–11.

McArthur DL, Chute DJ, Villablanca JP. Moderate and severe traumatic brain injury: epidemiologic, imaging and neuropathologic perspectives. Brain Pathol. 2004;14:185–194.

Mittl RL, Grossman RI, Hiehle JF, et al. Prevalence of MR evidence of diffuse axonal injury in patients with mild head injury and normal head CT findings. AJNR. 1994;15:1583–1589.

Multi-society Task Force on PVS. Medical aspects of the persistent vegetative state (in two parts). N Engl J Med. 1994;330:1499–1508,1572–1579.

194

REMEMBER THAT THERE IS USUALLY AN UPWARD DRIFT IN SOME INTRACRANIAL-PRESSURE MONITOR READINGS THE LONGER THEY HAVE BEEN IN PLACE

ELIAHU S. FEEN, MD
JOSE I. SUAREZ, MD

The normal intracranial pressure (ICP) ranges between 5 and 15 mm Hg (7 to 20 cm H_2O). ICP can be monitored invasively as well as non-invasively. One of the most sensitive indicators of elevated ICP is the neurologic exam—as the ICP rises above normal, the neurologic exam declines. A drop in the level of consciousness serves as one of the first signs of elevated ICP. It is well known that as ICP rises, certain neurologic signs develop. For example, pressure on the third cranial nerve causes a fixed, dilated pupil, and diffusely increased ICP can cause bilateral sixth cranial nerve palsies, with impaired lateral gaze. When ICP rises high enough to cause translocation of brain tissues from their normal neuroanatomic locations, classic herniation syndromes can develop. Neurologic signs, however, lack sufficient accuracy and specificity. Most importantly, the goal of neurologic monitoring is to identify and treat elevated ICP *before* neurologic damage, such as herniation occurs. In addition, in patients with traumatic brain injury, a deleterious rise in ICP is observed shortly after the injury for an extended period of time. As ICP rises, cerebral perfusion pressure (CPP) drops, since CPP is the difference between mean arterial pressure (MAP) and ICP. When CPP declines sufficiently, ischemia can result (secondary brain injury). Management in this area is controversial, but some guidelines suggest maintaining a CPP between 60 and 70 mm Hg in order to avoid secondary brain injury as a result of decreased cerebral blood flow.

Noninvasive methods of monitoring ICP include neuroimaging (especially computed tomography and magnetic resonance imaging) and neurovascular ultrasound. Neither of these methods provides good accuracy. Transcranial Doppler studies have not been found to provide precise predictions of when an ICP will become acutely and dangerously elevated. Therefore, direct (i.e., invasive) methods remain the preferred technique. These include intraventricular catheters, parenchymal catheters, subarachnoid bolts, epidural catheters, and lumbar drains (to measure the cerebrospinal fluid [CSF] pressure in the lumbar spinal space).

When a patient has an external intraventricular catheter placed into either the lateral ventricles or another part of the ventricular system of the brain, a pressure transducer can be connected to measure the fluid pressure of the CSF that drains. Intraventricular catheters are considered the gold standard of direct ICP monitoring, because fluid conveys pressure so well. Placement of intraventricular catheters carries with it up to a 6% risk of hemorrhage and up to about a 20% risk of infection, with the lowest reported infection rates of about 5%. Clinicians commonly use prophylactic antibiotics in conjunction with the placement of intraventricular catheters, but data are lacking about whether this practice reduces the infectious complications. Of the infections that do occur, most occur after at least 5 days of catheter placement. Some clinicians have recommended on this basis to replace catheters that are more than 5 days old.

Parenchymal catheters, such as the Camino or Codman Micro Sensor catheters, are inserted through a burr hole in the skull with depth catheters going through the dura into brain parenchyma. Measurement of the tissue pressure represents ICP measurement. However, many studies show that ICP is not uniform throughout the brain. So, the value of the ICP measured may reflect only the localized pressure in the area of the catheter. This is not a problem unique to parenchymal catheters, as intraventricular catheters also suffer from this issue, which may even be exacerbated if there is not freely circulating CSF to equally distribute pressure. Hemorrhagic and infectious complications appear to be about the same as with intraventricular catheters. One of the problems reported with parenchymal catheters is the phenomenon of "zero drift," in which the zero pressure baseline (to which the catheter is calibrated during initial placement) drifts. In Camino catheters one study indicated an average drift of up to 3 mm Hg of pressure. The longer the catheter remains in place, the greater the drift. This must be considered when trends in ICP are observed.

Subarachnoid bolts are fiberoptic pressure transducers placed through a burr hole but with only a saline-filled lumen exposed to the subarachnoid space through a tiny incision in the dura. Subarachnoid bolts carry a much lower risk of hemorrhagic complications and a lower infection rate, with reported rates of infection ranging only as high as about 7%. However, with subarachnoid bolts CSF cannot be analyzed, and the bolts are not as mechanically stable with respect to accurate ICP measurement as compared with intraventricular catheters or parenchymal catheters. Recommendations about the routine use of prophylactic antibiotics with the parenchymal catheters and subarachnoid bolts are lacking, but prophylactic antibiotics are commonly administered.

Epidural catheters are ICP-measuring of the epidural space devices inserted into the epidural space. Given the devices anatomic location between the dura and calvaria, infection and hemorrhagic complications are lower. However, the accuracy of the ICP measurement is compromised, since it is not directly measured. Lumbar drains can measure ICP and do provide CSF analysis while avoiding significant hemorrhagic complications and having a low infection rate. However, the accuracy of the ICP measurements is uncertain, because it is not clear in many brain-injured patients that the lumbar spinal cistern will accurately reflect the intraventricular pressure.

SUGGESTED READINGS

Czosnyka M, Pickard JD. Monitoring and interpretation of intracranial pressure. J Neurol Neurosurg Psychiatry. 2004;75:813–821.

Holloway KL, Barnet T, Choi S, et al. Ventriculostomy infections: the effect of monitoring duration and catheter exchange in 584 patients. J Neurosurg. 1996;85:419–424.

Mayhall CG, Archer NH, Lamb VA, et al. Ventriculostomy-related infections: a prospective epidemiologic study. N Engl J Med. 1984;310:553–559.

Paramore CG, Turner DA. Relative risks of ventriculostomy infection and morbidity. Acta Neurochir. 1994;127:79–84.

Piper I, Barnes A, Smith D, et al. The Camino intracranial pressure sensor: is it optimal technology? An internal audit with a review of current intracranial pressure monitoring technologies. Neurosurgery. 2001;49:1158–1165.

Suarez JI, ed. Critical Care Neurology and Neurosurgery. Totowa, New Jersey: Humana Press; 2004.

195

BE AWARE THAT INCREASING POSITIVE END-EXPIRATORY PRESSURE MAY RESULT IN INCREASING INTRACRANIAL PRESSURE

ELIAHU S. FEEN, MD
JOSE I. SUAREZ, MD

WATCH OUT FOR

Positive end-expiratory pressure (PEEP) can cause numerous physiologic changes. These changes may take place in the lungs, with respect to intrathoracic pressures and lung compliance, and in cardiac output. Clinical observation has also demonstrated for more than 30 years that PEEP can increase intracranial pressure (ICP). Animal and some human data have supported two theories about how this increase in ICP takes place. By increasing intrathoracic pressure, venous return is compromised. As a result, cerebral venous blood volume increases and causes elevation in ICP. Alternatively, in a case where increased PEEP reduces cardiac output, the mean arterial pressure (MAP) may go down and necessarily lower the cerebral perfusion pressure (CPP) and if the injured brain maintains autoregulation, a decreased CPP will result in arteriodilatation, which increases total cerebral blood volume (CBV). With increased CBV comes increased ICP.

It is important to note that increased PEEP does not always translate into increased ICP. Body position can interfere with the transmission of central venous pressure. For example, in patients sitting upright (at an angle of close to 90° degrees), the jugular vein will collapse in systole and fail to transmit increased intrathoracic pressure. Alternatively, for cases of brain injuries in which autoregulation is lost, decreased CPP may not alter ICP; however, decreased CPP may lead to other problems, such as ischemia. Some evidence has shown that in lungs with normal compliance, increased PEEP transmits to increased ICP, but in lungs with low compliance, it does not.

Making recommendations about PEEP in brain injury patients is difficult. No specific level of PEEP has yet been identified as ideal for brain injury patients. Additionally, data from the Adult Respiratory Distress Syndrome Network (ARDSNet) trial and other animal and human studies have demonstrated that some level of PEEP carries overall benefit for a wide variety of critically ill patients (with respect to the development of ARDS). We can safely say that clinicians must be aware that PEEP *can* increase ICP. Thus, in patients with known intracranial hypertension or even patients with any brain injury (who are at risk for low intracranial compliance), care must be taken to monitor patients closely. ICP monitoring and frequent neurologic examinations will represent extremely important elements of the care of these patients. If practitioners identify a correlation between PEEP and ICP elevations, they should exert their judgment and adjust the former to ameliorate the latter without compromising systemic oxygenation.

SUGGESTED READINGS

Burchiel KJ, Steege TD, Wyler AR. Intracranial pressure changes in brain-injured patients requiring positive end-expiratory pressure ventilation. Neurosurgery. 1981;8:443–439.

Caricato A, Conti G, Della Corte F, et al. Effects of PEEP on the intracranial system of patients with head injury and subarachnoid hemorrhage: the role of respiratory system compliance. J Trauma. 2005;58:571–576.

Cooper KR, Boswell PA, Choi SC. Safe use of PEEP in patients with severe head injury. J Neurosurg. 1993;63:552–555.

McGuire G, Crossley D, Richards J, et al. Effects of varying levels of positive end-expiratory pressure on intracranial pressure and cerebral perfusion pressure. Crit Care Med. 1997;25:1059–1062.

Shapiro HM, Marshall LF. Intracranial pressure responses to PEEP in head-injured patients. J Trauma. 1978;18:254–256.

196

Obtain a Computed Tomography Scan of the Head Immediately After Any Craniotomy or Intracranial Procedure if Patient's Neurologic Examination is Different from Preoperative Assessments

Jose I. Suarez, MD

Management of the critically ill patient after a craniotomy poses special challenges for the intensivist. Not only do practitioners have to manage the systemic alterations, but they must also understand how such alterations interact and affect brain functions. For instance, patients who develop intracerebral hemorrhage (ICH) after a craniotomy are more likely to experience hypertensive episodes both intraoperatively and in the first few hours postoperatively. Patients who undergo craniotomy for subdural hematoma (SDH) evacuation are more likely to experience recurrent SDH if they were coagulopathic before the surgical procedure was performed. Also the timing of neurological deterioration may vary depending on when they experience the intracranial complication. For instance, postoperative ICH will mostly present within 6 hours after surgery.

Neurologic Examination

Whenever possible, patients undergoing craniotomy should have a baseline neurologic examination prior to surgery. Such evaluation should include assessment of the level of consciousness; cranial nerves; motor strength; reflexes; coordination (i.e., finger-to-nose and heel-to-shin maneuvers); sensory perception (light touch and pain and temperature); and meningeal signs. Immediately after craniotomy the patient's neurological status should be reassessed and compared with the baseline. The two major limitations to the immediate postoperative neurologic examination are sedation and mechanical ventilation. Performing the Glasgow Coma Scale (GCS) before and after craniotomy is a very reliable way of assessing level of consciousness. As discussed in Chapter 192, GCS has been validated widely across medical and surgical specialties and can be performed in intubated patients using a predictive verbal score from the eye and the motor scores. It is of the utmost importance to act upon observed neurologic changes. The airway should be assessed and blood pressure evaluated. Patients with

GCS ≤8 should be intubated (if not done already). Extreme blood pressure levels (hypo- or hypertension) should be corrected. Seizures should be treated if present. Once the initial stabilization of the patient has been achieved, a head computed tomography (CT) scan should be the next step.

HEAD CT AND NEUROSURGICAL EVALUATION

Many of the immediate postcraniotomy complications are due to cerebral ischemia, ICH, seizures, and cerebral edema with or without elevated intracranial pressure (ICP). Therefore, head CT should be the first imaging study since it will identify most of these complications. If the head CT scan reveals no abnormalities, then an electroencephalogram (EEG) should be performed. EEG will be helpful to exclude nonconvulsive seizures that would be undetectable otherwise. Neurosurgical evaluation should be sought immediately after neurologic deterioration is detected (and before the head CT is obtained). This approach will guarantee that patients will be taken to the operating room promptly for repeat craniotomy if there is a neurosurgical target.

SUGGESTED READINGS

Basali A, Mascha EJ, Kalfas I, et al. Relation between perioperative hypertension and intracranial hemorrhage after craniotomy. Anesthesiology. 2000;93:48–54.

Higuchi Y, Iacono RP. Surgical complications in patients with Parkinson's disease after posteroventral pallidotomy. Neurosurgery. 2003;52:558–571.

Konig SA, Schick U, Dohnert J, et al. Coagulopathy and outcome in patients with chronic subdural hematoma. Acta Neurol Scand. 2003;107:110–116.

Rodrigue T, Selman WR. Postoperative management in the neurosciences critical care unit. In Suarez JI, ed. Critical Care Neurology and Neurosurgery. Totowa, NJ: Humana Press; 2004:433–448.

Taylor WAS, Thomas NWM, Wellings JA, et al. Timing of postoperative intracranial hematoma development and implications for the best use of neurosurgical intensive care. J Neurosurg. 1995;82:48–50.

197

CONSIDER LAST-DITCH MANEUVERS TO LOWER INTRACRANIAL HYPERTENSION IN IMPENDING HERNIATION

ELIAHU S. FEEN, MD
JOSE I. SUAREZ, MD

WHAT TO DO

Elevated intracranial pressure (ICP), or intracranial hypertension, is a common occurrence in critically ill neurologic patients and is associated with poor outcome. While much disagreement remains about the optimal treatment of elevated ICP, there is recognition of the most commonly employed techniques for lowering critically elevated ICP; hyperventilation followed by osmotherapy (administration of an osmotic diuretic, most commonly mannitol). Recent research supports the use of hypertonic saline (e.g., 3% saline solution) as an alternative or adjunctive agent to mannitol. These medical measures will hopefully temporize the elevated ICP while investigations as to the particular cause ensue. Of course, depending upon the cause, surgery may be necessary to definitively treat the elevated ICP.

WHAT TO DO NEXT

If these medical measures are not successful and a definitive surgical procedure is not an option, then for many practitioners the next step is usually general anesthesia. For many years barbiturate-induced coma was the accepted approach. Currently, propofol is recommended because of its short half-life, rapid washout time, and ability to allow for more rapid assessment of neurologic function. Keeping patients under generalized anesthesia for several days reduces cerebral metabolism and consequently reduces cerebral blood flow. It is through this mechanism that generalized anesthesia is thought to reduce the ICP. One important caveat to general anesthesia is the development of clinically significant hypotension. The latter can occur in up to 25% of patients treated with barbiturates and is certainly seen with propofol. Hypotension is associated with poor outcome in patients with neurologic injury.

Should metabolic coma not work, two more drastic measures have been advocated—hemicraniectomy and decompressive laparotomy. A substantial amount of evidence over the past 30 years has lent support to the use of decompressive hemicraniectomy for the treatment of intractably elevated ICP. In the case of unilateral cerebral edema (as determined by head computed tomography scanning), unilateral decompressive hemicraniectomy can be performed. In the case of bilateral cerebral edema, bilateral hemicraniectomy is often necessary (frontotemporal-parietal). An alternative surgical approach for the treatment of diffuse bilateral edema is bifrontal decompressive craniectomy. Case series and case reports document success with performance of early craniectomy (within 24 to 48 hours) as well as late craniectomy (after 24 to 48 hours). Some patients may have had unilateral mass lesions that were resected surgically and then developed localized reactive edema, which became refractory to standard treatments for intracranial hypertension. In some of these cases (where ipsilateral surgical resection had already been performed), success has been reported with a decompressive hemicraniectomy. Data from randomized, controlled trials are lacking. As a result, patient-selection protocols do not exist and the identification of risk factors predicting poor outcome remains uncertain. Nevertheless, the approach has become widespread, especially in certain specific circumstances, such as malignant cerebral edema due to middle cerebral artery occlusion. Of interest, the management of the bone flap varies between institutions. Some surgeons place the bone flap in the patient's abdomen for several weeks prior to reattachment, whereas others place the bone flap in (external) sterile environments at subzero temperatures for several weeks to months.

From the trauma literature, it has emerged that decompression of the abdomen results in lowering of the ICP. Not uncommonly, trauma patients frequently have both abdominal injuries and head injuries (and as a result have ICP monitoring). If such a patient developed the abdominal compartment syndrome, with elevation of intra-abdominal pressure (IAP), and then the patient was taken to surgery for abdominal decompression, it was coincidentally noted in some patients that the ICP was reduced afterward. From such cases trauma surgeons developed an approach to perform abdominal decompression as a method of lowering refractory intracranial hypertension, even in patients with normal intra-abdominal pressures. At this point only case series and animal data exist. In many of the patients from the case series, the ICP continued to remain elevated despite craniectomy. Consequently, abdominal decompression truly remains a last-ditch attempt to lower ICP—but one that has been shown to produce results in the most refractory of cases.

SUGGESTED READINGS

Albanese J, Leone M, Alliez J-R, et al. Decompressive craniectomy for severe traumatic brain injury: evaluation of the effects at one year. Crit Care Med. 2003;31:2535–2538.

Guerra WKW, Gaab MR, Dietz H, et al. Surgical decompression for traumatic brain swelling: indications and results. J Neurosurg. 1999;90:187–196.

Joseph DAK, Dutton RP, Aarabi B, et al. Decompressive laparotomy to treat intractable intracranial hypertension after traumatic brain injury. J Trauma. 2004;57:687–695.

Miglietta MA, Salzano LJ, Chiu WC, et al. Decompressive laparotomy: a novel approach in the management of severe intracranial hypertension. J Trauma. 2003;55:551–555.

Polin RS, Shaffrey ME, Bogaev CA, et al. Decompressive bifrontal craniectomy in the treatment of severe refractory posttraumatic cerebral edema. Neurosurgery. 1997;41:84–94.

Roberts I. Barbiturates for acute traumatic brain injury. Cochrane Database Syst Rev. 2000;CD000033.

Saggi BH, Bloomfield GL, Sugerman HJ, et al. Treatment of intracranial hypertension using nonsurgical abdominal decompression. J Trauma. 1999;46:646–651.

198

REMEMBER THAT PATIENTS UNDERGOING BARBITURATE COMA MUST HAVE ADEQUATE ELECTROPHYSIOLOGICAL MONITORING

JOSE I. SUAREZ, MD

High-dose barbiturates have been used for more than 60 years in critically ill neurologic patients. The most common application has been to lower elevated intracranial pressure (ICP) in patients with severe traumatic brain injury (TBI). Other uses include refractory status epilepticus, cerebral vasospasm after subarachnoid hemorrhage (SAH), comatose survivors of cardiac arrest, and patients with cerebral edema and elevated ICP from any etiology other than TBI. The most commonly used barbiturate is pentobarbital.

MECHANISM OF ACTION

High-dose barbiturates have various effects on the brain that may explain their apparently neuroprotective properties. It has been suggested that the most important property is that of coupling cerebral blood flow to regional cerebral metabolic demands. It is postulated that lowering cerebral metabolic requirements would lower cerebral blood volume, which in turn will result in lower ICP. Other mechanisms may include inhibition of free-radical-mediated lipid peroxidation and amelioration of glutamate release. High-dose barbiturates also suppress both clinical and electrical seizure activity.

DOSAGE, MONITORING, AND ADVERSE EFFECTS

A number of therapeutic regimens using pentobarbital have been used. One common strategy uses an initial loading dose of 10 mg/kg over 30 to 40 minutes followed by a maintenance drip of 0.5 to 2.0 mg/kg/h. The most reliable monitoring technique is continuous electroencephalogram (EEG) monitoring. Patients who undergo pentobarbital coma have no useful clinical examination; therefore, EEG is most helpful at titrating the therapy. Usually, the infusion rate of pentobarbital is titrated to a burst suppression pattern on the EEG record. There is no agreement regarding the depth of the EEG suppression that must be accomplished. However, many experts recommend an EEG burst suppression pattern of 5 to 10 seconds. There is also no general agreement on the duration of pentobarbital coma. Certainly the duration will depend on the condition being treated. For instance, patients with refractory ICP elevations will have to be treated as long as the abnormal intracranial compliance is present, which may be for several days. On the other hand, many patients with status epilepticus may need between 24 and 96 hours of treatment to control seizures. However, some patients with status epilepticus may also require days or weeks of treatment.

Pentobarbital coma is associated with a host of serious adverse effects. The most common side effects include respiratory depression and hypotension. The latter is an important issue since the beneficial effects of the therapy may be negated by the hypotensive effect. In fact, many treated patients will need extra cardiovascular support including vasopressors and pulmonary artery catheter insertion to monitor cardiac function and volume status. Other adverse effects of pentobarbital coma include ileus, decreased clearance of bronchial secretion leading to pneumonia, and liver dysfunction. All of these factors and the fact that there is no good evidence from randomized, controlled clinical trials that pentobarbital coma improves outcome in patients with various neurological pathologies have led many practitioners to consider this therapy as the last resort when other treatments have been exhausted. As such, pentobarbital coma should be used only in patients with elevated ICP refractory to medical and surgical therapy and status epilepticus refractory to other treatments including propofol and midazolam drips.

SUGGESTED READINGS

Brain Resuscitation Clinical Trial I Study Group. Randomized clinical study of thiopental loading in comatose survivors of cardiac arrest. N Engl J Med. 1986;314:397–403.

Eisenberg HM, Frankowski RF, Contant CF, et al. High-dose barbiturate control of elevated intracranial pressure in patients with severe head injury. J Neurosurg. 1988;69:15–23.

Finfer SR, Ferch R, Morgan MK. Barbiturate coma for severe, refractory vasospasm following subarachnoid hemorrhage. Intensive Care Med. 1999;25:406–409.

Goodman JC, Valadka AB, Gopinath SP, et al. Lactate and excitatory amino acids measured by microdialysis are decreased by pentobarbital coma in head-injured patients. J Neurotrauma. 1996;13:549–556.

Roberts I. Barbiturates for acute traumatic brain injury. Cochrane Database Syst Rev. 2000;(2):CD000033.

The Brain Trauma Foundation. The American Association of Neurological Surgeons. The Joint Section on Neurotrauma and Critical Care. Use of barbiturates in the control of intracranial hypertension. J Neurotrauma. 2000;17:527–530.

Ward JD, Becker DP, Miller JD, et al. Failure of prophylactic barbiturate coma in the treatment of severe head injury. J Neurosurg. 1985;62:383–388.

199

BE ALERT FOR CONVERSION OF NONHEMORRHAGIC (ISCHEMIC) STROKE TO HEMORRHAGIC STROKE

JOSE I. SUAREZ, MD

Ischemic stroke accounts for about 80% of all strokes. Many patients with an initial ischemic stroke will experience a hemorrhagic transformation. This may result in further neurological deterioration. As observed on autopsy studies, many patients will have some degree of hemorrhagic transformation, with 51% to 71% of cardioembolic and 2% to 21% of noncardioembolic ischemic strokes having hemorrhagic transformation. The incidence of hemorrhagic transformation seen on computed tomography (CT) scan ranges from a few percent to 40% of patients, depending on the criteria used.

WATCH OUT FOR

Although hemorrhagic transformation occurs frequently after ischemic stroke, it is often asymptomatic, part of the natural course of ischemic infarction, and may not alter the clinical outcome beyond what is to be expected based on the intrinsic characteristics of the ischemic infarct. Only symptomatic hemorrhagic transformation has clinical relevance. Different stroke trials have varying definitions of what constitutes symptomatic hemorrhagic transformation. In order to clarify this confusion, Berger et al. analyzed data from patients previously enrolled in the European Cooperative Acute Stroke Study (ECASS II) trial and found that clinically significant hemorrhagic transformation occurred mainly if greater than 30% of the infarcted area had dense homogenous-appearing hemorrhage with mass effect. In this case, patients had significantly increased risk of early neurologic deterioration and worse long-term outcome. In patients with smaller (<30%) homogenous hemorrhagic transformation with minimal mass effect, a worse short-term outcome was observed, but no effect on long-term clinical outcome was seen. In contrast, patients with small heterogeneous petechial hemorrhages did not have worse early or long-term outcome.

The mechanisms for hemorrhagic transformation vary depending on the clinical scenario; however, one of the essential requirements is breakdown of the blood–brain barrier (BBB). Certain factors at baseline may predict a higher rate of hemorrhagic transformation. These factors include hyperglycemia, increased patient age, embolic stroke mechanism, increased infarct size, edema formation, excessive hypertension, increased severity of stroke symptoms, and receiving anticoagulant or tissue-type plasminogen activator (tPA). Patients receiving tPA had about a 6.4% rate of symptomatic hemorrhagic transformation, as seen in the National Institute of Neurological Disorders and Stroke (NINDS) trial. One group of investigators found that tPA use facilitated dysregulation of extracellular proteolysis, resulting in BBB breakdown.

WHAT TO DO

Management of hemorrhagic transformation requires a multifaceted approach. First, the precipitating cause needs to be quickly identified and treated. The patient should have normoglycemia maintained, excessively elevated blood pressure should be gently lowered, and coagulopathy should be corrected promptly with administration of fresh frozen plasma. Generally, antiplatelet agents and anticoagulants should be held for at least a week depending on the size of the hemorrhagic transformation; however, solid data guiding this decision are lacking. Management of significant mass effect and edema associated with symptomatic hemorrhagic transformation should be reduced by instituting neuroprotective, pharmacologic, and surgical measures. Neuroprotective measures include maintaining normoglycemia and normothermia, as hyperglycemia and hyperthermia may worsen cerebral edema. If the patient becomes obtunded, a noncontrasted head CT should be performed immediately to exclude hydrocephalus or brain herniation.

If symptomatic hemorrhagic transformation occurs within the cerebellum, compression of the fourth ventricle can rapidly lead to obstructive hydrocephalus and death. Direct brain-stem compression with subsequent brain death may also occur. Thus, immediate neurosurgical intervention with a ventriculostomy and plan for possible posterior fossa decompression or cerebellectomy must occur. In addition, in patients with neurological deterioration and signs of impending herniation, immediate intubation should take place to protect the airway, and although very controversial, mild hyperventilation to keep the P_{CO_2} between about 30 and 34 mm Hg can be considered (this is a temporizing measure only). Additionally, 1 g/kg of mannitol, an osmotic agent, must be given immediately to help lower intracranial pressure. The serum osmolality should be maintained at a range of 310 to 320 mOsm/L. A hemicraniectomy should be considered in younger patients (<50 years) with large hemispheric stroke if conservative measures fail.

Another point that is very important is the correction of existing coagulopathy. Acute ischemic stroke patients are often treated with antithrombotic and antiplatelet agents. Thus, practitioners need to consider blood product transfusion (i.e., platelets, fresh frozen plasma, and cryoprecipitate) to correct potential coagulation abnormalities. In patients receiving intravenous unfractionated heparin, protamine sulfate (1 mg per 100 units of heparin given over the previous 4 hours) should be given, after consideration of protamine's risks. In addition, some early data on factor VIIa for treatment of coagulopathy has shown some benefit.

SUGGESTED READINGS

Berger C, Fiorelli M, Steiner T, et al. Hemorrhagic transformation of ischemic brain tissue: asymptomatic or symptomatic? Stroke. 2001;32:1330–1335.

Feen ES, Suarez JI. Raised intracranial pressure. Curr Treat Options Neurol. 2005;7(2):109–117.

Okada Y, Yamaguchi T, Minematsu K, et al. Hemorrhagic transformation in cerebral embolism. Stroke. 1989;20(5):598–603.

Wang X, Tsuji K, Lee SR, et al. Mechanisms of hemorrhagic transformation after tissue plasminogen activator reperfusion therapy for ischemic stroke. Stroke. 2004;35:2726.

200

Obtain a Head Computed Tomography Scan and Lumbar Puncture in Patients with Human Immunodeficiency Virus or Acquired Immunodeficiency Syndrome and New-Onset Mental Status Changes

ERIC M. BERSHAD, MD
JOSE I. SUAREZ, MD

Human immunodeficiency virus (HIV) and acquired immuno-deficiency syndrome (AIDS) patients may host a myriad of infectious, inflammatory, toxic, and neoplastic diseases that are not seen commonly in the immune-competent patient. Thus, it is important for the clinician to keep in mind the expanded differential diagnosis of mental status changes in the HIV patient. The etiology for mental status changes in general includes a vast differential of diseases in the categories of vascular, infectious, neoplastic, drugs, inflammatory, autoimmune, trauma, and endocrine or metabolic causes. In HIV/AIDS patients the differential must be expanded to include diseases and conditions related to immune dysfunction. The clinician should have a much lower threshold for suspecting a neurologic cause for mental status changes in the HIV/AIDS patient as compared with the immune-competent patient.

The initial workup for HIV/AIDS patients with new-onset mental status changes must include a contrasted head computed tomography (CT) scan to rule out intracranial mass lesions. A magnetic resonance imaging (MRI) with gadolinium is more sensitive for small intracranial lesions; however, the limited availability in some centers and the increased time to obtain images make CT scan a more practical initial imaging modality (*Table 200.1*).

In the HIV/AIDS patient it is important to obtain the head CT before performing a lumbar puncture (Fig. 200.1). A focal mass lesion may produce locally elevated intracranial pressure. A lumbar puncture done in this setting can result in a high pressure gradient between the lesion and lumbar cistern that forces the brain downward, resulting in fatal herniation. The most common mass lesions to consider are toxoplasmosis and primary central nervous system (CNS) lymphoma. The incidence of cerebral toxoplasmosis in HIV/AIDS patients ranges from 3% to 10% in the United States, while primary CNS lymphoma occurs in about 2% of patients.

TABLE 200.1	ETIOLOGIES OF MASS LESIONS IN HIV/AIDS PATIENTS
Infectious	Parasites: **Toxoplasmosis**, cysticercosis Fungi: *Cryptococcus*, *Candida*, aspergillosis, mucormycosis, coccidioidomycosis Bacteria: *Mycobacterium tuberculosis*, *Mycobacterium avium*, *Nocardia*, *Listeria*, *Treponema pallidum*
Neoplastic	**Primary CNS lymphoma**, glioma, metastatic neoplasm
Inflammatory	Progressive multifocal leukoencephalopathy (PML)
Vascular	Ischemic stroke, intracerebral hemorrhage

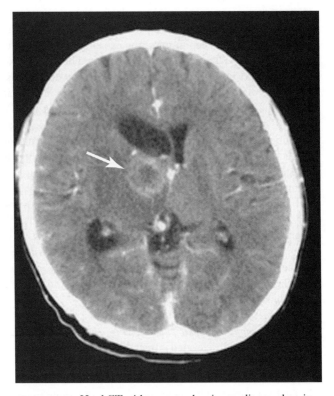

FIGURE 200.1. Head CT with contrast showing a solitary enhancing mass lesion (arrow) in the right basal ganglia later identified as a toxoplasmosis abscess. Primary CNS lymphoma may have a similar appearance. Reproduced with permission from a neuroradiology teaching file at University Hospitals of Cleveland. Courtesy of David Preston.

WHAT TO DO

Once an intracranial mass lesion has been found on imaging, it is important to determine the etiology. Based on the American Academy of Neurology (AAN) practice parameter on evaluation and management of intracranial mass lesions in AIDS, large lesions with mass effect threatening impending herniation require open biopsy with decompression. In all other cases, empiric therapy for toxoplasmosis should be instituted, unless there is only a single lesion seen and also negative toxoplasmosis serology. Patients treated for toxoplasmosis infections presumptively need to be carefully monitored clinically and radiographically over the first 10 to 14 days. The median time to response is 5 days. By day 14, 91% of patients with toxoplasmosis central nervous system infection exhibit a response. If no response is observed after empiric toxoplasmosis therapy, one should proceed with stereotactic brain biopsy.

In the absence of a brain mass lesion, a lumbar puncture should be done to exclude meningitis and encephalitis. *Cryptococcus* is the most common cause of meningitis in the HIV patient. HIV may directly result in aseptic meningitis. Other etiologies include Cytomegalovirus (CMV), varicella-zoster virus (VZV), Epstein-Barr virus (EBV), herpes simplex virus (HSV), *Listeria monocytogenes,* coccidioidomycosis, histoplasmosis, syphilis, tuberculosis, and lymphomatous meningitis.

When performing lumbar puncture, cerebrospinal fluid (CSF) should be sent for cell count, cell differential, Gram stain, protein, glucose, bacterial and fungal cultures, India ink stain, cryptococcus, and VDRL test (for syphilis). Polymerase chain reaction (PCR) should be sent for VZV, CMV, HSV, EBV, and tuberculosis. Furthermore, it is important to send CSF for cytology to assess for atypical lymphocytes as seen in lymphomatous meningitis.

SUGGESTED READINGS

Bradley W, ed. Neurology in Clinical Practice. New York: Butterworth-Heinemann; 2004:1581–1602.

Evaluation and management of intracranial mass lesions in AIDS. Report of the Quality Standards Subcommittee of the American Academy of Neurology. Neurology. 1998;50(1):21–26.

201

HAVE A LOW THRESHOLD FOR OBTAINING AN INITIAL AND REPEAT HEAD COMPUTED TOMOGRAPHY SCAN AFTER SUBARACHNOID HEMORRHAGE

ERIC M. BERSHAD, MD
JOSE I. SUAREZ, MD

Subarachnoid hemorrhage (SAH) is a neurologic emergency with a high mortality rate (50%). Morbidity results from extravasation of blood into the subarachnoid space, most commonly from a ruptured aneurysm. The resulting blood can lead to vasospasm and cerebral infarction, hydrocephalus, cerebral edema with brain herniation, seizures, and other complications. The typical presentation of SAH is a sudden-onset severe headache with nausea, vomiting, neck pain, photophobia, and brief loss of consciousness.

An immediate noncontrasted head computed tomography (CT) scan should be the first diagnostic test when suspecting SAH. The sensitivity of head CT approaches 100% within the first 12 hours and 93% within 24 hours after onset of symptoms. The amount of subarachnoid hemorrhage seen on head CT helps predict the subsequent chance of vasospasm and also the long-term outcome of the patient. A head CT can also assess for intraventricular hemorrhage, which portends a higher risk for hydrocephalus and cerebral edema (*Fig. 201.1*).

WHAT NOT TO DO

In the absence of the classic signs and symptoms, SAH may be misdiagnosed. The frequency of misdiagnosis may be up to 50% in patients presenting for their first visit to a physician. The main reasons for misdiagnosis include failure to obtain the appropriate imaging study (i.e., head CT) in 73% of cases and failure to perform, or correctly interpret the results of, a lumbar puncture in 23% of cases. Patients who are misdiagnosed are usually found to be less ill and have normal neurologic examination. However, it is important to realize that neurologic complications eventually occur in up to 50% of patients with delayed diagnosis and are associated with an increased risk of death and disability. Every patient presenting with a severe and unusual headache should be evaluated for SAH. Headache may be the only presenting complaint in up to 40% of patients and may abate completely

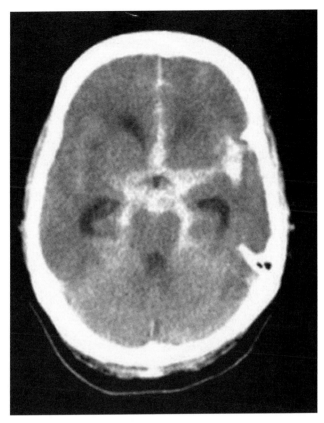

FIGURE 201.1. Head CT of subarachnoid bleed. This noncontrasted head CT shows a large amount of hyperintense signal, indicating acute subarachnoid blood in the basal cisterns. *(Continued)*

within minutes or hours (so-called sentinel or thunderclap headaches or "warning leaks"). Emergent evaluation of sentinel headaches is required since patients may experience a major SAH within 3 weeks.

Based on several factors, the clinician can categorize the severity of SAH to help predict outcome. The World Federation of Neurological Surgeons scale combines the score on the Glasgow Coma Scale and motor deficits to help prognosticate outcome, while the Head CT Grading Scale helps predict outcome based on the amount of SAH and presence or absence of intraventricular hemorrhage.

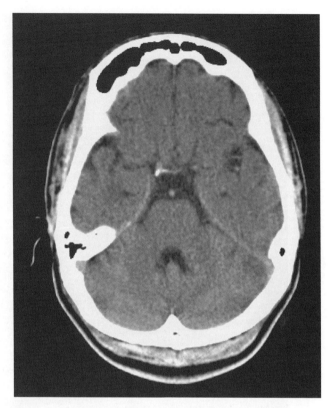

FIGURE 201.1. *(Continued)* This head CT is a normal study for comparison. Reproduced with permission, courtesy of David Preston, neuroradiology teaching file at University Hospitals of Cleveland.

WHAT TO DO

In patients with a clinical history suspicious for SAH and a negative head CT, a lumbar puncture should be done to assess for xanthochromia, a result of breakdown of red blood cells in the cerebrospinal fluid. Tubes 1 and 4 should be analyzed for cell count. This enables differentiation between an iatrogenic traumatic lumbar puncture, which produces elevated red blood cells in the first tube but not the last tube, versus a sustained red blood cell elevation, which is seen in true SAH.

Once the diagnosis of SAH is made, immediate steps should be taken to identify and secure ruptured aneurysms. The best initial diagnostic test is CT angiography, which is less invasive than standard digital subtraction angiography that requires invasive catheterization.

Once an aneurysm has been identified, it should be secured by either interventional neuroradiologic coiling or surgical clipping based on its intrinsic characteristics. This will help prevent rebleeding of the aneurysm, which carries a high mortality rate of 50%.

Once the aneurysm has been secured, the next step in the management of SAH patients is to monitor and treat the patients in the intensive care unit (ICU) setting. Common complications following aneurysmal SAH include symptomatic vasospasm (46%), hydrocephalus (20%), and rebleeding (7%). Other complications include seizures, deep venous thrombosis, pulmonary embolism, hyponatremia, neurogenic pulmonary edema, and metabolic and cardiac complications.

An immediate noncontrasted head CT should be done in any patient who develops mental status changes following SAH. This study will promptly diagnose rebleeding of the aneurysm, hydrocephalus, intraparenchymal hemorrhage, and/or cerebral edema.

The question may arise as to whether it is safe to use heparin or enoxaparin to prevent thromboembolic complications such as deep venous thrombosis and pulmonary embolism following SAH. A recent randomized double-blind study with 120 patients with aneurysmal SAH compared enoxaparin 20 mg subcutaneously daily versus placebo for 3 weeks after securing the aneurysm. The patients in the enoxaparin group had significantly lower incidence of cerebral vasospasm, cerebral infarction, and severe hydrocephalus. Furthermore, at 1-year follow-up, the patients who were treated with enoxaparin had improved overall outcome compared with placebo-treated patients. However, this conflicts with a previous randomized double-blind study of 170 patients with SAH that were treated with either enoxaparin 40 mg daily or placebo. In this study, there was no significant difference in long-term outcome (3 months) between the groups. Thus, it is still unclear whether or not anticoagulant agents should be used in SAH patients in the acute setting.

SUGGESTED READINGS

Siironen, J, Juvela S, Varis J, et al. No effect of enoxaparin on outcome of aneurysmal subarachnoid hemorrhage: a randomized, double-blind, placebo-controlled clinical trial. J Neurosurg. 2003;99(6):953–959.

Suarez JI, Tarr RW, Selman WR. Aneurysmal subarachnoid hemorrhage. N Engl J Med. 2006;354(4):387–396.

Wurm G, Tomancok B, Nussbaumer K, et al. Reduction of ischemic sequelae following spontaneous subarachnoid hemorrhage: a double-blind, randomized comparison of enoxaparin versus placebo. Clin Neurol Neurosurg. 2004;106(2):97–103.

202

BE ALERT FOR REBLEEDING IN PATIENTS WITH SUBARACHNOID HEMORRHAGE

NIRAV G. SHAH, MD

Subarachnoid hemorrhage (SAH) is a commonly misdiagnosed problem. Although SAH may produce minor symptoms (see *Table 202.1*), it is often fatal, and early surgical intervention can improve outcomes.

WATCH OUT FOR

The typical patient who develops a subarachnoid hemorrhage frequently has a positive personal or family history for SAH, a history of polycystic kidney disease, hypertension, alcohol abuse, or cigarette smoking. In addition, the incidence is more common in patients with heritable connective-tissue disease, especially fibromuscular dysplasia. A ruptured saccular aneurysm is the most common etiology of subarachnoid hemorrhage, followed by trauma, arteriovenous malformations, illicit drug use (especially cocaine), and vasculitides.

The most common presenting symptom of subarachnoid hemorrhage is headache of unusual severity. Patients typically describe their pain as "the worst headache of my life." Sometimes, the life-threatening bleed may be preceded by a small bleed and headache, which is called a sentinel headache. Other symptoms may include nuchal rigidity, diminished level of consciousness, aphasia, and bilateral weakness of the lower extremities. Signs that are apparent on physical examination include papilledema, third or sixth nerve palsy, nystagmus, left-side visual neglect, or retinal hemorrhage.

The most important study to obtain when suspecting a subarachnoid hemorrhage is a noncontrasted computed tomography (CT) scan of the head. Preferably, the study should be done with thin cuts about 3 mm in thickness in order to identify small collections of blood. The CT scan is most sensitive if obtained within 24 hours of the bleed. In one study, the percentage of positive scans went from 92% to 50% from day one to day seven. Of note is that if the underlying etiology of the subarachnoid bleed is a ruptured aneurysm, the location of blood on the CT scan does not accurately predict the location of the aneurysm. If the CT scan is negative but the clinical syndrome is still consistent with SAH, a lumbar puncture should be performed to identify blood in the cerebrospinal fluid.

TABLE 202.1	HUNT-HESS SCALE FOR GRADING SUBARACHNOID HEMORRHAGE
GRADE	NEUROLOGICAL STATUS
1	Asymptomatic; or minimal headache and slight nuchal rigidity
2	Moderate to severe headache; nuchal rigidity; no neurologic deficit except cranial nerve palsy
3	Drowsy; minimal neurologic deficit
4	Stuporous; moderate to severe hemiparesis; possible early decerebrate rigidity and vegetative disturbances
5	Deep coma; decerebrate rigidity; moribund appearance

WHAT TO DO

The treatment of subarachnoid hemorrhage includes active management of cerebral perfusion pressure, prophylaxis for vasospasm, anticonvulsive therapy to prevent seizures, and definitive therapy via surgery or endovascular repair. There is ongoing debate whether early surgery or endovascular repair portends a better prognosis compared with waiting 10 to 14 days for the improvement of edema prior to definitive therapy.

The three most common complications of subarachnoid hemorrhage are rebleeding, vasospasm, and hydrocephalus. Rebleeding is a significant risk in patients with an SAH and occurs with an incidence of approximately 3% to 6%. It most frequently occurs in the first 24 hours following a bleed with the highest risk in the first 6 hours. Rebleeding can present with altered mental status. Any changes in mental status after SAH warrants an emergent repeat CT scan. The factors that can most reliably predict the possibility of rebleeding are size of aneurysm and the Hunt-Hess Grade of the neurological status.

The second complication, vasospasm, is the leading cause of mortality in patients with ruptured aneurysms. The time of occurrence is usually between days three and seven but can be seen as far out as 14 days from subarachnoid hemorrhage. This should be suspected with any change in neurologic status or with any focal deficits. One method used to monitor for vasospasm is transcranial Doppler, which looks for changes in the velocity of blood flow as a precursor to actual symptomatic vasospasm. The risk of vasospasm is based on size of bleed, location, age, and neurologic status. Nimodipine, a calcium antagonist, has been used to significantly reduce the occurrence of vasospasm. Once vasospasm occurs after aneurysm clipping, treatment is optimized by use of the triple-H therapy, which includes hemodilution, induced hypertension, and hypervolemia.

Acute or chronic hydrocephalus is also a possible complication associated with subarachnoid hemorrhage. The etiology is thought to be secondary to occlusion of cerebrospinal fluid flow from debris or decreased cerebrospinal fluid production. Risk factors for the development of hydrocephalus include age at presentation, the location of the bleed, the size of the bleed, and concomitant intraventricular hemorrhage. The clinical presentation typically includes altered mental status with radiologic confirmation by CT scan. The treatment includes drainage of cerebrospinal fluid via ventriculostomy. Typically, about 50% of the patients with acute hydrocephalus have resolution of symptoms while the remaining patients have poorer outcomes with a high rate of mortality.

SUGGESTED READINGS

Edlow JA, Caplan LR. Avoiding pitfalls in the diagnosis of subarachnoid hemorrhage. N Engl J Med. 2000;342:29–36.
van Gijn J. Subarachnoid hemorrhage. Lancet. 1992;339:653.

203

REMEMBER THAT NEW ELECTROCARDIOGRAM CHANGES IN A PATIENT WITH A SUBARACHNOID BLEED MAY BE A SIGN OF PROGRESSION OF THE BLEED

AMISHA BAROCHIA, MD

Loss of consciousness is a common clinical occurrence in subarachnoid hemorrhage. However, the sudden death seen in these patients is thought to be the result of cardiac rhythm disturbances. Although the exact pathophysiology is unknown, there appears to be an imbalance in the autonomic nervous system, which leads to a catecholamine surge, changes in repolarization and depolarization, and subsequent ectopic foci. Hypokalemia secondary to increased circulating catecholamines, vomiting, and hypercortisolism may also contribute to the development of arrhythmias associated with a subarachnoid bleed.

WATCH OUT FOR

The most frequently observed electrocardiogram (ECG) changes in patients with subarachnoid bleeds include T wave inversions, ST-segment elevations or depressions, Q waves, U waves >0.1 mV, and QT prolongation. ECG changes secondary to subarachnoid bleeds may even mimic the changes seen in acute myocardial infarction. However, even though these latter changes may be associated with abnormal thallium perfusion scans in up to one-third of patients, they are not generally indicative of underlying myocardial ischemia. When autopsy specimens from patients with these ECG changes are examined, there is no correlation with the presence of coronary artery disease and the myocardium is intact on microscopic examination. ECG changes usually associated with a poor prognosis include pathologic Q waves, raised ST segments, P mitrale, QT prolongation >450 milliseconds, and tachycardia. However, one recent study did not find a relationship between the type or location of ECG change and mortality.

ECG changes are usually seen in the first 72 hours after a subarachnoid hemorrhage and usually resolve in a few days, but occasionally may persist for 4 to 8 weeks. If the patient rebleeds, the same ECG changes that occurred with the first episode are usually observed. Transient cardiac arrhythmias have been noted in >90% of patients in the acute phase of subarachnoid hemorrhage on Holter monitoring. The arrhythmia types include ventricular tachycardia, ventricular flutter, and *torsades de pointes*. There is no association between the patient's clinical condition and the occurrence of these arrhythmias, except that those patients who experienced arrhythmias tend to be older and have lower potassium levels. The severity, type, and lesion location generally do not correlate with the development of an arrhythmia.

In addition to ECG changes, echocardiographic changes have been noted in patients with subarachnoid bleed that have no relation to ECG changes in the same patient. Global or segmental wall motion abnormalities have been reported and are thought to be due to stunned myocardium, since the changes were found to be reversible. Unlike ECG abnormalities, echocardiogram findings do correspond to the degree of neurologic changes.

One final note is that is advisable to have patients with subarachnoid hemorrhage on continuous telemetry monitoring so that arrhythmias are detected and promptly treated, which can be lifesaving for the patient.

SUGGESTED READINGS

De Oliveira JJ, Silva SR. Signs of myocardial ischemia associated with subarachnoid bleed. Arq Bras Cardio. 1996;67(6):403–406.

Manninen PH, Ayra B, Gel B, et al. Association between electrocardiographic abnormalities and intracranial blood in patients following acute subarachnoid hemorrhage. J Neurosurg Anesthesiol. 1995;7(1):12–16.

204

CONSIDER THE USE OF THROMBOLYTIC AGENTS FOR TREATMENT OF ACUTE ISCHEMIC STROKE

NIRAV G. SHAH, MD

Acute ischemic stroke is the third leading cause of mortality in the United States and, when not fatal, can result in significant morbidity. The most effective way to decrease morbidity is to restore the blood flow to the ischemic area in a timely manner with thrombolytic therapy. Upon presentation to an emergency room, standard procedures such as establishing medical stability, obtaining a thorough history, and performing a physical examination and laboratory testing should be undertaken immediately. A quick diagnosis in the setting of ischemic stroke is associated with a reduction in morbidity. Following these measures, a computed tomography (CT) scan must be performed to differentiate between subarachnoid hemorrhage, intracerebral hemorrhage, and ischemic infarction. Other studies that may need to be performed based on the history of illness include lumbar puncture (encephalitis, subarachnoid hemorrhage), arterial blood gas (hypoxemia), cervical spine x-rays (trauma), magnetic resonance imaging (better anatomic definition), and cerebral arteriography (if considering intra-arterial thrombolysis).

WHAT TO DO

The indication for intravenous thrombolysis in the setting of acute ischemic stroke is predicated on the presentation and diagnosis occurring within 3 hours of symptom onset. The mortality benefit was demonstrated by the National Institute of Neurological Disorders and Stroke Recombinant Tissue Plasminogen Activator (tPA) Stroke Study. Tissue-type plasminogen activator is contraindicated in many patients including those with stroke or head trauma in the previous 3 months, a history of myocardial infarction in the previous 3 months, a history of gastrointestinal bleeding in the previous 3 weeks, and a major surgical procedure in the previous 2 weeks (although surgery is not an absolute contraindication). In addition, patients with thrombocytopenia or coagulopathy should be excluded from use of thrombolytic agents. Blood pressure must also be assessed. Patients with a blood pressure greater than 185/110 mm Hg should not receive tPA. The patient can receive a dose of intravenous (IV) 20 mg of labetotol times 2 doses given 10 minutes apart. If the blood pressure decreases below

185/110 mm Hg and remains, the patient can be considered for tPA. The overall benefit demonstrated by use of tPA was significant with close to 50% of patients having complete or near-complete recovery at 3 months and 1 year as compared with less than 30% in the group treated with placebo.

WATCH OUT FOR

While the use of tPA demonstrated a mortality benefit, there is also significant risk associated with it. The most significant risk is that of intracerebral hemorrhage, which occurred in approximately 6% of patients enrolled in the tPA trials. The risk of intracerebral hemorrhage is increased with CT-scan demonstration of mass effect prior to the use of thrombolytics, severity of neurologic status, age, and comorbidities including diabetes, thrombocytopenia, and cardiac disease. Other complications of tPA include systemic bleeding and angioedema (usually mild).

Thrombolytic therapy can also be provided through an intra-arterial method, almost always in conjunction with experienced neurointerventional radiology physicians. The agents that have been investigated are urokinase, tPA, and prourokinase. These agents demonstrated benefit with 75% of patients achieving total or partial recanalization of the occluded vessel. Intra-arterial thrombolytic therapy is administered on an incremental basis until the thrombus has resolved. The rate of complication of intracerebral hemorrhage is lower for intra-arterial than for intravenous administration of the agent. The risk factors associated with this complication were hyperglycemia, more severe neurologic status, lower platelet counts, and longer time to recanalization. Additional studies are being performed to evaluate the combined use of intravenous and intra-arterial thrombolytics in order to optimize the benefits of both.

SUGGESTED READINGS

Brott T, Bogousslavsky J. Treatment of acute ischemic stroke. N Engl J Med. 2000;343:710–722.

The National Institute of Neurological Disorders and Stroke rt-PA Stroke Study Group. Tissue plasminogen activator for acute ischemic stroke. N Engl J Med. 1995;333:1581.

205

CONSIDER ABSENCE OF WITHDRAWAL TO PAIN AT 24 HOURS AND ABSENCE OF EYE REFLEXES AT 72 HOURS POST–CARDIAC ARREST TO BE HIGHLY CORRELATED WITH PERMANENT COMA

AMISHA BAROCHIA, MD

Neurologic recovery after cardiac arrest occurs in only a small number of patients. One of the biggest challenges in the intensive care unit (ICU) is prognosticating outcomes in comatose patients and optimizing treatment decisions when a patient survives a cardiac arrest. The physical examination can help greatly in predicting death or poor outcome in comatose survivors of cardiac arrest.

When a cardiac arrest occurs, there is cessation of flow to the brain and other organs. The oxygen stores of the brain last for only approximately 20 seconds after arrest and the glucose and adenosine triphosphate (ATP) stores in the brain last less than 5 minutes. Neuronal death occurs after arrest and, depending on the extent, can result in a coma. During effective cardiopulmonary resuscitation, flow is restored, but it is almost always abnormal (e.g., a low flow state). With a shorter duration of arrest and resuscitation, the damage due to ischemic injury and hypoperfusion is expected to be less. When spontaneous circulation is restored, there is a brief period of cerebral hyperemia, followed by vasospasm and prolonged hypoperfusion.

The overall rate of a poor outcome in patients surviving a cardiac arrest who are comatose is approximately 77%. Poor outcomes were defined as severe cerebral disability, coma, vegetative state, or death (Glasgow-Pittsburgh Cerebral Performance Categories 3 through 5). Clinical exam findings can assist in determining the prognosis of comatose survivors of cardiac arrest. Decisions to withdraw care should not be made on the basis of these findings alone, but this information is often useful in helping the family make decisions about further care. The physical exam findings that were found to be most helpful in predicting poor outcome were related to motor and brain-stem function. The precision of the neurologic exam in predicting outcomes was found to be only moderately to substantially helpful. The positive likelihood ratios (LR) of various physical exam findings in predicting poor outcome are listed in *Table 205.1*.

Therefore, the absence of the pupillary and corneal reflexes at 24 hours and the absence of a motor response at 72 hours make it

TABLE 205.1	POSITIVE LIKELIHOOD RATIOS
AT TIME OF COMA ONSET	
Absent withdrawal to pain	LR 1.7
AT 24 HOURS	
Absent withdrawal to pain	LR 4.7
Absent pupillary response	LR 10.2
Absent motor response	LR 4.9
Absent corneal reflex	LR 12.9
AT 72 HOURS	
Absent pupillary response	LR 3.4
Absent motor response	LR 9.2
Seizure or myoclonus	LR 1.4

extremely likely that the patient will have a poor outcome. Levy et al., in an older study, found that none of the 210 patients who had all three of these findings ever regained an independent lifestyle. Although many clinicians believe that seizures or myoclonus portends a poor prognosis, this does not appear to be supported by the recent literature.

Finally, neuroprotective strategies for survivors of cardiac arrest hospitalized in the ICU include maintenance of cerebral perfusion and normoglycemia, control of seizures, and preventing hyperthermia. With regard to the latter, an elevation of 1° C leads to a 10% increase in brain oxygen consumption. Therefore, the avoidance of hyperthermia either by treating fever promptly or inducing mild hypothermia is felt to be beneficial.

SUGGESTED READINGS

Fischer C, Luaute J, Nemoz C, et al. Improved prediction of awakening or nonawakening form severe anoxic coma using tree-based classification analysis. Crit Care Med. 2006;34(5):1520–1524.

Koenig MA, Kaplan PW, Thakor NV. Clinical neurophysiological monitoring and brain injury from cardiac arrest. Neurol Clin. 2006;24(1):89–106.

Levy DE, Coronna JJ, Singer BH, Lapinski RH, et al. Predicting outcome from hypertoxic-ischamic coma. JAMA. 1985:253(10):1420–1426.

206

REMEMBER THAT FAILURE TO RECOGNIZE PITUITARY APOPLEXY CAN RESULT IN A NEUROLOGIC CATASTROPHE

ERIC M. BERSHAD, MD
JOSE I. SUAREZ, MD

Pituitary apoplexy refers to a clinical syndrome of abrupt severe headache, visual loss, ophthalmoplegia, and altered mental status due to hemorrhage or infarction within the pituitary gland, usually into an underlying pituitary adenoma.

CLINICAL SIGNS AND SYMPTOMS

In pituitary apoplexy, headache is universal and usually occurs abruptly and is severe in intensity. Meningeal signs including stiff neck, nausea, and vomiting may be present because of blood entering the subarachnoid space. Deterioration of visual fields is common because of compression of the proximate optic chiasm. The compression of crossed nasal retinal fibers, which represents the temporal visual fields, produces a characteristic bitemporal hemianopia. The proximity of the pituitary gland to the cavernous sinuses may result in opthalmoparesis and diplopia due to dysfunction of the third, fourth, and sixth cranial nerves and a Horner syndrome, ptosis, and miosis due to compression of the sympathetic plexus within the cavernous sinus. Some patients will complain of facial pain or altered sensation, which is related to trigeminal nerve compression. Hypotension may occur because of deficiency of adrenocorticotropic hormone (ACTH).

PRECIPITATING FACTORS

Pituitary apoplexy usually occurs without any specific provoking factor. Most patients are found to have an underlying pituitary adenoma. Several proposed pathophysiological mechanisms that may trigger the apoplectic event include (a) reduced blood flow in the pituitary gland related to either systemic hypoperfusion or transient elevated intracranial pressure; (b) acute increased blood flow; (c) stimulation of the pituitary gland by exogenous or endogenous sources; and (d) coagulopathic conditions. Some of the common clinical scenarios in which the previous conditions occur include surgical or procedural interventions, pregnancy, and acute systemic illnesses.

DIAGNOSIS

A magnetic resonance imaging (MRI) of the brain is the diagnostic modality of choice (see *Fig. 206.1*). This will usually show a pituitary adenoma with heterogeneous blood products within the suprasellar mass. Extension of blood and edema to surrounding tissue may be visualized. Noncontrasted computed tomography (CT) head scan has poor resolution compared with MRI in delineating the suprasellar contents but may be considered in some patients. A lumbar puncture is not sensitive or specific for pituitary apoplexy but may be useful in demonstrating subarachnoid blood if one suspects aneurysmal subarachnoid hemorrhage.

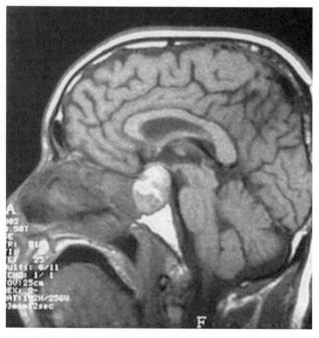

FIGURE 206.1. MRI of the brain showing hemorrhage into a pituitary adenoma (*arrow*). Unenhanced sagittal T1-weighted MRI demonstrating heterogeneous areas of high-intensity signals mixed with regions of lower signals, indicating subacute hemorrhage within a pituitary lesion. Reproduced from Verrees, M, Arafah B, Selman W. Pituitary tumor apoplexy: characteristics, treatment and outcomes. Neurosurg Focus. 2004;16(4) E6.

TREATMENT

Emergent neurosurgical consultation for definitive surgical treatment is mandatory. This will allow for prompt decompression of the pituitary gland and surrounding structures, thus salvaging visual and oculomotor function. Surgical resection via the transsphenoidal route is usually sufficient, although occasionally an intracranial route may be necessary. Endocrinologic disturbances occur frequently after pituitary apoplexy; thus comprehensive assessment of pituitary axis should be performed with the consultation of an endocrinologist. Intravenous hydrocortisone should be given immediately after the diagnosis of pituitary apoplexy has been made, as some patients develop adrenal crisis because of severe dysfunction of the pituitary gland.

PROGNOSIS

With expeditious neurosurgical intervention, most patients have excellent outcome. In one series of 37 patients, ocular paresis, visual field defects, and visual acuity resolved in 100%, 95%, and 88% of patients, respectively, after surgical intervention. In the same series, however, persistent hormonal disturbances occurred in the majority of patients. The most common deficiencies included growth hormone (88%), luteinizing hormone (76%), prolactin (67%), adrenocorticotropic hormone (66%), and estradiol (33%). Diabetes insipidus occurred in only 2% to 3% of the patients.

SUGGESTED READINGS

Biousse V, Newman NJ, Oyesiku NM. Precipitating factors in pituitary apoplexy. J Neurol Neurosurg Psychiatry. 2001;71(4):542–545.

Bradley W, ed. Neurology in Clinical Practice. Philadelphia: Butterworth-Heinemann; 2004:858–859.

Verrees M, Arafah BM, Selman WR. Pituitary tumor apoplexy: characteristics, treatment and outcomes. Neurosurg Focus. 2004;16(4):E6.

207

DO NOT PERFORM A LUMBAR PUNCTURE ON PATIENTS WITH POSTERIOR FOSSA MASSES

JOSE I. SUAREZ, MD

ANATOMY

The posterior fossa represents the area of the cranial vault located below the tentorium cerebella. The latter arises from the superior crest of the petrous portion of the temporal bone and roofs over the posterior fossa. The cerebellum overlies the posterior aspect of the brain stem and extends laterally under the tentorium to fill most of the posterior fossa. The most caudal aspect of the posterior fossa is the foramen magnum, through which the medulla exits the cranium and becomes the spinal cord.

TYPES OF LESIONS AND CLINICAL PRESENTATION

Mass lesions located in the posterior fossa mainly represent neoplasms, vascular lesions such as vascular malformations, and ischemic strokes with edema. Such mass lesions are classified according to their location within the posterior fossa (*Table 207.1*). The main areas where such lesions are found include the parenchyma (cerebellum and brain stem), the cerebellopontine angle, the fourth ventricle, and the foramen magnum. Because of the small anatomical space, these lesions can easily impinge upon the ventricular system (e.g., the fourth ventricle) and lead to obstructive hydrocephalus. Patients may present with headache, nausea, and vomiting, followed by altered sensorium. Posterior fossa lesions can also compress the brain stem, leading to various syndromes with multiple cranial nerve involvement with serious respiratory and cardiovascular consequences. Another important issue that needs to be recognized is that any occupying space in the posterior fossa has the potential to lead to cerebellar tonsillar herniation. The cerebellar tonsils are located in the most caudal and inferior aspect of the posterior lobe of the cerebellum. It can be easily appreciated that should there be tonsillar herniation, the foramen magnum becomes occluded and the cervicomedullary junction compressed. Respiratory failure and arrest with circulatory collapse ensues. Lastly, lesions that compress the upper brain stem may lead to the so-called upward herniation of the midbrain and the anterior cerebellar lobe clinically manifested by coma, hyperventilation, fixed pupils, and vertical gaze paralysis.

TABLE 207.1	TYPES OF POSTERIOR FOSSA MASS LESIONS ACCORDING TO ANATOMICAL LOCATION IN ADULTS
Intraventricular masses (fourth ventricle)	Metastasis Choroid plexus papilloma Subependymoma Dermoid/epidermoid tumors Hemangioblastoma
Cerebellopontine angle masses	Acoustic neuroma Meningioma Vascular ectasia/aneurysms Epidermoid tumors Metastasis
Intra-axial masses (brain stem and cerebellum)	Ischemic stroke with mass effect Intracranial hemorrhage Vascular malformation Metastasis Hemangioblastoma Exophytic glioma
Foramen magnum masses	Gliomas Fourth ventricular tumors (see above) Metastasis Hemangioblastoma

LUMBAR PUNCTURE IN PATIENTS WITH POSTERIOR FOSSA MASSES

Performing a lumbar puncture in patients with known or suspected posterior fossa masses is very risky. Lumbar puncture will upset the delicate balance between parenchyma, mass, cerebrospinal fluid (CSF), and blood volume and may precipitate herniation with disastrous consequences. Practitioners should refrain from performing a lumbar puncture under these circumstances. In those instances where obtaining CSF may be necessary (e.g., meningitis), direct sampling of the ventricular system is preferred. Many of these patients will require external ventricular drainage (most likely in the lateral ventricles) to alleviate hydrocephalus, facilitating CSF recovery. It is also important to realize that patients who undergo such external ventricular drainage may experience upward herniation if the posterior fossa pressure is elevated. Therefore, close neurologic monitoring of these patients is required.

SUGGESTED READINGS

Brazis PW, Masdeu JC, Biller J, eds. Localization in Clinical Neurology. 3rd ed. Boston: Little, Brown and Company; 1996:565–595.

Carpenter MB, ed. Core Text of Neuroanatomy. 4th ed. Baltimore: Williams & Wilkins; 1991:1,42–56.

Osborne AG, ed. Diagnostic Neuroradiology. St. Louis: Mosby; 1994:401–528.

208

EVALUATE FOR GUILLAIN-BARRÉ SYNDROME IN PATIENTS WITH ACUTE PARALYSIS OR RESPIRATORY FAILURE AND AREFLEXIA

JOSE I. SUAREZ, MD

Guillain-Barré syndrome (GBS) represents the most common cause of acute flaccid paralysis in otherwise healthy adults in the United States. GBS is more frequent in men as compared with women of all ages. There is a slight increase in the incidence of GBS in younger adults and in those older than 50 years of age.

Most patients will complain of a flulike illness about 1 to 3 weeks prior to initiation of symptoms. Other possible factors that may be associated with Guillain-Barré syndrome include infectious agents such as *Campylobacter jejuni*, Cytomegalovirus, Epstein-Barr virus, influenza virus, and human immunodeficiency virus; recent surgery; immunization; and systemic illnesses such as Hodgkin's disease and systemic lupus erythematosus. How these factors trigger or lead to Guillain-Barré syndrome is still unclear. However, mounting basic and clinical evidence supports an immune-mediated attack on the peripheral nervous system. Pathologic evaluation of peripheral nerves of GBS patients reveals perivascular infiltration by mononuclear cells along with demyelination and axonal loss.

CLINICAL PRESENTATION

The major clinical symptoms and signs include progressive limb weakness and areflexia (*Table 208.1*). Such weakness usually presents over a period of several hours to days. About half of patients will have ascending involvement of lower extremities followed by upper extremities. However, a variant presenting with descending paralysis starting in cranial nerves or upper limbs can be seen in about 14% of cases. Limb weakness does not usually progress beyond 4 weeks and half of the patients experience a nadir within 2 weeks. Frequently patients complain of limb paresthesias and dysesthesias concomitantly or preceding limb weakness that is sometimes accompanied by lower back pain. On physical examination practitioners encounter *areflexia* or *severely decreased myotatic reflexes* and usually symmetric limb weakness involving both distal and proximal muscles. On exam, the most common cranial nerves involved are facial, glossopharyngeal, and vagus nerves. Thus patients will have facial weakness (usually bilateral) and oropharyngeal

TABLE 208.1	DIAGNOSTIC CRITERIA FOR GUILLAIN-BARRÉ SYNDROME
FEATURES REQUIRED FOR THE DIAGNOSIS	Progressive motor weakness of more than one limb Areflexia

FEATURES STRONGLY SUPPORTIVE OF THE DIAGNOSIS

Clinical features	Symptoms and signs of motor weakness develop rapidly and cease to progress 4 weeks into the illness Symmetry is seldom absolute Mild sensory symptoms or signs Cranial nerve involvement (most common is facial nerve) Recovery usually begins 2 to 4 weeks after progression stops Presence of autonomic dysfunction Absence of fever at the onset of symptoms
Cerebrospinal fluid features	After the first week of symptoms, cerebrospinal fluid protein is elevated or has been shown to rise on serial lumbar punctures Counts of ≤ 10 leukocytes/mm^3
Electrodiagnostic features	Evidence of nerve conduction slowing or block at some point during the illness Distal latencies may be increased to as much as three times normal Conduction studies may not become abnormal until several weeks into the illness
Features casting doubt on the diagnosis	Marked, persistent asymmetry of weakness Persistent bladder or bowel dysfunction Bladder or bowel dysfunction at onset >50 mononuclear leukocytes/mm^3 in cerebrospinal fluid Presence of polymorphonuclear cells in cerebrospinal fluid Sharp sensory level
Features that rule out the diagnosis	Diagnosis of botulism, myasthenia, poliomyelitis, or toxic neuropathy Abnormal porphyrin metabolism Recent diphtheria infection Occurrence of purely sensory syndrome

From Asbury AK, Cornblath DR. Assessment of current diagnostic criteria for Guillain-Barré syndrome. Ann Neurol. 1990;27:S21–S24.

dysfunction manifested by dysphagia and dysarthria. Compromise of the cranial nerves innervating the extraocular muscles (i.e., III, IV, and VI cranial nerves) is less common and is usually part of a Guillain-Barré syndrome variant also known as Miller Fisher variant. The latter can present with ophthalmoparesis or ophthalmoplegia and areflexia followed by respiratory failure. The progression and severity of GBS are variable with 33% of patients requiring mechanical ventilation.

DIAGNOSIS

Suspicion of Guillain-Barré syndrome should be based on the clinical presentation and supported by cerebrospinal fluid and electromyographic findings (*Table 208.1*). All patients with suspected GBS require a lumbar puncture and an electromyogram (EMG). Both of these tests can help confirm the diagnosis or make the clinician suspect other conditions that can mimic GBS (*Tables 208.1 and 208.2*). Accurate diagnosis is important for effective treatment to be initiated promptly.

TABLE 208.2	DIFFERENTIAL DIAGNOSIS OF GUILLAIN-BARRÉ SYNDROME
CONDITION	**KEY PRESENTING CLINICAL FEATURES**
Acute intermittent porphyria	Asymmetric limb weakness progressing to quadriplegia after several attacks
Botulism	Nausea and vomiting preceding muscle weakness. Blurred vision, dysphagia, dysarthria, descending muscle paralysis, dilated pupils, dry mouth, constipation, and urinary retention
Critical illness myopathy	Patient with chronic obstructive pulmonary disease or asthma requiring mechanical ventilation and use of neuromuscular blockers and corticosteroids
Critical illness polyneuropathy	Patient with sepsis and difficulty weaning from the ventilator, diminished or absent reflexes
Electrolyte imbalance	Generalized muscle weakness, cardiac arrhythmias with or without rhabdomyolysis
Lambert-Eaton myasthenic syndrome	Symmetric proximal muscle weakness, hypoactive or absent deep tendon reflexes, dry mouth, blurred vision, orthostatic hypotension
Lead poisoning	Pure motor weakness, initially of extensors muscles, fasciculations, abdominal pain, constipation, anemia, renal failure
Motor neuron disease	Weakness, wasting, fasciculations
Myasthenia gravis	Fatigue worse toward the end of the day, fluctuating symptoms and signs, no sensory complaints
Organophosphate poisoning	Exposure to insecticides, petroleum additives, and modifiers of plastics followed by acute cholinergic crisis (muscle weakness, miosis, abdominal cramping)
Polymyositis	Proximal, symmetrical muscle weakness, elevated creatine kinase
Prolonged neuromuscular blocking	Patient with impaired renal or hepatic failure who had been on continuous neuromuscular blocking agents

TREATMENT

Management of the Guillain-Barré syndrome patient will depend on the severity and the rate of disease progression. In those patients with mild and nonprogressing symptoms, no specific treatment is necessary. However, in those patients with more severe compromise, admission to the intensive care unit (ICU) is indicated to evaluate respiratory status and to monitor for dysautonomia. Several randomized controlled clinical trials have supported the use of plamapheresis (200 to 250 mL of plasma/kg body weight for a total of 5 sessions) or immunoglobulin administration (400 mg/kg/d intravenous immunoglobulin [IVIg] for 5 days). Treatment should be initiated within 2 weeks of symptom onset to maximize response. Patients should also receive other supportive treatments such as mechanical ventilation (usually intubation is required when vital capacity is <15 cm^3/kg) and gastrointestinal and deep venous thrombosis prophylaxis. Dysautonomia manifested as intermittent episodes of bradycardia, tachycardia, and hypo- or hypertension may be severe and lead to death.

PROGNOSIS

Most patients recover satisfactorily over a period of weeks to months after initial presentation. Approximately 10% of patients are left with significant disability due to motor weakness. It should be noted that patients who require mechanical ventilation but are treated with plasmapheresis or IVIg within 2 weeks of symptom initiation are weaned off mechanical ventilation earlier than patients whose treatment was delayed, thus minimizing ventilator complications in the early-treatment group.

SUGGESTED READINGS

Asbury AK, Cornblath DR. Assessment of current diagnostic criteria for Guillain-Barré syndrome. Ann Neurol. 1990;27:S21–S24.

Ropper AH. The Guillain-Barré syndrome. N Engl J Med. 1992;326:1130–1136.

Suarez JI, ed. Critical Care Neurology and Neurosurgery. Totowa, NJ: Humana Press; 2004:481–492.

van der Merche FG, Schmitz PI. A randomized trial comparing intravenous immunoglobulin and plasma exchange in Guillain-Barré syndrome. N Engl J Med. 1992;326:1123–1129.

209

START EARLY PLASMAPHERESIS OR IMMUNOGLOBULINS IN GUILLAIN-BARRÉ PATIENTS

JOSE I. SUAREZ, MD

Guillain-Barré syndrome (GBS) is an acute inflammatory disease of the peripheral nervous system that is usually characterized by ascending paralysis with a paucity of objective sensory findings. The progression and severity of the disease vary. However, many patients will require intensive care within the first few days of presentation and about one-third of them will need mechanical ventilation.

WHAT TO DO

There are currently two therapeutic modalities recommended for GBS: plasma exchange and immunoglobulin administration (IVIg). The decision to treat GBS patients depends on the severity of the disease, rate of progression of symptoms, and duration of symptoms to time of presentation. Patients with mild symptoms (e.g., mild sensory complaints and very distal motor involvement) may need to be treated with supportive care alone. Patients who present within 2 weeks of onset of symptoms may require treatment. Patients presenting beyond 2 weeks should probably also be treated, but the evidence is less convincing.

Plasma exchange has been available longer than IVIg for GBS and the only one compared with conventional therapy. Statistically significant differences, favoring the plasma-exchange-treated group, were found in terms of improvement to 4 weeks, time to independent walking, and outcome at 6 months. Plasma exchange is particularly efficacious in those patients presenting within 7 days of symptom onset and in those requiring mechanical ventilation. One of the main disadvantages of plasma exchange is its availability (*Table 209.1*). Not all centers are well equipped and experienced to perform plasma exchange in all patients with GBS. About 10% of patients may experience recurrent symptoms within 1 to 2 weeks after treatment with plasma exchange. This may be because of a rebound production of antibodies. Further treatments with plasma exchange improve symptoms. The recommended amount of plasma exchange is 200 to 250 mL/kg of body weight every other day for a total of five treatments.

IVIg has never been compared with placebo. However, IVIg has been compared with plasma exchange in adequate randomized,

TABLE 209.1	ADVANTAGES AND DISADVANTAGES OF PLASMA EXCHANGE AND IVIg	
TREATMENT	ADVANTAGES	DISADVANTAGES
Plasmapheresis	Efficacious compared with placebo	Available in specialized centers; central-line-related complications; hypotension; coagulopathy; mild thrombocytopenia
Immunoglobulin therapy	Easily given (intravenously)	More expensive; headaches; fever; myalgias; anaphylactic reactions (especially IgA-deficient patients); hypercoagulable and hyperviscosity syndrome

controlled clinical trials. Such trials have shown that in patients with severe GBS, IVIg started within 2 weeks of symptom onset hastens recovery as much as plasma exchange. Also treatment with IVIg is more likely to be completed than plasma exchange. One great advantage is its ease of administration and potentially broader availability. IVIg appears to be superior to plasma exchange in those GBS patients who are serum IgG anti-GM1 positive. The recommended dose of IVIg is 400 mg/kg/day for 5 days.

WHAT NOT TO DO

The use of combination therapy (i.e., plasma exchange followed by IVIg) was advocated in the past. However, one randomized, controlled trial investigated the efficacy of plasma exchange alone, IVIg alone, and combination therapy within 2 weeks of symptom onset. The study showed that the combination of plasma exchange with IVIg did not confer significant advantage over each treatment alone. Currently combination therapy cannot be recommended.

SUGGESTED READINGS

Hughes RA, Raphael JC, Swan AV, et al. Intravenous immunoglobulin for Guillain-Barré syndrome. Cochrane Database Syst Rev. 2006;(1):CD002063.

Kuwabara S, Mori M, Ogawara K, et al. Intravenous immunoglobulin therapy for Guillain-Barré syndrome with IgG anti-GM1 antibody. Muscle Nerve. 2001;24:54–58.

Plasma Exchange/Sandoglobulin Guillain-Barré Syndrome Trial Group. Randomised trial of plasma exchange, intravenous immunoglobulin, and combined treatments in Guillain-Barré syndrome. Lancet. 1997;349:225–230.

The Guillain-Barré Syndrome Study Group. Plasmapheresis and acute Guillain-Barré syndrome. Neurology. 1985;35:1096–1104.

Van der Meche FG, Schmitz PI. A randomized trial comparing intravenous immunoglobulin and plasma exchange in Guillain-Barré syndrome. Dutch Guillain-Barré Study Group. N Engl J Med. 1992;326:1123–1129.

210

REMEMBER THAT PATIENTS WITH MYASTHENIA GRAVIS EXACERBATION USUALLY LOOK WELL UNTIL JUST BEFORE THEY REQUIRE INTUBATION

ELIAHU S. FEEN, MD
JOSE I. SUAREZ, MD

Myasthenia gravis is an autoimmune disease in which a patient primarily forms autoantibodies to the acetylcholine receptors on the postsynaptic membrane in the neuromuscular junction. Other kinds of autoantibodies also may play a role. In general for myasthenia gravis, the postsynaptic muscle membrane is distorted and the concentration of acetylcholine receptor proteins is reduced. As a result, the neurotransmitter acetylcholine released from the presynaptic nerve terminal—although it is released in normal concentration—has a muted effect. The muscle weakness that results can take several forms. In ocular myasthenia gravis, the weakness affects the extraocular muscles, with findings of diplopia and ptosis. In both bulbar myasthenia gravis (affecting primarily the bulbar muscles) and in generalized myasthenia gravis (affecting primarily the limb muscles), respiratory muscle involvement is common. Myasthenic crisis represents the exacerbation of myasthenia gravis to the point of requiring mechanical ventilation.

FACTORS CONTRIBUTING TO MECHANICAL VENTILATION

Many myasthenia gravis patients will complain of dyspnea frequently, especially with exertion. Exacerbations of myasthenia gravis present with two important risk factors for respiratory compromise. The first is that the muscle weakness impairs diaphragmatic accessory respiratory muscle function. As a result breaths are shallow. Consequently, to maintain adequate oxygenation, the respiratory rate climbs, which further exacerbates muscle fatigue. The shallow breaths also limit tidal volume, which impairs gas exchange. The second mechanism is that with pharyngeal dysfunction, the risk of aspiration rises. The development of aspiration pneumonia will further compromise both oxygenation and gas exchange because of shunting. The ominous danger of this situation is emergent respiratory failure. Once a patient develops extreme muscle fatigue, respirations will very rapidly become insufficient to maintain oxygenation. The accumulation of carbon dioxide

(CO_2) due to progressively inadequate gas exchange will cause hypercarbic respiratory failure. Careful monitoring of myasthenia gravis patients is necessary in order to avoid an emergent intubation as well as to avoid the complications of emergent respiratory failure and hypercarbia (such as hypoxia, hypotension, acidosis, and arrhythmias). As a myasthenia gravis patient shows signs of respiratory compromise, closer monitoring becomes essential. If such patients are not yet in an intensive care setting, it is necessary to place them in one.

BEDSIDE EVALUATION AND INDICATIONS FOR MECHANICAL VENTILATION

The most common bedside tests of respiratory strength are the measurement of vital capacity (VC) and negative inspiratory force (NIF). In normal adults VC is greater than 60 mL/kg, and the absolute value of the NIF is greater than 70 cm H_2O. Adults on the verge of intubation due to acute respiratory failure have a VC of about 15 to 20 mL/kg and an absolute value of NIF less than 20 cm H_2O. Myasthenia gravis patients should have their VC and NIF checked at least every 6 hours. A progression of these bedside pulmonary tests toward dangerously low levels may warrant intensive care unit (ICU) monitoring. In addition there is some evidence that myasthenia gravis patients with an abnormality on chest x-ray (such as an infiltrate, effusion, or atelectasis) are at higher risk than other patients of requiring intubation during their hospital course and should therefore be admitted directly to an ICU for close monitoring. It is important to remember that arterial oxygenation may remain high up to the point of respiratory collapse because of the pulmonary physiology of myasthenia gravis. Therefore, pulse oximetry and arterial blood gases may not be of help when deciding the need for intubation. Rather, a VC ≤ 15 mL/kg and NIF ≤ 20 cm H_2O should be used to intubate myasthenia gravis patients semielectively.

MANAGEMENT

Treatment of myasthenia gravis exacerbations acutely involves aggressive immunotherapy in the form of intravenous immunoglobulin (IVIg) or plasmapheresis. High-dose steroids are used by many clinicians acutely to improve the condition of patients. Cholinesterase inhibitors, while useful as chronic therapy for symptomatic relief, can be troublesome in the case of exacerbations where there is a concern for respiratory compromise. Many patients suffer side effects from these medications in the form of increased secretions. As a result this can further exacerbate respiratory difficulties. Additionally, while patients certainly need pulmonary toilet, incentive spirometers are not appropriate because this can fatigue patients, with a risk of expediting respiratory compromise that outweighs any benefit.

SUGGESTED READINGS

Mayer SA. Intensive care of the myasthenic patient. Neurology. 1997;48(Suppl): S70–S75.

Qureshi AI, Choudry MA, Akbar MS, et al. Plasma exchange versus intravenous immunoglobulin treatment in myasthenic crisis. Neurology. 1999;52:629–632.

Suarez JI, ed. Critical Care Neurology and Neurosurgery. Totowa, NJ: Humana Press; 2004.

Thomas CE, Mayer SA, Gungor Y, et al. Myasthenic crisis: clinical features, mortality, complications, and risk factors for prolonged intubation. Neurology. 1997;48:1253–1260.

211

AVOID USING INCENTIVE SPIROMETRY IN MYASTHENIA GRAVIS PATIENTS; USE INTRAPULMONARY PERCUSSIVE VENTILATION (IPPV) OR FLUTTER VALVE INSTEAD

ERIC M. BERSHAD, MD
JOSE I. SUAREZ, MD

WATCH OUT FOR

Myasthenia gravis is an autoimmune disease characterized by failure of neuromuscular transmission due to antibodies blocking postsynaptic nicotinic acetylcholine receptors. The resulting weakness may affect respiratory and bulbar musculature. Ineffective respiratory muscle strength results in small tidal volumes, with resulting atelectasis and hypercarbia. Weakness of bulbar muscles reduces cough and swallow effectiveness and thus reduces the ability to handle secretions. The combined weakness of respiratory and bulbar muscles predisposes patients to pulmonary and upper-airway infections.

Several methods of pulmonary conditioning can help improve pulmonary function by helping to clear mucus, reduce atelectasis, and prevent lung infections in intensive care unit (ICU) patients. Some of the options available include incentive spirometry (IS), chest physiotherapy with postural drainage, manual cough assist, percussion therapy, mechanical insufflation/exsufflation/intermittent positive pressure (IPPV) ventilation and intrapulmonary percussive ventilation (IPV). Incentive spirometry involves taking a maximal inspiration through a monitoring device to promote lung expansion and prevent atelectasis. IPPV is a patient-controlled, pneumatic, oscillating-pressure breathing device that loosens mucus by internally percussing the airway with high-frequency gas bursts. The patient can trigger the device by pressing a button during inspiration and releasing the button during expiration. Flutter-valve therapy is similar to IPPV in that oscillations of pressure are transmitted throughout the tracheobronchial tree to help loosen secretions, except that oscillations occur during expiration.

Despite the multiple modalities that can be used to improve pulmonary hygiene, the ideal method to use in patients with neuromuscular disease, including myasthenia gravis, is debatable. Recent data from the pediatric literature, however, suggests that IPV may have benefit over incentive spirometry in the neuromuscular population. In a small randomized study, 18 outpatients with chronic restrictive lung disease secondary to neuromuscular disease were allocated to receive either incentive spirometry or IPV twice daily for 6 months. The end point measured was antibiotic-free days. Investigators found that the number of antibiotic days was significantly higher in patients randomized to the IS group versus the IPV group (24/1,000 patient days vs. 0/1,000 patient days). Furthermore, 3 patients developed pneumonia or bronchitis in the incentive spirometry group, versus none of the patients in the IPV group. Additionally, the patients in the incentive spirometry group required more supplemental respiratory treatments and more frequent intensification of their respiratory therapy. No significant adverse events were reported in the IPV group. Investigators speculated that the ineffectiveness of incentive spirometry was due to the suboptimal respiratory muscle strength required to perform the inspiratory maneuver. Furthermore, incentive spirometry could possibly compromise already tenuous neuromuscular transmission by temporarily depleting acetylcholine reserves.

At this point, larger studies focusing on the myasthenia gravis population should be conducted to assess the role of IPV versus IS in the acute setting of hospitalization. Nevertheless, based on the current limited data available, it would seem prudent to include IPV or flutter-valve therapy and avoid incentive spirometry in the pulmonary regimen of myasthenic patients in the hospital setting, given the dubious efficacy of incentive spirometry in the neuromuscular population.

SUGGESTED READINGS

Langenderfer B. Alternatives to percussion and postural drainage. A review of mucus clearance therapies: percussion and postural drainage, autogenic drainage, positive expiratory pressure, flutter valve, intrapulmonary percussive ventilation, and high-frequency chest compression with the ThAIRapy Vest. J Cardiopulm Rehabil. 1998;(4):283–289.

Reardon CC, Christiansen D, Barnett ED. Intrapulmonary percussive ventilation vs incentive spirometry for children with neuromuscular disease. Arch Pediatr Adolesc Med. 2005;159(6):526–531.

212

REMEMBER THAT NOT ALL SEIZURES ARE CONVULSIVE AND OBVIOUS

JOSE I. SUAREZ, MD

Seizures are a common occurrence in the intensive care unit (ICU). The term *epilepsy* refers to recurrent seizures. Seizures presenting in the ICU can be somewhat simplistically classified into partial (or focal) and generalized. The most common focal seizures are motor and involve face or limb motor seizure activity without alteration of sensorium. Generalized seizures can be of various types: generalized tonic-clonic (generalized convulsions with loss of consciousness); complex partial (disturbed sensorium with common automatisms); and non-convulsive seizures (disordered sensorium or loss of consciousness).

WATCH OUT FOR

Critically ill patients experience seizures frequently regardless of whether they have underlying medical illnesses or have undergone a surgical procedure. Many medical and surgical complications increase the likelihood of seizures including hypoxia, cerebral ischemia, medications, drug withdrawal, infection, surgical injury, and metabolic derangements. Most seizures in the ICU occur in patients without prior history of seizures. In fact it has been reported that neurologic complications occur in about 12% of patients admitted to the ICU without prior intracranial pathology, and of these, 28% experience seizures. About 90% of seizures in the ICU are generalized tonic-clonic. However, about 10% of patients will have complex-partial or other nonconvulsive seizures including nonconvulsive status epilepticus (i.e., ongoing electrical seizures lasting more than 5 minutes). Patients with nonconvulsive seizures represent a difficult dilemma for intensivists. It has been estimated that the incidence of nonconvulsive status epilepticus may be 5% to 50% in patients in coma and the incidence of nonconvulsive seizures in general could be as high as 34%. The key point to learn from these data is that without monitoring (e.g., electroencephalography [EEG]), the diagnosis of nonconvulsive seizures and status epilepticus will be missed, to the detriment of the patient.

WHAT TO DO

The diagnostic test of choice to detect ongoing seizures in the ICU is the EEG (other than overt clinical manifestations). Even in patients who appear to have been successfully treated for overt status epilepticus, the incidence of subclinical or nonconvulsive seizures can be as high as 20%. Current recommendation is that unless patients return to their baseline level of consciousness after a seizure, an EEG, and preferably continuous EEG monitoring, should be performed. Continuous EEG monitoring should be performed for at least 24 hours to exclude nonconvulsive seizures. In fact, some investigators recommend continuous EEG monitoring in most ICU patients, particularly those with underlying neurologic injury or medical illnesses predisposing to seizures as mentioned earlier. Availability of continuous EEG monitoring may be a problem in nonspecialized centers. In such situations intensivists may want to obtain an EEG immediately after treatment of a seizure or in any patient with altered sensorium and repeat the EEG daily for the following 24 to 72 hours. However, it must be remembered that Intermittent EEGs may fail to detect many subclinical seizures and is not a replacement for continuous EEG.

SUGGESTED READINGS

Bleck TP, Smith MC, Pierre-Louis SJC, et al. Neurologic complications of critical medical illness. Crit Care Med. 1993;21:98–103.

Jordan KG. Continuous EEG and evoked potential monitoring in the neurosciences intensive care unit. J Clin Neurophysiol. 1993;10:445–475.

Towne AR, Waterhouse EJ, Boggs JG, et al. Prevalence of nonconvulsive status epilepticus in comatose patients. Neurology. 2000;54:340–345.

Varelas PN, ed. Seizures in Critical Care: A Guide to Diagnosis and Therapeutics. Totowa, NJ: Humana Press; 2005.

213

TREAT STATUS EPILEPTICUS AS A MEDICAL EMERGENCY

LAITH R. ALTAWEEL, MD

Status epilepticus is a medical emergency that requires immediate recognition and treatment. It is defined as a series of seizures that occur without recovery of underlying neurologic function. There are many causes of status epilepticus, which may be related to an underlying epileptic disorder or secondary to an acute neurologic insult (*Table 213.1*). In the ICU setting, up to 8% of patients experience this condition with an associated mortality that can be as high as 40%.

WATCH OUT FOR

There are many different presentations of status epilepticus. It can present with generalized bilateral involvement of skeletal muscles and loss of consciousness. It may begin as a focal seizure on one side, which then generalizes to the contralateral side, with loss of consciousness or, it may be nonconvulsive in nature. Status epilepticus can be confirmed by an electroencephalogram (EEG), but treatment should not be delayed pending an EEG result. The EEG can be used to confirm both clinically apparent and subclinical status epilepticus.

WHAT TO DO

When a patient is experiencing a seizure, fundamental principles of advanced life support need to be applied. The patient should receive supplemental oxygen and should be intubated if the airway is compromised. Blood pressure, heart rate, and oxygen saturation need to be assessed. Intravenous (IV) access should be obtained and serum chemistry profiles, complete blood count, and serum glucose level assessed. If the glucose level is low, dextrose 50% (D50) should be administered. Glucose in the absence of thiamine should not be given unless hypoglycemia is documented since it can precipitate Wernicke encephalopathy in thiamine-deficient patients. Alternatively, patients can be given 100 mg of thiamine before or with glucose administration. Once IV access is obtained, intravenous benzodiazepines, preferably lorazepam (0.1 mg/kg) should be administered. It is important to note that administration of benzodiazepines may further compromise the patient's mental and respiratory status. Therefore, preparation for intubation and mechanical ventilation should be done. If the seizure persists,

TABLE 213.1	CAUSES OF STATUS EPILEPTICUS
Prior seizure history	Subtherapeutic anticonvulsants
	Ethanol related
	Intractable epilepsy
No prior seizure history	Ethanol related
	Drug toxicity
	Central nervous system infection
	Head trauma
	Central nervous system tumor
Less common etiologies	Metabolic aberration
	Stroke

phenytoin 20 mg/kg should be given and repeat doses up to 30 mg/kg should be administered. The blood pressure, which may initially be elevated, can decrease with the administration of anticonvulsant therapy or after 15 to 30 minutes of continuous seizure activity due to impaired cerebrovascular autoregulation. Intravenous fluids and vasopressor support should be administered to maintain adequate blood pressure.

In status epilepticus cerebral injury results from prolonged electrical discharge that occurs. If seizures persist in spite of the previously described therapy, then the patient should receive intravenous phenobarbital, continuous infusion of intravenous benzodiazepine, or propofol. Continuing seizures that fail to respond should prompt an evaluation of the sodium level. Hyponatremia may cause status epilepticus that fails to respond to conventional anticonvulsant therapy. For these patients, empiric 3% saline may be indicated to stop the seizures. In addition, hypomagnesia may be the cause of seizures and status epilepticus in transplant patients because of the magnesium-depleting effect of most immunosuppression regimens. The experienced practitioner will realize that normal serum magnesium is not indicative of total body magnesium load. Many transplant centers administer IV magnesium empirically when any transplant patient seizures, regardless of serum levels.

SUGGESTED READINGS

Fink MP, Abraham E, Vincent JL, et al., eds. Textbook of Critical Care. 5th ed. Philadelphia: Elsevier Saunders; 2005:355–365.

Wyllie E, ed. The Treatment of Epilepsy: Practice and Principles. Philadelphia: Lippincott Williams & Wilkins; 2001:681–697.

214

KNOW THE POTENTIAL ADVERSE EFFECTS OF VALPROIC ACID

JOSE I. SUAREZ, MD

Valproic acid (Depakote) is useful in treating multiple seizure types including complex partial, generalized tonic-clonic, myoclonic, as well as status epilepticus. Valproic acid has multiple proposed mechanisms of action including blocking sodium channels, augmenting the action of glutamic acid decarboxylase, a γ-aminobutyric acid (GABA)–synthesizing enzyme, restricting GABA transaminase (GABA-T), an enzyme that degrades GABA, and blocking T-type calcium currents. Unlike some other anticonvulsant medications, it can be rapidly loaded, has little effect on blood pressure, and is available as an intravenous formulation. Thus, valproic acid may be especially useful in unstable intensive care unit (ICU) patients. Although valproic acid is very useful in treating status epilepticus, the clinician using it needs a thorough understanding of its potential adverse effects.

ADVERSE EFFECTS

The most important adverse effects of valproic acid include hepatotoxicity, pancreatitis, teratogenicity, thrombocytopenia, and hyperammonemia. Valproic acid carries a black-box warning for hepatotoxicity, pancreatitis, and teratogenicity. Serious hepatotoxicity usually occurs in young children rather than adults and occurs within the first 6 months of therapy; however, cases of hepatotoxicity have been reported in the older population. Preceding symptoms of malaise, weakness, anorexia, or vomiting may occur before serious or fatal hepatotoxicity is detected. Pancreatitis occurs rarely and appears to be an idiosyncratic effect. It may occur years after initiation of valproate therapy. Cases of rapidly fatal hemorrhagic pancreatitis have been reported in the literature. In addition, valproic acid has a strong teratogenic effect. Its use in pregnant patients is associated with a 1% to 2% rate of neural tube defects in offspring, which is much higher than the general population. High-dose folic acid supplementation should be given routinely to women of childbearing age who require valproate therapy. Thrombocytopenia may occur with valproate use and appears to be dose related. In a clinical trial of valproate monotherapy for epilepsy, 27% of patients had at least one value below 75×10^9/L when taking a dose of 50 mg/kg/day average. The incidence of thrombocytopenia increases significantly when plasma valproic acid levels exceeded about 110 to 135 mcg/mL. Finally, hyperammonemia may occur in patients taking valproate, even in the absence of abnormal liver-function tests. Patients who develop unexplained lethargy, nausea, vomiting, or mental status changes while taking valproate should have plasma ammonia levels checked. Underlying urea cycle disorders should be evaluated in patients found to have hyperammonemia in the setting of valproate use. Asymptomatic elevations of ammonia may occur.

MONITORING

Laboratory monitoring of patients initiated on valproate should include baseline complete blood count (CBC), liver-function tests (LFTs) and transaminases, and beta–human chorionic gonadotropin. Some clinicians repeat the CBC and liver tests 1 week after starting the drug. Subsequently, LFTs and transaminases should be performed several weeks after initiation of therapy and at monthly intervals at least for the first 6 months. CBC should also be checked periodically. It is not necessary to regularly check pancreatic enzyme levels or ammonia levels unless clinical symptoms develop.

SUGGESTED READINGS

Bradley W, ed. Neurology in Clinical Practice. Philadelphia: Butterworth-Heinemann; 2004:1953–1992.

Physician's Desk Reference. http://www.pdr.net/. New Jersey: Thomson Health; 2006.

215

LEARN THE CRANIAL NERVE EXAMINATION AS ONE CAN OBTAIN A LOT OF INFORMATION EVEN IN COMATOSE AND POORLY COOPERATIVE PATIENTS

ELIAHU S. FEEN, MD
JOSE I. SUAREZ, MD

FIRST CRANIAL NERVE: THE OLFACTORY NERVE

The olfactory nerve conveys the sense of smell to appropriate centers of the cerebral cortex via olfactory receptors located in the superior nasal septum. Smell is properly tested through the use of nonirritating volatile oils or liquids, for example, oil of wintergreen, oil of cloves, eucalyptus, oil of cinnamon, vanilla, or anise. One nostril is occluded while the patient inhales vigorously with the stimulant held close to the open nostril and with the patient's eyes closed. The fact that the patient can sense an odor is more important than being able to identify the particular stimulant. Even some bedside substances can be useful for rough, qualitative testing of smell, such as coffee grounds, lemon oil, or flavored toothpaste. Obviously a conscious patient is necessary for testing of the olfactory nerve. Some irritative substances may actually stimulate the trigeminal nerve and confuse the examiner, even though they are attractive to use in semiconscious or obtunded patients. Examples of the substances to be avoided are chloroform, menthol, camphor, ammonia, strong acetic acid, alcohol, and formaldehyde.

SECOND CRANIAL NERVE: THE OPTIC NERVE

The optic nerve conveys retinal fibers to the lateral geniculate bodies of the thalamus through the optic chiasm. From the lateral geniculate bodies, the optic radiation fibers travel to the primary visual cortex to begin the process of constructing vision based upon the visual stimulation of the retinal fibers. For the scope of this text, only the basic bedside clinical tests of vision are of concern. These fundamentally consist of confrontation testing and visual acuity testing. Visual acuity is tested in the conscious, cooperative patient by means of one of the easily available reading cards, such as the Snellen, Jaeger, or Rosenbaum reading cards. Confrontation testing consists most commonly of having a patient stare at a fixed point in the center of his or her vision (such as the examiner's nose, if the examiner is in front of the patient) and counting fingers of the examiner's hand, held in front of the patient. Ideally, each eye is tested independently by covering the contralateral eye with an opaque object. The examiner should hold up fingers of his or her own hand in each of four quadrants of the patient's scope of vision for each eye. It is important to remember that for the purpose of counting fingers, the fingers should be held up steadily and not moved or wiggled. Moving the fingers while asking the patient to count them will actually test the sense of visual movement and not object perception. In semiconscious, uncooperative or poorly communicative patients, visual confrontation testing may be performed at the bedside by flicking fingers close to each eye but without touching the eye. A blinking response indicates visual field perception. There are two caveats. First, the flicking should not be so vigorous as to induce air movement strong enough to stimulate the eyelashes or cornea, which would induce a blinking reflex. Second, this method can only grossly test visual perception without giving any definitive sense of quadrantanopsias. It can usually be done only in the field of the nasal retina.

The optic nerve, because it conveys light perception, is also involved in the pupillary light reflex (consensual pupillary constriction in response to light stimulation), but because of the involvement of the third cranial nerve in this reflex arc, this is treated in the next section.

THIRD CRANIAL NERVE (THE OCULOMOTOR NERVE), FOURTH CRANIAL NERVE (THE TROCHLEAR NERVE), AND SIXTH CRANIAL NERVE (THE ABDUCENS NERVE)

The oculomotor nerve subserves four of the six oculomotor muscles; the superior rectus, medial rectus, inferior rectus, and inferior oblique muscles. It also innervates the levator palpebrae superioris, which contributes to the elevation of the upper eyelid. There is a parasympathetic component to the innervation of the oculomotor nerve, which innervates the sphincter pupillae muscle and ciliary muscles. These latter muscles control pupillary size and are intimately involved in the pupillary light reflex and in accommodation to near vision. The trochlear nerve innervates the superior oblique muscle. The superior oblique muscle depresses the eye when it is adducted and has some rotatory effect. The abducens nerve innervates the lateral rectus muscle, which abducts the eye.

In a conscious patient testing of the oculomotor, trochlear, and abducens nerves consists basically of having the patient track a moving target, such as the examiner's finger. Each eye may be tested

independently. In poorly cooperative patients the examiner may observe spontaneous eye movements and use gross stimulation, such as
moving from one side of a patient's bed to the other while calling
or clapping, to observe for tracking eye movements. Some comatose
patients may have certain kinds of roving eye movements, which can
give information about which extraocular muscles are intact. Testing trochlear nerve function independently is difficult at the bedside,
most especially in an intensive care setting. The most common clinical presentation of acute isolated trochlear nerve palsy in an ambulatory patient is a head tilt—the patient presents with his or her head
tilted forward and to the contralateral side of the affected muscle. Increasing the head tilt in the direction of the palsied side may induce
vertical diplopia, which is part of the testing maneuver for trochlear
muscle weakness (Bielschowsky test). Obviously, this is somewhat difficult in many intensive care unit (ICU) patients. Examination of eye
movements must include observation of nystagmus and other eye-
movement abnormalities such as forced gaze in a particular direction
or opsoclonus (irregular oscillations of the eyes in both vertical and
horizontal directions), as these may help to localize neurologic lesions.

For patients who cannot cooperate (for example, comatose patients or those on sedation), the performance of oculocephalic maneuvers can elicit eye movements. The oculocephalic reflex depends
upon an intact vestibular system for its reliability. In a patient with an
intact oculocephalic reflex, turning the patient's head in a given horizontal direction will drive the eyes to the opposite side. This tests the
ipsilateral medial rectus (third cranial nerve) and the contralateral lateral rectus (sixth cranial nerve). Vertical eye movements can be tested
with a vertical motion of the head (with the head held in the midline
position). Isolation of a particular extraocular muscle abnormality is
difficult, though, because of the combination of extraocular muscle
function in the production of vertical eye movements. In addition to
eye movements, other clinical features will indicate oculomotor dysfunction. The presence of ptosis may suggest a lesion in the oculomotor
nerve.

Finally, testing of the pupillary light reflex is an absolutely essential
component of bedside cranial nerve testing. Light is conveyed through
the optic nerves to the midbrain and into the Edinger-Westphal nucleus. Efferent motor and parasympathetic fibers to the pupil are conveyed by the oculomotor nerve. There are multiple crossing points
along the pathway, so the pupillary light reflex is bilateral in nature.
It is tested with the swinging flashlight test, in which a bright light
is directed into each eye individually. The examiner must observe for

both the direct response and the consensual response. The pupil in a normal eye constricts in response to light shown directly into it; this is the direct response. The contralateral pupil should simultaneously (and equally) constrict if it is also normal, which represents the consensual response. An abnormality in one of the responses suggests a lesion somewhere along the pathway, which can involve both the optic nerve, the oculomotor nerve, or midbrain connections. In a conscious, cooperative patient, the accommodation reflex can also be tested. In the normal accommodation reflex, if a patient looks to a far object and then shifts his or her gaze to a near object, such as a hand held in front of the patient's face, the pupils constrict. The efferent limb of the reflex is conveyed by the oculomotor nerve.

FIFTH CRANIAL NERVE: THE TRIGEMINAL NERVE

The trigeminal nerve has both sensory and motor components. The sensory component conveys pain, temperature, and light touch sensation from the face region. In addition it carries taste from the oral mucosa and to some extent the tongue and proprioception from certain muscles of the face. The motor component primarily innervates several muscles coordinating mastication (chewing).

Clinical examination of the trigeminal nerve involves testing both its motor and sensory components. In an awake, cooperative patient, the motor limb may be examined by testing the strength of jaw movements. The examiner can try to open the patient's jaw against resistance, close the jaw against resistance, or resist the patient's effort to laterally displace his or her mandible (to the left or right). In a unilateral lesion of the motor component of the trigeminal nerve affecting the branches that innervate muscles of jaw opening or closing, an attempt to do this will result in deflection of the jaw to the side contralateral to the lesion.

Sensory examination is straightforward in an awake, cooperative patient. There are three branches of the trigeminal nerve innervating sensation of the face—the ophthalmic, maxillary, and mandibular branches. These three branches roughly divide the anterior, central face into three sensory zones, from top to bottom, respectively. Touching the patient's face with either a soft or sharp object will indicate intact sensation through the trigeminal nerve on each respective side. Traditionally the patient is stimulated on the forehead for the ophthalmic branch, on the cheek lateral to the nose for the maxillary branch, and on the chin or jaw for the mandibular branch (on each side of the face).

Uncooperative or unconscious patients may require reflex testing of the trigeminal nerve, as careful observation for lateral deflection may be inadequate and a sensory exam unreliable. The jaw reflex (also called masseter reflex or mandibular reflex) is elicited by placing the examiner's finger on the middle of the chin and tapping with a reflex hammer over that finger. A relaxed or slightly open jaw is necessary. For an intact reflex the jaw will suddenly and momentarily close in response to the tapping. The corneal reflex is arguably the most famous trigeminal reflex. Corneal sensation is conveyed by the trigeminal nerve. Stroking the cornea gently with a nonabrasive object (such as a wisp of cotton) or washing the cornea with sterile, saline flush will stimulate the afferent limb of the reflex. The seventh cranial nerve (facial nerve) conveys the efferent limb of the corneal reflex. The efferent limb consists of two parts in most patients—a direct corneal reflex and a consensual reflex. The direct reflex consists of the ipsilateral closing of the eye (i.e., ipsilateral to the side of the stimulus). The consensual reflex involves simultaneous closure of the contralateral eye. Not all patients will normally evince the consensual response.

Other reflexes may be especially useful in comatose patients. In these cases the sensory limb of the reflex arc is conveyed by the trigeminal nerve. Stimulation of the cornea may cause pupillary constriction or dilatation followed by constriction (bilateral due to the nature of pupillary innervation, as described earlier). Tickling the nasal mucosa with, for example, a cotton swab may cause sneezing or facial muscle contraction, especially in the vicinity of the nose (the sternutatory reflex).

SEVENTH CRANIAL NERVE: THE FACIAL NERVE

The facial nerve has primarily motor function to innervate the muscles of the face (excepting the muscles of mastication, which are innervated by the trigeminal nerve) and platysma of the upper, anterior neck to give facial expression. There is some sensory function, in particular taste, over the anterior two-thirds of the tongue. Variable portions of the external auditory meatus have superficial sensation conveyed by the facial nerve in some individuals. Parasympathetic input to the lacrimal (tear) glands, the several salivary glands, and mucous-secreting glands is also conveyed by the facial nerve.

Clinical testing of the facial nerve in awake, cooperative patients involves asking them to raise their eyebrows, squeeze their eyes shut, smile or frown, blow out their cheeks, whistle, and contract the chin muscles by retracting the angles of the mouth downward (for testing of the platysma). Uncooperative or unconscious patients may be observed carefully for the performance of these actions spontaneously. As well, a facial droop or an asymmetry of the nasolabial folds and size of the palpebral fissures will give some clue to asymmetric facial tone. If a patient is lying with his or her eyelids closed, asymmetry in the ease with which the eyelids are passively pulled open by an examiner may give some indication of a lesion in one of the facial nerves (ophthalmic branch).

The most reliable reflexes testing the facial nerve are those with a sensory limb along the trigeminal nerve, namely the corneal and sternutatory reflexes. There are various reflexes noted in some patients that involve stimulation of eye closure, puckering of the mouth, or lower facial muscle flexion, but these are too variable to be generally reliable.

Eighth Cranial Nerve: The Vestibulocochlear Nerve

The eighth cranial nerve consists of two separate nerve bundles that combine into a single nerve trunk, namely the acoustic nerve and the vestibular nerve. The acoustic nerve conveys the sensation of sound, as derived from the receptor cells in the organ of Corti. The vestibular nerve conveys the sensation of balance and head position in space, as derived from the receptor cells in the semicircular canals.

Bedside testing of the acoustic nerve in an intensive care setting is necessarily inexact. For awake, cooperative patients, testing air and bone conduction of sound through the Rinne and Weber tests may be appropriate. The details are beyond the scope of this text. It is important to note, though, that almost immediately after each acoustic nerve enters the brain stem, there is fiber crossing. Thus, sound conduction from the brain stem up to the cortex is bilateral, and unilateral acoustic nerve lesions may be missed on simple sound testing.

The most common symptom of vestibular dysfunction is vertigo and one of the most common signs on exam is positional nystagmus. Careful testing of awake, cooperative patients in terms of peripheral motor functions, muscle tone, postural reflexes, and eye movements can contribute to the delineation of a vestibular problem, but again this is well beyond the scope of this text. For our purposes, the most important clinical test of vestibular function is in comatose patients for whom caloric testing may be necessary. As discussed in the section on the cranial nerves controlling eye movements, the oculovestibular reflex tests eye movements based upon the stimulation of the vestibular system. In the clinic, patients can be placed on rotating chairs to stimulate the vestibular system. Awake, cooperative patients can undergo caloric testing as well, which is often uncomfortable for them.

At the bedside of comatose patients, in preparation for caloric testing, each external auditory meatus should be examined to be sure it is free of cerumen or other substances. The tympanic membrane should be examined with the use of an otoscope for any evidence of perforation. Should perforation be found, it is advisable to avoid testing that side. However, where testing is absolutely necessary, an antiseptic solution may be used. For a supine patient the head is placed at a 30-degree angle above the horizontal plane. This head position will put the lateral semicircular canal in the vertical plane. Ice water is recommended (at $0°$ to $5°C$). The examiner should instill a minimum of 10 mL over a maximum of 30 to 40 seconds. One common practice, though, is to instill about 60 mL over 30 seconds and then observe for another 30 seconds. The examiner observes for any eye movements. The reason the external auditory canal is filled with cold (or in some variations of the test, warm) water is to stimulate endolymph flow within the semicircular canals. A response to cold-water caloric testing in a normal patient consists of a rotatory nystagmus of the eyes, with a slow phase to the side ipsilateral to the cold-water stimulation. (Warm water produces a slow phase to the side contralateral to the stimulation.) Caloric testing is a very strong stimulus, and failure to produce eye movements suggests a lesion in the vestibular system (on the appropriate side), the ocular motor system, or in the brain-stem connections that link these together. Absence of this reflex is a common test in confirming brain death.

NINTH CRANIAL NERVE (THE GLOSSOPHARYNGEAL NERVE) AND TENTH CRANIAL NERVE (THE VAGUS NERVE)

The glossopharyngeal nerve supplies some minimal muscular function to the arch of the soft palate, the afferent limb of part of the reflex of salivation, and taste sensation to the posterior third of the tongue and part of the pharynx. For clinical purposes the most important innervation of the glossopharyngeal nerve is the afferent limb of the gag reflex. Stroking the posterior pharyngeal tissue, including the area of the tonsils, with a soft or blunt device, such as a cotton swab or tongue blade, will elicit elevation and constriction of the muscles of the pharynx as well as retraction of the tongue. This motor response, however, is carried through the vagus nerve. A lesion of the glossopharyngeal nerve will cause unilateral impairment in the gag reflex, so that stimulation to the side ipsilateral to the lesion will fail to elicit a response.

The vagus nerve has multiple functions throughout the body, as its anatomic course and name ("wandering") suggest. The motor control of the vagus involves the muscles of the soft palate, pharynx, and larynx. Coordination of swallowing and phonation are under vagal control primarily. For clinical purposes, sensory functions of the vagus include a small area of skin sensation in the external auditory meatus and pinna in some individuals and taste over certain regions of the deep pharynx. (Some other sensory functions of the vagus lack clinical utility since they are difficult to test, such as sensory innervation of the meninges and taste over the epiglottis.) The vagus also conveys a large amount of parasympathetic innervation to the viscera, as well as carrying some general sensory information from the viscera.

When a patient has difficulty with swallowing and slurred speech, this may be an indication of vagal dysfunction (for a lower motor neuron lesion). A hoarse or raspy voice, as opposed to other phonation abnormalities, represents the most typical manifestation of vagal nerve lesions through the laryngeal branches. To definitively prove a vocal cord palsy requires laryngoscopy. The gag reflex is also necessary in the examination of vagal function. A unilateral vagus lesion that causes palatal and pharyngeal weakness will produce an ipsilateral droopy soft palate. Upon contraction of the palatal and pharyngeal muscles (either voluntarily or through stimulation of the gag reflex in comatose patients), the uvula and soft palate will be pulled to the side contralateral to the lesion.

ELEVENTH CRANIAL NERVE: THE SPINAL ACCESSORY NERVE

The spinal accessory nerve, entirely a motor nerve for all practical purposes, innervates most of the fibers of the sternocleidomastoid muscle and a minority of the fibers of the trapezius muscles. The rest of the innervation from these muscles comes from cervical spinal nerves. As a result, complete lesions of the spinal accessory nerve produce weakness as opposed to complete paralysis. Clinical examination of the sternocleidomastoid involves having the patient turn his or her head fully to one side against resistance. This requires contraction of the sternocleidomastoid muscle contralateral to the side to which the head is turned. Weakness of head turning will suggest a lesion. The trapezius muscle elevates the shoulder, retracts the head, and assists in the elevation of the arm above the horizontal position. Clinical examination of these functions requires awake, cooperative patients. The examiner has the patient shrug his or her shoulders against resistance. Again, weakness may suggest a lower motor neuron lesion of the spinal accessory nerve.

TWELFTH CRANIAL NERVE: THE HYPOGLOSSAL NERVE

The hypoglossal nerve innervates almost all of the muscles that control tongue movement. Observations of tongue movement, even in uncooperative or unconscious patients, will give insight into lingual paresis. Unilateral lesions of the hypoglossal nerve will produce ipsilateral weakness in the tongue. The fibers of the lingual muscles that protrude the tongue are angled in such a way that unilateral lesions of the nerve cause the tongue to deviate to the ipsilateral side. When the tongue cannot be examined in this way or tongue movements are restricted by endotracheal tubes or the like, some clinical features suggest hypoglossal nerve lesions if the lesions are *chronic*. Chronic hypoglossal nerve lesions produce atrophy of the lingual muscles and fasciculations of the muscles, which are visible upon inspection of the tongue.

Of note, while the full spectrum of cranial nerve abnormalities is well beyond the scope of this text, some vitamin deficiencies produce typical changes in the mucosa of the tongue. For example, the tongue of Wernicke (thiamine deficiency) appears smooth and shiny but reddened with some atrophy present.

SUGGESTED READINGS

Brazis PW, Maseu JC, Biller J. Localization in Clinical Neurology. 4th ed. Philadelphia: Lippincott Williams & Wilkins; 2001.
Campbell WW, ed. DeJong's the Neurologic Examination. 6th ed. Philadelphia: Lippincott Williams & Wilkins; 2005.

216

DO NOT SQUEEZE THE TOENAILS OR ADMINISTER A PAINFUL STIMULUS TO THE FOOT TO TEST RESPONSE TO PAIN IN COMATOSE PATIENTS AS THIS MAY TRIGGER A SPINAL REFLEX THAT MAY BE SEEN EVEN IN BRAIN-DEAD PATIENTS

JOSE I. SUAREZ, MD

The evaluation of the comatose patient using the Glasgow Coma Scale (GCS) requires testing the respective modalities of eye opening, verbal response, and motor response. In testing motor response, it is important to precisely characterize the degree of motor responsiveness. This helps to characterize the degree of coma and it may also have prognostic value when assessing a patient after hypoxic or ischemic injury.

WATCH OUT FOR

One specific element in the motor exam that often creates confusion for the examiner (and the family) is the interpretation of the patient's response to a painful stimulus in the lower extremity. The confusion relates to the issue of differentiating between a purposeful withdrawal response to pain versus a simple spinal reflex withdrawal to pain. The importance of this differentiation is that a purposeful withdrawal response to pain may be a good prognostic sign in patients with hypoxic-ischemic injury, whereas a spinal reflex withdrawal may be seen in brain-dead patients. It is important to realize that brain-dead patients may exhibit a variety of movements that are spinally mediated and do not imply intact brain-stem or cortical function. Among the possible movements are extensor plantar responses, jerks of the fingers, toe flexion, and a Lazarus sign, which involves flexion of the arms at the elbow, adduction of the shoulders, lifting of the arms, dystonic posturing of the hands, and crossing of the hands. Furthermore, a triple-flexion response with dorsiflexion at the ankle, knee, and hip may be seen with distal lower-extremity pain stimulation, which may appear at first glance to be a purposeful withdrawal response but is actually a spinal cord reflex.

The ways to differentiate between a spinal cord reflex and a true withdrawal response involve observing the character of the withdrawal response to pain. A spinal cord reflex will usually have a stereotyped amplitude and duration. The amplitude of reflexic movement is usually proportional to the stimulus intensity. Furthermore, a spinal reflex such as the triple-flexion response is usually more easily elicited by distal lower-extremity stimulation, especially the foot or toenail beds. Thus, it is better to test for withdrawal response in the lower extremity by using a more proximal stimulation such as squeezing the calf or thigh.

SELECTED READINGS

Saposnik G, Maurino J, Saizar R, et al. Spontaneous and reflex movements in 107 patients with brain death. Am J Med. 2005;118(3):311–314.

Teasdale G, Jennett B. Assessment and prognosis of coma after head injury. Acta Neurochir (Wien). 1976;34(1–4):45–55.

217

DO NOT ASCRIBE AN INCREASED SERUM LACTATE LEVEL TO RENAL INSUFFICIENCY

SUSANNA L. MATSEN, MD

Lactic acid levels are a useful adjunct in assessing perfusion in the intensive care unit (ICU). Lactate levels >2 mEq/L may reflect tissue ischemia. However, lactate levels may be confounded by various circumstances and are also prone to misinterpretation. When using lactate levels in clinical management, it is important to understand the physiology behind lactate production and the commonly held misconceptions about lactic acidosis.

When cells face insufficient oxygen to carry out their metabolic functions, they convert from aerobic to anaerobic metabolism. Without an available oxygen molecule, pyruvate is instead converted to lactate, contributing to an anion-gap acidosis. In other words, rather than yielding the complete 36 adenosine triphosphate (ATP) molecules for each mole of glucose, metabolism is halted at lactate, rendering only 2 ATP. The clearance of lactate (in the setting of adequate tissue perfusion) occurs in the liver, through one of two mechanisms. It may combine with oxygen with the end result being carbon dioxide, water, and bicarbonate:

$$CH_3CHOHCOO^- + 3 O_2 \Rightarrow 2 CO_2 + 2 H_2O + HCO_3^-$$

Alternatively, lactate may be processed in the Cori cycle in the liver, where lactate is converted to pyruvate, then to glucose in the process of gluconeogenesis.

There are two types of lactic acidosis, A and B. Type A was described earlier: lactate resulting from inadequate oxygen to complete aerobic metabolism. Type B, on the other hand, stems from insufficient clearance. If the patient suffers from liver failure, he or she may not be able to clear the lactate by converting it to pyruvate. Thus, a persistently high lactate in the setting of liver failure may *not* be indicative of ongoing ischemia, but simply of the inability to resolve the lactic acidosis metabolically.

Of note, lactic acidosis should *not* be ascribed to renal insufficiency. The kidney filters lactic acid only at a threshold of 6 to 8 mEq/L; at lower levels lactate is cleared hepatically as described previously. In addition, Lactated Ringer solution does *not* contribute to lactic acidosis and may be given in the setting of ischemia without concern for confounding the picture. Isotonic with plasma, Lactated Ringer contains a balanced solution of sodium (130 mEq/L), chloride (109 mEq/L), potassium (4 mEq/L), and calcium (3 mEq/L) with a lactate buffer to render a pH of 6.4. Although a small amount of lactate is contained within this fluid, its isotonicity renders this lactate clinically inconsequential. In fact, Lactated Ringer is preferred over 5% dextrose solution in the setting of critical illness: the latter has been shown to contribute to higher postoperative lactate levels as the added glucose is metabolized to lactate during periods of ischemia.

Interpretation of lactic acid levels may be further confounded by lag time in laboratory processing. If a sample sits for a period of time prior to processing, the measured lactate may be spuriously elevated. As the blood remains within the tube, the red cells continue their metabolism, using the oxygen dissolved within the serum. As this is depleted, the red cells convert to anaerobic metabolism, yielding a further elevation in lactate.

SELECTED READINGS

Marino PL, ed. The ICU Book. 2nd ed. Philadelphia: Lippincott Williams & Wilkins; 1998:196–198,230–231,592–600.

Souba WW, Fink MP, Jurkovich GJ, eds. American College of Surgeons Principles and Practice. New York: WebMD; 2004:1171–1178.

218

DO NOT TREAT LACTIC ACIDOSIS WITH BICARBONATE

PRASERT SAWASDIWIPACHAI, MD

Lactic acidosis is one type of anion-gap metabolic acidosis. It occurs when aerobic tissue metabolism converts to anaerobic metabolism, which produces a significant amount of lactic acid.

Lactic acidosis occurs at the cellular level (mitochondria) when the oxygen delivery to the tissue is inadequate or the cells cannot utilize the oxygen. Many causes of lactic acidosis are recognized, with the most common being due to low oxygen delivery from shock (septic, hypovolemic, cardiogenic, neurogenic), severe anemia, and severe hypoxemia. It also can occur from exposure to drugs (e.g., metformin, antiretroviral therapy, acetaminophen, salicylates, cocaine, valproic acid, salfasalazine, isonicotinic acid hydrazide, fluorouracil), toxins, and sugar alcohols (sorbitol, xylitol, fructose).

WATCH OUT FOR

Many systemic diseases can also be complicated with lactic acidosis including diabetes mellitus, alcoholism, pancreatitis, cancer, infections, vitamin B_1 deficiency, short gut syndrome, and malabsorption syndrome. Certain rare congenital inborn errors in metabolism (e.g., Von Gierke disease, methylmalonic aciduria, pyruvate dehydrogenase deficiency) can also be responsible for lactic acidosis.

The best treatment of lactic acidosis is to treat the underlying causes. This often includes volume expansion, correcting anemia, increasing cardiac performance, and correcting hypoxemia. If the cause is detected and treated promptly, the lactic acidosis should gradually subside. The severity of acidemia (arterial pH) can be used to follow the effectiveness of the intervention.

Alkali therapy (especially sodium bicarbonate) should not be given in lactic acidosis. Although it may initially correct the deranged lab value, it actually worsens the clinical condition. The exogenous bicarbonate will result in a significant amount of CO_2, which can move freely between the compartments (including across the blood–brain barrier) while the bicarbonate does not. This creates disequilibrium of strong ions. Many studies both in animal and human cells have confirmed the increase in intracellular acidosis by bicarbonate therapy. Bicarbonate administration is widely accepted in acidosis associated with chronic loss of bicarbonate (e.g., renal tubular acidosis, pancreatic transplantation, diarrhea) but not in lactic acidosis.

One final thought is that mild to moderate systemic acidosis is not as deleterious as once thought. The growing use of permissive hypercapnia in patients with acute respiratory distress syndrome has shown that many adult patients have no change in cardiac contractility even when systemic pH is as low as 7.15.

SUGGESTED READING

Forsythe SM. Sodium bicarbonate for the treatment of lactic acidosis. Clinical investigations in critical care. Chest. 2000;117:260–267.

219

REMEMBER THAT POSTOPERATIVE HYPERTENSION CAN BE A RESULT OF INCREASED PCO$_2$

MELVIN K. RICHARDSON, MD

Postoperative hypertension is common and can be difficult to manage. When other vital signs are normal, including normal pulse oximetry and normal respiratory rate, it is common to assume that the hypertension is due to poorly treated pain and should be treated with opioids. This may be a dangerous approach.

Hypoventilation is a not uncommon postoperative occurrence. Frequent causes of hypoventilation include residual effects of inhaled anesthetics and opioids, as well as persistent neuromuscular blockade, suboptimal ventilation due to pain or surgical site factors, and coexisting chronic obstructive pulmonary disease (COPD). As hypoventilation worsens, it can lead to carbon dioxide retention and hypercarbia. As hypercarbia worsens, direct cardiac and vascular depression occurs, and in order to compensate for this depression, hypercarbia can also stimulate catecholamine release. There is a linear correlation between increases in PaCO$_2$ and increases in heart rate and cardiac output. The overall effect of the catecholamine release is hypertension, along with increased pulse pressure, stroke volume, myocardial contractility, and heart rate. Treating hypertension with opioids, therefore, may worsen the situation, as opioids may lead to further hypoventilation, hypercarbia, hypertension, and eventually respiratory insufficiency or failure.

WHAT NOT TO DO

It cannot be overly stressed that the O$_2$ saturation on the pulse oximeter is not an adequate measure of ventilatory status. While the pulse oximeter is considered the standard of care in the postoperative setting and is able to noninvasively measure peripheral oxygen saturation, it is an estimate only of arterial oxygenation. This is a nonlinear relationship, and as illustrated in the oxyhemoglobin dissociation curve, an oxygen saturation of 90% to 100% can reflect an extremely wide range of values for the PaO$_2$, from 60 mm Hg to >100 mm Hg. The pulse oximeter is therefore a poor indicator of ventilatory status, as it can be misleading about the PaO$_2$ value and can be poorly reflective of the underlying respiratory effort, including the PaCO$_2$. Further, as the PaCO$_2$ increases, it shifts the oxyhemoglobin dissociation curve to the right, reflective of increased oxygen unloading. In managing a postoperative patient with hypertension, therefore, it is important to assess the full clinical picture for other signs of respiratory depression, including dyspnea, shallow respirations, use of respiratory muscles, paradoxical motions of the chest and abdomen, cyanosis, and obtundation, to determine adequacy of ventilation, likelihood of hypoventilation/hypercarbia, and the full differential for the hypertension.

SUGGESTED READINGS

Dubbink DA. Physiologic Effects of Hyper- and Hypocarbia. In Faust RJ, ed. Anesthesiology Review. 3rd ed. Philadelphia: Churchill Livingstone, 2002:26–27.

Wilson WC and Benumof JL. Respiratory Physiology and Respiratory Function during Anesthesia. In Miller RD, ed. Anesthesia. 6th ed. Philadelphia: Churchill Livingstone, 2005:679–722.

Brian JE. Carbon dioxide and the cerebral circulation. Anesthesiology. 1998:88:1365–1386.

220

Do not use a normal arterial blood gas to rule out a pulmonary embolism

David N. Hager, MD

Venous thromboembolic disease affects 200,000 persons in the United States annually. Among affected persons, almost half suffer symptomatic pulmonary embolism (PE). Without treatment, 30% of patients will die within 1 year. However, despite its high incidence, PE is a difficult diagnosis to make. Clinical presentations vary and the symptoms are often nonspecific. Though an abnormal arterial blood gas can be informative, normal indices of oxygenation and ventilation do not rule out PE.

RISK FACTORS

The major risk factors for PE are the same as those for venous thrombosis. Broadly defined, these include a prior thromboembolic event, neoplastic disease, immobility, recent surgery or trauma, estrogen replacement therapy (especially in the context of tobacco use), and a family history of hypercoaguability such as activated protein C resistance, hyperhomocysteinemia, proteins C and S deficiency, antithrombin III deficiency, and factor V Leiden.

SIGNS AND SYMPTOMS

PE most commonly presents as a triad of dyspnea (70% to 80%), pleurisy, and tachypnea (RR >20). Among those patients enrolled and proven to have PE in the Prospective Investigation of Pulmonary Embolism Diagnosis (PIOPED) study, 97% exhibited one of these three symptoms. A less common presentation is hemodynamic compromise, which may be severe enough to cause syncope. The elderly often present with symptoms consistent with unresolving pneumonia or heart failure despite appropriate therapy. On clinical exam an enhanced second heart sound, tachycardia, and jugular venous distention may be appreciated. A normal chest radiograph is consistent with PE, as are other findings such as pleural effusion, Westermark sign (a focal loss of peripheral vascular markings), and even focal infiltrates. Tachycardia and nonspecific ST-T wave changes are the most common abnormal finding on an electrocardiogram (ECG). The frequently discussed $S_1Q_3T_3$ pattern is present in less than 12% of patients with PE.

Hypoxia (PaO_2 <80 mm Hg), hypocapnia (PaCO_2 <35 mm Hg), and an elevated alveolar-arterial oxygen difference (P[A−a]O_2 >20 mm Hg) are the most common arterial blood gas abnormalities in patients with PE. However, in a group of subjects suspected of having PE, these indices did not effectively discriminate between those ultimately proven to have PE and those who did not. Further, among individuals without prior lung disease, these indices will often fall within normal limits even in the presence of PE. For these reasons, arterial blood gas data contribute little to the diagnosis or exclusion of PE.

DIAGNOSIS

Because of the nonspecific nature of the clinical findings associated with PE and the risks and limited availability of invasive pulmonary angiography (the definitive test), approaches to diagnosis should include a combination of (a) a clinical estimation of the likelihood of PE prior to further radiographic testing, and (b) the results of further radiographic testing. As demonstrated in the PIOPED study, this combination approach is more successful at diagnosing and excluding PE than clinical assessment or radiographic assessment alone. Though the interpretation of ventilation/perfusion (V/Q) imaging and computed tomographic (CT) angiography is beyond the scope of this chapter, all clinicians should be able to determine if a patient's clinical presentation is consistent with a high, intermediate, or low probability of PE.

> *High probability* is defined as an 80% to 100% chance of having had a PE. Such patients have (a) unexplained dyspnea, tachypnea, and/or pleurisy, (b) an unexplained gas exchange abnormality or x-ray abnormality, and (c) a risk factor for hypercoaguability.
>
> *Intermediate probability* is defined as a 20% to 79% chance of having had a PE. Most simply, such patients are defined as not meeting criteria for high or low probability.
>
> *Low probability* is defined as a 1% to 19% chance of having had a PE. Such patients may have dyspnea, tachypnea, pleurisy, x-ray abnormalities, or gas exchange abnormalities. However, in these patients, such findings can be attributed to a different condition. Typical risk factors for hypercoaguability are not present.

The clinical impression can then be combined with the radiologist's interpretation of a V/Q scan, CT angiogram, or both. Each radiographic test has limitations. V/Q studies are very difficult to interpret in the context of coexisting lung disease such as pneumonia, emphysema, or fibrosis and take a long time to complete compared with a CT angiogram. However, V/Q has been more thoroughly evaluated and, in otherwise normal lungs, is more sensitive to peripheral emboli. CT angiography can be performed quickly and usually detect emboli in the large central and segmental pulmonary arteries if present. However, some reports suggest that the sensitivity of CT angiography may be as low as 70%. Further, the resolution of CT scanner at different centers varies widely, intravenous contrast is required (which may pose risks) and the expertise of radiologists also varies.

These imaging limitations emphasize the important role of the clinical impression in the workup of a suspected PE. If the clinical impression and radiographic assessment both suggest a low probability of PE, the evaluation can be stopped. If both suggest a high probability of PE, anticoagulation should be continued or initiated. However, if both the clinical impression and radiographic assessment suggest intermediate probability, or if one or the other suggests high probability, invasive angiography should be pursued. For the patient in whom the clinical probability of PE is low and the radiographic assessment suggests intermediate probability (or vice versa), some investigators have advocated the use of lower-extremity duplex ultrasound imaging to rule out venous thrombosis. If such testing is negative, anticoagulation therapy may be withheld without further evaluation provided close follow-up is available.

D-DIMER

There has been much emphasis on the use of d-dimer assays in the evaluation of deep venous thrombosis and PE in the last several years. It is frequently suggested that a positive d-dimer is nondiagnostic, but that a negative result rules out venous thrombosis and/or PE. However, studies assessing the utility of d-dimer testing in the diagnosis of thromboembolic disease show that the results of d-dimer tests are subject to not only the type of test used (latex agglutination or enzyme-linked immunosorbent assay [ELISA]) but also the prevalence of thromboembolic disease in the study population, patient age, length of hospitalization, and even location in the hospital (floor vs. emergency department). For these reasons, d-dimer testing remains of little utility, especially when the clinical impression suggests a high probability of PE.

SUGGESTED READINGS

Hyers TM. Venous thromboembolism. Am J Respir Crit Care Med. 1999;159:1–14.

Tapson VF, Carroll BA, Davidson BL, et al. The diagnostic approach to acute venous thromboembolism. Am J Respir Crit Care Med. 1999;160:1043–1066.

Value of the Ventilation/Perfusion Scan in Acute Pulmonary Embolism. Results of the Prospective Investigation of Pulmonary Embolism Diagnosis (PIOPED). JAMA. 1990;263:2753–2759.

221

REMEMBER THAT ARGATROBAN INCREASES INTERNATIONAL NORMALIZED RATIO BUT DOES NOT AFFECT COAGULATION IN THE EXTRINSIC SYSTEM

KELLY GROGAN, MD

Heparin-induced thrombocytopenia (HIT) is an adverse drug reaction characterized by thrombocytopenia and a high risk for venous and arterial thrombosis. It is defined as a decrease in platelet count during or shortly following exposure to heparin. There are two classifications of HIT: a benign form, called type I, and an immune-mediated form, called type II, which is associated with an increased risk for potentially catastrophic thrombosis. Type I affects 10% of patients exposed to heparin and is classified by a rapid, mild decrease in platelet count (100 to 150,000/μL) in the first 1 to 4 days of exposure that resolves despite continued heparin use and is thought to be due to a direct interaction between heparin and platelets. It does not require any medical treatment and does not appear to have any major clinical consequences.

Type II HIT, in patients receiving heparin for the first time, presents as a more severe thrombocytopenia (80% with nadirs between 20 and 100,000/μL) that occurs between 4 and 14 days after therapy is initiated. Patients who have received heparin in the past and have been sensitized may show a decrease in platelet count that may occur within hours and up to 3 days after exposure. After discontinuation of the heparin, the platelet count starts to rise after 2 to 3 days and usually returns to normal within 4 to 10 days. The antibody disappears within 2 to 3 months after cessation of heparin therapy. Platelets of sensitized patients are capable of aggregation and release reactions at 2 months after recovery without evidence of circulating antibody in the serum, suggesting that a major portion of the antiplatelet antibody is membrane bound. Although HIT does not invariably recur during subsequent re-exposure to heparin, future exposure to heparin must be approached with extreme caution.

TREATMENT OF HIT

In patients who have tested serologically positive or who are strongly suspected of having HIT based on clinical data, heparin should be stopped immediately and an alternative form of antithrombotic therapy commenced. Two direct thrombin inhibitors (DTIs), lepirudin and argatroban, are approved in the United States for heparin-induced thrombocytopenia.

Direct Thrombin Inhibitors. Four parenteral DTIs have been approved by the Food and Drug Administration in North America: lepirudin and argatroban for the treatment of heparin-induced thrombocytopenia, bivalirudin as an alternative to heparin in percutaneous coronary intervention, and desirudin as prophylaxis against venous thromboembolism in hip replacement.

To briefly review, thrombin is central in the clotting process: it coverts soluble fibrinogen to fibrin; activates factors V, VIII, and XI, which generates more thrombin; and stimulates platelets. Furthermore, by activating factor XIII, thrombin favors the formation of cross-linked bonds among the fibrin molecules, stabilizing the clot. The coagulation cascade is regulated by natural anticoagulants, such as tissue factor pathway inhibitor, the protein C and protein S system, and antithrombin.

The DTIs also have an antiplatelet effect secondary to their effect of reducing the thrombin-mediated activation of platelets. Since DTIs do not bind to plasma proteins, these agents should produce a more predictable response than does unfractionated heparin and should be more effective than low-molecular-weight heparins because they inhibit fibrin-bound thrombin.

Argatroban. Antihirudin antibodies develop in 40% to 74% of patients receiving lepirudin after 4 days or more of treatment. Of note, fatal anaphylaxis has been described with lepirudin, particularly in patients who are treated again within 3 months of a previous exposure to this agent. In contrast, argatroban does not appear to be immunogenic.

Argatroban is a small-molecule direct thrombin inhibitor that, unlike lepirudin, is not immunogenic. It is a univalent competitive inhibitor of thrombin and binds only to the catalytic site of thrombin via a noncovalent bond to form a reversible complex. Argatroban has a plasma half-life of 39 to 52 minutes and is extensively metabolized by the liver into four mostly inactive metabolites. Renal dysfunction, age, and gender do not alter the elimination half-life of the drug.

Currently argatroban is approved in the United States for the prophylaxis and treatment of thrombosis in patients with HIT. The recent recommended dose of argatroban in the treatment of HIT for patients in the intensive care unit (ICU) is 0.5 μg/kg/min and the dose should be adjusted to maintain the activated partial thromboplastin time (aPTT) at 1.5 to 3.0 times the patient's baseline, with the maximum infusion rate at 10 μg/kg/min. A general guideline is to increase the infusion rate by 20% and recheck the aPTT in 4 hours. If supratherapeutic, it is recommended to decrease the infusion rate by 50% and recheck the aPTT in 4 hours. Argatroban increases the aPTT and activated clotting time (ACT) in a dose-dependent manner.

Monitoring Argatroban Clinical Activity. The best method to monitor therapy with DTIs has not been clearly established. The anticoagulation effect of direct thrombin inhibition is typically monitored using the activated partial thromboplastin time. Although dose-dependent increases also occur in the prothrombin time (PT) and international normalized ratio (INR), these are *not* dependable markers of activity. It must be stressed that an elevated PT does not mean there is a clinically significant alteration in the extrinsic pathway. The ecarin clotting time better reflects the actual plasma concentration of DTIs, but this test is not widely available. Recombinant hirudins and argatroban can be monitored with the use of the aPTT and bivalirudin with the ACT.

Since direct thrombin inhibitors also increase the PT and INR, a reliable means to monitor warfarin therapy during coadministration of a direct thrombin inhibitor is important. Efforts to characterize argatroban's effect on the INR during concurrent warfarin therapy have been reported. In one study, argatroban 1 to 2 μg/kg/min and warfarin 2.5 to 5.0 mg/day were administered concurrently to healthy subjects over 6 days. Because of its short half-life, argatroban was temporarily discontinued daily to simulate warfarin monotherapy. Within 4 hours of stopping the argatroban, mean INRs decreased almost twofold although mean functional factor X levels remained unchanged. Subsequent in vitro studies using plasma from warfarin-treated patients demonstrated a linear relationship between the INR in the presence versus absence of exogenous argatroban.

This underscores the importance of postponing warfarin initiation pending substantial resolution of HIT (platelets greater than 100,000/dL) to avoid warfarin-induced microvascular thrombosis. This complication appears to be caused by depletion of the vitamin K–dependent natural anticoagulant, protein C. This complication is usually seen when the INR rises above 3.5 as this represents a surrogate marker for protein C depletion.

A chromogenic-based method can be used to determine factor X levels as a monitor of the oral anticoagulation from warfarin without effect from argatroban. Also, patients receiving argatroban cannot be evaluated for potential coagulation abnormalities with routine functional (clot-based) assays for fibrinogen, factor levels, or protein C. Argatroban acts as an inhibitor in these assays, causing a dose-dependent false decrease of fibrinogen and factor levels, and a false increase of protein C.

SUGGESTED READINGS

Di Nisio M, Middeldorp S, Buller HR. Drug therapy: direct thrombin inhibitors. N Engl J Med. 2005;353:1028–1040.

Schmitt BP, Adelman B. Heparin-associated thrombocytopenia: a critical review and pooled analysis. Am J Med Sci. 1993;305:208–215.

Warkentin TE, Heddle NM. Laboratory diagnosis of immune heparin-induced thrombocytopenia. Curr Hematol Rep. 2003;2:148–157.

222

CHECK SERIAL METHEMOGLOBIN LEVELS IN PATIENTS ON INHALED NITRIC OXIDE

TIMOTHY M. MOORE, MD, PhD

Inhaled nitric oxide acutely and locally relaxes constricted pulmonary vascular smooth muscle, resulting in decreased pulmonary vascular resistance, but it generally does not cause hemodynamic changes outside the lung. Additionally, inhaled nitric oxide may improve arterial oxygenation in hypoxemic patients by reducing intrapulmonary shunt and improving ventilation-perfusion matching. In both pediatric and adult patients, inhaled nitric oxide has been studied and used as a treatment modality in the intensive care unit (ICU) setting for a large number of clinical conditions in which reduction of pulmonary vascular resistance and/or improvement in arterial oxygenation is desired, including persistent pulmonary hypertension of the newborn; congenital diaphragmatic hernia; premature infant respiratory failure; respiratory distress syndrome (adults and children); cystic fibrosis; sickle cell disease; primary pulmonary hypertension; postoperative congenital heart disease; one-lung ventilation during thoracic surgery; postpneumonectomy; lung transplantation ischemia/reperfusion injury; and perioperative pulmonary hypertension associated with cardiac transplantation and left ventricular assist device implantation. Multiple outcome parameters have been measured to show inhaled nitric oxide treatment efficacy for the various clinical conditions listed above, but results have varied, yielding both positive and negative findings. However, it is safe to say that there is currently no evidence that inhaled nitric oxide therapy improves long-term morbidity or mortality rates for any clinical condition studied, and any short-term benefits of instituting inhaled nitric oxide therapy must be weighed against the known acute and potential long-term toxic effects of inhaled nitric oxide. The current Food and Drug Administration (FDA)–approved use for inhaled nitric oxide (marketed as INOmax) is for the treatment of term and near-term (>34 weeks) neonates with hypoxic respiratory failure associated with clinical or echocardiographic evidence of pulmonary hypertension, where it improves oxygenation and reduces the need for extracorporeal membrane oxygenation. Thus, all other off-label indications for inhaled nitric oxide are regulated at the institutional level.

Because of the short half-life of nitric oxide, sustained pulmonary vasodilatation requires continuous delivery of inhaled nitric oxide via commercially available systems that accurately deliver inspired concentrations between 1 and 80 parts per million (ppm). These systems must be able to deliver a constant concentration of inhaled nitric oxide to patients while minimizing the generation of nitrogen dioxide (NO_2), a direct toxin and environmental pollutant, as well as continuously monitor inspired NO, NO_2, and O_2 concentrations. Clinically significant levels of NO_2 are unlikely to occur when inhaled nitric oxide is delivered by an efficient delivery system at concentrations of 20 ppm or less. Inhaled NO is usually delivered during mechanical ventilation into the inspiratory limb of the ventilatory circuit by either pulse or continuous modes, although it may be administered to spontaneously breathing patients with a close-fitting mask.

WHAT TO DO

FDA-recommended dosing for inhaled nitric oxide is 20 ppm for neonates, with treatment duration as clinically indicated for up to 14 days. For other uses, dosing is usually titrated to the desired pulmonary systolic and diastolic pressures (assessed with a pulmonary arterial catheter) and/or arterial blood oxygenation (measured by continuous O_2 saturation and/or arterial blood gases). There is little evidence to suggest that concentrations of 40 ppm or less are toxic even for extended periods, but it is important to note that nontitrated weaning off or sudden withdrawal of inhaled nitric oxide therapy has been shown to produce severe, life-threatening rebound hypoxemia and pulmonary hypertension. Additional complications or side effects of inhaled nitric oxide therapy may include peroxynitrite ($ONOO^-$) formation leading to cellular membrane lipid peroxidation, altered pulmonary inflammatory responses, altered surfactant function, genotoxic alterations, inhibition of platelet function, and alteration of iron- and heme-based protein function such as cyclo-oxygenase and cytochromes.

WATCH OUT FOR

Methemoglobinemia is a potentially very dangerous complication of inhaled nitric oxide treatment, and inhaled nitric oxide is contraindicated in patients with congenital or acquired methemoglobin reductase deficiency. The danger with methemoglobinemia lies in its insidious nature of development, with development and progression occurring despite normal arterial blood gas measures. It is a functional anemia where nitrates accumulate during inhaled nitric oxide therapy and lead to methemoglobin formation, characterized by oxidation of ferrous iron to ferric iron, which in turn prevents O_2 release into the tissues (i.e., shifts the oxyhemoglobin dissociation curve to the left).

Hypoxia secondary to methemoglobinemia is therefore refractory to correction by O_2 therapy and if not detected and treated can be rapidly fatal. Normal methemoglobin, reported as a fraction of normal hemoglobin, is <2%. Cyanosis is appreciated when methemoglobin levels approach 15% to 20%, with progressive, multiorgan hypoxic symptoms developing with increasing methemoglobin fractions. Death occurs when methemoglobin levels reach 70%. However, in the critically ill, ventilated patient receiving inhaled nitric oxide, it is difficult to say what level of methemoglobin correlates with what degree of tissue hypoxia, since the patient may be also be in a hypoperfused state and more severe tissue hypoxia could result at lower methemoglobin fractions.

Thus, institution of inhaled nitric oxide therapy requires concomitant methemoglobin monitoring. Clinically significant levels of methemoglobin are unlikely to result unless inhaled nitric oxide concentrations over 20 ppm are administered, but methemoglobin should be measured every 4 hours after instituting inhaled nitric oxide delivery and daily thereafter, since inadvertently high NO concentrations may be delivered. High methemoglobin levels (>5%) may provoke changes in dosing, but the overall risks and benefits of altering dosing must be considered given the overall clinical picture, particularly in light of the known possible detrimental effect of rapid off weaning of inhaled nitric oxide. Decreasing dosing alone will not rapidly correct methemoglobinemia. High levels alone may warrant treatment, whereas increased levels plus additional clinical findings of tissue hypoxia such as electrocardiogram (ECG) changes, lactic acidosis, change in neuro exam, and so on mandate treatment. The standard treatment for methemoglobinemia is intravenous (IV) infusion of methylene blue at 1 to 2 mg/kg of a 1% solution over 5 minutes. The dose may need to be repeated but should not exceed 1.5 times the initial dose. Methylene blue will rapidly convert ferric iron back to its ferrous state, which will refacilitate O_2 off loading into the tissues. Ascorbic acid treatment may be used for patients who are resistant to methylene blue.

SUGGESTED READINGS

Germann P, Braschi A, Della Rocca G, et al. Inhaled nitric oxide therapy in adults: European expert recommendations. Intens Care Med. 2005;31:1029–1041.

Griffiths MJD, Evans TW. Inhaled nitric oxide therapy in adults. N Engl J Med. 2005;353(25):2683–2695.

Haddad E, Lowson SM, Johns RA, et al. Use of inhaled nitric oxide perioperatively and in intensive care patients. Anesthesiology. 2000;92(6):1821–1825.

Maimo G, Redick E. Recognizing and treating methemoglobinemia. A rare but dangerous complication of topical anesthetic or nitrate overdose. Dimens Crit Care Nurs. 2004;23(3):116–118.

Weinberger B, Laskin DL, Heck DE, et al. The toxicology of inhaled nitric oxide. Toxicol Sci. 2001;59:5–16.

223

REMEMBER THAT TROPONIN LEVELS ARE INACCURATE AS A MEASURE OF CARDIAC DAMAGE IN RENAL INSUFFICIENCY

BRADFORD D. WINTERS, MD, PhD

The measurement of cardiac troponins has become a commonly used biochemical marker for myocardial injury and infarction. Unfortunately, there are several factors that may make the interpretation of troponin values difficult, including spurious elevations that are not indicative of myocardial injury after further evaluation. One of the major clinical confounders, particularly in critically ill patients, is renal insufficiency. Patients with chronic renal insufficiency are known to be at higher risk for developing accelerated atherosclerotic coronary artery disease (CAD), so the ability to interpret biochemical markers for myocardial disease in this population is of great importance. For patients with acute renal insufficiency or failure, there is no similar incremental risk of CAD directly attributable to the renal failure, but myocardial events are nevertheless common in these patients.

Troponins are protein molecules that participate in the regulation of contractile function of the myocardial sarcomeres and are released into the general circulation when myocardial injury occurs much as creatinine kinase–MB (CK-MB) is under similar conditions. There are two troponins: I and T. Elevated troponin T has been shown to correlate with an increased risk of future acute coronary syndromes. For troponin I, this relationship is not as clear, with the study results being contradictory. Some hospitals measure and report troponin I, but many hospital laboratories report troponins as a combined value. The problem with this is that troponin T has been shown to lack specificity for making the diagnosis of an acute coronary event in patients with end-stage renal disease. The exact values for the upper normal limit of troponins may vary from hospital lab to hospital lab based on the assay used. Where the cutoff is set for any particular lab test will determine its specificity and sensitivity and should be optimized using receiver operator curve (ROC) analysis. The preponderance of data suggests that higher thresholds are required for using cardiac troponins to define outcomes for renal patients suspected of having an acute coronary syndrome. ROC analysis suggests that for nonrenal patients, the upper limit should be approximately 0.1 μg/L while for renal patients the upper limit should be approximately 0.5 μg/L, though these values are not absolute. In comparison, most of the data on CK-MB suggest that values for this analyte do not need to be significantly adjusted for renal patients.

Since troponin levels rise over a 6- to 8-hour period post-myocardial injury and remain elevated for up to 10 days, it is imperative to follow the values sequentially. If there is a definite rise and then fall over this time frame, then an acute myocardial event has likely occurred especially if in context with a suspicious clinical scenario. CK–MB values generally rise more slowly but fall more quickly. These are usually measured on a q8h basis from the time of the suspected event for a period of 24 hours with the second and third values being most predictive. The CK–MB fraction is usually reported as a percent of the total CK, with values of greater than 3% being indicative of myocardial injury assuming the total CK is greater than approximately 200. Percentages higher than 3 in face of low total CK are generally considered spurious.

The evidence in support of requiring higher troponin thresholds for patients with renal disease for diagnosing and prognosticating acute coronary syndromes is primarily based on patients with end-stage renal disease on chronic dialysis therapy. While there are limited data on critically ill patients, it seems reasonable to consider intensive care unit (ICU) patients who are on dialysis for renal failure similar to the chronic renal failure patient in terms of the use of troponins as biomarkers though there is evidence that the longer a patient is on dialysis, the higher his or her troponins may be. The greater difficulty comes in interpreting troponins in critically ill patients with lesser degrees of renal insufficiency, some native glomerular filtration, and who are not on dialysis. In this situation, there are virtually no data and even less consensus on thresholds despite the concern that troponins may be falsely elevated even when the renal failure is incomplete. Reliance on the clinical scenario and other tests including CK–MB and echocardiography are necessary in this situation. Given that thresholds and assays vary from institution to institution and some use troponin I and/or troponin T as the analyte in their lab test, clinicians should familiarize themselves with the reference values at their hospital and whether allowances are made for renal insufficiency.

A final note is that a myriad of commercial assays are available to measure troponin level. Up to a 20-fold variation in troponin values may be seen depending on the assay used.

SUGGESTED READINGS

Bueti J, Krahn J, Karpinski M, et al. Troponin I testing in dialysis patients presenting to the emergency room: does troponin I predict the 30 day outcome? Nephron Clin Pract. 2006;103:129–136.

Kanderian AS, Francis GS. Cardiac troponins and chronic kidney disease. Kidney Int. 2006;69:1112–1114.

Van Lente F, McErlean ES, DeLuca SA, et al. Ability of troponins to predict adverse outcomes in patients with renal insufficiency and suspected acute coronary syndromes: a case-matched study. J Am Coll Cardiol. 1999;33:471–478.

224

Ask the Laboratory for a Synergy Panel in Resistant Pseudomonas Infections

Harjot K. Singh, MD
Sara E. Cosgrove, MD

The use of combination therapy (double coverage) in the management of Gram-negative infections is a controversial practice. Reasons to consider combination therapy include (a) broadening empiric coverage in the event that the causative organism is resistant to one agent, (b) prevention of emergence of resistance during therapy, and (c) obtaining synergistic activity between two agents that is greater than would be expected from the sum of the activities of the individual agents.

Broadening empiric coverage should be considered in patients who are critically ill as data suggest that inappropriate empiric therapy can lead to adverse patient outcomes. Agents from two different classes of antibiotics should be used. Review of the local antibiogram is important to assess whether combination therapy is needed and what agents should be used. For example, if the usual empiric therapy regimen for a penicillin-allergic patient is a fluoroquinolone, but 40% of *Pseudomonas* isolates in a unit are known to be resistant to fluoroquinolones, addition of a second agent such as an aminoglycoside may effectively broaden empiric coverage if *Pseudomonas* is suspected. In all cases in which combination therapy is chosen for empiric coverage, therapy should be narrowed on the basis of microbiologic data.

WHAT TO DO

Prevention of emergence of resistance is often cited as a reason for combination therapy in the management of definitive infections with Gram-negative organisms; however, emergence of resistance on therapy is uncommon, occurring in 5% to 10% of Gram-negative infections. In most circumstances, long-term combination therapy is not needed and may be harmful as it increases toxicity from adverse drug reactions. It can be considered in the treatment of a deep-seated infection (such as pneumonia or severe osteomyelitis) when the organism being treated is already resistant to one or more classes of antibiotics. Discontinuing one of the agents after 5 to 7 days of therapy when the bacterial burden has decreased is an option. In all cases, attention should be given to appropriate dosing of antibiotics and to obtaining follow-up cultures if the patient is failing therapy. Of note is that when organisms that produce inducible beta-lactamases (e.g., *Enterobacter*, *Serratia*, *Citrobacter*) are treated with beta-lactam agents, emergence of resistance on therapy can occur in ~20% of cases. Monotherapy with beta-lactam agents is best avoided for treatment of serious infections in these patients if other agents are available.

Although in vitro synergy exists between antipseudomonal penicillins and aminoglycosides for *Pseudomonas aeruginosa* and other Gram-negative rods, no definitive evidence exists that combining these agents in humans leads to enhanced outcomes. A study by Hilf et al. in 1989 suggested that combination therapy was superior to monotherapy in patients with *Pseudomonas* bacteremia, but 84% of patients receiving monotherapy received only an aminoglycoside. Aminoglycosides should not be used as monotherapy for infections caused by *Pseudomonas* except for uncomplicated urinary tract infections. More recent studies have not shown a difference in mortality when patients received appropriate monotherapy for bacteremia due to Gram-negative rods, including *Pseudomonas*; these studies have been summarized in a recent meta-analysis examining patients with sepsis due to Gram-negative bacteria.

Synergy between drug combinations other than beta-lactam and aminoglycosides is less predictable and has unclear clinical significance. Synergy testing with two antibiotics is of significant value only when treating a highly resistant Gram-negative organism that is resistant to one or both of the drugs in the combination. Formal synergy testing is recommended if using combination therapy in this setting, although such testing is not within the purview of many microbiology laboratories.

SUGGESTED READINGS

Comber KR, Basker MJ, Osborne CD, et al. Synergy between ticarcillin and tobramycin against *Pseudomonas aeruginosa* and Enterobacteriaceae in vitro and in vivo. Antimicrob Agents Chemother. 1977;11:956–964.

Fish DN, Piscitelli SC, Danziger LH. Development of resistance during antimicrobial therapy: a review of antibiotic classes and patient characteristics in 173 studies. Pharmacotherapy. 1995;15:279–291.

Hilf M, Yu VL, Sharp J, et al. Antibiotic therapy for *Pseudomonas aeruginosa* bacteremia: outcome correlations in a prospective study of 200 patients. Am J Med. 1989;87:540–546.

Ibrahim EH, Sherman G, Ward S, et al. The influence of inadequate antimicrobial treatment of bloodstream infections on patient outcomes in the ICU setting. Chest. 2000,118:146–155.

Kaye KS, Cosgrove S, Harris A, et al. Risk factors for emergence of resistance to broad-spectrum cephalosporins among *Enterobacter* spp. Antimicrob Agents Chemother. 2001;45:2628–2630.

Paul M, Benuri-Silbiger I, Soares-Weiser K, et al. Beta lactam monotherapy versus beta lactam-aminoglycoside combination therapy for sepsis in immunocompetent patients: systematic review and meta-analysis of randomised trials. BMJ. 2004;328:668–672.

225

Obtain Blood Used for Mixed Venous Oxygen Testing from the Distal Pulmonary Artery Catheter Port

Ala' S. Haddadin, MD

Analysis of mixed venous blood provides valuable information in evaluating the oxygen supply-demand axis. Mixed venous oxygen saturation (SvO_2) is the O_2 saturation of blood in the pulmonary artery after the venous effluent from various organs has mixed thoroughly in the right ventricle (normal $SvO_2 = 70\%$ to 80%, normal mixed venous oxygen pressure [PvO_2] = 35 to 45 mm Hg). Normally, blood from the inferior vena cava is more fully saturated (5% to 7%) than blood from the superior vena cava due to highly saturated blood from the renal vein entering the inferior vena cava, but the reverse is true in shock states because of redistribution of flow away from the splanchnic, renal, and mesenteric beds.

The SvO_2 can be measured intermittently by slowly withdrawing a sample of blood from the distal port of the unwedged pulmonary artery catheter or continuously with a fiberoptic pulmonary artery catheter that measures O_2 saturation by reflectance oximetry. Intermittent sampling of SvO_2 is accomplished by discarding the initial 3 mL of blood and then withdrawing a sample *very slowly* in order to avoid contamination with capillary blood, which may artifactually increase the oxygen content.

The value of mixed venous blood analysis is best understood in the framework of tissue O_2 delivery-supply dynamics. Oxygen delivery is the product of cardiac output and arterial O_2 content, the latter being determined by the hemoglobin and arterial O_2 saturation (SaO_2). Each organ receives a variable percentage of the total amount, a flow that may be luxuriant, just adequate, or insufficient to satisfy the aerobic metabolism demand. The O_2 tension (PvO_2) and saturation of the venous effluent reflect the balance between supply and demand. Normally, peripheral oxygen consumption is independent of the oxygen delivery. Therefore, as cardiac output and oxygen delivery decline, peripheral extraction increases to keep consumption constant. This results in decreased mixed venous oxygen saturation. Under normal conditions, the SaO_2–SvO_2 difference is 20% to 25%, yielding an SvO_2 of 65% to 75% when arterial blood is well oxygenated. Increased SvO_2 is seen in a variety of conditions. In sepsis, SvO_2 is often normal, but in some cases there is extreme peripheral vasodilatation, and cardiac output increases disproportionately to metabolic demands, resulting in increased SvO_2. Cirrhosis is one of the more common causes of marked increase in SvO_2, with values usually >85%. A number of vasodilating agents and left-to-right shunts (either intracardiac or peripheral) also result in increased SvO_2. Wedging of the catheter and mitral regurgitation (which tend to bring the catheter tip into contact with arterialized blood) are additional factors that raise the SvO_2. Finally, agents that interfere with mitochondrial cytochrome activity (e.g., cyanide) may produce an elevated SvO_2 value owing to inability of the tissues to utilize oxygen.

The continuous measurement of O_2 saturation in mixed venous blood is performed with specialized pulmonary artery catheters (more expensive than regular ones) equipped with fiberoptic bundles that can transmit light to and from the catheter tip. The optical detection of SvO_2 is performed by reflection spectrophotometry. Wavelengths of light similar to those used in pulse oximetry are passed along the fiberoptic bundles in the pulmonary artery catheter and out from the catheter tip. The light beam is transmitted through the circulating blood and the light that comes in contact with hemoglobin in the circulating erythrocytes is reflected back to the catheter tip. This light is then transmitted back through the catheter to a photodetector and microprocessor that record the average SvO_2 at 5-second intervals. A >5% variation in SvO_2 that persists for longer than 10 minutes is considered a significant change. Perhaps the most rational use of the fiberoptic pulmonary artery catheter is in the management of patients with cardiac dysfunction, in whom rapid changes in the cardiac output maybe expected to occur on the basis of the underlying disease process or in response to a therapeutic intervention.

WATCH OUT FOR

It must be stressed that a normal or high SvO_2 does not necessarily mean adequate oxygen delivery (as in sepsis), and the need to further augment cardiac output in this setting is controversial. A normal SvO_2 may be associated with different levels of cardiac output depending on the underlying aerobic metabolism. In essence, the SvO_2 helps us define the appropriateness of measured cardiac output. In one recent study, the mixed venous oxygen saturation correlated well with decreased morbidity after cardiac surgery when therapy was targeted to keep SvO_2 >70% and a lactate level <2 mg/dL. However, no benefit was shown in another study that involved a more heterogeneous group of critically ill patients when goal-directed hemodynamic therapy was based on SvO_2.

DETERMINANTS OF SvO$_2$

$$S\bar{v}O_2 = SaO_2 - (VO_2/Q \times Hb \times 13)$$

VO_2 is oxygen consumption; Q is cardiac output; Hb is hemoglobin. (Low SvO$_2$ <60% indicates an abnormality of one or more of the factors on the right-hand side of the above equation.)

SUGGESTED READINGS

Gattinoni L, Brazzi L, Pelosi P, et al. A trial of goal-oriented hemodynamic therapy in critically-ill patients: SvO$_2$ Collaborative Group. N Engl J Med. 1995;333:1025.

Polonen P, Ruokonen E, Hippelainen M, et al. A prospective, randomized study of goal-oriented hemodynamic therapy in cardiac surgical patients. Anesth Analg. 2000;90:1052.

Vaugh S, Puri VK. Cardiac output changes and continuous mixed venous saturation measurement in the critically ill. Crit Care Med. 1988;16:495.

CHECK THYROID FUNCTION IN CRITICALLY ILL PATIENTS

MEGHAN C. TADEL, MD

Both hypothyroidism and hyperthyroidism can contribute to life-threatening situations during the care of critically ill patients. Although the most severe forms of these diseases, myxedema coma and thyroid storm, generally occur in patients with previously diagnosed thyroid disorders, they can rarely be the presenting episode of thyroid abnormality in a patient undergoing the extreme stresses of trauma, infection, perioperative periods, or recovery from anesthesia.

HYPOTHYROIDISM

Although up to 90% of intensive care unit (ICU) patients have been found to have abnormal thyroid function tests (most commonly low triiodothyronine [T_3]), the vast majority of them are found to have sick euthyroid syndrome, also known as nonthyroidal illness syndrome. Because of this complicating factor it has been very difficult to quantitate the true incidence of hypothyroidism in ICU patients, but estimates range from 5% to 30% of patients admitted to medical ICUs.

Signs and symptoms of hypothyroidism exist along a continuum. Patients may exhibit some symptoms while lacking others, and the most severe symptoms are present only when a patient has progressed to myxedema coma. Possible manifestations of hypothyroidism include hypoglycemia, hypothermia (or cold intolerance), hypotension, hypoventilation, hyponatremia, bradycardia, electrocardiogram changes (T-wave inversions and eventually J waves), gastrointestinal atony, bladder atony, skeletal muscle myopathy, doughy nonpitting edema, fatigue, lethargy, and altered level of consciousness. Perhaps the most ubiquitous sign of hypothyroidism is a pericardial effusion, which is present in up to 30% of hypothyroid patients; pleural and peritoneal effusions can be seen as well. Medications that have been associated with hypothyroidism include lithium, amiodarone, aminoglutethimide, interferon alpha, thalidomide, betaroxine, and stavudine.

Critically ill patients who demonstrate any number of the aforementioned stigmata of hypothyroidism should be tested for thyroid function as early as possible as this minimizes the likelihood of values being abnormal because of sick euthyroid syndrome. There are many tests available for screening and diagnosis of thyroid dysfunction and some controversy surrounds the order in which these tests should be completed. The most common method, which provides >90% sensitivity for detection of hypothyroidism, is a combination of thyrotropin and either free thyroxine (T_4) or total T_4 and free T_4 index. In primary hypothyroidism (which accounts for 95% of hypothyroidism), thyrotropin levels will be elevated outside the normal range of 0.5 to 5.0 mU/L and in most cases of clinical hypothyroidism will actually be elevated above 20 mU/L. In secondary, or central, hypothyroidism, which is due to adenohypophyseal or pituitary dysfunction, the thyrotropin will be very low or undetectable. In either situation, free T_4 will be below the normal range. Total T_4 levels are not helpful because only free hormone is active and total T_4 levels may be low in the face of normal free T_4 in situations of altered protein binding or decreased proteins available for binding. The free T_4 index takes into account binding and protein availability by multiplying the total T_4 by a factor determined by T_3 resin uptake.

WHAT TO DO

Treatment of hypothyroidism must encompass supportive measures, in addition to thyroid hormone replacement. Hormone replacement can be accomplished via oral or parenteral supplementation of thyroid hormone in the form of either T_3 or T_4. Because intravenous supplementation of thyroid hormone, in particular T_3, has been associated with life-threatening arrhythmias, specifically ventricular tachyarrhythmias, it has been argued that this be reserved for patients demonstrating only the most severe symptoms of hypothyroidism—myxedema coma or hypotension and bradycardia not responsive to other therapies. Because of this concern, there is no consensus on therapy but several generally accepted regimens of thyroid hormone repletion are most commonly recommended. In mild cases, where a patient can tolerate oral (PO) medications, they can be started at a dose of 50 μg/day (elderly should start at 25 μg/day) with titrations of 50 μg/day of T_4 every 3 to 4 weeks with monitoring of thyrotropin level to determine when therapeutic doses have been reached. The usual ending dose is 50 to 200 μg/day. Patients who cannot tolerate oral medications or who are demonstrating significant symptoms from hypothyroidism can be given 200 to 500 μg intravenously (IV) as a single bolus to help replete the thyroxine circulating volume, then 100 μg 24 hours later and then 50 μg daily, with further titrations every 3 to 4 weeks based on thyrotropin levels. If IV T_4 is given, it can be supplemented with IV T_3 at the dose of 25 μg for a young, noncardiac patient, 12.5 μg for an elderly or cardiac patient; the single dose of T_3 may be repeated once at 12 hours. The rationale for supplementing T_3 in addition to T_4 is that there are concerns given that T_3 is the more active form of thyroid hormone, although 90% of T_3 is made via peripheral conversion from T_4 and in a hypothyroid state, peripheral conversion of T_4 to T_3 is reduced. It should be noted when converting from an IV to a PO, the dose should be doubled as the bioavailability is 50%.

HYPERTHYROIDISM

Hyperthyroidism, or as it is commonly called, thyrotoxicosis, is rarely diagnosed in the ICU setting, but decompensation of chronic hyperthyroidism in these critically ill patients can be life threatening. The most common cause of thyrotoxicosis, accounting for up to 90% of cases in the United States, is Graves disease, which occurs in anywhere from 0.02% to 0.4% of the population. Signs and symptoms of thyrotoxicosis include supraventricular tachyarrhythmias (sinus tachycardia and atrial fibrillation most commonly), agitation (although lethargy can be seen in the elderly), fine tremors, anxiety, heat intolerance, increased perspiration, and weight loss, often in spite of an increased appetite. When thyrotoxicosis progresses to its most severe form, thyroid storm, the previous symptoms are accompanied by fever, severe agitation or coma, and high-output cardiac failure. The medication most commonly associated with thyrotoxicosis is chronic amiodarone therapy because of its high iodine content. The other diagnosis to consider, particularly in a patient with no known history of thyrotoxicosis, is that of thyrotoxicosis factitia, which is caused by ingestion of supratherapeutic doses of thyroxine.

The laboratory test most useful in diagnosing thyrotoxicosis is free T_4 or total T_4 and T_4 index. By definition, free T_4 or T_4 index will be elevated in thyrotoxicosis. It has been traditionally argued that thyrotropin levels provide little or no insight into hyperthyroidism. However, now that sensitive thyrotropin tests are available that can detect levels of thyrotropin as low as 0.01 mU/L (normal range 0.5 to 5.0 mU/L), it is argued that a value below 0.1 mU/L is indeed diagnostic of primary thyrotoxicosis with appropriate negative feedback of thyrotropin release.

WHAT TO DO

Thyrotoxicosis should be managed with supportive measures as well as antithyroid medications. The two available medications that suppress thyroxine production are methimazole and propylthiouracil (PTU). There is some disagreement as to which therapy is preferred because methimazole is thought to have a more rapid onset of action and has a better side-effect profile; however, PTU has been traditionally preferred because it demonstrates inhibition of peripheral conversion of T_4 to T_3, which is the more active form of thyroid hormone. There is also little consensus as to the optimal dosing of these medications but most protocols are within the range of PTU 100 to 200 mg two or three times a day or methimazole 10 to 60 mg per day. Both medications are available only in enteral formulations and if a patient cannot have PO medications they can be given via nasogastric tube.

These medications primarily affect production of thyroxine, which means they can take weeks to affect the available pool of thyroid hormone. In the meantime, additional therapies can be of benefit. Propranolol in either IV or PO formulation can be titrated to effect for improvement of tachyarrhythmias and agitation. Although other selective beta-blockers have been shown to be helpful, particularly in patients with bronchoconstrictive lung disease, propranolol is generally favored because it demonstrates some minimal inhibition of peripheral T_4-to-T_3 conversion. Iodide, given as Lugol's solution either PO or as an enema, has an instantaneous inhibition of release of thyroid hormone from the gland. However, this therapy should be instituted only after either methimazole or PTU therapy has begun to prevent an increase in thyroxine production. Via the same mechanism, the gallbladder dyes iopanoic acid and ipodate, which both contain high levels of iodide, can also be given. These dyes also act to decrease peripheral T_4-to-T_3 conversion. In the short term amiodarone has also been used because of its high iodine content and inhibition of T_4-to-T_3 conversion, but as noted earlier in chronic therapy this medication can cause thyrotoxicosis. Finally, in life-threatening cases, plasmapheresis and other forms of direct removal of thyroxine from circulation have been used, including cholestyramine for gastrointestinal binding of thyroxine, although no tested protocol exists for any of these methods.

SUGGESTED READINGS

Goldman L, ed. Cecil Textbook of Medicine. 22nd ed. Philadelphia: WB Saunders; 2004:1392–1405.

Larsen P, ed. Williams Textbook of Endocrinology. 10th ed. Philadelphia: WB Saunders; 2003:346–365.

227

USE AN EMPTY LAB TUBE TO CHECK THE VIABILITY OF A STOMA

B. ROBERT GIBSON, MD

While stoma placement is typically considered a minor procedure, complications following it are frequent and potentially devastating. The complication rate has been reported to vary from 25% following colostomy to 75% following end ileostomy. These complications include retraction, prolapse, hernia, fistula, ulceration, stenosis, bleeding, and necrosis.

Stomal ischemia is more common with end stomas than with loop stomas. Causes of compromised blood flow are varied and usually related to surgical technique around the time of stoma formation. A too-tight abdominal stoma site may cause extrinsic compression of the blood vessels feeding the distal bowel. Tension on the vascular pedicle due to progressive abdominal distention or inadequate mobilization may lead to progressive ischemia of the stoma. Excessive intraoperative dissection of the bowel mesentery can lead to compromised distal arterial blood supply. Blood vessels may also become kinked as the bowel mesentery traverses the abdominal wall.

Ideally, a clear stoma appliance will be in place prior to patient arrival in the intensive care unit (ICU). This not only allows for collection and measurement of stoma effluent but also allows for bedside visual inspection of the bowel mucosa without necessitating a dressing or appliance change. Immediately postoperatively, it is common for bowel edema to be present at the stoma site. While a frequent cause of concern for patients and staff, some duskiness is to be expected. Typically, the stoma appearance improves and the duskiness resolves within 48 hours.

If there is no improvement in the stomal appearance within 48 hours, or if the stoma becomes black, the depth of stomal necrosis must be assessed to rule out an impending abdominal catastrophe. A simple technique for bedside examination of the stomal mucosa is as follows: Remove the rubber top and adhesive paper label of a glass blood collection tube and after lubrication gently place the bottom-closed end into the stoma. Then, shine a flashlight through the open mouth of the tube to illuminate the mucosa. In a noncompromised stoma, the reassuring pink color of viable bowel is typically apparent just below skin level.

If there is further concern regarding necrosis of the stoma, a flexible endoscope inserted gently into the stoma can better define the limits of necrosis. Necrosis that does not involve a large, continuous segment of bowel or is confined to the mucosa may be managed expectantly. Typically this type of lesion heals by secondary intention without perforation. If this is the case, the clinician must be aware of an increased risk of fistula formation or stenosis as the segment of necrosis heals. Necrosis that extends below the level of the fascia or is circumferential requires emergency surgery.

SUGGESTED READINGS

Deitch EA, ed. Tools of the Trade and Rules of the Road: A Surgical Guide. Philadelphia: Lippincott–Raven Publishers; 1997:186–202.
Nyhus LM, Baker RJ, Fischer JE, eds. Mastery of Surgery. 3rd ed. Boston: Little, Brown and Company; 1997:1366–1377.

228

Never retest low serum glucose; treat immediately and then prevent further episodes

Kathleen A. Williams, MSN, RN, CRNP
Sherita Hill Golden, MD, MHS

Maintaining euglycemia in the inpatient setting has been shown in multiple studies to decrease morbidity and mortality across multiple types of patient populations. One of the leading barriers to achieving optimal glucose control is the fear of hypoglycemia on the part of both patients as well as care providers. This fear is understandable. Hypoglycemia can cause behavioral changes, seizures, permanent neurological injury, and even death. Prompt and appropriate recognition, treatment, and prevention of hypoglycemia is therefore of critical importance.

Current methods for inpatient glucose monitoring include laboratory analysis of serum, point-of-care testing with portable bedside glucometers, and ongoing commercial investigations of continuous subcutaneous and serum glucose monitoring systems for inpatient use. The most accurate is laboratory analysis of a serum value. However, these values often take considerable time to obtain. Bedside glucometers, when used within the manufacturer's guidelines, can provide a rapid assessment of the patient's glycemic control. Appropriate training of staff using and interpreting blood glucose values obtained by bedside monitoring is critical to patient safety. Some conditions that alter the accuracy of glucometer readings may include the following:

1. The skin site may be inadequately prepared.
2. The arterial or venous lines may not be adequately cleared before blood is drawn and placed on the glucometer strip.
3. Conditions of decreased peripheral blood flow may not reflect the true physiological state. Examples of decreased blood flow include severe dehydration, hypotension, shock, and peripheral vascular disease or peripheral vasoconstriction due to vasoactive drugs.
4. Acetaminophen levels greater than 8 mg/dL may produce elevated glucose results
5. At glucose values above 200 mg/dL, low hematocrits (<20%) may cause elevated glucose readings compared with a whole blood reference.
6. At glucose values above 200 mg/dL, high hematocrits may cause reduced glucose value compared with a whole blood reference.

WHAT TO DO

Glucose monitoring orders should be written with notification parameters for both hypo- and hyperglycemia. If notification is given that a patient has a glucose value of <60 mg/dL, immediate treatment is required. If the patient is awake and able to swallow without risk for aspiration, the patient should be given 15 g of fast-acting carbohydrate (4 oz of juice or nondiet soda, 8 oz of milk, or a packet of graham crackers). If the patient is not able to take anything by mouth, he or she should be given 25 to 50 mL of 50% dextrose (D50) intravenously (IV). For those patients who are unable to swallow and lack IV access, initial treatment should consist of glucagon 1 mg intramuscularly and with establishment of IV access. Glucose values should be rechecked within 20 minutes of the initial administration of glucose or glucagon to assess response. Continued frequent monitoring is required for the duration of action of any hypoglycemic agent given. This is especially important if the causative agent is either intermediate or long-acting insulin or a sulfonylurea.

WHAT NOT TO DO

It is important to note that some diabetic patients may demonstrate hypoglycemic unawareness. Hypoglycemic unawareness is defined as the loss of hypoglycemic warning symptoms such as diaphoresis, tachycardia, and shaking due to defects in hormonal counterregulation. These are patients who will have low glucose readings but present without obvious symptoms. This lack of symptoms has caused the nursing and medical staff to disbelieve the glucose result and delay treatment, waiting for a repeat result to verify. This delay in treatment can result in a prolonged hypoglycemic event with subsequent neurologic injury. The transient increase in glucose from the administration of a single dose of D50 or oral intake of 15 g of fasting-acting carbohydrates is significantly less likely to cause harm to the patient as compared with the risk associated with prolonged hypoglycemia.

Patients at particular risk for hypoglycemic unawareness include those who have been maintained with intensive insulin therapies in the outpatient setting, those with near-normal glycosylated hemoglobin (HgbA1c), and those with autonomic neuropathy from the diabetes. Patients who are intubated, sedated, or otherwise lack the ability to self-report hypoglycemic symptoms (e.g., stroke) are also at a very high risk for unrecognized prolonged hypoglycemia.

Hypoglycemia is considered a preventable complication of antihyperglycemic therapy. In a recent study of 24 inpatient hypoglycemic events, 22 were considered preventable. Inadequate management response to a change in the course of care was the most common cause (82%) and inappropriate disease management, defined as inappropriate medication selection and inadequate monitoring selection, occurred in 50% of the events. Of note, exclusive use of the sliding scale regimen (which is still frequently being ordered as a hyperglycemia treatment modality) accounted for 26% of the hyperglycemic events in the same study.

To prevent hypoglycemia, the care provider should follow the American Association of Clinical Endocrinologists (AACE) Inpatient Glycemic Control Guidelines recommendations, which include the following:

1. Appropriate selection of patients for the use of IV insulin
2. Provision of IV insulin or addition of insulin in the total parenteral nutrition (TPN) bag to meet the requirements for insulin created by the use of TPN. This will avoid having a long-acting subcutaneous insulin continuing to have an effect if the TPN is stopped.
3. Use of a programmed subcutaneous insulin regimen that includes a basal–nutritional–correction component
4. Daily revision of the scheduled insulin regimen based on clinical condition and the response to previous therapy
5. Adjustment of insulin therapy with any change in renal function
6. Recognition of the risk for hypoglycemia with sudden changes in nutrition and the subsequent need for insulin adjustment and hypoglycemia prevention—including the use of D10 to mitigate the loss of either TPN or enteral feeding
7. Importance of close and accurate glucose monitoring at the bedside

SUGGESTED READINGS

Furnary AP, Gao G, Grunkemeier GL, et al. Continuous insulin infusion reduces mortality in patients with diabetes undergoing coronary artery bypass grafting. J Thorac Cardiovasc Surg. 2003;125:1007–1021.

Krinsley JS. Association between hyperglycemia and increased hospital mortality in a heterogeneous population of critically ill patients. Mayo Clin Proc. 2003;78:1471–1478.

van den Berghe G, Wouters P, Weekers F, et al. Intensive insulin therapy in the critically ill patient. N Engl J Med. 2001;345:1359–1367.

D-DIMER LEVELS CAN RULE OUT BUT NOT RULE IN PULMONARY EMBOLISM IN POSTOPERATIVE PATIENTS

HARI NATHAN, MD

D-dimer is a degradation product of cross-linked fibrin. A normal level of d-dimer is typically less than 500 ng/mL. In a patient with pulmonary embolism (PE), deep venous thrombosis (DVT), or other clot burden, elevated d-dimer levels reflect the body's endogenous fibrinolysis. In addition, d-dimer levels may also be raised in myocardial infarction, pneumonia, sepsis, and cancer; during the second and third trimesters of pregnancy; and after surgery. Elevated d-dimer levels may persist up to 3 months after surgery.

When DVT or PE is suspected in a postoperative patient, normal d-dimer levels argue against the diagnosis. The negative predictive value of the test varies from 85% to 99%, depending on the assay used and the pretest probability of PE. Elevated d-dimer levels, while consistent with PE, by no means confirm the diagnosis in postoperative patients. Thrombus in locations other than the pulmonary arterial bed (as in DVT or clot at the site of surgery) can explain d-dimer elevations, as can any of the factors listed previously. Therefore, if the clinical suspicion of PE is low, a normal d-dimer level is helpful in ruling out the diagnosis. When the clinical suspicion of PE is high, further investigation is mandated regardless of the d-dimer level.

SUGGESTED READINGS

Goldhaber SZ. Pulmonary embolism. Lancet. 2004;363:1295–1305.

Thompson BT, Hales CA. Clinical manifestations of and diagnostic strategies for acute pulmonary embolism. In: Rose BD, ed. UpToDate. Waltham, MA: UpToDate; 2006.

REMEMBER THAT DIABETIC KETOACIDOSIS OFTEN BEGINS WITH AN ANION-GAP METABOLIC ACIDOSIS

NIRAV G. SHAH, MD

Diabetic ketoacidosis (DKA) is a common diagnosis encountered in the hospital setting with an estimated incidence of 4.6 to 8 episodes per 1,000 patients with diabetes. It is a disorder that typically occurs after a precipitating event that causes an increase in catecholamines and is typified by the triad of hyperglycemia, metabolic acidosis, and ketosis. The importance of prompt diagnosis and treatment is evident by the severity of lab derangements and clinical deterioration that occurs if it is left untreated.

WATCH OUT FOR

The typical intensive care unit (ICU) patient with DKA is a known diabetic with insulin deficiency who has an event that causes an increase in growth hormone, glucagon, cortisol, or catecholamines, or an omission or deficiency of insulin. Occasionally, it may also be the presenting diagnosis for a new-onset diabetic patient. An underlying cause should always be excluded in the patient with DKA. The most common underlying etiologies include infection, myocardial infarction, stroke, and pancreatitis.

The physiology of DKA is fairly straightforward. The hyperglycemia in DKA results from gluconeogenesis and glycogenolysis in the liver and a reduced utilization of glucose by peripheral tissues. This, in turn, releases the inhibitory effect on glucagon, which when combined with low insulin levels results in more hepatic gluconeogenesis and glycogenolysis. Glucose levels can routinely run as high as 800 mg/dL. This level of hyperglycemia leads to dehydration and other electrolyte abnormalities because of the ensuing osmotic diuresis. Total-body stores of sodium, potassium, chloride, phosphorus, and magnesium are reduced by the polyuria that accompanies the diuresis. The serum potassium may be artificially elevated secondary to the profound acidosis. In addition, a factitious hyponatremia may occur in the setting of hyperglycemia. Therefore, the serum sodium must be corrected by increasing the sodium level by 1.6 mEq for each 100-mg/dL increase in serum glucose.

The treatment for DKA addresses two major goals: correcting the insulin deficiency and electrolyte abnormalities and treating the underlying cause. Therefore, the initial management is intravenous insulin therapy and aggressive intravenous fluid resuscitation. Insulin therapy should begin with a 10- to 20-unit bolus of regular insulin intravenously followed by a continuous infusion of 5 to 10 U/h that can be titrated to response. Intravenous fluid therapy should start with 2 to 3 liters of normal saline followed by 0.45% normal saline. Once the serum glucose reaches approximately 240 mg/dL, a combination of 5% glucose with 0.45% normal saline should be initiated. Throughout this course, careful attention should be paid to the level of serum potassium. Once the level is normal, or less than 5.5 mEq/L, replacement of potassium should begin at a rate of 10 mEq/h and should be increased to 40 to 80 mEq/h if the serum potassium is less than 3.5 mEq/L or if bicarbonate therapy is administered, though replacement of bicarbonate is not routinely suggested.

Of note, the metabolic acidosis of DKA is frequently severe with serum bicarbonate measurements less than 10 to 15 mEq/L and arterial pH ranging between 6.8 and 7.3. The metabolic acidosis is an anion-gap type and is present secondary to the inability to measure ketones in the blood. Beta-hydroxybutyric acid is the main ketone present in DKA. The anion-gap acidosis resolves as ketone production slows with the initiation of insulin and intravenous fluid therapy. In fact, with the administration of normal saline (154 mEq of both sodium and chloride) a hyperchloremic non–anion-gap metabolic acidosis may develop. This has no adverse effects and will gradually improve as renal acid excretion is enhanced in the days following admission with careful observation of chloride load.

Complications of DKA and/or inadequate therapy can be devastating. These include hypoglycemia, hypokalemia, cerebral edema (primarily in the pediatric population), and adult respiratory distress syndrome.

SUGGESTED READINGS

Kitabchi AE, Umpierrez GE, Murphy MB, et al. Management of hyperglycemic crises in patients with diabetes. Diabetes Care. 2000;24:131–153.

Rose BD, Post TW. Clinical Physiology of Acid-Base and Electrolyte Disorders. 5th ed. New York: McGraw-Hill; 2001:809–815.

231

CONSIDER OBTAINING A SERUM B-TYPE NATRIURETIC PEPTIDE LEVEL IN THE ACUTELY DYSPNEIC PATIENT

LAWRENCE OSEI, MD

B-type natriuretic peptide (BNP) is a 32-amino-acid polypeptide cardiac neurohormone specifically secreted from the ventricles in response to volume expansion and pressure overload. BNP was originally identified in extracts of porcine brain. It is present in minute amounts in human brain, but the clinically important source originates in the cardiac ventricles. The levels of B-type natriuretic peptide are elevated in patients with left ventricular dysfunction and the levels correlate with both the severity of symptoms and the prognosis.

The presenting features of acute cardiogenic and noncardiogenic pulmonary edema are similar and can be clinically difficult to distinguish. Common causes of cardiogenic pulmonary edema include cardiac ischemia with or without myocardial infarction, exacerbation of chronic systolic or diastolic heart failure, and dysfunction of the mitral or aortic valve. Volume overload should also be considered. A typical history of paroxysmal nocturnal dyspnea or orthopnea suggests cardiogenic pulmonary edema. However, a silent myocardial infarction or occult diastolic dysfunction may also manifest as acute pulmonary edema, with few clues provided by the history.

In contrast, noncardiogenic pulmonary edema is associated primarily with other clinical disorders, including pneumonia, sepsis, aspiration of gastric contents, and major trauma associated with the administration of multiple blood-product transfusions. In a patient presenting with acute dyspnea, measuring serum BNP levels may be able to help differentiate between cardiogenic and noncardiogenic pulmonary edema.

In one recent study by Maisel et al., BNP levels by themselves were more accurate than historical or physical findings or laboratory values in identifying congestive heart failure as the cause of dyspnea. The diagnostic accuracy of BNP at a cutoff of 100 pg/mL was 83.4%. The negative predictive value of BNP at levels of less than 50 pg/mL was 96%. The authors concluded that used in conjunction with other clinical information, BNP levels were useful in excluding the diagnosis of congestive heart failure.

SUGGESTED READINGS

Maisel A, Krishnaswamy P, Nowak RM, et al. Rapid measurement of B-type natriuretic peptide in the emergency diagnosis of heart failure. N Engl J Med. 2002;347(3):161–167.

Mueller C, Scholer A, Laule-Kilian K, et al. Use of B-type natriuretic peptide in the evaluation and management of acute dyspnea. N Engl J Med. 2004;350(7):647–654.

232

CONSIDER HYPOMAGNESEMIA AS A CAUSE OF REFRACTORY HYPOKALEMIA

ANTHONY D. SLONIM, MD, DRPH

Hypomagnesemia and hypokalemia are both common electrolyte disturbances in the intensive care unit (ICU) setting. Magnesium and potassium have important interactions to consider when treating deficiencies of either ion. Magnesium is intimately involved in a number of biochemical reactions in the body, particularly those involving adenosine triphosphate (ATP). The ionized form of magnesium in the serum is metabolically active but represents only a small component of the total-body magnesium. Furthermore, the relationship between the ionized and serum concentrations, and the serum and intracellular (cytoplasmic) concentrations are not clear. Therefore, total serum concentrations may not be representative of active ion.

Magnesium intake through the diet is usually sufficient for maintaining appropriate serum concentrations unless there is insufficient absorption or increased losses either through the gastrointestinal tract or urine. When hypomagnesemia occurs, the storage pool in the bone, muscle, and soft tissues is often sufficient for maintaining appropriate serum concentrations.

The symptoms of hypomagnesemia include arrhythmias (atrial fibrillation and flutter, ventricular tachycardia, and supraventricular tachycardia), electrocardiogram changes (prolonged QT, increased PR, and widening QRS), neurologic changes (seizures, altered mental status), and other electrolyte problems (hypophosphatemia, hypokalemia).

The treatment of hypomagnesemia is dependent upon the underlying cause. When magnesium is administered parenterally, the reabsorption at the level of the kidney is reduced and a large component of the administered dose will be excreted in the urine. Hypokalemia coexists with hypomagnesemia approximately 50% of the time. The mechanism for this is related to the ATP-dependent inhibition of luminal potassium channels in the distal nephron. When magnesium is deficient, the ATP is less effective and potassium is secreted into the tubular fluid, leading to a refractory hypokalemia. Therefore, magnesium (even in the setting of a normal serum value and considering its large therapeutic window) should be administered empirically in the setting of hypocalcemia or hypokalemia.

SUGGESTED READING

Dacey MJ. Hypomagnesemic disorders. Crit Care Clin. 2001;17:155–173.

233

BE AWARE THAT ENTERAL FEEDS CAN LOWER PHENYTOIN LEVELS

TIMOTHY M. MOORE, MD, PhD
FARAMARZ ZARFESHANFARD, RPh

Phenytoin (Dilantin) is an anticonvulsant drug, which can be useful in the treatment of seizures and epilepsy. The primary site of action appears to be the motor cortex where spread of seizure activity is inhibited, possibly by promoting sodium efflux from neurons and stabilizing the threshold against hyperexcitability caused by excessive stimulation or environmental changes capable of reducing membrane sodium gradient. Loss of posttetanic potentiation prevents cortical seizure foci from detonating adjacent cortical areas. Phenytoin reduces the maximal activity of brain-stem centers responsible for the tonic phase of tonic–clonic (grand mal) seizures.

Phenytoin exhibits nonlinear, dose-dependent, Michaelis-Menten pharmacokinetics. At therapeutic levels, phenytoin enzyme hepatic metabolism reaches its capacity and its pharmacokinetics changes from first order to zero order, at which time a small increase in the daily dose will result in a disproportionately higher level. Because of its capacity-limited metabolism, phenytoin half-life and time to reach steady state are concentration dependent. The higher the concentration, the longer the half-life and the longer the time it takes to reach steady state. The plasma half-life in humans after oral administration of phenytoin averages 22 hours, with a range of 7 to 42 hours. After intravenous (IV) administration, the half-life ranges between 11 and 15 hours. The difference in half-life is due to slower absorption and varying bioavailability of phenytoin formulations. Drug interactions may increase or decrease phenytoin half-life. Estimation of time to reach steady state cannot be based on half-life. Serum level determinations should be obtained after treatment initiation, dosage change, or addition or subtraction of an interacting food or drug to the regimen. Trough levels provide information about clinically effective serum level range and are obtained just prior to the patient's next scheduled dose. Peak levels indicate an individual's threshold for emergence of dose-related side effects and are obtained at the time of expected peak concentration. For Dilantin capsules, peak serum levels occur 4 to 12 hours after administration. For Dilantin Infatabs and Dilantin suspension, peak serum levels occur 1.5 to 3 hours after administration. The timing of levels is dependent on the clinical situation as well as route of administration and dosage form. In the acute setting, it is advisable to check non-steady-state phenytoin levels to avoid subtherapeutic or toxic levels prior to reaching steady state. Suggested sampling time after oral load is in 24 hours. Because of slow absorption of oral formulations, timing is not critical for level monitoring, but trough levels are suggested. Suggested sampling time for IV maintenance is also a trough level (or just prior to the next dose). Though beyond the scope of this review, detailed pharmacokinetic equations are available to help dose and monitor phenytoin treatment. (See suggested readings.)

Optimum control without clinical signs of toxicity occurs more often with total serum levels between 10 and 20 $\mu g/mL$ and free levels of between 1 and 2 $\mu g/mL$, although some mild cases of tonic-clonic (grand mal) epilepsy may be controlled with lower serum levels of phenytoin. In most patients maintained at a steady dosage, stable phenytoin serum levels are achieved. There may be wide interpatient variability in phenytoin serum levels with equivalent dosages. The patient with large variations in phenytoin plasma levels, despite standard doses, presents a difficult clinical problem. Unusually high levels result from liver disease, congenital enzyme deficiency, or drug interactions resulting in metabolic interference. Plasma protein binding is decreased in renal failure and hypoalbuminemia. Patients with unusually low levels may be noncompliant or hypermetabolizers of phenytoin. However, in the ICU setting in patients receiving enteral feeds, unusually or persistently low serum phenytoin levels may actually be attributable to a known interaction with enteral feeding.

Although it has been widely reported that serum phenytoin levels are lowered in patients receiving concomitant enteral feeding, the exact mechanism underlying this interaction is unknown. The majority of studies have suggested that there is some physical incompatibility between phenytoin and certain components in enteral feeding formulas causing decreased bioavailability of the drug. Other proposed mechanisms include binding of phenytoin to the feeding tube lumen, pH interaction of feeds and drug, increased metabolism or clearance of the drug after prolonged use of enteral feeds, and interaction of phenytoin and other drugs being administered via the enteric tube. A small number of studies have refuted the existence of an interaction between phenytoin and enteral feeding altogether. Interestingly, these studies were prospective but were also performed in healthy volunteers rather than in an ICU patient population. Ethical and logistic considerations limit the ability to perform prospective, controlled, randomized trials in appropriate patients.

The predominantly recommended method for reducing this inter-action between enteral feedings and phenytoin is to stagger phenytoin administration with feeding time. When continuous feeds are required, it has been recommended to hold feeds 1 to 2 hours prior to phenytoin dosing, flush the feeding tube with at least 20 cm^3 free water or saline before and after administration, and resume feeding 1 to 2 hours after dosing. It should be noted that there is no clear evidence that this strategy increases absorption. Other strategies to achieve and main-tain seizure control in the tube-fed patient include simply adjusting the phenytoin dosage while on continuous feeds without interrupting the feeds regimen, changing phenytoin administration to intravenous, changing the antiseizure medication regimen, and changing the enteral feeding formula. An alternative strategy is to use the injectable prod-uct down the feeding tube. This strategy has been shown to increase the rate of absorption but not the extent of absorption. It is important to note that implementation of any or all of these recommendations should be made only upon careful consideration of the overall clinical condition of the critically ill patient. It is also especially important to remember that if a correction is made to increase serum phenytoin lev-els in the patient receiving enteral feeds, a correction must likely also be made during weaning off feeds to limit the possibility of phenytoin toxicity secondary to overdose.

SUGGESTED READINGS

Au Yeung SCS, Ensom MH. Phenytoin and enteral feedings: does evidence support an interaction? Ann Pharmacother. 2000;34:896–905.

Dipiro JT, Spruill WJ, Blouin RA, et al. Concepts in Clinical Pharmacokinetics. 4th ed. Bethesda, MD: The American Society of Health-System Pharmacists; 2005.

Doak KK, Haas CE, Dunnigan KJ, et al. Bioavailability of phenytoin acid and phenytoin sodium with enteral feedings. Pharmacotherapy. 1998;18(3):637–645.

Gilbert SJ, Hatton J, Magnuson B. How to minimize interaction between pheny-toin and enteral feedings: two approaches—a strategic approach. Nutr Clin Pract. 1996;11:28–30.

Kitchen D, Smith D. Problems with phenytoin administration in neurol-ogy/neurosurgery ITU patients receiving enteral feeding. Seizure. 2001;10:265–268.

Levy RH, Mattson RH, Meldrum BS, Perucca E, eds. Antiepileptic Drugs. 5th ed. Philadelphia: Lippincott Williams & Wilkins; 2002.

Murphy JE, ed. Clinical Pharmacokinetics Pocket Reference. 2nd ed. Bethesda, MD: The American Society of Health-System Pharmacists; 2000.

Winters ME. Basic Clinical Pharmacokinetics. 4th ed. Philadelphia: Lippincott Williams & Wilkins; 2003.

CONSIDER EARLY ENTERAL FEEDING

BRYAN A. COTTON, MD

If the gut works, use it!

As with other basic principles in patient care, this simple maxim of nutrition has sometimes been inexplicably ignored as our technological and pharmacological advances have exponentially increased over the past several decades. However, to ignore this simple idea is often to the detriment of the patient. Numerous studies have demonstrated a correlation with poor nutritional status and poor postoperative outcome. The current literature supports the preferential use of enteral feeding over parenteral nutrition (total parenteral nutrition, TPN) in intensive care unit (ICU) patients whenever possible. The reasons for this include not only the beneficial effects of enteral support but also the detrimental effects of TPN.

BENEFICIAL EFFECTS OF ENTERAL FEEDING

Several recent studies have demonstrated that gut mucosal dysfunction, in the form of increased permeability and villous sloughing, occurs early in the absence of enteral feedings. In the critically injured patient, several authors have demonstrated improvements in the catabolic state, specifically through improved nitrogen balance, when enteral nutrition is utilized instead of TPN. Physiological advantages of enteral nutrition over TPN include its stimulation of gallbladder emptying and release of pancreatic secretions, as well as maintenance of gut-associated lymphoid tissue (GALT) and mucosal immune function. The improved gut mucosal integrity noted with enteral feedings is likely responsible for the decreased bowel perforation rate, improved intestinal anastomotic healing, and decreased septic complications. In addition, enteral feeding is significantly less expensive (even when excluding the costs associated with TPN complications) than parenteral formulations.

DETRIMENTAL EFFECTS OF PARENTERAL NUTRITION

The intestinal mucosa and submucosa is an area of intense metabolic and immunologic activity, especially in the critically ill and severely injured patient. Utilization of TPN in these patients further compromises an already tenuous situation, with loss of mucosal mass and weight, increased villous sloughing, and disturbed mucosal enzyme activity. TPN use has been shown to decrease IgA in the gut, as well as in upper respiratory secretions. From a metabolic standpoint, TPN causes metabolic acidosis, hyperglycemia, hyperlipidemia, and significant electrolyte disturbances. In addition, TPN has been associated with hepatic steatosis and cellular injury leading to liver dysfunction and failure. Systemically, the effects of TPN include impairment of leukocyte chemotaxis, impaired phagocytosis, and an attenuated inflammatory response. Other authors, however, have shown TPN-associated alterations may actually potentiate the systemic inflammatory state by allowing increased bacterial translocation and increasing free-radical formation. Some studies have demonstrated higher mortality, especially among the critically ill, in those receiving parenteral nutrition compared with enteral feeding, with TPN almost doubling the risk of dying. Of note, the risks of TPN toxicity can be reduced by the addition of low-rate (sometimes referred to as trophic) tube feedings (10 to 30 mL/h).

WHEN AND HOW TO GIVE ENTERAL FEEDINGS

Several authors have investigated the impact and timing of early enteral nutrition. In the trauma and burn setting, delays of as little as 24 hours have been demonstrated to impact morbidities and outcomes. In fact, no evidence exists to support withholding enteral feedings in those patients with an open abdomen. Among the emergency surgery population, enteral feedings should be utilized early in the postoperative period. Although tube feedings are routinely held because of concerns of bowel-wall edema and nonperistalsis, this is not supported by the literature. With the exception of bowel obstruction and proximal enteric fistulae, early enteral nutrition has been demonstrated to be tolerated and of benefit even among those presenting with significant peritonitis and premorbid malnutrition. Early enteral support is also recommended following surgery for gastrointestinal malignancies and even in cases of severe pancreatitis, with evidence of attenuated organ dysfunction and improved outcomes.

When possible, the postpyloric position should be utilized for enteral feeding, with the nasojejunal location preferred in pancreatitis. Although many patients experience gastroparesis and some evidence suggests increased risk for aspiration, numerous studies support safety and tolerance of the gastric route. Most importantly, aggressive attention to placing enteral access (whether surgical or nasal route) should be considered prior to completion of the operative procedure. It is at this time that placement is most likely to be successful from a technical standpoint and best tolerated with regard to patient comfort.

One final note is that some experienced clinicians who believe in early and aggressive enteral feedings do not support the use of high-volume enteral feedings during the initial phase of active resuscitation from shock or sepsis or in high-dose pressor use.

SUGGESTED READINGS

Jabbar A, McClave SA. Pre-pyloric versus post-pyloric feeding. Clin Nutr. 2005;24:719–726.

Kaur N, Gupta MK, Minocha VR. Early enteral feeding by nasoenteric tubes in patients with perforation peritonitis. World J Surg. 2005;29:1023–1027.

Marik PE, Pinsky M. Death by parenteral nutrition. Intens Care Med. 2003;29:867–869.

Simpson F, Doig GS. Parenteral vs. enteral nutrition in the critically ill patient: a meta-analysis of trials using the intention to treat principle. Intens Care Med. 2005;31:12–23.

235

BE ALERT FOR OVERFEEDING

JASON SPERRY, MD
HEIDI L. FRANKEL, MD

Providing inadequate caloric supplementation during times of critical illness is associated with negative effects. Equally as detrimental is the administration of excessive calories, or overfeeding. Overfeeding is associated with significant metabolic disorders including hyperglycemia, elevated serum triglycerides, and subsequent hepatic steatosis. In addition, overfeeding may cause a significant increase in CO_2 production that can be deleterious to those with respiratory insufficiency and may make ventilator weaning challenging (or impossible).

WHAT TO DO

To avoid overfeeding, accurate estimates of energy and caloric requirements of critically ill patients are required. Critically ill patients typically undergo a period of catabolism, which can be associated with significant body protein loss, depending on the severity of critical illness and the length of the catabolic process. Calculation of nitrogen balance can quantify the extent of catabolism and evaluate the efficacy of supplemental nutrition in these patients. Nitrogen balance is calculated by subtracting total nitrogen losses (urine, stool, insensible losses) from nitrogen intake (1 g nitrogen per 6.25 g of protein). The primary mode of nitrogen excretion is urinary, and 24-hour urine collection for urinary urea nitrogen (UUN) is the most common means of measurement. Fecal and insensible losses are typically small but estimated. UUN can be a poor estimate of overall nitrogen losses in burn patients, when urine output is low (<1L/d), in patients with acute or chronic renal failure and in patients with enteric fistulas where exceedingly high losses occur in the fistulae output.

Alternatively, nutritional assessment can be accomplished via indirect calorimetry, where O_2 consumption and CO_2 production are measured and a respiratory quotient (RQ) is calculated at the patient's bedside. An RQ of 0.7 is typical of fat oxidation and an RQ of <0.7 suggests ketosis, lipolysis, and underfeeding. An RQ ≥ 1.0 exemplifies primary carbohydrate metabolism and possible overfeeding. Because of the accuracy of measurements required for indirect calorimetry, it is generally limited to those who are on ventilatory support. Since changes in minute ventilation, cardiac output, fraction of inspired oxygen, and acid-base status can affect CO_2 production and O_2 uptake, indirect calorimetry must also be performed, with the patient at a relative steady state for maximal accuracy.

SUGGESTED READINGS

Brandi LS, Bertolini R, Santini L, et al. Effects of ventilator resetting on indirect calorimetry measurement in the critically ill surgical patient. Crit Care Med. 1999;27(3):531–539.

Dickerson RN, Tidwell AC, Minard G, et al. Predicting total urinary nitrogen excretion from urinary urea nitrogen excretion in multiple-trauma patients receiving specialized nutritional support. Nutrition. 2005;21(3):332–338.

Hunter DC, Jaksic T, Lewis D, et al. Resting energy expenditure in the critically ill: estimations versus measurement. Br J Surg. 1988;75(9):875–878.

Long CL, Schaffel N, Geiger JW, et al. Metabolic response to injury and illness: estimation of energy and protein needs from indirect calorimetry and nitrogen balance. J Parenter Enteral Nutr. 1979;3(6):452–456.

Mann S, Westenskow DR, Houtchens BA. Measured and predicted caloric expenditure in the acutely ill. Crit Care Med. 1985;13(3):173–177.

236

BE ALERT FOR THE DEVELOPMENT OF REFEEDING SYNDROME

WILLIAM S. HOFF, MD

Phosphate (PO_4^{2-}) is the most abundant intracellular anion, the majority of which is found in bones. As a result, the measured serum PO_4^{2-} does not accurately reflect the total-body content of PO_4^{2-}. Biologically, PO_4^{2-} is an important component of cell membranes (e.g., phospholipids), enzyme systems, and bone matrix (e.g., hydroxyapatite). Phosphate is also a component of adenosine triphosphate (ATP), an important source of cellular energy. Synthesis of 2,3-diphosphoglycerate (2,3-DPG) also depends on PO_4^{2-}.

WATCH OUT FOR

Hypophosphatemia is the hallmark electrolyte abnormality associated with the refeeding syndrome. Concomitant serum abnormalities include hypokalemia, hypomagnesemia, and hyperglycemia. Refeeding syndrome is rare, occurring in 0.8% of hospitalized adults. However, the mortality in hospitalized patients who develop severe hypophosphatemia (serum PO_4^{2-} <1 mg/dL) is 30%. Risk factors for refeeding syndrome include prolonged malnutrition, gastrointestinal losses (e.g., vomiting, nasogastric suctioning, diarrhea), chronic alcohol abuse, abdominal surgery, and metastatic cancer.

Refeeding syndrome typically occurs when either enteral or parenteral nutrition is initiated in a patient with one of the high-risk factors listed. The sudden introduction of carbohydrate stimulates a release of insulin, which results in an intracellular shift of PO_4^{2-}, potassium, and magnesium. This transcellular shift frequently occurs in the presence of reduced body stores of these key electrolytes. Refeeding syndrome should be suspected in the presence of any of the electrolyte disorders noted earlier. A common manifestation in the intensive care unit (ICU) patient is respiratory failure secondary to diaphragm and intercostal muscle weakness as a result of ATP depletion. This clinical presentation may be acute respiratory failure in a spontaneously breathing patient or inability to wean a patient from mechanical ventilation. Deficiency of 2,3-DPG resulting in impaired O_2 off-loading at the cellular level may result in dyspnea and fatigue, further compromising respiration. Although less specific in the ICU population, patients may also present with generalized skeletal muscle weakness secondary to depleted ATP stores. Other less common clinical findings include ventricular dysrhythmias, left ventricular dysfunction, confusion, lethargy, and gait disturbances.

The key to treatment of refeeding syndrome is anticipating development of the condition in patients at risk. In this group of patients, nutrition should be introduced gradually, for example, beginning with a one-half nutrition goal of 5,040 kilocalories and increasing by 840 kilocalories every 24 to 48 hours, with careful attention to serum electrolytes (1 calorie $= 4.186$ kJ). Active treatment depends on the degree of hypophosphatemia. Moderate hypophosphatemia ($PO_4^{2-} = 1$ to 2.5 mg/dL) may be managed with oral or enteral replacement. Severe or symptomatic hypophosphatemia mandates intravenous replacement; a typical intravenous replacement regimen is sodium phosphate Na_2PO_4 0.16 to 0.32 mmol/kg administered over 4 to 6 hours. Intravenous replacement should be done cautiously in hypercalcemia. Serum electrolytes should be monitored closely during intravenous replacement therapy. Ionized calcium levels should also be monitored as overzealous dosing of PO_4^{2-} may result in hypocalcemia.

SUGGESTED READINGS

Fink MP, Abraham E, Vincent JL, eds. Textbook of Critical Care. 5th ed. Philadelphia: Elsevier Saunders; 2005:71–73.

Khardori R. Refeeding syndrome and hypophosphatemia. J Int Care Med. 2005;20:174–175.

Marinella MA. Refeeding syndrome and hypophosphatemia. J Int Care Med. 2005;20:155–159.

237

CONSIDER USING ELEMENTAL OR SEMIELEMENTAL FEEDS IN PATIENTS WITH ALBUMIN LESS THAN 2.5 GRAMS PER DECILITER

RONALD W. PAULDINE, MD

WATCH OUT FOR

Enteral feeding formulas can be categorized based on their protein source. Intact protein feeds contain protein that has not been hydrolyzed and include Ensure, Osmolite, Jevity, and Promote. Semielemental feeds contain hydrolyzed proteins (small peptides) as their source of nitrogen and include Peptamen, Alitraq, and Perative. Elemental formulas utilize free amino acids (FAA) as their source of nitrogen and include Vivonex and F.A.A. Not all patients can utilize intact protein feeds. In patients with hypoalbuminemia (albumin <2.5) there is significant gut edema and an impairment of gut cell–wall proteins necessary for nutrient absorption. Use of elemental or semielemental formulas is associated with better amino acid absorption and insulin responses compared with intact protein formulas. Semielemental formulas may be better tolerated than either intact or elemental formulas with regard to diarrhea. Because elemental formulas are hypertonic they may also have a higher incidence of nausea, vomiting, and abdominal distension.

In general, critically ill patients are hypercatabolic and mildly hypermetabolic. The goals of metabolic support strategies are to preserve organ function, body cell mass, and protein synthesis. Of note, providing high levels of nonprotein calories does not prevent protein catabolism. Overfeeding can lead to increased production of carbon dioxide and interfere with weaning from mechanical ventilation. Current recommendations suggest initiating nutritional support with total calories of approximately 84 to 105 kilocalories/kg/d with protein content of 1.2 to 1.5 g/kg/d. Adjustment of nonprotein calories is based upon indirect calorimetry (metabolic cart) to ensure patients are not over- or underfed. Assessment of total protein needs and utilization should be based on laboratory parameters (e.g., prealbumin, transferrin) and nitrogen balance (urine urea nitrogen [UUN]).

Critically ill patients with ongoing systemic inflammatory response syndrome, with sepsis, or requiring vasopressors may be at particular risk of gastrointestinal complications with enteral feeds. In these patients, parenteral nutrition should be considered, although when gut function is assessed to be present, enteral feeds are much preferable to the parenteral option. Complications of enteral nutrition include high gastric residuals, diarrhea, constipation, abdominal distension, vomiting with aspiration, and pneumonia. Assessment of gastric residuals can be used to assess tolerance of enteral feeds. These can be checked at 1 and 4 hours and then every 8 hours to evaluate whether or not a plateau has been reached. Usually, residuals will plateau at 20% to 50% of the volume infused by 3 to 13 hours after initiation of feeds. Failure to reach a plateau suggests that the infusion should be stopped or slowed down.

WHAT TO DO

Patients receiving enteral feeds are at risk for developing either diarrhea or constipation. Diarrhea can be addressed by methods including transitioning to semielemental formulas, decreasing osmolality by dilution of the formula and addition of antidiarrheal agents including kaolin-pectin, bismuth or salicylate, or deiodinized tincture of opium (DTO). The importance of first ruling out an infectious cause of diarrhea cannot be overstated. *Clostridium difficile* is a commonly missed diagnosis when new onset diarrhea is erroneously attributed to tube feeds. Constipation can be treated by removal of antidiarrheal therapy (if present), correcting dehydration by the addition of free-water flushes, adding fiber if using intact formulations, or adding laxatives or enemas. Clinical assessment should always include careful attention to signs and symptoms suggestive of intolerance to enteral feeds including abdominal distension, pain, nausea, and/or vomiting.

SUGGESTED READINGS

Griffiths RD, Bongers T. Nutrition support for patients in the intensive care unit. Postgrad Med J. 2005;81:629–636.
Mechanick JI, Brett EM. Nutrition support of the chronically critically ill patient. Crit Care Clin. 2002;18:597–618.

238

CONSIDER ENTERAL FEEDINGS IN PANCREATITIS AND ENTEROCUTANEOUS FISTULAE

CHRISTOPHER J. SONNENDAY, MD, MHS

Classic surgical teaching has historically dictated that minimization of enteric flow by withholding enteral feeds is essential to the management of patients with disruption of the normal continuity of the gastrointestinal tract (i.e., enterocutaneous fistula). The use of parenteral nutrition thus became fundamental to the treatment of enterocutaneous fistulae, as well as to the management of severe acute pancreatitis, where enteral feeds that stimulate pancreatic exocrine were believed to contribute to exacerbation of the complex course of that disease. However, with a preponderance of evidence in favor of the benefits of enteral nutrition in critical illness, clinicians have sought ways to provide enteral nutrition even in these disease states where it was previously thought to be deleterious.

WHAT TO DO

In the case of proximal enterocutaneous fistulae (e.g., esophageal, gastric, duodenal, proximal jejunum), distal jejunal feeds are always preferable to parenteral nutrition and should be the mainstay of therapy. The nutritional requirements for patients with enterocutaneous fistula may be excessive because of the significant gastrointestinal (GI) protein losses and catabolism associated with these conditions. It may be prudent to maintain the patient on parenteral nutrition until enteral feeds are advanced and optimized. Optimal caloric support is frequently not possible for 4 to 5 days following initiation of enteral feeds, and parenteral nutrition can bridge that gap in critically ill patients. In the case of a more proximal fistula, it is often possible to cannulate the distal limb of the fistula itself to feed the distal small bowel. Such procedures often require expert interventional radiologists and should not be performed without the guidance of an experienced GI surgeon.

Enterocutaneous fistulae involving the distal small bowel may present more difficult challenges in establishing adequate enteral nutrition. If at least 4 feet of small bowel from the ligament of Treitz exist prior to the fistula site, the stomach or duodenum may be fed with low-residue elemental or semielemental formulas that are most likely to be absorbed in the proximal gut (i.e., before it reaches the fistula). Establishing a means to supply enteral nutrition whenever it is safe and feasible should be part of the comprehensive management of an enterocutaneous fistula.

A similar paradigm shift away from parenteral nutrition has also occurred in the management of severe acute pancreatitis. Traditional teaching has argued that enteral feeding would stimulate the pancreas, exacerbating the retroperitoneal inflammation that drives the disease state. However, two recent prospective trials and at least two meta-analyses have shown patient outcomes (including mortality, need for surgical intervention, and hospital length of stay) to be at least equivalent between patients fed via enteral versus parenteral routes. In addition, infectious complications and cost are lower among patients treated with enteral nutrition. While all prospective trials to date have been small and based at a single center, the evidence is growing that enteral nutrition is not harmful and limits the risk of central-line infections associated with parenteral nutrition.

Each of the prospective trials for enteral feeding in pancreatitis have used nasojejunal tubes placed either endoscopically or under fluoroscopic guidance as their delivery method for enteral feeds. Early percutaneous gastrojejunostomy tubes should be considered in patients projected to have a lengthy clinical course. While most experts recommend feeding distal to the ligament of Treitz as a way to minimize pancreatic stimulation, both animal studies and anecdotal reports in humans suggest that gastric feedings may be possible without adverse effects. However, this has not been studied prospectively and a jejunal route for enteral nutrition should be achieved whenever possible. In patients with severe acute pancreatitis who require percutaneous or surgical interventions, attention should be paid to interruptions in enteral nutrition for procedures and diagnostic studies. If enteral nutrition is frequently interrupted, a transition period of parenteral nutrition should be necessary. Any patient who requires a laparotomy for debridement and drainage should have a feeding jejunostomy surgically placed, if possible.

WATCH OUT FOR

Both of these groups of patients require vigilant monitoring to ensure that nutritional supplementation is adequate. Frequent biochemical monitoring of serum markers such as albumin, prealbumin, transferrin, and lipid profiles is essential. Measurement of urine urea nitrogen excretion should be performed weekly in the most critically ill patients as they navigate the catabolic phase of their illness. Metabolic cart studies may be necessary to assist in the estimates of energy requirements in these patients whose clinical condition, and therefore metabolic needs, change rapidly. Studies have shown that a dedicated nutrition service can improve the outcomes of these patients and serious consideration should be given to obtaining consultation from them.

SUGGESTED READINGS

Dudrick SJ, Maharaj AR, McKelvey AA. Artificial nutritional support in patients with gastrointestinal fistulas. World J Surg. 1999;23:570–576.
Heinrich S, Schafer M, Rousson V, et al. Evidence-based treatment of acute pancreatitis: a look at established paradigms. Ann Surg. 2006;243:154–168.

239

Use the Metabolic Cart Only When Patients Are on Low Vent Settings

Anthony D. Slonim, MD, DrPH

Appropriate nutritional support improves the care of the critically ill patient by improving wound healing, and by reducing inflammation, infections, and the rate of complications. In addition, it has been shown to reduce overall ventilator days and intensive care unit (ICU) length of stay. Traditional approaches to the assessment of nutrition in the ICU have included a number of metabolic formulas. The most well known of these is the Harris-Benedict equation, which measures the resting energy expenditure (REE) and then "adjusts" that value based upon the overall stressors of the patient. The Harris-Benedict equation is represented by the following formulas:

$$REE \text{ (men)} = 66 + (13.7 \times \text{weight in kilos})$$
$$+ (5 \times \text{height in centimeters}) - (6.8 \times \text{age})$$
$$REE \text{ (women)} = 655 + (9.6 \times \text{weight in kilos})$$
$$+ (1.8 \times \text{height in centimeters}) - (4.7 \times \text{age})$$

In the presence of invasive monitoring such as the pulmonary artery catheter, where accurate values for oxygen consumption are available, the Weir equation may allow a better approximation of energy expenditure.

$$\text{energy expenditure} = (3.94 \times \text{oxygen consumption})$$
$$+ (1.11 \times \text{carbon dioxide production})$$

These values directly use the components of the respiratory quotient (CO_2 production/O_2 consumption) to impute the energy expenditure.

Apart from the use of a calculated assessment of nutritional value, there may be opportunities to improve upon the assessment of the metabolic status for patients hospitalized in the ICU. It is likely that the metabolic status of the ICU patient changes as his or her condition changes. The ability to keep track of these changes and to modify therapy may be important in improving the overall outcome of the patient. Indirect calorimetry provides an important opportunity to objectively measure the metabolic needs of the patient and to match the provision of nutritional support to the patient's demand. This is important particularly with complex patients who may need both enteral and parenteral support to achieve nutritional goals.

<table>
<tr><td>

WATCH OUT FOR

</td><td>

Indirect calorimetry is a simple bedside procedure that provides accurate measurements for oxygen consumption, carbon dioxide production,

</td></tr>
</table>

and resting energy expenditure when the ability to detect these measurements from pulmonary artery catheterization is not available. While simple, there are a number of important caveats that can affect the obtained measurements. First, there cannot be any air leaks from the system since these leaks will cause inaccuracies in the measurements of oxygen consumption and carbon dioxide production and will adversely affect the calculations for respiratory quotients and resting energy expenditure. Second, a fraction of inspired oxygen (F_{IO2}) of >0.6 can also make these measurements inaccurate. Third, patients need to be in a steady state with little fluctuation (<10%) in oxygen consumption or carbon dioxide production. This limitation is often overcome by experienced clinicians by increasing the interval of measurement for the patient to 30 minutes.

SUGGESTED READINGS

Fink MP, Abraham E, Vincent JL, et al. Textbook of Critical Care. 5th ed. Philadelphia: Elsevier Saunders; 2005:1895–1897.

Irwin RS, Rippe JM. Intensive Care Medicine. 5th ed. Philadelphia: Lippincott Williams & Wilkins; 2003.

240

USE A DEDICATED, UPPER-BODY, SINGLE-LUMEN CENTRAL VENOUS CATHETER FOR ADMINISTRATION OF PARENTERAL NUTRITION

LISA MARCUCCI, MD

Although the use of parenteral nutrition was one of the milestone breakthroughs in the care of critically ill patients, serious morbidities are associated with its use. One troublesome complication is total parenteral nutrition (TPN) catheter-related sepsis, which is associated with poorer outcomes in patients, including longer intensive care unit (ICU) stays, longer hospital stays, and higher mortality. To this end, some hospitals have developed entire care teams dedicated to the management of central venous lines used for TPN, including insertion procedure, skin site inspection, dressing changes, and evaluation of possible infection. Given the potential morbidities, numerous studies have been done to determine the best protocols for catheter care used for TPN.

From an accumulating body of research regarding how to reduce risks of infection, including TPN catheter tip infection, site infection, bacteremia, and catheter colonization, the following facts seems clear: (a) TPN should be initiated through a new catheter inserted via a clean stick, not a catheter changed over a wire; (b) TPN catheters should be inserted via subclavian (preferably) or internal jugular veins, not via femoral veins; (c) TPN should have its own dedicated lumen used for nothing else; and (d) a team dedicated to TPN central-line care should be assembled to lower catheter infection rates. A 2003 study by Dimick et al. showed that single-lumen subclavian catheters dedicated to TPN use and cared for by a dedicated team had a fivefold decrease in infection compared with other catheters that were used for multiple reasons. One final note is that because the realities of care in seriously ill patients do not always allow for the placement of a dedicated TPN line, one port of a newly placed multiple-lumen catheter can be designated for exclusive administration of TPN if no other options exist.

SUGGESTED READINGS

Clark-Christoff N, Watters VA, Sparks W, et al. Use of triple-lumen subclavian catheters for administration of total parenteral nutrition. J Parenter Enteral Nutr. 1992;16:403–407.

Dimick JB, Swoboda S, Talamini MA, et al. Risk of colonization of central venous catheters: catheters for total parenteral nutrition vs other catheters. Am J Crit Care. 2003;12:328–335.

Kemp L, Burge J, Choban P, et al. The effect of catheter type and site on infection rates in total parenteral nutrition patients. J Parenter Enteral Nutr. 1994;18:71–74.

241

BE ALERT FOR HYPOPHOSPHATEMIA IN THE INTENSIVE CARE UNIT PATIENT ON DIALYSIS

ADAM R. BERLINER, MD
DEREK M. FINE, MD

Outpatients on chronic dialysis usually have trouble with hyperphosphatemia, requiring high doses of oral phosphorus binders to block absorption of dietary phosphate. In the intensive care setting, the opposite situation—hypophosphatemia—is often encountered in patients on dialysis for several reasons including higher frequency of dialysis and relative malnutrition. It is critical to check the serum phosphate level daily in the intensive care unit (ICU) patient on hemodialysis. A level that may have been quite high prior to dialysis can plummet to critical values if unmonitored. Severe (<1.5 mg/dL) hypophosphatemia can cause diaphragmatic weakness, apnea, cardiac instability, rhabdomyolysis, or hemolysis.

Conventional intermittent hemodialysis is intrinsically very effective at phosphate removal, but the overall treatment time (usually 2 to 4 hours) is often not enough to cause profound hypophosphatemia, since extracellular stores are rapidly repleted from intracellular reserve. In the ICU setting it is common to use sustained, high-intensity dialysis, usually in the form of a continuous renal replacement therapy such as continuous venovenous hemofiltration (CVVH) or continuous venovenous hemodiafiltration (CVVHDF). A retrospective study showed that CVVHDF curbs hyperphosphatemia better than intermittent hemodialysis, but at an increased risk of hypophosphatemia. In addition to continuous renal replacement therapy, other risk factors for hypophosphatemia in the ICU include parenteral nutrition, diarrhea, and profound renal phosphate wasting due to tubular cell injury.

WHAT TO DO Intermittent intravenous repletion with sodium phosphate is recommended for serum phosphate <1.5 mg/dL. Dosing regimens are not standardized. One small study of seven patients noted good results from 15 mmol intravenous sodium phosphate over 2 hours for serum phosphates of 1.56 to 2.1 mg/dL (0.5 to 0.7 mmol/L). The authors of this study calculated a volume of distribution for phosphate ranging from 0.21 to 0.87 L/kg and went on to postulate that doses closer to 25 mmol should be given for values closer to 1.09 mg/dL (0.35 mmol/L) or less. Once corrected, chronic maintenance phosphate supplementation, either orally or in parenteral nutrition, should be given when phosphate is chronically low in order to prevent reoccurrence of critical hypophosphatemia.

One final note is that standard dialysate contains no phosphate. Phosphate-enriched dialysate can be considered in refractory cases, though it is usually not required.

SUGGESTED READINGS

French C, Bellomo R. A rapid intravenous phosphate replacement protocol for critically ill patients. Crit Care Resusc. 2004;6:175–179.

Subramanian R, Khardor R. Severe hypophosphatemia: pathophysiologic implications, clinical presentations, and treatment. Medicine. 2000;79:1–8.

Tan HK, Bellomo R, et al. Phosphatemic control during acute renal failure: intermittent hemodialysis versus continuous hemodiafiltration. Int J Artif Organs. 2001;24(4):186–191.

242

KNOW THE DRUGS THAT MUST BE REDOSED AFTER DIALYSIS

EDWARD T. HORN, PHARMD

Acute renal failure is a common disease encountered in critically ill patients, with reported incidences of 5% to 10%. Hemodialysis and continuous venovenous hemodialysis (CVVHD) are commonly used in intensive care unit (ICU) patients to treat acute renal failure, and there are data to suggest that increasing the dose of dialysis can improve mortality outcomes in these patients. It is common sense that as the dose of dialysis is increased, clearance will increase, and therefore medications will need to be dosed more frequently. When considering this issue, one must evaluate various drug characteristics that will require more frequent dosing and close monitoring for therapeutic failure.

WHAT TO DO

When evaluating drug regimen adjustments in acute renal failure patients on hemodialysis or CVVHD, one must first consider whether or not the drug is significantly cleared through the kidneys. If the drug has less than 30% of its dose cleared renally, then dialysis is unlikely to play a significant role in its elimination. Other drug characteristics that play a significant role in determining the effect of dialysis on the need to redose a medication include protein binding, volume of distribution (Vd), molecular size, and molecular charge.

With respect to protein binding, only the unbound, or free, concentration is available to be dialyzed out of the blood. Drugs that are >80% bound are unlikely to be cleared by dialysis. Many physiologic derangements can influence drug binding, such as acidosis, uremia, hypoalbuminemia, and hyperbilirubinemia. Drug interactions can also cause displacement of bound drug through competition for binding sites (sulfamethoxazole and trimethoprim are classic culprits of this). While free drug is more available to exert its pharmacologic activity, it is also available to be cleared as well.

Volume of distribution can be considered synonymous with plasma protein binding in that only free drug available in the blood can be cleared by hemodialysis or CVVHD. Drugs with large volumes of distribution or increased lipophilicity or tissue binding will have relatively small concentrations in the serum compared with the

TABLE 242.1	MEDICATIONS AND ADJUSTED DOSAGES		
MEDICATION	CRCL <10ML/MIN (ESRD NOT HD)	HEMODIALYSIS	CVVHD
Amikacin	16 mg/kg IV ×1; then start regimen based on levels	16 mg/kg IV ×1; then dose based on levels	16 mg/kg IV ×1; then dose based on levels
Ampicillin	2 g q8h	2 g q8h	1–2 g q8–12h
Cefazolin	1 g q24h	1 g q24h immediately after dialysis	1–2 g q12h
Cefepime	0.5 g q24h	500 mg q24h 1 g q24h (*Pseudomonas*)	1–2 g q12h
Ceftriaxone	No dosage adjustment	No dosage adjustment	No dosage adjustment
Ciprofloxacin	IV: 400 mg q24h PO: 500 mg q24h	IV: 400 mg q24h after dialysis PO: 500 mg q24h immediately after dialysis	IV: 400 mg q12–24h PO: 250–500 mg q12–24h
Clindamycin	No dosage adjustment	No dosage adjustment	No dosage adjustment
Gatifloxacin	400 mg once; then 200 mg q24h	200 mg q24h immediately after dialysis	400 mg once; then 200 mg q24h
Gentamicin	4 mg/kg IV ×1; then start regimen based on levels	4 mg/kg IV ×1; then dose based on levels	4 mg/kg IV ×1; then dose based on levels
Meropenem	0.5 g q24h	500 mg q24h after dialysis	1 g q8h
Oxacillin	No dosage adjustment	No dosage adjustment	No dosage adjustment
Piperacillin	3–4 g q12h	3 g q12h after dialysis[a]	4 g q8h
Piperacillin/ tazobactam	2.25 g q8h	2.25 g q8h	2.25–3.375 g q6h
Tobramycin	See gentamicin	See gentamicin	See gentamicin
Vancomycin	10–15 mg/kg for one dose; then check level in 24 hours	Loading dose 15–20 mg/kg; then check levels post-hemodialysis	15–20 mg/kg q36–48h (confirm by dosing by levels)

IV, intravenously; PO, by mouth
[a] Dose to be given immediately after dialysis and then every 3 hours.

total-body concentration. In general, drugs with Vd >0.7 L/kg will be less likely to be effectively dialyzed with hemodialysis. This is because of the usual short duration of hemodialysis, which allows for a redistribution phenomenon to occur where drug from the tissues will distribute back to the serum after the cessation of hemodialysis. Clearance of these types of drugs will be increased with CVVHD because of the slow, continuous nature of this modality that allows for a continuous removal of drug from the serum. An example that illustrates this is the vancomycin dosing differences between hemodialysis and CVVHD. Vancomycin has a Vd of 0.7 L/kg and usually requires dosing once per week with regular hemodialysis schedules (4 hours per day, 3 times per week). With CVVHD, vancomycin doses are usually required every 36 to 48 hours.

Molecular weight also needs to be considered when examining the influence of dialysis on drug clearance. Solutes, including drugs, that have a molecular weight less than 500 d are readily cleared by hemodialysis, where as CVVHD can clear molecules that are much larger. This is because of the high-flux filters that CVVHD machines utilize and that have the capacity to remove solutes that have a molecular size up to 30 kd. Again, vancomycin illustrates this difference nicely. It has a molecular weight of about 1,450 d; thus it is not removed well by hemodialysis but is removed fairly well by CVVHD.

Taking all of this into account, it is clear that many of the drugs that require close monitoring for dosing in dialysis patients are antibiotics. Unfortunately, the only agents in this class that are able to be monitored adequately through obtaining serum concentrations are the aminoglycosides (gentamicin, tobramycin, and amikacin) and vancomycin. *Table 242.1* details some important antibiotic dosing information in hemodialysis and CVVHD. When information is not available in textbooks or handbooks, a search of primary literature is necessary as the data around this issue are constantly evolving.

SUGGESTED READINGS

Bugge JF. Pharmacokinetics and drug dosing adjustments during continuous venovenous hemofiltration or hemodiafiltration in critically ill patients. Acta Anaesthesiol Scand. 2001;45:929–934.

Joy MS, Matzke GR, Armstrong DK, et al. A primer on continuous renal replacement therapy for critically ill patients. Annal Pharmacother. 1998;32(3):362–375.

Schiffl H, Lang SM, Fischer R. Daily hemodialysis and the outcome of acute renal failure. N Engl J Med. 2002;346:305–310.

Uchino S, Kellum JA, Bellomo R, et al. Acute renal failure in critically ill patients: a multinational, multicenter study. JAMA. 2005;294(7):813–818.

Veltri MA, Neu AM, Fivush BA, et al. Drug dosing during intermittent hemodialysis and continuous renal replacement therapy: special considerations in pediatric patients. Pediatr Drugs. 2004;6(1):45–65.

243

REMEMBER THAT CONTINUOUS VENOVENOUS HEMODIALYSIS CAN OBSCURE A TEMPERATURE SPIKE

FRANK ROSEMEIER, MD

In the normal person, body core temperature is tightly regulated around a set value of 37° C ± 0.2° by hypothalamic thermoreceptors, despite fluctuation in heat uptake, heat production, and heat loss. Diurnal variations of ± 0.5° C occur with the minimum value in the morning and maximum in the evening.

In critical care patients, this normal thermoregulation can be compromised by several factors and can cause perturbations of both hyper- and hypothermia. For instance, not every fever is caused by infection. Both exogenous (e.g., bacteria) and endogenous pyrogens can set the "thermostat" at a higher value. Infection, inflammation, and necrosis activate macrophages, which in turn release interleukin 1 and interleukin 6 and increase prostaglandin metabolism. An initial but temporary temperature rise following surgery is classically thought to be part of an inflammatory response. Suspicion for an infective cause is raised by sustained, recurrent, and/or prolonged period of temperature typically >38.3° C.

In addition, thermoregulation is compromised by a combination of central nervous system processes (dysregulation of the autonomic nervous system, inability to engage skeletal muscles in shivering and heat production) and administration of drugs such as acetaminophen, nonsteriodal anti-inflammatory drugs (NSAIDs), opioids, propofol, and neuromuscular blockers. Room-temperature intravenous fluids and cold blood or blood products also contribute to induced hypothermia. Environmental factors such as exposure to laminar airflow and cold room temperature (which is thermoneutral and comfortable to work in for the clothed staff, yet too low for the patient covered by a thin blanket) contribute further to heat loss.

WATCH OUT FOR

One particular environmental factor that is notorious for lowering core temperature is continuous venovenous hemodialysis (CVVHD). This is a form of renal replacement therapy often encountered in critically ill patients with acute renal failure in which solute is separated from blood across a semipermeable membrane as a result of a diffusion gradient. Both the afferent limb and efferent limb are connected to a large vessel such as the patient's femoral, subclavian, or internal jugular vein using a large-bore, double-lumen catheter (e.g., Shiley or Davol catheter). Most of the CVVHD machines in use today do not have an external heating source. Hence, blood is cooled through convective heat loss in the extracorporeal circuit as the blood tubing is exposed. Room-temperature dialysate in countercurrent to the blood flow increases conductive heat loss. Large temperature drops of >1° C can be observed, rendering the normothermic patient hypothermic and masking a fever in the infected patient.

SUGGESTED READINGS

Fink MP, Abrahams E, Vincent J-L, et al., eds. Textbook of Critical Care. 5th ed. Philadelphia: Elsevier Saunders; 2005:1151–1158.

Miller RD, ed. Miller's Anesthesia. 6th ed. Philadelphia: Elsevier-Churchill Livingstone; 2005:1571–1592.

244

CLAMP THE DIALYSATE LINE IN CONTINUOUS VENOVENOUS HEMODIALYSIS IMMEDIATELY IF IT BECOMES PINK TINGED

ANTHONY D. SLONIM, MD, DRPH

Acute renal failure is a commonly occurring problem in the care of intensive care unit (ICU) patients. One method of improving the care of these complex patients is to use continuous renal replacement therapies (CRRTs), of which continuous venovenous hemofiltration with dialysis (CVVHD) is one of the more common forms. This technique has the same indications as traditional dialysis (hyperkalemia, refractory acidosis, fluid overload, and symptomatic azotemia), but CVVHD supposedly is a gentler, more physiologic procedure to achieve solute and fluid clearance and may be particularly useful for those patients with hemodynamic instability. While this is the commonly accepted dogma in critical care, it is important to recognize that there is currently no literature that demonstrates a survival advantage in CRRT when compared with intermittent hemodialysis.

A simplified, schematized version of the mechanics of CVVHD is shown in *Figure 244.1*. There are several steps to be completed when initiating CVVHD. First, the placement of a double-lumen, large-bore central venous catheter (e.g., Shiley) for access is accomplished. Next, blood from this catheter is withdrawn at approximately 150 to 200 mL/min by a pump and passed through a filter with multiple layers of a semipermeable membrane. This membrane allows for the diffusion of fluid and solute across the membrane with the resulting formation of a filtrate that is normally clear in appearance. Finally, the blood flows back to the patient from the other end of the filter by a venous return line that in most systems has a trap for clots and an air detector. This line is reconstituted with a crystalloid solution that mimics the composition of plasma. It is a necessity that the blood flow in the dialysis circuit continues without stagnation so that clots do not form. Anticoagulation is usually administered either through the use of heparin or citrate-containing replacement fluids to ensure an adequate blood flow.

WATCH OUT FOR

It is important to note that the filter used in CVVHD maintains a barrier between the blood column and the dialysis column. This filter has

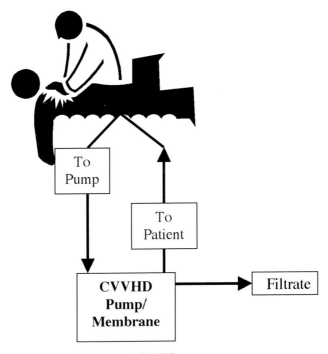

FIGURE 244.1. Schematic of CVVHD

a number of characteristics that allow it to meet threshold criteria for filtration. Several complications can occur related to the filter, and it requires appropriate monitoring of the device by the provider. Filters typically last at least 3 days. Dialysis filters have an intrinsic failure rate. The longer a filter is in use, the higher the likelihood it will fail over time. One method of monitoring a filter's function is through the use of plasma-free hemoglobin. Plasma-free hemoglobin increases when erythrocyte breakdown products begin to accumulate and signals the provider that a filter change may be necessary. Changing the circuit before the filter becomes dysfunctional is important. Another filter complication that can occur is a breech in the continuity of the membrane. This complication will usually manifest itself as a pink-tinged or frank blood in the filtrate. If this occurs, it is important to immediately clamp the dialysis catheter flowing from the patient and assess the integrity of the filter. If the membrane in the filter ruptures, the semipermeable membrane will no longer separate the blood column from the filtrate column and the patient can receive a high concentration of deleterious solution through the venous line. For this reason, it is imperative to clamp the tubing immediately if the fluid becomes pink tinged.

SUGGESTED READINGS

Critical Care Medicine Tutorials. Renal Replacement Therapy. http://www. ccmtutorials.com/renal/RRT/index.htm

Fink MP, Abraham E, Vincent JL, et al. Textbook of Critical Care. 5th ed. Philadelphia: Elsevier Saunders; 2005:1151–1158.

245

DO NOT USE CONTINUOUS VENOVENOUS HEMODIALYSIS IN THE SETTING OF ANGIOTENSIN-CONVERTING ENZYME 2 AND VICE VERSA

ANTHONY D. SLONIM, MD, DRPH

Kinins are a group of peptides that have strong vasodilating properties. They are formed from large precursor molecules named kininogens by the action of proteolytic enzymes called kallikreins, which are formed in the liver. Kallikreins exist peripherally as prekallikreins, which become activated through a number of different mechanisms including exposure to Hageman factor (factor XII) from the coagulation system and artificial surfaces including dialysis membranes. Rapid deactivation occurs for most kinins after formation to prevent the body from having an overwhelming response to these powerful substances.

Bradykinin, however, is an example of a kinin that has a longer half-life. It is formed from its precursor kallidin, which is a product of low-molecular-weight kininogen in the tissues. Bradykinin is a physiologically active product that has several functions. It can act on the vascular endothelium to reduce smooth muscle tone and cause vasodilatation. It is also active during acute inflammation as a signal to the generation of arachidonic acid–derived products such as prostaglandins and leukotrienes. In addition, bradykinin becomes activated during activation of the clotting cascade and tissue repair mechanisms. Finally, there is a potential role for bradykinin in hypertension since it is involved in the conversion of prorenin to renin and levels appear to be reduced in patients with hypertension.

WHAT TO DO

It is important for the clinician to note that hypersensitivity reactions that cause alterations in blood pressure have been described in patients treated with polyacrylonitrile dialysis membranes (commonly used in continuous dialysis treatment) who are concurrently taking angiotensin-converting enzyme (ACE) inhibitors for their hypertension. The suspected hypersensitivity reaction occurs because bradykinin is produced and its degradation is inhibited in the setting of ACE administration, leading to a longer half-life and thereby magnifying its effects on the cardiovascular system and leading to hypotension. Several strategies exist for reducing this bradykinin response to the dialysis membrane including changing the pH of the rinsing solution, thereby altering its charge and activation. Another approach is to use alternative dialyzers since not all membranes evoke the same level of response. In animal studies, it appears as though the response is related to the dose of the ACE inhibitor. So, an additional one option may be to reduce or eliminate the ACE inhibitor dose and use alternative methods of blood pressure control for these patients.

SUGGESTED READINGS

Amore A, Guarnieri G, Atti M, et al. Use of alkaline rinsing solution to prevent hypersensitivity reactions during hemodialysis: data from a multicentre retrospective analysis. J Nephrol. 1999;12:383–389.

Krieter DH, Grude M, Lemke HD, et al. Anaphylactoid reactions during hemodialysis in sheep are ACE inhibitor dose-dependent and mediated by bradykinin. Kidney Int. 1998;53:1026–1035.

Schulman G, Ikizler TA, Hakim R. Angiotensin-converting inhibitors and hemodialysis membranes. Semin Dial. 1999;12:S88–S91 .

Wakasa M, Akizawa T, Kinugasa E, et al. Plasma bradykinin levels during hemodialysis with PAN DX and polysulfone membranes with and without concurrent ACE inhibitor. Clin Nephrol. 1995;44:S29–S32.

246

DO NOT GIVE FLUDROCORTISONE TO PATIENTS ON DIALYSIS

ANTHONY D. SLONIM, MD, DRPH

At times of stress or after major traumatic injury, the hypothalamic-pituitary-adrenal axis provides an important mechanism to support the body through diurnal rhythms. The hypothalamus releases corticotropin-releasing factor, which stimulates the anterior pituitary gland to produce adrenocorticotropic hormone (ACTH). The ACTH then stimulates the cortex of the adrenal gland to release glucocorticoids and mineralocorticoids. Glucocorticoids primarily affect carbohydrate and protein metabolism. These chemicals include cortisol, cortisone, and hydrocortisone. Mineralocorticoids primarily affect sodium and water metabolism.

Mineralocorticoids lead to the retention of sodium and secretion of potassium. In addition, calcium, phosphorous, and bicarbonate are also reabsorbed. These actions are primarily mediated by the renin-angiotensin-aldosterone system. Angiotensin 2 produced by this system leads to aldosterone production, which is a naturally occurring mineralocorticoid. Fludrocortisone is the pharmacological form of mineralocorticoids and is used to provide mineralocorticoid effects in conditions like syncope, orthostatic hypotension, and Addison disease.

WHAT NOT TO DO

Patients with end-stage renal disease and a low glomerular filtration rate often require dialysis to appropriately remove urea, fluid, and electrolytes from their body in the absence of functioning kidneys. The administration of fludrocortisone to this group of patients may be relatively contraindicated for a number of reasons, including the exacerbation of hypertension and the extrarenal absorption of many of the electrolytes that dialysis is attempting to remove. These agents lead to sodium reabsorption and therefore fluid retention. The sodium reabsorption occurs from sites that are remote from the kidney, including the sweat glands and gastrointestinal tract. In addition, calcium and phosphorous retention can occur with this agent. Patients on dialysis are often taking calcium and phosphorous binders to improve the excretion of these elements. The administration of mineralocorticoids may worsen the retention of these electrolytes and lead to an increase in the medications necessary to control the underlying renal failure.

SUGGESTED READINGS

Furuya R, Kumagai H, Sakao T, et al. Potassium lowering effect of mineralocorticoid therapy in patients undergoing hemodialysis. Nephron. 2002;92:576–581.

Vlassopoulos D, Sonikian M, Dardioti V, et al. Insulin and mineralocorticoids influence on extrarenal potassium metabolism in chronic hemodialysis patients. Ren Fail. 2001;23:833–842.

247

AVOID THE SUBCLAVIAN VEIN FOR CENTRAL ACCESS OF ANY TYPE IN A DIALYSIS PATIENT OR POSSIBLE DIALYSIS PATIENT

MICHAEL J. MORITZ, MD

There are almost 300,000 hemodialysis patients in the United States today, and the number increases by about 4% to 5% annually. The median age of the dialysis patient in the United States has risen to 65 years. The aging population and the relative scarcity of renal transplants (about 10,000 done annually in the United States) means that dialysis will be required for longer periods of time and in many patients will be lifelong. In parallel, the critical nature of the vascular access in hemodialysis patients is amplified by longer dependence on this access for dialysis. Provision of vascular access is the greatest problem in dialysis today, with the solution involving the patient, nephrologist, surgeon, and interventional radiologist.

In the optimal situation, the patient presents early enough that the surgeon can place a permanent access in advance of dialysis. However, more commonly, patients present with an acute need for dialysis that requires temporary dialysis access via percutaneous catheters. As the majority of these patients will go on to require chronic dialysis, it is vital that the temporary-access catheter not compromise the anatomy required for permanent-access procedures. The preferred sites for temporary-access catheter placement are the internal jugular veins and the femoral veins; the subclavian veins should be avoided.

WHAT NOT TO DO

Temporary percutaneous dialysis access catheters are placed via central veins. They are very large in diameter compared with other venous catheters and can be associated with cannulated vein and an increased risk of thrombosis or stenosis of the vein, which can occur acutely or can present much later. The venous damage can be at the site of entrance into the vein or more centrally. In studies examining damage from short-term use (2 to 4 weeks), dialysis catheters placed by the subclavian route resulted in venous stenosis or thrombosis in 50% to 70% of veins, in contrast to a 0% to 10% incidence in catheters placed by the internal jugular route. Although the risk of injury to the vein is less than with dialysis catheters, in dialysis patients the subclavian vein should be avoided for placement of smaller-bore central venous catheters such as triple-lumen catheters, TPN (total parenteral nutrition) lines, or catheters that permit pulmonary artery catheters to be threaded through them.

Permanent accesses are arterial-to-venous connections, either as a fistula (direct artery-to-vein anastomosis) or via a bridge prosthetic graft between artery and vein. The best, longest-lasting permanent accesses are placed in the extremities, and upper extremities are preferred over lower extremities for reasons of infection, edema, and patient comfort. Permanent accesses create high flow through the vessels of the extremity, and the success of the access is highly dependent on adequate venous outflow from the access to the right atrium. Compromise of venous return results in access failure or edema of the access extremity to a degree that can be profound and limb threatening. Thus, subclavian vein stenosis or thrombosis (even if clinically silent) results in loss of all potential access sites in the ipsilateral upper extremity. Placement of a permanent access in such an extremity will result in immediate clinical symptoms of venous insufficiency (edema, cellulitis) and usually requires undoing the arteriovenous connection.

Patients who require a permanent dialysis access after prior subclavian venous puncture should be screened for patency of the central veins. Screening with Doppler ultrasound is noninvasive and is sensitive for veins that are easily visualized (e.g., jugular or axillary veins), but it is not sensitive for detection of venous stenosis or thrombosis of intrathoracic central veins such as subclavian and brachiocephalic (innominate) veins. If there is any reason to suspect problems with more central veins, a more sensitive study such as magnetic resonance imaging (MRI) or venography would be indicated.

Finally, patients with central venous occlusion may have spontaneous recanalization after 3 to 6 months, although the vein will never be completely normal. Patients with symptomatic stenosis of central veins can be treated with angioplasty and stent placement. The results overall are not as good as for arterial disease but can be helpful in patients with few or disappearing dialysis access alternatives.

SUGGESTED READINGS

Bander SJ, Schwab SJ. Central venous angioaccess for hemodialysis and its complications. Semin Dial. 1992;5:121–128.

Ciniochowski GE, Worley E, Rutherford WE, et al. Superiority of the internal jugular over the subclavian access for temporary hemodialysis. Nephron. 1990;54: 154–161.

Criado E, Marston WA, Jaques PF, et al. Primary venous outflow obstruction in patients with upper extremity arteriovenous dialysis access. Ann Vase Surg. 1994;8:530–535.

National Kidney Foundation. DOQI clinical practice guidelines for vascular access and anemia of chronic renal failure. Am J Kidney Disease. 1997;30(suppl 3):7–240.

Schillinger F, Schillinger D, Montagnac R, et al. Post catheterisation vein stenosis in haemodialysis: comparative angiographic study of 50 subclavian and 50 internal jugular accesses. Nephrol Dial Transplant. 1991;6:722–724.

248

USE CAUTION WHEN USING MILRINONE IN RENAL FAILURE

YING WEI LUM, MD

MECHANISM OF ACTION

Milrinone is a selective inhibitor of type III cyclic adenosine mono-phosphate (cAMP) phosphodiesterase isozyme in cardiac and vascular smooth muscle. Its inhibitory action on phosphodiesterase results in increased cAMP levels, which in turn increases contractility in cardiac muscle and stimulates vasodilatation in blood vessels. This causes an increase in cardiac output and decrease in pulmonary wedge pressure. These hemodynamic changes are obtained without excessive changes in heart rate or increase in myocardial oxygen consumption.

INDICATION

The use of milrinone has been best studied in patients with congestive heart failure. It appears to be very efficacious in nonhypotensive pa-tients with acute nonischemic cardiomyopathy, despite treatment with diuretics. These patients benefit from an enhancement in contractil-ity and afterload reduction. Duration of therapy should last for 48 to 72 hours. There are no studies to date that support its use for a longer period. Long-term oral therapy with milrinone has been associated with increased mortality.

DOSE

The recommended dose in patients with normal renal function is 50 μg/kg bolus followed by a continuous infusion at 0.375 to 0.75 μg/kg/min. Since milrinone is excreted mainly through the kidneys, its dose in patients with renal impairment should be adjusted accordingly (by surface area):

> Creatinine clearance (CrCl) 50 mL/min/1.73 m^2: Administer 0.43 μg/kg/min.
> CrCl 40 mL/min/1.73 m^2: Administer 0.38 μg/kg/min.
> CrCl 30 mL/min/1.73 m^2: Administer 0.33 μg/kg/min.
> CrCl 20 mL/min/1.73 m^2: Administer 0.28 μg/kg/min.
> CrCl 10 mL/min/1.73 m^2: Administer 0.23 μg/kg/min.
> CrCl 5 mL/min/1.73 m^2: Administer 0.2 μg/kg/min.

An immediate improvement in hemodynamic function is seen within 5 to 15 minutes after initiation of therapy. The mean half-life of milrinone is approximately 2.4 hours and patients reach a steady-state plasma milrinone concentration (of 200 ng/mL) within 6 to 12 hours of a continuous maintenance infusion of 0.50 mcg/kg/min. The impact of the half-life of milrinone is clinically important as providers must recognize that the effects of the drug cannot be turned off rapidly like many of the other commonly used inotropic agents such as epinephrine.

CAUTION

Milrinone decreases atrioventricular nodal conduction time, allowing a potential for increased ventricular response rates (up to 3.8%) for patients with supraventricular arrhythmias. Ventricular arrhythmias (ventricular ectopy, sustained and nonsustained ventricular tachycardia) have also been reported in up to 12% of patients. Life-threatening ventricular arrhythmia appears related to the presence of other underlying factors such as a pre-existing arrhythmia and metabolic abnormalities. Extreme caution must be used in patients with renal compromise. Fatal ventricular arrhythmias developed in six of nine patients in a recent study of the pharmacokinetics of milrinone in patients on continuous venovenous hemofiltration (CVVH). These patients were oliguric (<400 mL/d) and had a serum creatinine of more than 2.0 mg/dL. All patients received 0.25 μg/kg/min of milrinone and developed a mean steady-state concentration of 845 ng/mL, four times higher than that of patients with normal renal function. The high protein-binding affinity of milrinone and decreased urinary excretion could have contributed to this high concentration, thereby leading to the increased incidence of ventricular arrhythmias.

SUGGESTED READINGS

The Milrinone Source. http://milrinone.com/

Taniguchi T, Shibata K, Saito S, et al. Pharmacokinetics of milrinone in patients with congestive heart failure during continuous venovenous hemofiltration. Intens Care Med. 2000;26(8):1089–1093.

249

DECREASE THE DOSE OF GANCICLOVIR IN RENAL INSUFFICIENCY

ANGELA D. SHOHER, MD

Ganciclovir is an antiviral agent similar to acyclovir. It is active against all herpes viruses but is especially effective for Cytomegalovirus (CMV). Ganciclovir is often used in the intensive care unit (ICU) to prevent CMV disease in transplant patients and is also effective for chronic suppression of CMV retinitis in immunocompromised patients. It is an acyclic guanine nucleoside analog that acts by inhibiting viral DNA synthesis. One form used in ICU patients is valganciclovir, which is the L-valyl ester prodrug of ganciclovir. Valganciclovir is well absorbed, is hydrolyzed to ganciclovir rapidly, and produces levels comparable to intravenous (IV) ganciclovir. The plasma half-life is about 2 to 4 hours in patients with normal renal function. More than 90% of ganciclovir is eliminated unchanged by renal excretion. The half-life may be significantly increased in patients with severe renal failure and thus requires dosing based on renal function.

WHAT TO DO

For the treatment of CMV retinitis in a patient with normal renal function (creatinine clearance >70), the recommended dosage for induction is 5 mg/kg intravenously every 12 hours for 2 to 3 weeks. Maintenance dosing after the induction period is 5 mg/kg intravenously once per day 7 days a week or 6 mg/kg once per day 5 days a week. Oral ganciclovir is not predictably absorbed, so for patients taking oral valganciclovir, the recommended dose is 900 mg by mouth twice a day. Reinduction is recommended for patients who experience progression of CMV retinitis while on maintenance dosing. To prevent CMV disease in transplant patients with normal renal function, the dosage is also 5 mg/kg every 12 hours for 2 to 3 weeks, followed by daily dosing for intravenous maintenance. The oral maintenance regimen is also 1,000 mg three times a day with food. Oral valganciclovir maintenance is 900 mg per day. For patients in renal failure, see *Table 249.1* for dosing guidelines.

The side effects of ganciclovir include myelosuppression, which can cause neutropenia (worse when not dose reduced for renal failure), anemia, and thrombocytopenia. Neutropenia occurs in 15% to 40% and thrombocytopenia in 5% to 20% of patients. The myelosuppressive effects can be fatal but usually reverse within 1 week of cessation. Oral valganciclovir may also cause gastrointestinal symptoms such as

TABLE 249.1		GANCICLOVIR DOSING IN RENAL FAILURE		
CREATININE CLEARANCE	INDUCTION (MG/KG)	DOSING INTERVAL (HOURS)	MAINTENANCE (MG/KG)	DOSING INTERVAL (HOURS)
50–69	2.5	12	2.5	24
25–49	2.5	24	1.25	24
10–24	1.25	24	0.625	24
<10	1.25	3 times a week after dialysis	0.625	3 times a week after dialysis

nausea and diarrhea as well as headache. Central nervous system effects of ganciclovir occur in 5% to 15% of patients and can range from behavioral changes to coma. Approximately one-third of patients must stop using either ganciclovir or valganciclovir secondary to these side effects.

SUGGESTED READINGS

Katzung BG, ed. Basic & Clinical Pharmacology. 9th ed. New York: McGraw-Hill; 2004:823–844.

Wickersham RM, Gremillion S, eds. Drug Facts & Comparisons Pocket Version. 10th ed. St. Louis: Wolters Kluwer Health, Inc.; 2005:963–1010.

250

REMEMBER THAT TRIMETHOPRIM-SULFAMETHOXAZOLE (BACTRIM) CRYSTALS CAN PRECIPITATE IN THE KIDNEY AND CAUSE RENAL DAMAGE AND FAILURE

PRAVEEN KALRA, MD

Bactrim is an antibiotic drug formed by combining the sulfonamide sulfamethoxazole (5 parts) with trimethoprim (1 part). This combination (SMX-TMP) has in vivo activity against both Gram-positive and Gram-negative aerobic organisms. It has minimal activity against anaerobic organisms. Sulfonamides are structural analogs of para-aminobenzoic acid (PABA) and competitively inhibit the bacterial enzyme dihydropteroate synthetase that is responsible for incorporation of PABA into dihydrofolic acid, resulting in a decrease in the amount of metabolically active tetrahydrofolic acid.

Trimethoprim is a bacteriostatic lipophilic weak base structurally related to pyrimethamine. It binds and reversibly inhibits the enzyme dihydrofolate reductase and, like sulfonamide, selectively blocks the conversion of dihydrofolic acid to tetrahydrofolic acid, thus leading to depletion of folate, which results in interference of bacterial nucleic acid production. The individual effects of each component drug are magnified in combination and together may provide bactericidal effects.

SMX-TMP is rapidly absorbed after oral administration, with the bioavailability estimated at 90% to 100%. Sulfamethoxazole is primarily metabolized in the liver by acetylation to inactive metabolites that retain the toxicity of the parent compound. Trimethoprim is also metabolized in the liver, with 10% to 20% metabolized to inactive metabolites by o-demethylation ring N-oxidation and alpha-hydroxylation. Sulfamethoxazole is excreted renally by glomerular filtration with some tubular secretion. Excretion is increased in alkaline urine. Trimethoprim is 40% to 60% excreted within 24 hours primarily by tubular secretion. Excretion is increased in acid urine and decreased in alkaline urine.

WATCH OUT FOR

Although Bactrim is generally an effective antibiotic, its administration must be accompanied by knowledge of its toxicity. Hematological side effects include agranulocytosis, aplastic anemia, thrombocytopenia, leukopenia, hemolytic anemia, and methemoglobinemia. Largely because of the sulfonamide moiety, Bactrim has been associated with severe dermatological sequelae including erythema multiforme, Stevens-Johnson syndrome, and toxic epidermal necrolysis. Again, largely because of the sulfonamide component, use of Bactrim has been associated with hypoglycemia; it is structurally similar to the sulfonylureas, thus mimicking the effect of oral hypoglycemic agents. In addition, arthralgias and myalgias have been reported with the use of Bactrim.

Although rare, the renal effects of SMX-TMP can be striking. With only therapeutic doses, the development of crystalluria, interstitial nephritis, and renal failure has been reported, particularly in patients with pre-existing renal impairment. Sulfamethoxazole is relatively insoluble in acid urine and will cause crystal formation when the pH is <5.5. Most commonly, crystals are needle shaped or rosettes. The presence of sulfonamide crystals can be confirmed at the bedside by the lignin test. This is performed by placing one drop of urine on a paper and adding one drop of 10% hydrochloric acid. The appearance of yellowish-orange color is considered a positive test.

The best strategy to prevent the formation of crystals and the ensuing renal damage is by maintaining fluid intake above 3 L/d and by monitoring the urine for crystals if there is an unexplained decrease in renal function. If crystals are seen, the drug should be discontinued if possible with consideration given to alkalinizing the urine. Management of established renal insufficiency includes volume management, dialysis support if necessary, adjustment of drug doses, and avoidance of further exposure to nephrotoxins.

SUGGESTED READINGS

Perazella MA. Crystal induced renal failure. Am J Med. 1999;106(4):459–465.
Vree T, Martea M, Hekster YA, et al. Deterioration of the kidney function by high doses of cotrimaxozole in man. Pharm World Sci. 1987;9(2):117–124.

251

BE AWARE THAT LIPID-BASED AMPHOTERICIN PRODUCTS ARE ASSOCIATED WITH LESS RENAL TOXICITY THAN REGULAR AMPHOTERICIN BUT CAN STILL CAUSE RENAL INJURY

JOHN J. LEWIN III, PHARMD

Amphotericin B is a polyene antifungal agent that acts by binding directly to ergosterol on the fungal cell membrane, resulting in disruption of membrane integrity and cell death. Amphotericin B has activity against a very wide range of clinically important yeasts and molds. Resistance to amphotericin B is rare and has been reported in only a few species (*Candida lusitaniae, Candida guilliermondii, Aspergillus terreus*, and *Fusarium* species). Amphotericin B has been the gold standard for the treatment of invasive fungal diseases for many years. Despite the more recent advent of newer antifungal agents with broad spectrums of activity (e.g., caspofungin and voriconazole), amphotericin B remains the standard treatment for many severe infections.

WATCH OUT FOR

Amphotericin B is often associated with numerous side effects including nephrotoxicity and an infusion-related phenomenon marked by hypotension, fever, chills, and rigors. In an effort to alleviate these side effects, three different lipid-based products have been developed: liposomal amphotericin B (L-AMB), amphotericin B lipid complex (ABLC), and amphotericin B colloidal dispersion(ABCD). It is important to note that these products should not be considered interchangeable, as each has different pharmacokinetic and physiochemical characteristics (see *Table 251.1*).

Amphotericin B–related nephrotoxicity occurs presumably as a result of its vasoconstrictive effects, as well as direct effects on the epithelial cell membranes and tubular dysfunction. Other renal toxicities associated with amphotericin B include potassium- and magnesium-wasting syndromes as well as renal tubular acidosis. As a result, a reversible decline in glomerular filtration rate (GFR) and a rise in serum creatinine up to as high as 2.5 mg/dL is not uncommon during a course of therapy. However, the resultant reduction in renal blood flow and GFR can also precipitate necrosis and acute renal failure (ARF) in some patients. Patients at greatest risk for developing ARF

TABLE 251.1 SELECTED CHARACTERISTICS OF AMPHOTERICIN B PRODUCTS

	AMPHOTERICIN B	LIPOSOMAL AMPHOTERICIN B	AMPHOTERICIN B LIPID COMPLEX	AMPHOTERICIN B COLLOIDAL DISPERSION
Trade name	Fungizone	AmBisome	Abelcet	Amphotec
Usual dose	0.7–1 mg/kg/d	3–5 mg/kg/d	5 mg/kg/d	4 mg/kg/d
V$_d$(L/kg)	2–4	0.1–0.4	131	4
Plasma half-life (hours)	24–48	8.7–11.2	19.7–23.5	22.2
Clearance (mL/hr/kg)	40.6	9.4	17.8	105
Cost per day[a]	1 mg/kg/d	5 mg/kg/d	5 mg/kg/d	4 mg/kg/d
	$17.64	$1,318.80	$840.00	$392.00

V$_d$, volume of distribution.

[a] Cost calculated based on a 70-kg patient using average wholesale price 2005.

are the critically ill and patients receiving concomitant nephrotoxins (e.g., cyclosporine, aminoglycosides). Numerous studies consistently suggest that lipid-based amphotericin products are associated with at least 50% less renal toxicity as compared with conventional amphotericin B. However, it is still important to note that nephrotoxicity and renal failure can still develop with the lipid-based products; therefore, close monitoring of urine output, electrolytes, blood urea nitrogen, and serum creatinine is warranted in all patients.

Intravascular volume expansion with isotonic crystalloid solutions is indicated in all patients receiving amphotericin B products, as it may ameliorate the decline in GFR. A 500-mL bolus of 0.9% sodium chloride solution prior to each dose is recommended, provided the clinical situation permits. In many cases, aggressive electrolyte replacement and correction of acid-base disorders may be warranted.

SUGGESTED READINGS

Costa S, Nucci M. Can we decrease amphotericin nephrotoxicity? Curr Opin Crit Care. 2001;7(6):379–383.

Deray G. Amphotericin B nephrotoxicity. J Antimicrob Chemother. 2002;49(suppl 1): 341.

Herbrecht R, Natarajan-Arne S, Nivioix Y, et al. The lipid formulations of amphotericin B. Expert Opin Pharmacother. 2003;4(8):1277–1287.

252

HAVE A HIGH LEVEL OF SUSPICION FOR DRUG-INDUCED ACUTE INTERSTITIAL NEPHRITIS

ADAM R. BERLINER, MD
DEREK M. FINE, MD

Drugs cause the vast majority of acute interstitial nephritis (AIN), particularly in hospitalized patients. The seminal characterization of drug-induced AIN was a 1978 series of 13 patients treated with methicillin, in which AIN was accompanied by fever, rash (usually maculopapular), and peripheral eosinophilia (the classic triad of AIN), which occurred in 58%, 100%, and 100% of patients, respectively. However, methicillin use is no longer common, and the reliance on this group of signs to diagnose AIN in the context of more modern, diverse drugs may lead to missed diagnoses. Indeed, the complete triad is seen in only 5% of nonmethicillin AIN. A study of 150 AIN cases illustrates how certain signs and symptoms may be poorly sensitive for diagnosis of AIN (Fig. 252.1).

Of note, interstitial nephritis from nonsteroidal anti-inflammatory drugs (NSAIDs) may sometimes present with bland urinary sediment but heavy proteinuria, even in the nephritic range.

Dozens of drugs are known to cause AIN and theoretically any drug can be blamed.

- Drugs commonly associated with AIN include penicillin derivatives, cephalosporins, aminoglycosides, sulfa-containing drugs (including furosemide and torsemide), rifampin, allopurinol, mesalamine, NSAIDs, and proton pump inhibitors.
- The time from first drug dose to evidence of AIN may be only a few days (particularly upon re-exposure) or as long as 2 to 3 weeks.
- In some cases, one dose of a medication may be sufficient to cause AIN.
- Prior tolerance of a given drug does *not* rule it out as a cause of AIN in the present.

Renal biopsy is the gold standard for diagnosis of AIN and shows inflammatory interstitial infiltrates, with or without interstitial eosinophils. It is important to note that even biopsy can give unexpected results. In one series of 32 patients with acute renal failure, only 44% thought to have AIN on clinical grounds actually had it on biopsy. Conversely, acute interstitial nephritis is frequently

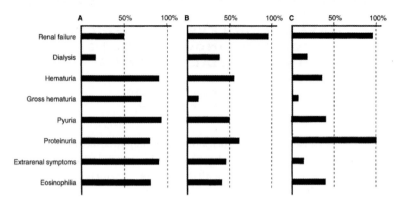

FIGURE 252.1. Approximated frequency with which clinical manifestations occur during the course of methicillin-induced AIN (**A**), AIN induced by drugs other than methicillin (**B**), or AIN induced by NSAIDs and associated with a nephritic syndrome (**C**). Proteinuria was considered positive when it was at least 0.5 g/L or positive by dipstick. Data are derived from case reports and analysis of cases. Reused with permission from Rossert J. Drug-induced acute interstitial nephritis. Kidney Int. 2001;60:804–817.

found on biopsy when prebiopsy suspicion is low. In addition, the urine may be examined with either Hansel stain or Wright stain for eosinophiluria (considered positive when >1% of urinary leukocytes show positive staining). In one series of 200 patients with urinary eosinophils, the sensitivity, specificity, and positive predictive value for AIN (with renal biopsy the gold standard) were only 40%, 72%, and 38%, respectively. Eosinophiluria can also be seen in prostatitis, rapidly progressive glomerular nephritis, bladder cancer, and renal atheroembolic disease. Renal ultrasound is very nonspecific and usually shows normal-sized kidneys, occasionally enlarged, with increased echogenicity.

WHAT TO DO

Other than discontinuing the suspected drug, treatment is limited. Supportive care of renal failure with dialysis if needed is the mainstay of therapy. Earlier cessation of an offending drug holds better hope for return to baseline renal function, since tubular atrophy and interstitial fibrosis increase with time. In one series of biopsy-proven AIN, resolution of acute renal failure within 2 weeks was associated with a lower residual serum creatinine (1.4 mg/dL) than longer-resolving acute renal failure (3.4 mg/dL).

Corticosteroids can be considered after discussion with a nephrologist, though preferably with biopsy-proven AIN. Corticosteroid-treated patients in the 1978 methicillin study tended to return to a lower serum creatinine, and in greater numbers, than untreated patients. This, however, was a small retrospective study, and only 8 of the 14 patients had biopsy-proven AIN. A larger retrospective study of corticosteroids for AIN found no benefit.

SUGGESTED READINGS

Galpin J, et al. Acute interstitial nephritis due to methicillin. Am J Med. 1978;65: 756–765.
Michel DM, Kelly CJ. Acute interstitial nephritis. J Am Soc Nephrol. 1998;9(3): 506–515.
Rossert J. Drug-induced acute interstitial nephritis. Kidney Int. 2001;60:804–817.

253

CONSIDER RHABDOMYOLYSIS IN THE PATIENT WHO DEVELOPS OLIGURIC RENAL FAILURE AFTER A PROLONGED SURGERY WHERE MUSCLE COMPRESSION MAY HAVE OCCURRED

WILLIAM R. BURNS III, MD

Oliguria, characterized by an hourly urine output below 0.5 cc per kilogram of body weight or a daily urine output less than 400 cc, is a common clinical problem. Early recognition and successful diagnosis are required to promptly initiate appropriate therapy and to limit the risk of renal failure. While there are a number of potential causes for this condition, one important etiology to consider (especially in postoperative patients and trauma victims) is rhabdomyolysis, a condition that often progresses to myoglobinuric acute renal failure.

Rhabdomyolysis is defined by an excessive breakdown of striated muscle. When this occurs, cellular materials (including a number of muscle-specific enzymes) are released into the bloodstream. Elevated blood levels of creatine kinase, as well as lactate dehydrogenase or aldolase, are often used to confirm the diagnosis. Myoglobin, an oxygen-carrying hemeprotein found in muscle cells, also enters the bloodstream during rhabdomyolysis. Following excessive muscle injury, the blood is unable to bind and clear the increased myoglobin load, which is then excreted by the kidneys. When urinary myoglobin becomes elevated, patients develop dark, tea-colored urine characteristic of myoglobinuria.

Most clinicians are able to recognize the common risk of rhabdomyolysis in trauma scenarios with extremity ischemia, reperfusion injury, compartment syndrome, crush injury, substantial blunt trauma, or electrical injury. Identification in postoperative patients, on the other hand, is more difficult. Positioning during prolonged surgical procedures has been well described in association with rhabdomyolysis and myoglobinuric renal failure. Whether related to nonsupine positions (lithotomy or lateral decubitus) or suboptimal padding (hard tables or back boards), muscle compression of any etiology impairs perfusion and ischemic injury is likely to occur. Morbidly obese are also at increased rate of developing significant muscle injury because of excessive pressure and often extended operative times. Likewise, muscle injury from malignant hyperthermia and prolonged paralysis (often in conjunction with steroid use) can result in rhabdomyolysis. Therefore, specific at-risk populations should be routinely screened to ensure prompt diagnosis. The astute clinician will also recognize that the inciting event for rhabdomyolysis can be as minimal as compressions delivered by sequential compression devices.

Patients with myoglobinuria are at increased risk of acute renal failure. A routine urinalysis is an effective screening test, revealing occult blood but no erythrocytes. This is because of the detection of myoglobin's heme molecules in the absence of hematuria. Identification of urinary myoglobin is also used to confirm the diagnosis. The association of myoglobinuria and acute renal failure is most attributed to an obstructive process, but other mechanisms, some independent of myoglobin, play a role as well. In an acidic environment (pH <5), myoglobin will precipitate and form casts that impair filtration and damage the nephron. Reactive oxygen species, which are also generated in rhabdomyolysis, can initiate direct toxic effects on the renal tubules. In addition, a number of vasoactive agents released during rhabdomyolysis cause renal arteriolar constriction and subsequent ischemic injury. Regardless of the exact mechanism of injury, early diagnosis and prompt initiation of therapy are critical to limiting renal damage.

While strategies to prevent, limit, and recognize muscle injury have improved, successful treatment of rhabdomyolysis remains critical in preventing myoglobinuric renal failure. The hallmarks of therapy are reversal of shock, minimization of ongoing muscle damage, and aggressive volume resuscitation. After an initial crystalloid fluid bolus, infusion rates are usually titrated to maintain a robust hourly urine output (often as high as 200 cm^3). Dosing of medication often needs to be reduced and nephrotoxic agents should be discontinued whenever possible. Additional therapies include the use of mannitol bicarbonate, and diuretics although these remain controversial. Mannitol is felt to be of benefit because of a number of physiologic effects including volume expansion, renal vasodilatation, and hydroxyl radical scavenging. Although controversial Bicarbonate administration can be used to alkalinize the urine, which may limit myoglobin precipitation and the resultant tubular obstruction with myoglobin casts. Therapies such as plasmapheresis and hemofiltration are very effective at clearing circulating heme pigments but do not seem to slow the progression to renal failure.

SELECTED READINGS

Anema JG, Morey AF, McAninch JW, et al. Complications related to the high lithotomy position during urethral reconstruction. J Urol. 2000;164:360–363.

Khurana RN, Baudendistel TE, Morgan EF, et al. Postoperative rhabdomyolysis following laparoscopic gastric bypass in the morbidly obese. Arch Surg. 2004;139:73–76.

Slater MS, Mullins RJ. Rhabdomyolysis and myoglobinuric renal failure in trauma and surgical patients: a review. J Am Coll Surg. 1998;186:693–716.

254

AIM FOR 2 MILLILITERS PER KILOGRAM PER HOUR OF URINE OUTPUT IN RHABDOMYOLYSIS

AWORI J. HAYANGA, MD
ELLIOTT R. HAUT, MD

Rhabdomyolysis is a syndrome characterized by muscle necrosis and the release of intracellular muscle constituents into the circulation. The severity of illness ranges from asymptomatic elevations of serum muscle enzymes to life-threatening cases associated with severe electrolyte imbalances, acute renal failure, disseminated intravascular coagulation, and death.

The classic presentation of rhabdomyolysis includes myalgias, pigmenturia due to myoglobinuria, and elevated serum muscle enzymes. The most commonly measured enzyme is serum creatinine kinase (CK), which is typically greater than 10,000 IU/L. It should be noted that serum CK levels may remain elevated in the absence of myoglobinuria since myoglobin is cleared from the serum more rapidly than CK. Since serum and/or urine myoglobin levels often take at least hours (if not days) to obtain results, these should not be relied upon to make the diagnosis. Rhabdomyolysis can be reliably diagnosed with the combination of the urine dipstick that is positive for heme (because of urine myoglobin) and urine microscopy showing an absence of red blood cells. Other abnormal electrolyte findings include hyperkalemia, hyperphosphatemia, hypocalcemia, and metabolic acidosis.

Rhabdomyolysis has many varied etiologies, which are difficult to categorize. Direct mechanical injury resulting in rhabdomyolysis can be caused by trauma, electrocutions, prolonged immobilization, ischemic limb injury, and crush injuries. Other cases can be caused by heatstroke and exertional rhabdomyolysis following vigorous exercise (e.g., strong-man triathlons). In addition, rhabdomyolysis can be caused by drugs and toxins, which can exert either direct myotoxicity (e.g., statins) or cause indirect muscle damage (e.g., alcohol or cocaine). Infections, inflammatory disorders, endocrine, and metabolic etiologies are also included in the long list of differential diagnoses. Genetic causes must be considered if no other cause is readily apparent.

The most important goal of treatment in rhabdomyolysis is preservation of renal function. Plasma volume expansion with intravenous isotonic saline should be given as soon as possible, even while trying to establish the cause of the rhabdomyolysis. As an example, saline infusion may be started before reperfusion of the trapped body part in the case of severe crush injury. The time to adequate fluid volume restoration directly influences the rate of renal failure. Massive amounts of fluids (well over 10 L) are often required to compensate for the amount of fluid sequestered by necrotic muscle. Urine output is the most important early marker of adequate hydration and many experienced physicians aim for 2 mL/kg/h.

Controversy still exists about the use of mannitol and alkalinization of the urine as additional possible therapies to help prevent renal failure. While some physicians have very strong beliefs regarding the utility of these maneuvers, most agree that neither approach should be used in patients with oliguria. There is no clear evidence that alkalinization is beneficial and there is a risk that alkalinization may worsen hypocalcemia. Likewise, there is no good evidence of the benefit of mannitol use. Saline diuresis seems to be the primary therapeutic action. Monitoring with serial measurements of serum potassium, calcium, phosphate, and creatinine is recommended. It should be noted that hypocalcemia should not be corrected unless the patient is symptomatic to avoid worsening the common rebound hypercalcemia seen during the recovery phase.

Acute renal failure secondary to rhabdomyolysis is managed expectantly and renal replacement therapy begun to control hyperkalemia and/or volume overload. Rhabdomyolysis-induced renal failure behaves somewhat differently than renal failure from other causes. Serum creatinine rises to a higher level more quickly, yet the patients have a better prognosis for recovery of renal function.

SUGGESTED READINGS

Melli G, Chaudhry V, Cornblath DR. Rhabdomyolysis: an evaluation of 475 hospitalized patients. Medicine (Baltimore). 2005;84(6):377–385.

Sauret JM, Marinides G, Wang GK. Rhabdomyolysis. Am Fam Phys. 2002;65(5):907–912.

255

DO NOT ATTEMPT TO CONVERT OLIGURIC TO NONOLIGURIC RENAL FAILURE WITH DIURETICS

BRANDON R. BRUNS, MD
HEIDI L. FRANKEL, MD

Oliguria, recently defined as urine output of less than 0.3 mL/kg/h for a 24-hour period, is a common problem in the intensive care unit (ICU). Oliguria is an important harbinger of acute renal failure. Nearly 70% of ICU patients who develop acute renal failure are oliguric. Classically, renal failure has been ascribed to three causes: prerenal, renal, and postrenal.

PRERENAL

- Absolute decrease in intravascular volume
  - Hemorrhage
  - Fluid sequestration (e.g., pancreatitis, after an exploratory laparotomy, burns, diarrhea, and vomiting)
- Renal perfusion impairment
  - Thrombosis of renal vasculature
  - Emboli to the renal artery
  - Abdominal compartment syndrome
  - Dissection of a renal artery
- Relative decrease in intravascular volume
  - Vasodilatation associated with sepsis
  - Severe right-sided heart failure
  - Cirrhosis
  - Nephrosis

RENAL

- Acute tubular necrosis
  - Myoglobin
  - Aminoglycosides
  - Intravenous contrast
- Acute interstitial nephritis, which can be caused by a wide variety of drugs (e.g., antibiotics)

POSTRENAL

- Prostatic hypertrophy

- Ureteral obstruction
- Foley catheter malfunction

Other than the avoidance of unnecessary toxins or attention to the appropriate volume resuscitation of the ICU patient, there are few modalities that can prevent incipient acute renal failure. In general, patients with nonoliguric renal failure are easier to manage than patients with oliguric renal failure. However, the use of loop diuretics in an attempt to convert from oliguric to nonoliguric renal failure is associated with an increased mortality and a decreased rate of recovery of renal function. Similarly, agents such as dopamine and fenoldopam have been unsuccessful.

A new renal failure grading system—RIFLE—uses glomerular filtration rate (GFR) criteria or urine output to predict whether acute renal failure will result in chronic deficits. The categories include *r*isk, *i*njury, *f*ailure, and the subcategories of *l*oss and *e*nd-stage renal disease. In general, the longer it takes for renal function to return, the less the chance it ever will. After 6 months of acute renal failure, there is little hope for recovery. Thus, whereas avoidance of nephrotoxins (and intravenous contrast) is critical in those with incipient or acute renal failure of short standing, there is little need to withhold these therapies in those with chronic renal failure; thus the old saying "You can't kill a nephron twice."

Treatment for acute renal failure involves resolution of the underlying cause, for example, restoring intravascular volume in a trauma patient or removal of an offending nephrotoxic agent. Other options include mechanical means of renal replacement—dialysis. Recovery from the effects of renal failure depends on the severity of the underlying damage.

SUGGESTED READINGS

Bell M, Liljestam E, Granath F, et al. Optimal follow-up time after continuous renal replacement therapy in acute renal failure patients stratified by the RIFLE criteria. Nephrol Dial Transplant. 2005;20:354–360.

Civetta JM, Taylor RW, Kirby RR. Critical Care. 3rd ed. Philadelphia: Lippincott–Raven Publishers; 1997:2081–2091.

Fink MP, Abraham E, Vincent JL, eds. Textbook of Critical Care. 5th ed. Philadelphia: Elsevier Saunders; 2005:1139–1149.

256

CONSIDER N-ACETYLCYSTEINE OR SODIUM BICARBONATE PROPHYLAXIS ALONG WITH ADEQUATE HYDRATION TO COMBAT CONTRAST-INDUCED NEPHROPATHY

MICHAEL J. MORITZ, MD

Contrast-induced nephropathy is the third most common cause of in-hospital acute renal failure and has been reported to occur in between 6% and 15% of patients receiving intravenous contrast dye. Iodinated contrast is used for arteriography (including cardiac catheterization) and venography and is administered intravenously (IV) for contrast-enhanced computed tomography (CT) scans. All iodinated contrast agents used for intravascular radiography have potential nephrotoxicity. The mechanism of renal injury is unknown but may include oxidative injury, a prerenal component from the diuretic effect of the contrast agent, and other etiologies. Nephrotoxicity depends on patient factors and increases with the following: renal insufficiency; diabetes or myeloma as the etiology of chronic renal insufficiency; dehydration; and increasing age. Nephrotoxicity is also a function of the specific agent, with an increased incidence with the older, ionic, higher-osmolarity agents and a decreased incidence with newer, more expensive, nonionic, lower-osmolarity agents.

WHAT TO DO

To reduce the risk of contrast-induced nephrotoxicity, patients should be adequately hydrated before exposure to contrast. Varying regimens have been used. One common regimen consists of 0.45% saline pre-exposure at 1 mL/kg/h for 12 hours for inpatients or 2 mL/kg/h for at least 4 hours for outpatients and postexposure at 75 mL/h for 12 hours. In addition to hydration, consideration should be given to administering N-acetylcysteine (NAC), especially in patients with renal insufficiency. One recent meta-analysis showed that NAC (which is relatively inexpensive and has few side effects if taken by mouth) reduced the risk of contrast-induced nephrotoxicity in patients with pre-existing chronic renal insufficiency. However, in this analysis, single doses varied widely, with oral doses of 400 to 1,500 mg and IV doses of 50 to 150 mg/kg given at varying intervals and durations. Some clinicians say that if oral dosing is used, apparently more than one pre-exposure dose is needed. One common regimen consists of pre-exposure NAC 600 mg orally for two doses at least 4 hours apart and postexposure two doses 12 hours apart. For oral administration, NAC is best administered in a strongly flavored drink such as a carbonated cola or Fresca to partially mask the disagreeable odor and taste. In emergencies, IV administration of 150 mg/kg in 500 mL of 0.9% saline over 30 minutes pre-exposure and 50 mg/kg in 500 mL of 0.9% saline over 4 hours postexposure has been used, although IV use is more common for the treatment of acetaminophen overdose. Intravenous NAC has a higher risk of anaphylactoid reactions than does oral administration and the physician must consider the risk-to-benefit ratio of using IV NAC for renal prophylaxis.

Perhaps a better choice than using IV NAC for contrast prophylaxis is administering a sodium bicarbonate infusion of 3 amps (total 150 milliequivalents sodium bicarbonate which is usually 150 cc) in 850 cc of D5W (dextrose 5% water) for a total net volume of 1 L. A recent randomized, controlled trial has shown the effectiveness of reducing contrast-induced nephropathy with the use of sodium bicarbonate in patients with both normal renal function and renal insufficiency pre–contrast administration. In this study patients received a bolus of 3 mg/kg/h for 1 hour before iopamidol contrast followed by an infusion of 1 mL/kg/h for 6 hours after the procedure. Contrast-induced nephropathy occurred in 1.7% of patients in the bicarbonate group, as compared with 13.6% in the control group of sodium chloride infusion. Use of sodium bicarbonate may have an advantage over NAC in the urgent setting because the pretreatment time is only 1 hour.

One final note is that NAC or sodium bicarbonate is not needed with magnetic resonance imaging contrast agents. These contrast agents are not iodine based, but rather use a metal with magnetic properties (e.g., iron or the rare earth gadolinium) and have different toxicities.

SUGGESTED READINGS

Alonso A, Lau J, Jaber BL, et al. Prevention of radiocontrast nephropathy with N-acetylcysteine in patients with chronic kidney disease: a meta-analysis of randomized, controlled trials. Am J Kidney Dis. 2004;43:1–9.

Fishbane S, Durham JH, Matzo K, et al. N-acetylcysteine in the prevention of radiocontrast-induced nephropathy. J Am Soc Nephrol. 2004;15:251–260.

MacNeill BC, Harding SA, Bazari H, et al. Prophylaxis of contrast-induced nephropathy in patients undergoing coronary angiography. Catheter Cardiovasc Interv. 2003;60:458–461.

Merten GJ, Burgess WP, Gray LV, et al. Prevention of contrast-induced nephropathy with sodium bicarbonate: a randomized controlled trial. JAMA. 2004;291:2328–2334.

257

REMEMBER THAT TRANSFUSION-RELATED ACUTE LUNG INJURY IS NOT DOSE DEPENDENT

ALA' S. HADDADIN, MD

Transfusion-related acute lung injury (TRALI) is a syndrome of sudden-onset noncardiogenic pulmonary edema occurring during or a few hours after transfusion of a blood product. TRALI is believed to occur in approximately 1 in every 5,000 transfusions and it usually occurs after administration of products containing large amounts of plasma, although it has been reported to occur after administration of as little as 50 mL of whole blood or any plasma–containing blood products including packed red blood cells and intravenous immunoglobulins. Leukoagglutination and pooling of granulocytes in the recipient's lungs may occur, with the release of the contents of leukocyte granules that results in injury to cellular membranes, endothelial surfaces, and potentially to lung parenchyma. In most cases, leukoagglutination results in mild dyspnea, hypoxia, hypovolemia, hypotension, fever, chills, and pulmonary infiltrates within about 6 hours of transfusion and spontaneously resolves. Occasionally, more severe lung injury occurs as a result of this phenomenon and acute respiratory distress syndrome (ARDS) results. TRALI has a reported mortality rate of 5% to 8% (the third most common cause of transfusion-related mortality). Host factors such as infection, lung disease, and recent surgery may contribute to the incidence and severity of TRALI. Laboratory findings include hemoconcentration, hypoalbuminemia, and neutropenia or neutrophilia. Typically, chest radiograph reveals bilateral infiltrates.

WHAT TO DO

Treatment is largely supportive. The transfusion should be stopped if the reaction is recognized in time. The patient should be given supplemental oxygen and ventilatory support as necessary (required in approximately two-thirds of cases), ideally using the same low-tidal-volume lung-protective strategies that are employed in ARDS. The pulmonary edema is noncardiogenic, and hence diuretics are not warranted. Glucocorticoids have been used, but there are no data to support this practice. Prevention is the most important measure, including avoiding unnecessary transfusions and increased use of red cells containing less plasma. Plasma derived from multiparous women has been identified as a significant source of antileukocyte antibodies, and it has been proposed that these "femme fatales" be excluded from the donor pool.

SUGGESTED READINGS

Looney MR, Gropper MA, Matthay MA. Transfusion-related acute lung injury: a review. Chest 2004;126:249–258.

Siliman CC, Boshkov LK, Mehidzadehkashi Z, et al. Transfusion-related acute lung injury: epidemiology and a prospective analysis of etiologic factors. Blood 2003;101:452–464.

Toy P, Popovsky MA, Abraham E, et al. Transfusion related acute lung injury: definition and review. Crit Care Med 2005;33(4):721–726.

258

KNOW THE SIGNS OF A TRANSFUSION REACTION

EUGENIE S. HEITMILLER, MD

SIGNS AND SYMPTOMS

An acute hemolytic transfusion reaction occurs when immunologic incompatibility between the donor and the recipient results in lysis of red blood cells. Most hemolytic transfusion reactions are due to the transfusion of ABO-incompatible packed red blood cells secondary to clerical or system errors. The severity of the reaction is relative to the amount of incompatible blood received, the type of incompatibility, and the length of time before treatment is initiated. These include chills, anxiety, dyspnea, rash, nausea, fever or rise in temperature of 1°C or more from baseline, hypertension or hypotension, headache, and chest and flank pain. In a deeply sedated or anesthetized patient, hemoglobinuria, hypotension, and coagulopathy may be the only signs. A hemolytic transfusion reaction is usually manifested during the transfusion and can occur after receiving as little as 10 mL of incompatible blood.

An increased temperature during a transfusion may be the first sign of a hemolytic transfusion reaction, or it may be a sign of bacterial contamination of the blood product. Fever with hypotension is characteristic of bacterial contamination. A Gram stain of the blood product is helpful to confirm the diagnosis. Bacterial contamination may occur from contamination at the phlebotomy site during blood collection, from an unrecognized infection in the donor, or from improper storage. The risk of infection has been reported as 1 in 2,000 to 10,000 units for platelets and from 1 in 250,000 to 1,500,000 for packed red blood cells

WHAT TO DO

If a transfusion reaction is suspected, the transfusion should be stopped immediately. The blood tubing should be disconnected and normal saline solution hung with new intravenous (IV) tubing to produce a urine output of 1 to 2 mL/kg/h to reduce the risk of acute renal failure. Although controversial, some clinicians use diuretics to increase urine output. Newer biologic agents are being developed that target complement intermediates or proinflammatory cytokines and may be effective agents in the treatment of severe hemolytic transfusion reactions when available.

If a patient develops urticaria during a transfusion with no other signs or symptoms, it is not necessary to stop the transfusion. Administration of an antihistamine (i.e., Benadryl) may help to decrease the urticaria, which is usually due to transfused allergens that interact with the patient's mast cells, resulting in degranulation of the mast cells. In addition, patients who receive repeated transfusions are more likely to experience febrile nonhemolytic transfusion reactions, which can be treated with acetaminophen.

It is the responsibility of the clinician to know his or her institution's protocol for testing blood and urine samples in suspected cases of hemolytic transfusion reaction.

SUGGESTED READINGS

American Society of Anesthesiologists. Practice Guidelines for Perioperative Blood Transfusion and Adjuvant Therapies. http://www.asahq.org/publicationsAndServices/practiceparam.htm#blood

Blajchman BA, Beckers EA, Dickmeiss E, et al. Bacterial detection of platelets: current problems and possible resolutions. Transfus Med Rev 2005;19(4):259–272.

Davenport RD. Pathophysiology of hemolytic transfusion reactions. Semin Hematol 2005;42(3): 165–168.

Goodnough L. Risks of blood transfusion. Anesthesiol Clin North Am 2005;23:241–252.

Yazdanakhsh K. Review: complement receptor 1 therapeutics for prevention of immune hemolysis. Immunohematology 2005;21(3):109–118.

259

HAVE A HIGH THRESHOLD IN TRANSFUSING PLATELETS, ESPECIALLY IN NONBLEEDING PATIENTS WHO ARE NOT PREOPERATIVE

MICHAEL J. HAUT, MD

Platelet transfusion has made a significant contribution to the care of certain patient populations. These groups include those undergoing high-dose chemotherapy (e.g., for acute leukemia or stem cell transplant) and patients sustaining major trauma. Platelets for transfusion are obtained either by centrifugation of units of whole blood (random donor platelets) or by pheresis. In general, units available in the United States are leukoreduced. Leukoreduction reduces the incidence of platelet transfusion reactions and may reduce the incidence of alloimmunization.

WHAT TO DO

Considerable effort has gone into determining what the trigger should be for the transfusion of platelets and how many platelets should be transfused. Historically, the platelet transfusion trigger for patients with chemotherapy-induced thrombocytopenia was $20 \times 10^9/\mu L$. However, several recent large studies have suggested that $10 \times 10^9/\mu L$ is acceptable. A large retrospective study has shown that the most significant predictor of bleeding in thrombocytopenic patients is not the platelet count but a history of bleeding in the previous 5 days. These data suggest that attention should be focused on providing aggressive platelet therapy for active bleeding rather than on prophylactically transfusing platelets. Such an approach may not be appropriate in trauma patients, in whom hypothermia, acidosis, and other factors may affect the function of the patient's own platelets and the platelets that are transfused. Specific situations requiring platelet transfusions in thrombocytopenic patients include the presence of bleeding and the need to perform invasive procedures such as lumbar puncture, bronchoscopy, and surgery.

In the asymptomatic medical patient, transfusion should be given when the platelet count is 10×10^9 platelets$/\mu L$ or when the patient is bleeding and the platelet count is $20,000 \times 10^9/\mu L$ or less. In many institutions, either one pheresis single-donor pack (equal to 6 units of platelets) or 6 units of random-donor platelets is used. More recently, many institutions have opted to give 4 units of random-donor platelets, which is effective in many situations.

WATCH OUT FOR

A major problem after platelet transfusion is the development of alloantibodies. This results in suboptimal rise, or no rise at all, in platelet count after platelet transfusion. This can happen after either random-donor or single-donor platelets, and often occurs after only a few platelet transfusions. To achieve adequate hemostasis after a patient has developed autoantibodies, HLA-matched platelets should be transfused. When this does not raise the platelet count, platelets can be cross-matched. In patients for whom HLA-matched platelets do not raise the platelet count, hemostasis can sometimes be achieved with epsilon-aminocaproic acid.

SUGGESTED READINGS

Hoffman R, Benz E, Shattil SI, et al. Hematology: Basic Principles and Practice, 4th ed. New York: Churchill Livingstone, 2005:2433–2440.

Slichter SJ. Relationship between platelet count and bleeding risk in thrombocytopenic patients. Transfus Med Rev 2004;18(3):153–167.

Spahn DR, Rossaint R. Coagulopathy and blood component transfusion in trauma. Br J Anaesth 2005;95(2):130–139.

Strauss RG. Pretransfusion trigger platelet counts and dose for prophylactic platelet transfusions. Curr Opin Hematol 2005;12(6):499–502.

260

DO NOT ADMINISTER PLATELETS IN IMMUNE THROMBOCYTOPENIC PURPURA

LAITH ALTAWEEL, MD

Immune thrombocytopenic purpura (ITP) is an autoimmune disorder characterized by low platelet count and mucocutaneous bleeding. The estimated incidence is 100 per 1 million persons per year. ITP can be a primary disorder or secondary to an underlying disorder and can have an acute (6 months or less) or chronic presentation. ITP in children and adults is very different. In children, the incidence is equal between boys and girls, who are usually in good health until they present with petechiae or purpura a few days or weeks after an acute infectious illness. In more than 70% of the cases, the illness resolves within 6 months. In adults, the illness is more chronic and insidious, and is more common in women.

The pathophysiology is related to autoantibodies against platelets, which then undergo accelerated clearance in the spleen. The diagnosis of ITP remains one of exclusion. Disorders that ITP occurs secondary to include systemic lupus erythematosus, antiphospholipid syndrome, immunodeficiency states such as common variable hypogammaglobulinemia and immunoglobulin A deficiency, lymphoproliferative disorders (chronic lymphocytic leukemia, large granular lymphocytic leukemia, and lymphoma), infection with human immunodeficiency virus and hepatitis C virus, and drugs such as heparin and quinidine.

WATCH OUT FOR Marked splenomegaly is not common in ITP, and should prompt a search for an alternative diagnosis. The profile of the complete blood count should be normal except for a low platelet count and possibly low hemoglobin in the setting of hemorrhage. The blood smear should be evaluated to rule out pseudothrombocytopenia, inherited giant platelets, and other hematologic disorders. Large immature platelets are often seen in ITP. For patients older than 60 years of age, a bone marrow aspiration is recommended.

Patients with platelet counts of greater than $50,000/mL^3$ are usually diagnosed incidentally. For counts between $10,000/mL^3$ and $30,000/mL^3$, petechiae or ecchymoses develop spontaneously, and platelet counts less than $10,000/mL^3$ can result in spontaneous internal hemorrhage.

WHAT TO DO The initial treatment of ITP consists of corticosteroid treatment, and a response is seen in most patients within three weeks. For very low platelet counts and patients refractory to corticosteroids, intravenous immune globulin can be used. For urgent treatment, as might occur with internal bleeding or a need for emergency surgery, intravenous corticosteroids and intravenous immunoglobulin should be given. In addition, antifibrinolytic therapy with aminocaproic acid or activated factor VII can also be administered.

Chronic treatment is only necessary for patients with platelet counts less than 30,000 platelets/mm^3. Aside from continued medical therapy with corticosteroids, danazol, dapsone, and intravenous immunoglobulin, a surgical option may be necessary. Splenectomy, whether laparoscopic or open, is the surgical treatment for chronic ITP. Approximately two thirds of patients have a response after surgery. Prior to surgery, patients need to be immunized for the encapsulated organisms including pneumococcus, *Haemophilus influenzae* type b, and meningococcus. For those who do not respond to splenectomy, optimal medical therapy with combination therapy as noted before is attempted with a goal of maintaining platelet count greater than 30,000/mm^3. If the platelet count does not respond to surgical or standard medical therapy, treatment with immunosuppressive agents, such as azathioprine or cyclophosphamide, may need to be initiated. Finally, there are a number of investigational therapies available for cases that are refractory to standard therapeutic approaches.

SUGGESTED READINGS

Cines D, Blanchette V. Immune thrombocytopenic purpura. N Engl J Med 2002;346:995–1008.

Guidelines for the investigation and management of idiopathic thrombocytopenic purpura in adults, children and in pregnancy. Br J Haematol 2003;120:574.

261

DO NOT ADMINISTER PLATELETS IN TYPE 2 HEPARIN-INDUCED THROMBOCYTOPENIA

LAITH ALTAWEEL, MD

Heparin is an important anticoagulant in both medical and surgical patient populations. One of the most serious complications of its use is the development of heparin-induced thrombocytopenia (HIT). There are two types of HIT: type 1 and type 2. Type 1 is a non–immune-mediated reduction in the platelet count that occurs a few days after starting heparin, causes a mild thrombocytopenia, and normalizes with continued heparin use. Type 2 HIT is considerably more dangerous than type 1, is immune mediated, and often results in thrombosis.

WATCH OUT FOR

Type 2 HIT results in a reduction of platelets by at least 50%. HIT is seen in approximately 3% to 5% of patients exposed to unfractionated heparin and 1% of those exposed to low-molecular-weight heparin. In heparin-naïve patients, the condition usually presents 5 days after the initiation of heparin therapy. In patients exposed to heparin within the prior 100 days, HIT may develop sooner, often within 24 hours of heparin initiation. Heparin of bovine origin is more likely than porcine heparin to cause HIT type 2. The development of HIT does not depend on the quantity or dose of exposure. HIT type 2 has been demonstrated in patients exposed to minute amounts of heparin as may be found in heparin flushes and heparin-coated catheters. Discontinuation of heparin does not eliminate the risk for complications. HIT-associated thrombosis may occur up to 4 to 6 weeks after the discontinuation of heparin.

The platelet count is important in considering a diagnosis of HIT type 2. HIT should be considered whenever the platelet count drops by more than 50% at 5 to 10 days after the onset of heparin treatment in naïve patients. It is important to note that the platelet count may still be normal in patients whose baseline platelet count is high. Profound thrombocytopenia is unusual and often warrants a search for an alternative diagnosis. Patients who have received heparin in the recent past have a rapid onset of HIT type 2, usually within 24 hours of heparin exposure.

The laboratory confirmation is made by solid-phase assays or platelet activation assays. Solid-phase assays, such as the solid-phase enzyme-linked immunosorbent assay (ELISA), tend to be very nonspecific. Platelet activation assays, such as serotonin release assays (SRAs), are more specific but are also technically demanding. Another method of testing platelet activation assay is the platelet aggregation test, which is less demanding technically but also less sensitive than SRA and solid-phase ELISA. The results from laboratory data must be considered within the context of the pretest clinical probability.

The most common clinical presentation includes thrombosis, usually in the deep venous system of the lower limbs. Venous thrombosis in the arms can occur particularly at sites of indwelling venous catheters. Other sites can develop thrombosis including the cavernous sinus, adrenal cortex, and skin lesions at sites of cutaneous heparin injections. Other presentations include disseminated intravascular coagulation, myocardial infarction, mesenteric infarction, renal artery thrombosis, stroke, and transient global amnesia. Therefore, it is critical that the clinician have a high index of suspicion for this condition and empirically discontinue heparin or use alternative forms of anticoagulation if HIT is present.

WHAT TO DO

The treatment of HIT type 2 consists of discontinuing heparin when the platelet count drops or when thrombosis develops while the patient is on heparin. After discontinuing the heparin, the patient who needs continued anticoagulation can be started on a thrombin inhibitor, such as argatroban or lepirudin. It is important to remember that low-molecular-weight heparin can cross-react with HIT antibodies and should not be used. Once the patient is on a thrombin inhibitor, warfarin can be started if continued anticoagulation is indicated for the patient's care. It must be realized that starting warfarin in the acute setting may result in acute skin necrosis and additional thrombosis. Because the risk of thrombosis persists for several weeks after discontinuation of heparin, patients should be anticoagulated for 30 to 60 days after the diagnosis is made. Platelet transfusion should be avoided because this increases the severity of thrombosis.

SUGGESTED READINGS

Davoren A, Aster R. Heparin-induced thrombocytopenia and thrombosis. Am J Hematol 2006;81:36–44.

Warkentin T, Kelton J. Temporal aspects of heparin-induced thrombocytopenia. N Engl J Med 2006;344(17):1286–1292.

262

REMEMBER THAT RETICULOCYTE COUNT IS NOT ACCURATE AFTER BLOOD TRANSFUSION

ANTHONY SLONIM, MD, DrPH

The presence of both an adequate number of erythrocytes and circulating blood volume is essential for the delivery of oxygen and substrates to the cells in the body. An inadequate number of erythrocytes results in anemia and compromises oxygen delivery by reducing the oxygen content of the blood. Oxygen content is comprised of two subcomponents. The contribution of oxygen bound to hemoglobin represents a considerably larger component of the oxygen delivery than the dissolved component, which highlights the relative importance of hemoglobin to overall oxygen delivery. The numerical equation for this relationship is

$$O_2 = (hbg \times \%sat \times 1.32) + (PaO_2 \times 0.0032)$$

WATCH OUT FOR

There are a number of types and causes of anemia that affect intensive care unit (ICU) patients, and the initial workup for this condition is important in correcting the underlying dysfunction. For example, the ICU patient may present with acute blood loss from a bleeding duodenal ulcer or diverticulosis. In this case, the administration of packed red blood cell transfusions and the treatment of the underlying cause are of importance. If, for example, the patient had a malignancy such as lymphoma, the anemia may result from an overcrowded marrow and insufficient erythrocyte production. Understanding the context of the anemia will not only allow for appropriate therapy and the correction of any underlying oxygen deficits, but will also provide an opportunity to appropriately treat the underlying condition.

The initial classification of anemia is improved with the use of the reticulocyte count. The reticulocyte count represents the number of immature erythrocytes that are present in the peripheral blood pool. They can be identified by the use of a specific stain on the peripheral smear and their number provides an estimate of bone marrow functioning. It is important to remember that normal erythrocytes have an average lifespan of approximately 120 days. As these cells are cleared from the circulation by the spleen, they are replaced by reticulocytes from the bone marrow. The normal reticulocyte count is 1% to

2%, which represents the normal turnover of erythrocytes from the circulation.

The reticulocyte count increases severalfold within the first 2 weeks after the onset of anemia. This assumes that there is an adequate store of iron and erythropoietin to stimulate production of erythrocytes in the bone marrow when the hemoglobin drops below 10g/dL. It is important to note that the reticulocyte count needs to be corrected for the number of circulating erythrocytes. This is done with the use of the following formula:

$$\text{Corrected reticulocyte count} = \text{Actual reticulocyte count}$$
$$\times (\text{Actual hemoglobin or [hematocrit]})/$$
$$(\text{Normal hemoglobin [or hematocrit]})$$

This formula also highlights one of the major problems with checking the reticulocyte count after a transfusion. The reticulocyte count might be expected to decrease after a blood transfusion because the bone marrow no longer needs to provide the same level of peripheral erythrocytes. The corrected reticulocyte count as displayed in the equation will be altered because the actual hemoglobin will be artificially elevated, thereby providing an inappropriate ratio of actual to normal hemoglobin to allow for the corrected reticulocyte count. Once in the periphery, the reticulocyte usually requires an additional 1 to 2 days to reach full maturation and function. Therefore, an additional correction known as the reticulocyte production index can be performed to account for this additional maturation.

SUGGESTED READING

Kasper DL, Braunwald E, Fauci AS, et al., eds. Harrison's Principles of Internal Medicine,16th ed. New York: McGraw-Hill, 2005.

263

Consider Leukocyte-Depleted Blood in Patients Who Are Immunosuppressed

MEHMET OZCAN, MD
PRAVEEN KALRA, MD

Leukocytes in allogenic blood products have been shown to cause several transfusion-related adverse reactions and complications. Leukocyte depletion of cellular blood products has been shown to reduce risks such as alloimmunization against donor leukocyte antigens, transmission of cytomegalovirus (CMV), and febrile nonhemolytic transfusion reaction. Immunosuppressed patients and potential recipients of organ transplants are especially vulnerable to those adverse effects and deserve consideration of administration of leukocyte-depleted blood products when indicated.

WATCH OUT FOR

Alloimmunization against donor leukocyte antigens may potentially cause rejection of solid-organ transplants via cross-immunization. This is mediated by the HLA-antigen system. Matching of HLA antigens is most important for kidney and heart transplants and least important for liver transplants. Therefore, using leukocyte-depleted blood products to prevent HLA alloimmunization is most logical for potential recipients of kidney and heart transplants. In liver transplantation, leukocytes in the intraoperatively administered blood have been suggested as a contributor of acute cellular rejection via an inflammatory cascade, although there are no randomized, controlled trials to support the benefit of leukocyte depletion for this indication. Overall, there is reasonable evidence for the benefit of using leukocyte-depleted blood products to prevent graft rejection in future recipients of kidney transplants, whereas the data are insufficient regarding heart transplants. Leukocyte-depleted blood products are not indicated for liver transplant candidates, at least for the purpose of preventing HLA alloimmunization.

CMV infection is a major cause of morbidity and mortality in the immunosuppressed patients. Allocating CMV-negative blood products for those patients is challenging because up to 80% of blood donors are seropositive. Because CMV is transmitted by leukocytes, leukocyte-depleted blood has been suggested as an alternative to CMV-seronegative blood. Even with CMV-seronegative blood, there is up to a 4% chance of seroconversion of the recipient. Although leukocyte-depleted blood is not absolutely CMV safe, its risk is comparable to that of seronegative blood. There is not a clear consensus on whether serologic testing for CMV should be abandoned if universal leukocyte reduction is implemented. In summary, both serologic testing and leukocyte depletion are effective but somewhat imperfect ways to reduce the risk of CMV transmission to the immunosuppressed.

The term "leukocyte-depleted" or "leukoreduced" refers to a unit of blood product containing less than 5×10^6 leukocytes. There are approximately 10^9 leukocytes in a unit of whole blood. Packed red blood cell (PRBC) units contain roughly half that number (5×10^8). "Washed" and "frozen-deglycerolized" PRBCs typically have 10^7 and 5×10^6 leukocytes per unit, respectively. As for platelets, apheresis single-donor units contain 5×10^8 leukocytes, whereas random donor concentrates contain 5×10^7 leukocytes per unit. Fresh-frozen plasma and cryoprecipitate do not contain any cellular elements including leukocytes.

Leukocyte depletion is most commonly achieved by filtration. Leukocyte filters (third-generation filters with a pore size <40 μm) achieve a 1,000-fold decrease in leukocyte counts of cellular blood products (i.e., <10 leukocytes per μL of PRBC). Leukocyte filtration can be performed pre- or poststorage. However, prestorage filtration is the preferred method because it prevents the release of metabolites from leukocytes during blood product storage, which may also be responsible for alloimmunization. Another disadvantage of poststorage filtration is a risk of hypotension at the time of transfusion, probably due to the activation of the bradykininogen/kininogen system during filtering. This hypotension from poststorage filtering can be more pronounced in patients using angiotensin-converting-enzyme inhibitors.

Perhaps the biggest concern regarding the use of universal leukocyte depletion is financial: it costs about $100 to leukofilter one unit of blood. In the United States, universal leukocyte depletion of all cellular blood products would cost an additional hundreds of millions of dollars annually (2004 estimate).

SUGGESTED READINGS

Bordin JO, Heddle NM, Blajchman MA. Biologic effects of leukocytes present in transfused cellular blood products. Blood 1994;84:1703–1721.

Dzik WH. Leukoreduction of blood components. Curr Opin Hematol 2002;9:521–526.

Shapiro MJ. To filter blood or universal leukoreduction: what is the answer? Crit Care 2004;8(Suppl 2):S27–S30.

264

ADMINISTER OCTREOTIDE IN VARICEAL BLEEDING WHILE WAITING FOR ENDOSCOPY

MADHAVI MEKA, MD

Cirrhosis affects 3 of 1,000 adults in North America and is responsible for more than 30,000 deaths annually. A major consequence of cirrhosis is variceal bleeding, which contributes significantly to the morbidity and mortality associated with cirrhosis. Obstruction to the portal venous blood flow as seen in cirrhosis, Budd-Chiari syndrome, portal venous thrombosis, portal fibrosis, and other infiltrative diseases causes portal hypertension. Eventually, varices develop to decompress the hypertensive portal vein and return blood to the systemic circulation. Varices usually develop when the portal venous pressure rises above 12 mm Hg (normal value is <5 mm Hg).

WHAT TO DO

Various modalities of treatment have been used over the years for treating varices. Previously, vasopressin and terlipressin, which directly constrict the mesenteric arterioles and reduce the portal venous flow, were used in medical management, but they are falling out of favor somewhat due to their ischemic effects on heart, brain, bowel, and limbs. Today, more commonly used drugs in the medical management of variceal bleeds include somatostatin and octreotide. These drugs inhibit the release of vasodilator hormones such as glucagon and indirectly cause splanchnic vasoconstriction. Octreotide is a long-acting synthetic analogue of somatostatin. An intravenous injection of 50-μg bolus followed by continuous infusion of 50 μg/h has been shown to cause significant decrease in the portal pressure. The effect of a single dose of octreotide on reducing portal pressure is effective but short-lived ($t_{1/2}$ is 3 h in patients with liver disease).

Endoscopic therapy is a mainstay of invasive treatment for bleeding varices. There are two therapeutic options available with endoscopy: sclerotherapy and ligation. Octreotide in combination with sclerotherapy has been shown to be superior to sclerotherapy alone in that it decreases the incidence of early rebleeding. A similar effect is observed when octreotide is used in combination with variceal ligation. In addition, octreotide reduces the bleeding and aids in better visualization of the varices during endoscopy when used prior to the procedure. Most hepatologists recommend continuing it for at least 24 to 48 hours after endoscopy to reduce the risk of rebleeding.

It is important to note that octreotide has effects on other hormones such as insulin, vasoactive intestinal peptide, and growth hormone. Side effects of octreotide include nausea, diarrhea, vomiting, constipation, stomach upset, gas, bloating, dizziness, headache, light-headedness, fatigue, flushing, and dry mouth. Pain and irritation have been reported at the injection site.

SUGGESTED READINGS

D'Amico G, Criscuoli V. Meta-analysis of trials for variceal bleeding. Hepatology 2002;36(4 pt 1):1023–1024.

D'Amico G, Polit, G, Morabito A. Octreotide compared with placebo in a treatment strategy for early rebleeding in cirrhosis. A double blind, randomized pragmatic trial. Hepatology 1998;28(5):1206–1214.

265

CONSIDER BLEEDING AROUND A CHEST TUBE TO BE A SIGN OF BLEEDING IN THE CHEST CAVITY UNTIL PROVEN OTHERWISE

DAVID J. CAPARRELLI, MD

Establishing adequate drainage of the mediastinum and pleural cavities at the time of surgery plays an extremely important role in the post-operative care of patients at risk for intrathoracic or mediastinal hemorrhage. Adequate drainage allows early recognition of surgically correctable bleeding and the prevention of life-threatening complications such as cardiac tamponade and tension pneumothorax. Traditionally, such drainage has been achieved with large-bore plastic chest tubes. Typically a combination of straight and right-angle tubes measuring between 28 French (F) and 32F in diameter are used after open cardiac surgery (e.g., coronary artery bypass), whereas straight tubes alone are most often used after elective thoracic procedures (e.g., lobectomy). However, these rigid tubes can be quite painful, damage bypass grafts, impair ventilation, and cause cardiac arrhythmias. For these reasons, many surgeons have recently adopted the use of smaller (19F or 24F), more flexible, fluted Silastic drains. Clinical data have demonstrated that these drains cause less pain and are as effective as their more rigid predecessors. Currently, in cardiac surgery, many advocate the use of one rigid chest tube in the mediastinum (32F) in conjunction with flexible Silastic drains (19F) to drain the pleural spaces. Typically, the mediastinal tube is removed on postoperative day one, whereas the Silastic drains remain in place until drainage is deemed appropriately low (usually 100 cc/24 h) for removal. For noncardiac thoracic procedures, where re-expansion of the lung and the management of air leaks are more of a priority than risk of hemorrhage, large-bore rigid chest tubes still predominate.

WATCH OUT FOR

Regardless of the type of tube chosen, early recognition of significant intrathoracic hemorrhage is vital in the care of cardiac and thoracic surgical patients. In the early postoperative period, frequent monitoring of both the quantity and the quality of the chest tube output is essential. Often chest tube output will be high (>100 cc/h) over the first few hours as efforts are made to warm the patient and correct residual coagulopathy. Ongoing bleeding despite repletion of coagulation factors (usually with fresh-frozen plasma) and platelet transfusions is suggestive of surgically correctable hemorrhage. If chest tube output is low and/or there is significant clot forming in the tubes, one must be concerned with undrained ongoing hemorrhage in any patient with persistent transfusion requirements. Moreover, significant bleeding *around* a chest tube should be considered a sign of hemorrhage in the chest cavity until proven otherwise; the chest tube may well allow capillary drainage around the tube, even if the lumen of the tube is not draining, perhaps due to a blockage.

When evaluating an intensive care unit patient in a situation in which intrathoracic or mediastinal hemorrhage is a concern, physical exam can play a role but usually takes a back seat to more objective data. Muffled heart sounds or decreased breath sounds over one hemithorax may indicate fluid around the heart or lung, but these findings are neither sensitive nor specific. Furthermore, evaluation of jugular venous distension can be hindered by central venous access in the neck. Hypotension and a decreasing cardiac output in the context of increasing central venous pressure may suggest cardiac tamponade physiology; however, these findings are also consistent with ventricular failure, for which the treatment is very different. Therefore, prompt accurate diagnosis of the primary problem is extremely important. All patients being evaluated for intrathoracic hemorrhage should have a stat chest radiograph (CXR). An enlarged cardiac silhouette or widened mediastinum may be indicative pericardial effusion, but CXR provides no information on this fluid that is physiologically significant. Opacification of the pleural space on CXR is a good indication of pleural effusion; however, the character of the fluid cannot be determined by this modality. Evaluation of the heart and mediastinum is best undertaken by transthoracic echocardiography. Not only can this modality effectively diagnose pericardial effusion, it also provides data with regard to the physiologic significance of the effusion (e.g., right ventricular collapse). Although very sensitive and specific for intrathoracic hemorrhage, computed tomography (CT) scan is not a diagnostic modality often used in the acute setting. However, in a stable patient who is several days to weeks out from surgery, CT scan can be very useful in identifying significant intrathoracic or mediastinal fluid collections. Such information can help to guide interventions such as pericardial window, thoracentesis, and video-assisted thoracoscopic decortication.

WHAT TO DO

Once the diagnosis is entertained that there is new or ongoing hemorrhage in the chest, the surgical team should be notified immediately. Significant undrained fluid in the mediastinum after cardiac surgery can be evacuated at the bedside by pericardiocentesis or in the operating room through a subxiphoid pericardial window or redo sternotomy. Similarly, fluid in the pleural spaces can be drained by thoracentesis, tube thoracostomy (chest tube insertion), or in the operating room via an open or thoracoscopic approach. Thoracentesis is usually reserved for the stable patient who is several days to weeks out from surgery with a large pleural effusion (unresponsive to diuretics) and persistent shortness of breath or fever. In the early postoperative period, tube thoracostomy is most appropriate for drainage of pleural fluid, and a large-bore (28F to 32F) tube is recommended. Typically, smaller chest tubes (e.g., 20F) can be used when the indication for chest tube placement is pneumothorax without associated pleural effusion. When persistent bleeding from a chest tube occurs (particularly after a bedside insertion) hemorrhage from the chest wall or intercostal vessel must be considered. This invariably requires more definitive treatment, such as repeat thoracotomy or an interventional radiology procedure.

SUGGESTED READINGS

Braunwald E, ed. Heart Disease: A Textbook of Cardiovascular Medicine. Philadelphia: WB Saunders, 1997:229–230, 1731–1732.

Obney JA, Barnes MJ, Lisagor PG, Cohen DJ. A method for mediastinal drainage after cardiac procedures using small Silastic drains. Ann Thorac Surg 2000;70:1109–1110.

Yang SC, Cameron DE, eds. Current Therapy in Thoracic and Cardiovascular Surgery. Philadelphia: Mosby, 2004:532–535.

266

START A PROTON PUMP INHIBITOR INFUSION FOR GASTRIC AND DUODENAL BLEEDING

HARI NATHAN, MD

Upper gastrointestinal bleeding from the stomach or duodenum may be the primary reason for intensive care unit admission or may be a subsequent complication in an already critically ill patient. Upper gastrointestinal bleeding carries a mortality rate of approximately 12%. After control of the airway as warranted, initial resuscitation, and placement of a nasogastric tube, attention must be turned to identifying the cause of the bleeding. Potential etiologies include vascular abnormalities (e.g., arteriovenous malformations, Dieulafoy's lesions, or varices), traumatic injury (e.g., Mallory-Weiss tears), gastritis or duodenitis, and peptic ulcers.

Initial localization and control of bleeding may be achieved by endoscopy or angiography with embolization. Uncontrollable hemorrhage may require surgical intervention. Gastric acid potentiates bleeding by causing ongoing tissue damage, inhibiting platelet aggregation, and promoting clot lysis. Inhibition of gastric acid secretion may therefore be an important adjunct to prevent further bleeding. The efficacy of this strategy has been demonstrated in upper gastrointestinal bleeding from peptic ulcers. Intravenous proton pump inhibitor (PPI) therapy has been shown to reduce the risk of rebleeding from peptic ulcers (odds ratio 0.49) after initial hemostasis (e.g., by endoscopic therapy). Intravenous PPIs also reduce the need for surgery (odds ratio 0.61). It should be noted, however, that PPI therapy has not demonstrated any consistent mortality benefit. In addition, it should also be noted that H_2-receptor antagonists have failed to show any benefit in preventing rebleeding.

To briefly review, proton pump inhibitors covalently bind and irreversibly inhibit the H^+,K^+-ATPase responsible for parietal cell acid production. Most studies of PPIs in upper gastrointestinal bleeding have evaluated omeprazole, which is unavailable in intravenous form in the United States. Intravenous agents in the class that are available in the United States include pantoprazole, lansoprazole, and esomeprazole. The suggested pantoprazole dosage regimen is an intravenous bolus of 80 mg followed by a continuous infusion of 8 mg/h for 72 h. The patient should then be placed on 40 mg intravenously twice daily as maintenance therapy.

SUGGESTED READINGS

Irwin RS, Rippe JM, eds. Irwin and Rippe's Intensive Care Medicine, 5th ed. Philadelphia: Lippincott Williams & Wilkins, 2003:1089–1093.

Leontiadis GI, Sharma VK, Howden CW. Proton pump inhibitor treatment for acute peptic ulcer bleeding. Cochrane Database Syst Rev 2006(1):CD002094.

267

REMEMBER THAT BLEEDING ASSOCIATED WITH DIRECT THROMBIN INHIBITORS IS NOT CORRECTABLE WITH PROTAMINE, FRESH-FROZEN PLASMA, OR PLATELETS

MICHAEL B. STREIFF, MD

Thrombocytopenia is a common occurrence among hospitalized patients, particularly among patients in the intensive care unit (ICU). When a patient is diagnosed with, or suspected of having, heparin-induced thrombocytopenia (HIT) type 2, ICU caregivers should be familiar with a clear treatment plan. In addition to discontinuation of all heparin products, therapy for HIT may include alternative intravenous anticoagulants, specifically argatroban or lepirudin. It is important to understand alternatives for therapy and how to manage these and their potential complications.

1. Therapy for patients with HIT consists of the following:
   a. Eliminate *all* exposure to heparin
   b. Place a sign above the patient's bed and on the chart indicating heparin allergy
   c. Start a direct thrombin inhibitor (DTI)
      i. Argatroban dosing (half-life 45 min, with normal hepatic function)
         1. For ICU patients or patients with mild hepatic insufficiency (see *Table 267.1*), begin argatroban at 0.5 μcg/kg/min, and check the first activated partial thromboplastin time (aPTT) in 4 h (target aPTT ratio 1.5 to 2.5)
         2. Monitor aPTT every 4 h until two consecutive aPTT values are in the therapeutic range, then check aPTT 12 h later and, if still therapeutic, then at least daily
         3. Dose adjustments (argatroban)
            a. If argatroban is subtherapeutic, increase the infusion rate by 20% and recheck the aPTT in 4 h
            b. If supratherapeutic, decrease the infusion rate by 50% and recheck the aPTT in 4 h
               i. If aPTT ratio is >3.0, hold the infusion 30 min
               ii. If aPTT ratio is >4.0, hold 1 h before restarting at the lower rate
            c. After any dose adjustment, more frequent aPTT testing is warranted (e.g., every 4 h until aPTT is therapeutic

TABLE 267.1	ARGATROBAN DOSING IN HEPATIC INSUFFICIENCY	
TOTAL BILIRUBIN	AST/ALT	PERCENTAGE OF STANDARD INFUSION RATE
1.8–3.6 mg/dL	150–600 IU/L	25
>3.6 mg/dL	>600 IU/L	Avoid, use lepirudin

AST, aspartate aminotransferase; ALT, alanine aminotransferase.

for two consecutive tests, then 12 h later, then at least daily)

d. Special note: Argatroban also increases the ratio of prothrombin time to international normalized ratio (PT/INR); however, the aPTT should be used for dose adjustments (prolongation of the PT is an issue with warfarin cotherapy; see later comment)

ii. Lepirudin dosing (half-life 80 min)

1. For patients with normal renal function (>60 mL/min), begin lepirudin at 0.1 mg/kg/h continuous infusion and check the first aPTT in 6 h (target aPTT ratio 1.5 to 2.5)

2. For patients with renal insufficiency refer to *Table 267.2* for dosing or use argatroban

3. Monitor aPTT every 6 h until two consecutive values are in the therapeutic range, then check the aPTT 12 h later and, if still therapeutic, at least daily thereafter

4. Dose adjustments (lepirudin)

a. If lepirudin is subtherapeutic, increase the infusion rate by 20% and recheck the aPTT in 6 h

b. If supratherapeutic, decrease the infusion rate by 50% and recheck the aPTT in 6 h

i. If aPTT ratio is >3.0, hold the infusion 1 h, then restart at the lower rate

TABLE 267.2	LEPIRUDIN DOSING FOR RENAL INSUFFICIENCY
CREATININE CLEARANCE (ML/MIN)	PERCENTAGE OF STANDARD INFUSION RATE
45–60	50
30–44	25
15–29	10
<15	Use argatroban

ii. If aPTT ratio is >4.0, hold 2 h, then restart at the lower rate

c. After any dose adjustment, more frequent aPTT testing is warranted (e.g., every 6 h until two consecutive aPTT values are therapeutic, then 12 h later, then at least daily)

d. Special note: Approximately 50% of patients treated with lepirudin for more than 5 days develop antibodies to lepirudin that generally increase its plasma half-life; therefore the need to make dose reductions is common after 5 to 7 days of therapy; adjust according to the aPTT

d. Warfarin dosing

i. Do not start warfarin until the patient's platelet count has returned to the normal range and the patient is on a therapeutic dose of a direct thrombin inhibitor (DTI)

ii. Start warfarin at a dose that is appropriate for the patient's clinical situation (no more than 5 mg; probably 2.5 mg is more appropriate for most ICU patients with HIT)

iii. Argatroban will increase the INR disproportionally in patients on warfarin; at infusion rates of 2 μg/kg/min, it generally doubles the INR; therefore, when the patient's INR is double the intended target range in the setting of therapeutic argatroban therapy (INR 4 to 6 for intended range 2 to 3), the argatroban infusion may be discontinued with close follow-up of the aPTT and INR (every 4 h to make sure the patient is therapeutic on warfarin [INR 2.0 or more]) when all traces of argatroban effect are gone (e.g., aPTT ratio is normal)

2. Management of DTI-associated bleeding

DTIs are not reversible with protamine: Generally, because argatroban and lepirudin have short half-lives, discontinuation of the infusion can be used in most situations to reverse the anticoagulant effect; if life-threatening bleeding occurs or an urgent surgical procedure is necessary, recombinant human factor VIIa (NovoSeven, Novo Nordisk, Princeton, NJ) has been used with some success in normalizing hemostasis in patients being treated with a DTI: The use of fresh-frozen plasma and/or platelet concentrates is less likely to be beneficial.

SUGGESTED READINGS

Warkentin TE. Heparin-induced thrombocytopenia: pathogenesis and management. Br J Haematol 2003;121:535–555.

Warkentin TE, Greinacher A. Heparin-induced thrombocytopenia and cardiac surgery. Ann Thorac Surg 2003;76:2121–2131.

268

Attempt to Decrease Phlebotomy

Elliott R. Haut, MD

Blood transfusion is commonly used to treat anemia in intensive care units (ICUs). By ICU day three, 95% of all ICU patients have an abnormal hemoglobin level. After a 1-week stay in the ICU, patients have an 85% chance of being transfused. According to the American Red Cross, 14 million units of packed red blood cells (PRBCs) are transfused every year in the United States. Blood component therapy can be a lifesaving measure in many patients and these transfusions have a sound physiologic rationale: to increase hemoglobin and oxygen-carrying capacity. However, blood transfusion poses significant risks including viral transmission, hemolytic transfusion reaction, volume overload, and the uncommon but devastating clerical error leading to an ABO-incompatible transfusion. Transfusion of PRBCs in the intensive care unit is associated with increased nosocomial infections, diminished organ function scores, and ICU mortality.

As stated above, hemoglobin levels decrease in ICU, even in non-bleeding patients. A large percentage of this blood loss is associated with phlebotomy, which accounts for 30% of all blood transfused in the ICU. The number of blood draws and the volume of blood drawn correlate with worse ICU organ dysfunction scores. Attempts to decrease red blood cell loss from phlebotomy in the ICU can be wide ranging.

WATCH OUT FOR

Fewer numbers of samples can be drawn if practitioners are careful to order only what labs are truly necessary. There are many indications for specific lab tests in the ICU. The number of lab tests performed obviously varies according to patient-specific factors (e.g., diagnosis, severity of illness, comorbidities). However, other, patient-independent factors also influence the number and type of labs performed. These include the presence of arterial lines, admission to a teaching versus nonteaching ICU, and written or unwritten "protocols" for ordering certain labs. Not every patient needs every test every day, especially chronically critically ill patients.

ICU practitioners can reduce blood waste when drawing diagnostic samples from indwelling lines by reinfusing blood that is normally discarded. This can be accomplished by using a system such as the SAFESET Blood Sampling System (Hospira) or the Venous

Arterial blood Management Protection (VAMP) system (Edwards Lifesciences). This type of closed system connects to an arterial or venous line and makes it easy to reinfuse the initially drawn-off diluted sample, which would otherwise be discarded. The use of smaller "pediatric tubes" and point-of-care testing can lead to less blood waste by using smaller blood volumes for diagnostic testing.

As with many issues in the ICU, blood conservation is multifactorial. Other aspects to reducing blood loss include using adjuncts such as pharmacologic hemostasis (i.e., aprotinin, factor VIIa) and red blood cell salvage techniques such as an intraoperative cellsaver. Research into blood substitutes is ongoing to decrease the need for PRBC transfusions.

ICU physicians can also help patients to increase red cell mass. This can sometimes be accomplished by the administration of exogenous erythropoietin. Erythropoietin may improve hemoglobin levels and decrease blood transfusions in specific patient populations, such as those with renal failure and possibly for those transferred to long-term acute care facilities. In patients who have concomitant iron deficiency, enhanced nutritional support with supplemental iron and vitamin C may be beneficial.

Another important way to avoid exposure to PRBCs is to only order appropriate PRBC transfusions. The commonly quoted goal of a hemoglobin level of 10 g/dL has been used for many years with very little data to support this number. Lower transfusion triggers are safe and may actually improve patient outcomes. There is a widely held misconception that states "give one, give two," meaning that all patients who receive a transfusion should get at least two units of blood. This adage is entirely unfounded. Some patients really only need one unit of PRBCs.

SUGGESTED READINGS

Barie PS, Hydo LJ. Learning to not know: results of a program for ancillary cost reduction in surgical critical care. J Trauma 1996;41(4):714–720.

Fowler RA, Rizoli SB, Levin PD, et al. Blood conservation for critically ill patients. Crit Care Clin 2004;20(2):313–324.

Nguyen BV, Bota DP, Melot C, et al. Time course of hemoglobin concentrations in nonbleeding intensive care unit patients. Crit Care Med 2003;31(2):406–410.

Vincent JL, Baron JF, Reinhart K, et al. Anemia and blood transfusion in critically ill patients. JAMA 2002;288:1499–1507.

269

CONSIDER THE USE OF FACTOR VIIA TO TREAT MEDICAL BLEEDING IN A SURGICAL OR TRAUMA PATIENT

SUNEEL KHETARPAL, MD
ANDREW J. KERWIN, MD

The primary initial goal in the care of the trauma patient has always been control of hemorrhage. Under most circumstances this can be achieved by surgical control or more recently by other adjuncts such as angiography. However, in the massively injured patient a second form of bleeding commonly referred to as nonsurgical bleeding can pose a significant threat to life. The etiology of this nonsurgical bleeding is multifactorial; it results from a significant decrease in hemostatic components (platelets, fibrinogen, and coagulation factors) as well as unfavorable conditions for enzyme kinetics such as acidosis, hypothermia, and hypocalcemia. The end result is that the patient develops diffuse bleeding that cannot be controlled by surgical methods.

WATCH OUT FOR

The primary treatment of nonsurgical bleeding is prevention. Early recognition of predisposing factors such as hypothermia, correction of acidosis by improved resuscitation, and replacement of blood and blood products can help protect against the development of coagulopathy in trauma patients. However, coagulopathic bleeding may still be present in as much as 35% of severely traumatized individuals and its incidence increases with the severity of trauma. The treatment of such individuals has traditionally been supportive. Recently, there have been an increasing number of cases supporting the use of recombinant factor VII in the therapy of this uncontrolled nonsurgical bleeding.

Recombinant factor VIIa (rFVII) (NovoSeven; Novo Nordisk A/S, Denmark) has been approved by the U.S. Food and Drug Administration in the treatment of bleeding episodes in hemophilic patients with inhibitors to factor VIII or factor IX. The first reported use of this factor in a trauma patient was in 1999. The principle behind the use of this factor in the trauma patient is the cell-based model of coagulation. This suggests that rFVII enhances hemostasis at the site of injury. Tissue factor exposed at the site of injury forms a complex with factor VII, which in turn initiates the coagulation cascade by activating factor X and factor IX. Factor X complexes with its cofactor, factor V, which activates prothrombin to produce thrombin. Whereas this can contract fibrinogen to fibrin clot, it also accelerates the coagulation cascade by activating factor V, factor VIII, factor XI, and additional platelets. This last acceleration causes a large amount of thrombin to be formed, which changes fibrinogen to insoluble fibrin, resulting in hemostasis. This clot should be localized and, at least theoretically, should avoid any systemic hypercoagulability.

Since the first reported use of factor VIIa for trauma in 1999, there has been an increasing number of successful cases. In these cases, the dose varied from 40 to 140 μg/kg. In 2005, a multicenter randomized, controlled trial from Europe, South Africa, and Canada showed that use of the drug was (1) safe with no increase in thrombogenic activity and (2) helped to reduce the number of transfusions in severely injured trauma patients. The study did not show a mortality benefit. Furthermore, the study suggested a dose of between 100 and 200 μg/kg given intravenously over 5 min, followed by repeated doses of 100 μg/kg $\times$ 2 at hourly intervals if there is ongoing evidence of bleeding. The cost of the drug is significant, averaging approximately $1,000/mg (resulting in an average cost per dose of $10,000 to $20,000). Although this cost may initially seem prohibitive, use of the drug may be cost effective if it significantly decreases the need for blood and blood products and massive transfusions can be eliminated. Further work is necessary to establish the optimal timing, dose, and indication for factor VIIa. However, it is clear that there must be ongoing resuscitation to correct hypothermia and acidosis, and there must be significant fibrinogen for the drug to work. Finally, factor VIIa is not meant, nor will it work, as a substitute for sound surgical management in the trauma patient.

SUGGESTED READINGS

Boffard KD, Riou B, Warren B, et al. NovoSeven Trauma Study Group. Recombinant factor VIIa as adjunctive therapy for bleeding control in severely injured trauma patients: two parallel randomized, placebo-controlled, double-blind clinical trials. J Trauma 2005;59(1):8–15; discussion 15–18.

Kenet G, Walden R, Eldad A, et al. Treatment of traumatic bleeding with recombinant factor VIIa. Lancet 1999;354(9193):1879.

Mohr AM, Holcomb JB, Dutton RP, et al. Recombinant activated factor VIIa and hemostasis in critical care: a focus on trauma. Crit Care 2005;9(Suppl 5):537–542.

270

CONSIDER ANGIOGRAPHY AS AN ADJUNCT IN CONTROLLING SOLID-ORGAN BLEEDING AFTER DAMAGE CONTROL SURGERY

MICHAEL D. GROSSMAN, MD

Patients typically enter the intensive care unit (ICU) with an open abdomen following trauma "damage control" surgery or treatment or prevention of abdominal compartment syndrome. Damage control surgery is performed when excessive bleeding results in the lethal triad of acidosis, hypothermia, and coagulopathy. Obtaining control of bleeding in the operating room usually involves packing and occasionally the use of balloon occlusion catheters. Surgery is terminated before the completion of the procedure in order to return the patient to the ICU. This ICU resuscitation phase of rewarming and reversal of coagulopathy is referred to as the second phase of damage control surgery. On return to the ICU, resuscitation will only be successful if both medical and surgical bleeding has been adequately controlled.

In general, inability to correct hypothermia, acidosis, and coagulopathy with ongoing requirement for transfusion indicates the presence of ongoing surgical bleeding. Reexploration and repacking may be attempted, even in the ICU. Consideration of angiographic embolization or placement of balloon occlusion catheters is appropriate in certain cases.

Embolization represents an acceptable primary form of therapy in many solid-organ injuries in which the goal is to avoid laparotomy and/or loss of an organ. In addition, for high-grade liver injury, bleeding pelvic fracture, and retroperitoneal bleeding, embolization reduces the overall blood loss associated with a more invasive operative approach that interrupts the compressive effects of natural tissue planes. Once the abdomen is open, in the setting of phase II damage control, the role of angiography is more specific.

WHAT TO DO

Success of angioembolization is more likely when coagulation can be corrected (international normalized ratio is ≤2.0). Because damage control patients are physiologically unstable, highly selective embolization is often avoided in favor of options that are more expeditious. For example, embolization of the right hepatic artery in a hypotensive bleeding damage control patient may be chosen as opposed to a segmental branch occlusion in a more stable patient. Hypogastric (internal iliac) artery occlusion may be preferable to selective occlusion of a pudendal artery branch. In certain cases clinical judgment may dictate that it is worth sacrificing a paired organ such as the kidney to avoid reoperating on an unstable patient who would require a nephrectomy to control hemorrhage. Embolization under these circumstances may result in necrosis of viable tissue leading to fever or late infection, bile leaks (liver), or renovascular hypertension.

Although angioembolization has provided exponential improvement in the options available for controlling control traumatic intraabdominal hemorrhage, clinicians must be careful not to ask too much of their radiology colleagues. Transport of an unstable, hypotensive, hypothermic, acidemic patient to the interventional radiology suite should only be done when the trauma surgeon is present and directing the overall approach to care. The adage that "the ICU is a philosophy, not a physical location" can be life-saving in these patients who require ongoing resuscitation.

One final comment is that although bleeding may be from sources that can be addressed by reoperation and direct surgical repair (i.e., suture ligation), bleeding often results from diffuse oozing secondary to coagulopathy or bleeding from sites not easily amenable to surgical repair. Differentiation of these entities can be complex and requires a thorough understanding of the injuries encountered and how they were managed surgically. Options for medical hemorrhage control include administration of coagulation factors in the form of fresh-frozen plasma, platelets, cryoprecipitate, and factor VII in addition to correction of hypothermia.

SUGGESTED READINGS

Gourlay D, Hoffer E, Routt M, et al. Pelvic angiography for recurrent traumatic pelvic arterial hemorrhage. J Trauma 2005;59(5):1168–1174.

Mohr AM, Lavery RF, Barone A. Angiographic embolization of liver injuries: low mortality, high morbidity. J Trauma 2003;55(6):1077–1082.

Rotondo MF, Zonies DH. The damage control sequence and underlying logic. Surg Clin North Am 1997;77(4):761–777.

271

CONSULT SURGERY EMERGENTLY IF A PATIENT WITH A BLEEDING PEPTIC ULCER REBLEEDS AFTER ENDOSCOPIC CONTROL

LEE ANN LAU, MD
HEIDI L. FRANKEL, MD

Peptic ulcer bleeding is a significant concern, with an incidence reported at 100 to 150 per 100,000 population per year. Approximately 5% of all intensive care unit (ICU) patients develop upper gastrointestinal bleeding, usually due to peptic ulcer disease or erosive gastritis. Most patients will not require endoscopy for diagnosis or treatment.

SIGNS AND SYMPTOMS

In the ICU patient, the diagnosis of bleeding due to peptic ulceration is made by bloody/coffee-ground nasogastric aspirate, emesis, or melena. Upper endoscopy is warranted when the bleeding is associated with decreasing hematocrit and/or hemodynamic instability. If active bleeding or signs of recent bleeding are identified during endoscopy, hemostatic therapies can be performed, including epinephrine injection to cause vasospasm, placement of clips to directly occlude the vessel, or heater probe application to coagulate the vessel. Nonsteroidal anti-inflammatory drug/aspirin treatment should be stopped in patients diagnosed with upper gastrointestinal bleeding. In addition, acid reduction must be instituted because lower gastric pH may cause clot lysis. Evidence supports the use of intravenous proton pump inhibitor in this setting. Despite aggressive endoscopic and medical management, rebleeding occurs in 15% to 20% of patients; therefore surgical consultation is imperative in all patients requiring urgent upper endoscopy.

The clinical factors that increase rebleeding risk include: age greater than 60 years, medical comorbidities (especially cardiopulmonary disease or liver disease), and initial presentation consistent with severe hemorrhage (frank hematemesis or copious melena, low hematocrit or coagulopathy, shock, and need for >5 units of packed red blood cells). The endoscopic findings linked to rebleeding include arterial bleeding ("spurting") from the ulcer base, visible vessel in the ulcer bed, adherent clot in the ulcer bed, and ulcers located on the lesser curvature or the posterior duodenum due to proximity to major vessels (left gastric artery and gastroduodenal artery, respectively). Technically, bleeding from these locations is more challenging to control endoscopically.

WHAT TO DO

Because endoscopy is a successful diagnostic and therapeutic tool, it is the first-line treatment for upper gastrointestinal bleeding. However, surgical intervention must be considered whenever there is endoscopic failure to stop hemorrhage. If the patient is physiologically unable to tolerate the hemodynamic stress of a significant bleed, if endoscopic therapy is not immediately available, or if the ulcer characteristics suggest additional endoscopic treatment will fail (especially large ulcers), the patient should undergo immediate surgery on rebleeding rather than additional endoscopy. Interventional therapy with embolization is also an option. Most patients, however, should undergo a second endoscopic attempt at hemostasis. With endoscopic retreatment, approximately one third of patients will still eventually need operative intervention.

SUGGESTED READINGS

Lau JY, Sung JJ, Lam YH, et al. Endoscopic retreatment compared with surgery in patients with recurrent bleeding after initial endoscopic control of bleeding ulcers. N Engl J Med 1999;340(10):751–756.

Lau JY, Sung JJ, Lee KK, et al. Effect of intravenous omeprazole on recurrent bleeding after endoscopic treatment of bleeding peptic ulcers. N Engl J Med 2000;343(5):310–316.

Schoenberg MH. Surgical therapy for peptic ulcer and nonvariceal bleeding. Langenbecks Arch Surg 2001;386(2):98–103.

272

CALL FOR A SENGSTAKEN-BLAKEMORE OR MINNESOTA TUBE WHEN A CIRRHOTIC PATIENT HAS AN UPPER GASTROINTESTINAL BLEED

ANTHONY D. SLONIM, MD, DRPH

Cirrhotic liver disease is a condition that is caused by chronic scarring and fibrosis of the hepatic parenchyma. The causes of cirrhosis are quite varied and include alcohol abuse, metabolic diseases (α-1 antitrypsin deficiency, Wilson disease), biliary disorders (bile duct obstruction, sarcoidosis, cystic fibrosis), toxins (carbon tetrachloride, hypervitaminosis A), and infections (hepatitis A, B, or C). Regardless of the etiology, the pathophysiology and clinical findings are similar. The liver becomes enlarged on clinical examination until late in the course. There may be jaundice, hyperbilirubinemia, transaminitis, or overt liver failure. With noninvasive imaging, the liver appears nodular and may elicit stigmata of portal hypertension including splenomegaly, esophageal varices, and reversal of portal blood flow. A definitive diagnosis is usually made by liver biopsy.

Upper gastrointestinal bleeding is a common intervening finding in patients with cirrhosis and can occur from the more traditional types of lesions including gastritis, Mallory-Weiss tears, and peptic ulcer disease. An important and critical complication of portal hypertension that is responsible for nearly one third of all deaths in patients with cirrhotic liver disease is variceal bleeding. The bleeding from esophageal varices can be abrupt and massive. With the occurrence of a variceal bleed, traditional approaches to hemodynamic stabilization need to be implemented including the use of two large-bore intravenous access devices, isotonic saline infusions and blood to maintain intravascular volume, and identification of the underlying etiology. For emergent variceal bleeding, most patients can be cared for with endoscopic and pharmacologic interventions, although each of these interventions will fail between 15% and 20% of the time. When endoscopic and pharmacologic interventions fail, the use of balloon tamponade may be used as a temporizing measure to control bleeding.

Balloon tamponade had its origins in the early 1930s. The placement of a tube with four ports, an esophageal and gastric ports for aspiration of gastrointestinal contents, and an esophageal and gastric balloons that when filled with air and lodged against the bleeding site can lead to tamponade of a bleeding varix. These tubes are available under a number of names, including the Sengstaken-Blakemore tube and the Minnesota tubes, but the conceptual approaches and applications are similar regardless of the specific tube used.

Before placement of this tube, the airway should be protected by endotracheal intubation. The tamponade tube is then inserted through the nares and into the stomach in much the same way as a nasogastric tube. A radiograph is obtained to verify position below the diaphragm. Then, the gastric balloon is inflated with 30 to 50 mL of air and a radiograph is repeated to again verify that the balloon is below the diaphragm. The tube is pulled back until tension is felt and traction is placed to assure that the balloon applies pressure to the esophagogastric junction with a counterweight device. If there is an esophageal balloon present, it is inflated and the esophageal and gastric ports are then placed to suction to remove any debris, secretions, or blood from below the balloon and to prevent regurgitation. There is controversy regarding how long the tamponade balloons can remain inflated without undue risk of gastric or esophageal perforation. The classic recommendation is 24 hours, although many practitioners leave the balloon inflated longer if need be while definitive treatment is being arranged. Ultimately, it must be remembered that balloon tamponade is a temporizing measure only and the patient will need a decompressive procedure to reduce the pressure in the portal circulation by either a transjugular intrahepatic portosystemic shunt procedure or systemic shunt.

SUGGESTED READING

Sharara AI, Rockey DC. Gastroesophageal variceal hemorrhage. N Engl J Med 2001; 345:669–681.

273

TREAT LOSS OF DOPPLER SIGNALS IN A FREE FLAP AS A SURGICAL EMERGENCY

MAZEN BEDRI, MD

SURGICAL TECHNIQUE

The use of autologous free tissue transplantation was pioneered in the 1950s and has since been an important rung in the "reconstructive ladder" commonly described in plastic surgery. This reconstructive ladder is based on the concept of using the simplest technique possible to provide adequate closure or coverage, with increasingly complex techniques employed as needed. The free flap is generally considered the highest and most complex rung of this ladder. Both functional and aesthetic considerations influence a surgeon's decision to utilize a free flap, often in the setting of postoncologic reconstruction of the head and neck or breast, after traumatic loss of soft tissue, or in facial reanimation procedures. Depending on the nature of the defect, the flap may include innervated muscle, as well as myocutaneous, fasciocutaneous, or osseocutaneous components.

Preoperative evaluation of a patient for a potential free flap reconstruction must consider the patient's general clinical status and the quality and condition of both the donor and recipient sites. The patient's nutritional status and age, as well as associated comorbidities such as diabetes, peripheral vascular disease, and cardiovascular disease, are important factors to be weighed when making the assessment. The effect of tobacco use on flap viability is controversial, although it is not an absolute contraindication to creating a free flap. Patients with multiple comorbidities warrant preoperative medical risk stratification.

Specific to the surgical sites, factors to consider are the length of the vascular pedicle, the quality and caliber of recipient vessels, the size match of donor and recipient vessels, the volume and geometry of the flap tissue, and the general condition of the recipient site (prior irradiation, vascular disease, traumatic injury, and infection can affect flap survival).

The most important determinant in graft survival is intraoperative technique. In addition to prophylactic antibiotics, most microvascular surgeons administer either a one-time bolus of 5,000 U of heparin prior to graft harvest or a lower-dose bolus of heparin followed postoperatively by a continuous low-dose infusion. Topical lidocaine or papaverine is used for vasodilation. Surgical technique should emphasize the delicate handling of vasculature to prevent vasospasm and thrombosis. Excessive traction and drying should be avoided. Vessels should be 1 to 3 mm in diameter, and the ends should be trimmed of loose adventitia. Alignment of the donor and recipient vessels is of utmost importance and is facilitated by ensuring adequate pedicle length (2 to 3 cm), appropriate matching of vessel caliber, and the meticulous placement of interrupted sutures symmetrically and circumferentially. The anastomoses should be free of tension but also of redundancy to prevent kinking and twisting. Flap ischemia time should be minimized, although ischemia times shorter than 3 to 4 hours should not contribute to the risk of flap loss. On insetting the flap, the vascular pedicle should be inspected to ensure the vascular pedicle is not compromised by kinking, twisting, or compression. Postoperatively, patients are often maintained on heparin, dextran, or aspirin, although studies do not conclusively show benefit of any particular regimen.

How Graft Viability Is Monitored

Many methods of flap monitoring have been described and used with varying degrees of success, including laser Doppler, transcutaneous and intravascular measurement of oxygen tension, and temperature monitoring. However, diligent clinical assessment with hourly exams in the initial postoperative period remains the standard in postoperative care for free flaps. Free flaps with a cutaneous component should be visually inspected for color, which should be similar to the color of the surrounding recipient bed. The flap should be warm to touch, with relatively normal turgor and a capillary refill of 1 to 2 seconds. Arterial occlusion is suggested by a pale color, cool temperature, and sluggish or absent capillary refill. Problems with venous outflow are suggested by congestion, often with darkening of color, warmth and edema, and brisk capillary refill. Bedside Doppler is helpful in the assessment of blood flow, although a signal may be falsely reassuring in the setting of venous compromise, or if the signal is from surrounding tissue. A pinprick may also be useful in evaluation of the flap and should produce two to three drops of bright red blood. Brisk venous bleeding or absence of bleeding suggests venous or arterial compromise, respectively.

A unique challenge in monitoring flap viability is posed by the buried flap, in which clinical assessment is impossible and surface Doppler is unreliable. The temporary placement of implantable Doppler probes can facilitate postoperative care.

LOSS RATE OF FLAPS, WHAT TO DO IF LOSS OF SIGNAL OCCURS, RATE OF SALVAGE WITH RE-EXPLORATION

The overall success rate of free flaps has increased significantly since the technique was initially introduced (currently 95% to 99%). Some clinical series have associated certain factors with higher failure rates, including free flaps with an osseous component, previously irradiated recipient sites, or the use of vein grafts. The use of medicinal leeches with proper antibiotic prophylaxis has been described with some success in the setting of venous congestion due to inadequate outflow. However, the most common cause of flap failure is venous thrombosis, with early re-exploration rates as high as 15% in some series. Almost 80% of such failures occur within the critical period of the first two postoperative days. With the timely detection and management of vascular compromise—within 6 to 8 hours—salvage rates in recent series have ranged from 60% to 75%.

The detection of vascular compromise should prompt immediate mobilization of the operative team. Re-exploration may begin with intravenous administration of heparin, followed by an inspection of the anastomosis site for kinking or twisting, hematoma, or any other extrinsic compression. Intravascular thrombosis necessitates takedown of the anastomoses and embolectomy with a Fogarty catheter. Persistent failure to freely irrigate suggests thrombosis of the microvasculature and may respond to high-dose infusions of streptokinase, urokinase, or recombinant tissue plasminogen activator while the flap is completely disconnected to avoid systemic dosing. The flap is then re-anastomosed and inset, followed by maintenance on heparin or dextran. Failure to re-establish circulation necessitates removal of the nonviable flap.

SUGGESTED READINGS

Jones NF. Intraoperative and postoperative monitoring of microsurgical free tissue transfers. Clin Plast Surg 1992;19(4):783–797.

Townsend C, ed. Sabiston Textbook of Surgery, 17th ed. Philadelphia: WB Saunders, 2004:2186–2188.

274

REMEMBER WHEN REVIEWING DOPPLER ULTRASOUND RESULTS THAT THE SUPERFICIAL FEMORAL VEIN IS A COMPONENT OF THE DEEP VENOUS SYSTEM

PATRICK SCHANER, MD

Doppler ultrasound of the veins is a widely used test to search for the presence of deep vein thrombosis (phlebitis) that requires anticoagulation and that may result in pulmonary embolism. This test is often ordered for a patient with signs or symptoms of a suspected pulmonary embolism (pleuritic chest pain, tachypnea, tachycardia, hypocapnia, hypoxia, hypotension) or deep vein thrombosis (leg swelling, calf pain, positive Homan sign) or for a fever workup. Commonly, a preliminary reading that identifies which veins may be harboring clots is placed in the chart or reported verbally by the technician. The decision to anticoagulate a patient hinges on these results. In this setting, it is important to know the venous anatomy of the leg and the risk of pulmonary embolism for phlebitis of the relevant veins.

The venous drainage of the leg is comprised of two systems: the deep veins and the superficial veins. The two chief superficial veins are the greater and lesser saphenous veins. Other superficial veins are the superficial epigastric, superficial circumflex iliac, and external pudendal veins and surface varicosities. Components of the deep venous system include the soleal sinusoids, anterior and posterior tibial, common femoral, profunda femoral, superficial femoral, circumflex femoral, and iliac veins. The deep veins course in proximity to the major arteries (venae comitantes). Clots in the deep system put a patient at much higher risk of pulmonary embolism and usually require anticoagulation (20% of patients with clots in the superficial system also have coexisting clots in the deep system).

It is important to remember when reviewing the location of blood clots on the Doppler report that the superficial femoral vein that accompanies the superficial femoral artery is a major *deep* vein. This vein is "superficial" only relative to the profunda (i.e., deep) femoris vein but is a major deep structure despite the superficial appellation. Clots in the more proximal veins (such as the superficial femoral) have a greater risk of life-threatening embolism than those more distal, and a finding of a clot here should never be dismissed as inconsequential.

SUGGESTED READINGS

April EW. Anatomy. Media, PA: Harwal, 1984:381–382.

Ernst CB, Stanley JC, eds. Current Therapy in Vascular Surgery. St. Louis: Mosby, 1995:875–876.

Moore KL, Dailey AF, eds. Clinically Oriented Anatomy, 4th ed. Philadelphia: Lippincott Williams & Wilkins, 1999:524–526.

275

POST A SIGN OUTSIDE OF THE DOOR OF PATIENTS WHO HAVE RECEIVED A TAGGED WHITE BLOOD CELL SCAN WARNING OF THE PREGNANCY RISK

TONYA N. WALKER, MD
ELIZABETH A. MARTINEZ, MD, MHS

A tagged white blood cell (WBC) scan is a nuclear medicine study used to diagnose and localize areas of infection and/or inflammation. It can be helpful when an occult infection such as pyelonephritis, abdominal abscess or osteomyelitis is suspected. A major component of the immune system's defense mechanism is the activation and upregulation of white blood cells. These cells can be found in large numbers in areas where there is active inflammation and/or infection; the ability to "tag" these cells allows the detection of such foci in the evaluation of patients with a suspected source of infection.

To perform a tagged WBC scan, a sample of the patient's WBCs is mixed with the radioactive material indium oxine, isotope 111 (^{111}In). The tagged sample is then reinfused intravenously to the patient. If there is an area of active inflammation/infection, a scanner will detect localized areas of these tagged white cells and convert them into an image viewed on a screen or recorded on film. The scan takes approximately 1 to 2 hours and requires patient transport to the nuclear medicine suite.

There are several special considerations when deciding whether a tagged WBC scan is the appropriate diagnostic tool. False-negative results can occur due to antibiotic use or chronic infection, and because WBCs are usually found in the spleen and liver, a true infection in these organs can be missed with the scan. False-positive results can occur due to bleeding and the presence of tubes, drains, or catheters in the body. Because the patient has to wait 6 to 24 hours to be scanned after the reinfusion, this study may not always be the best option for the critically ill patient.

The radiation dose of interest for patients undergoing a nuclear medicine scan is the radiation absorbed dose (rads). Dose limits are expressed in sieverts (Sv) of photons or electron exposure, where 1 millisievert (mSv) = 0.1 rad. The average annual radiation exposure from natural sources to an individual in the United States is approximately 3 mSv. One chest x-ray exposes a patient to an additional 6 mSv (0.6 rad), whereas a transatlantic flight exposes an individual to 0.25 mSv (0.025 rad). One tagged WBC scan provides an effective dose of 7.2 mSv (0.72 rad) to the patient undergoing the study. This is equivalent to slightly more than a typical chest x-ray and about 30 transatlantic flights. Those individuals, visitors, or caregivers exposed to the patient would be exposed to 10 to 100 times less than this.

WATCH OUT FOR

Once a patient returns to the care area from a tagged WBC study, the radiation emitted from the patient presents two types of risks: the risk to the patient and the risk to groups exposed to the patient. As indicated previously, the risk to the patient is minimal. Exposed groups include ward staff and visitors. The medical, nursing, and ancillary staff caring for a "radioactive" patient can be, and in many instances are, women of childbearing age. These women may also be pregnant while on the ward with the patient. It is important to inform visitors and hospital staff of the slightly increased radiation risk by posting a sign outside the patient's door. According to the U.S. Nuclear Regulatory Commission, *direct abdominal/pelvic exposure* at the level of 2 rads (20 mSv) is the amount of radiation considered to be the lowest exposure level for possible damage to fetuses. This is many times higher than the likely radiation exposure a nurse or physician would sustain from caring for a patient who had a tagged WBC scan. However, because most pregnant women would likely want **no** extra radiation if it could be avoided (it must be remembered that radiation effects on a fetus are cumulative), it seems prudent and reasonable to post a warning sign.

Two days after the WBC scan is complete, the sign indicating increased radiation exposure may be removed because virtually all radioactivity has dissipated.

SELECTED READINGS

Lowe SA. Diagnostic radiography in pregnancy: risks and realities. Austr N Z J Obstet Gynaecol 2004;44:191–196.

MedLine Plus Medical Encyclopedia. WBC (nuclear) scan. http://www.nlm.nih.gov/medlineplus/ency/article/003834.htm

Mountford PJ. Risk assessment of the nuclear medicine patient. Br J Radiol 1997;70:671–684.

United States Nuclear Regulatory Commission, Office of Public Affairs. Fact Sheet. Biological Effects of Radiation, December 2003.

276

Obtain an Echocardiogram to Rule Out Bacterial Endocarditis in Gram-Positive Bacteremia

Mike Faulkner, MD

Bacterial endocarditis is an uncommon condition with significant morbidity and mortality. The classic clinical triad of bacteremia, valvular pathology, and peripheral embolic phenomena unfortunately only presents in a minority of affected individuals. Cardiac imaging with echocardiography has enhanced the ability to diagnose infective endocarditis, currently comprising one of the major criteria in the Duke clinical criteria for diagnosis of the disorder (*Fig. 276.1*).

WHAT TO DO

In patients with low clinical suspicion and low initial risk (fever, previous heart murmur, no peripheral stigmata), transthoracic echocardiography (TTE) is a reasonable initial screening test. TTE is noninvasive and has an excellent specificity for vegetations (98%). Unfortunately, TTE has relatively poor sensitivity for diagnosing infective endocarditis, detecting approximately 60% of native valve infections and 20% of prosthetic valve infections. It poorly resolves lesions less than 2 mm or lesions of the left heart. In addition, a significant number of patients may suffer from conditions such as chronic obstructive pulmonary disease or obesity that make imaging technically difficult. The limited resolution of TTE also hinders diagnosing complications of infective endocarditis such as valvular leaflet perforations, perivalvular abscesses, and intracardiac fistulae.

Transesophageal echocardiography (TEE) may be indicated as an initial imaging technique in high-risk patients (prosthetic valves, congenital heart disease, previous endocarditis, new murmur, heart failure, or other stigmata of endocarditis) or in patients with moderate to high clinical suspicion of infective endocarditis. TEE is a more invasive technique, but it allows placement of the echo transducer closer to the valvular structures of the heart. Sensitivity of TEE has been reported to be greater than 90% in detecting vegetations. Detailed imaging of complications from infective endocarditis such as perivalvular abscess is also enhanced by the transducer's proximity to cardiac structures.

Bacteremia with Gram-positive organisms such as *Streptococcus viridans* and *Streptococcus bovis* are uncommonly seen in patients without infective endocarditis. The presence of these pathogens in two

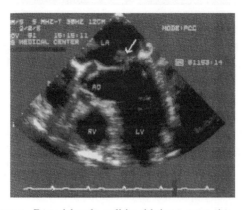

FIGURE 276.1. Bacterial endocarditis with large vegetation on the mitral valve (*arrow*). (Reprinted with permission from Aurigemma GP, Tighe DA. Echocardiography in the intensive care unit. In: Irwin RS, Rippe JM. Irwin & Rippe's Intensive Care Medicine, 5th ed. Philadelphia: Lippincott Williams & Wilkins, 2003:91.)

separate blood cultures defines a major criterion in the Duke clinical criteria for the diagnosis of infective endocarditis.

Staphylococcus aureus infection has increased dramatically over the last 30 years and is now the most common organism found in all types of infective endocarditis. Risk factors for infection include intravenous (IV) drug abuse, indwelling central venous catheters, and the presence of conditions such as malignancy, renal failure, diabetes, alcoholism, and steroid use. Infection with this organism tends to follow an aggressive course, often resulting in perivalvular extension. More than 50% of valve infections involving IV drug abuse involve the tricuspid valve.

Infection with streptococcal organisms tends to follow a more subacute presentation. Left-sided structures are affected most often, with mitral valve involvement more common than aortic valve infection. *S. viridans* is responsible for 50% to 60% of subacute infections. Enterococci are the third-most-common cause of infective endocarditis and have high rates of antimicrobial resistance. The nonenterococcal group D streptococci (especially *S. bovis*) are associated with gastrointestinal pathologies such as colon cancer and polyps. Infection with group B streptococci is most common in pregnant women or in elderly patients with chronic diseases. Embolic complications are common and treatment of these infections with antibiotics alone is often unsuccessful.

Prosthetic valve infections make up 15% to 20% of infective endocarditis. Early (<2 months after surgery) cases usually result from perioperative contamination by organisms such as *Staphylococcus epidermidis* or *S. aureus* and often involve mechanical valves. Late prosthetic valve infections can result from transient bacteremia from dental or gastrointestinal sources. These later infections are often seen in bioprosthetic valves implanted for longer than 1 year.

SUGGESTED READINGS

Bayer AS, Bolger AF, Taubert KA, et al. Diagnosis and management of infective endocarditis and its complications. Circulation 1998;98:2936–2948.

Durack DT, Lukes AS, Bright DK. New criteria for diagnosis of infective endocarditis: utilization of specific echocardiographic findings: Duke Endocarditis Service. Am J Med 1994;96:200–209.

Mylonakis E, Calderwood SB. Infective endocarditis in adults. N Engl J Med 2001;345(18):1318–1330.

Sachdev M, Peterson GE, Jollis JG. Imaging techniques for diagnosis of infective endocarditis. Cardiol Clin 2003;21:185–195.

DIAGNOSE TAMPONADE BASED ON CLINICAL FINDINGS AND NOT ECHOCARDIOGRAM

JAY WELLER, MD

SIGNS AND SYMPTOMS

Cardiac tamponade occurs when increased intrapericardial pressure for any reason (e.g., blood, fluid, air) impedes venous filling of the right ventricle. Symptoms may include tachycardia, tachypnea, dyspnea, orthopnea, and diaphoresis. Beck's triad of elevated central venous pressure (CVP), systemic hypotension with decreased pulse pressure, and distant/muffled heart sounds describes the classic clinical signs, but one or more findings is frequently absent. Electrocardiography may reveal decreased amplitude or electrical alternans. Ultimately, as intrapericardial pressure (IPP) dictates intracardiac chamber pressures, diastolic filling pressures equilibrate (i.e., $CVP = PADP = PCWP = IPP$, where PADP is the pulmonary artery diastolic pressure, and PCWP is the pulmonary capillary wedge pressure). The hemodynamics of tamponade physiology are uniquely susceptible to wide respiratory variations. In particular, pulsus paradoxus is an exaggeration of the normal physiologic decrease in systemic arterial blood pressure with spontaneous inspiration. In the post–cardiac surgery patient, compression may be isolated to a single chamber of the heart (e.g., due to loculated blood clot), making the classic signs and symptoms less useful; a high degree of clinical suspicion is required to make the diagnosis.

Increased availability has led to an increase in reliance on perioperative echocardiography for the diagnosis of cardiac tamponade. Echo findings may include presence of a pericardial effusion, right atrial collapse during systole, right ventricular collapse during diastole, and inferior vena caval plethora. Echocardiographic correlates of pulsus paradoxus may be seen, including respiratory variation in both left and right ventricular filling as evidenced either by Doppler inflow patterns or by variations in septal wall motion. Right atrial collapse lasting longer than one third of systole has a 94% sensitivity and 100% specificity for the diagnosis of tamponade. In the post–cardiac surgery patient, transthoracic imaging may be technically limited, necessitating a transesophageal study (*Figure 277.1*).

Immediate hemodynamic management goals for the patient with pericardial tamponade are to keep the patient "full, fast, and tight." Because right ventricular filling is impeded by increased intrapericardial

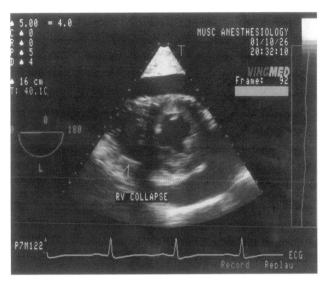

FIGURE 277.1. Transesophogeal echocardiogram showing a large amount of fluid in the pericardial see causing right ventricular collapse (arrow).

pressure, hypovolemia and vasodilation are poorly tolerated. The restrictive nature of tamponade physiology prevents compensatory increases in stroke volume, leaving cardiac output heavily dependent on heart rate. As discussed previously, the patient with pericardial tamponade is particularly susceptible to respiratory variation in systemic blood pressure. Conversion from spontaneous ventilation (with its inspiratory augmentation of venous return to the right ventricle) to positive-pressure ventilation (with increased intrathoracic pressure inhibiting venous return) can lead to catastrophic hemodynamic collapse.

Definitive treatment of pericardial tamponade requires drainage of the fluid filling the pericardial sac. For the patient in extremis, percutaneous drainage should be considered. In the case of penetrating thoracic trauma, emergency department thoracotomy may be indicated. Echocardiography may be useful in guiding needle placement. When the effusion is loculated or posterior, percutaneous drainage may not be feasible. Because of its sympathomimetic properties, ketamine is generally considered to be the induction agent of choice when general anesthesia is required for surgical drainage. For the acutely symptomatic patient, it may be wise for the surgeon to prep and drape prior to induction of general anesthesia. Spontaneous ventilation can be maintained through the induction phase to sustain hemodynamics until the effusion is drained.

SUGGESTED READINGS

Otto C, ed. Textbook of Clinical Echocardiography, 2nd ed. Philadelphia: WB Saunders, 2000:218–222.

Thomas S, Kramer J, eds. Manual of Cardiac Anesthesia, 2nd ed. New York: Churchill Livingstone, 1993:129–136.

278

CONSIDER PULSUS ALTERNANS AS A SIGN OF IMPENDING TAMPONADE

MELISSA CAMP, MD

Cardiac tamponade occurs when fluid accumulates in the pericardial space and leads to impaired diastolic filling due to increased pericardial pressure. The pericardium is relatively inelastic and in the acute setting an accumulation of 100 to 200 cc of fluid can cause tamponade physiology. In intensive care unit patients the most common scenarios involving tamponade include after cardiothoracic surgery, after central line placement with inadvertent puncture of the superior vena cava or right atrium, and after blunt or penetrating chest trauma. Of note, following cardiothoracic surgery, tamponade may also result from a small clot compressing the filling of the heart.

SIGNS AND SYMPTOMS

Early signs of tamponade include tachycardia and elevated central venous pressure, followed by hypotension and decreased cardiac output. Beck's triad describes the classic findings of jugular venous distention, muffled heart sounds, and hypotension. If a pulmonary artery catheter is present, the equalization of filling pressures may be evident with right atrial pressure = right ventricular end-diastolic pressure = pulmonary artery diastolic pressure = pulmonary artery wedge pressure = left ventricular end-diastolic pressure. It should be noted that pressure equalization may not be evident postcardiac surgery because the pericardium has invariably been opened. Pulsus paradoxicus, the decrease in systolic blood pressure of greater than 10 to 15 mm Hg on inspiration, is also observed in tamponade. Pulsus paradoxicus is a result of systemic venous return during inspiration causing rapid right ventricular filling, which compresses and impairs left ventricular filling.

Electrical alternans is one of the findings on the electrocardiogram that is suggestive of cardiac tamponade. With each beat, the amplitude of the QRS complex varies from large to small. Electrical alternans is due to a change in the QRS axis from a "bobbing" movement of the heart within a large pericardial effusion (*Fig. 278.1*).

Emergent treatment of cardiac tamponade is pericardiocentesis using an 18-gauge spinal needle. A needle with an electrocardiogram lead attached with an alligator clip for monitoring of needle position

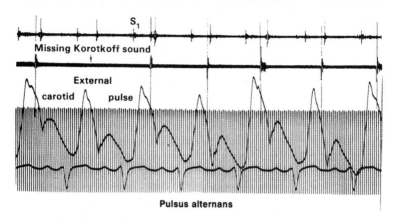

FIGURE 278.1. Pulsus alternans in the carotid artery. (Reprinted with permission from Constant J. Bedside Cardiology, 5th ed. Philadelphia: Lippincott Williams & Wilkins, 1999:52.)

is inserted 0.5 cm to the left of the xiphoid at an angle of 45 degrees and directed posteriorly while being aimed toward the left shoulder and continuously aspirated. The needle will produce a QRS complex inversion once the epicardium of the pericardial sac is contacted. The needle should be advanced until the pericardial space is entered and fluid or blood is aspirated. If the needle is advanced too far, touching the myocardium, ST-segment elevation will be observed. If ST elevation occurs, the needle should be withdrawn back into the pericardial space. Once the pericardial effusion is drained and tamponade relieved, diastolic filling will be improved. As a result, cardiac output and blood pressure will increase.

The best imaging study (although not 100% sensitive) to confirm diagnosis of a suspected pericardial effusion is an echocardiogram; it can also guide pericardiocentesis.

SUGGESTED READINGS

Chen H, Sonnenday C, Lillemoe K, eds. Manual of Common Bedside Surgical Procedures. Philadelphia: Lippincott Williams & Wilkins, 2000:90–94.

Lanken P, ed. The Intensive Care Unit Manual. Philadelphia: WB Saunders, 2001:615–626.

Longo M, Jaffe C. Images in clinical medicine—electrical alternans. N Engl J Med 1999;341:2060.

279

DO NOT USE A NEGATIVE FOCUSED ASSESSMENT WITH SONOGRAPHY FOR TRAUMA (FAST) EXAM TO RULE OUT BOWEL INJURY OR INJURY TO THE RETROPERITONEUM OR AS THE ONLY TEST IN PENETRATING TRAUMA

BRENDAN G. CARR, MD
PATRICK K. KIM, MD

Focused assessment with sonography for trauma (FAST) is a noninvasive ultrasound procedure that is a quick, reliable exam used to detect free intraperitoneal fluid in the injured patient. Initially used in Europe as a diagnostic modality, the ease of use and ability to evaluate the injured patient in the resuscitation area has led to its widespread use. The FAST exam aids in the triage of injured patients directly to the operating room without obtaining further imaging studies. The traditional FAST exam consists of the following four views (one pericardial and three abdominal) (*Fig. 279.1*):

1) Subxiphoid view (to evaluate the pericardium)
2) Right upper quadrant view (hepatorenal recess or Morrison's pouch)
3) Left upper quadrant view (splenorenal recess)
4) Suprapubic view

For decades, the standard for evaluation of the abdomen in unstable blunt trauma was diagnostic peritoneal lavage (DPL). This invasive modality is sensitive but nonspecific and reliance on DPL results in high rates of nontherapeutic laparotomies. Computed tomography (CT) has largely replaced DPL in the evaluation of the stable blunt trauma patient and is highly sensitive and specific. However, CT requires transport of the patient to the radiology suite, with the inevitable delay in obtaining and evaluating the images.

In contrast, ultrasound is available at the bedside, readily learnable by nonradiologists, and very quick to perform (2 to 4 minutes). In the blunt trauma population, reported sensitivity and specificity approximate 83.3% and 99.7%, respectively. More important, in the evaluation of hypotensive trauma patients, the sensitivity and specificity of ultrasound approach 100% in experienced hands.

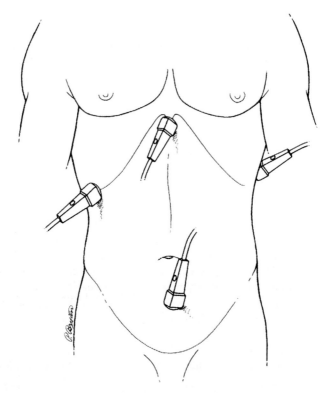

FIGURE 279.1. Transducer positions for focused assessment with sonography for trauma (FAST): (1) pericardial area, (2) right and (3) left upper quadrants, and (4) pelvis. (Reprinted with permission from Rozycki GS, Ballard RB, Feliciano DV, et al. Surgeon-performed ultrasound for the assessment of truncal injuries: lessons learned from 1540 patients. Ann Surg 1998;228(4):557–567.)

WATCH OUT FOR

The sensitivity of the FAST exam depends on multiple factors including the volume of hemoperitoneum, patient positioning, and ultrasonographer experience. Although there is substantial variability, about 500 cc of intraperitoneal fluid is necessary to enable ultrasonographic visualization (*Fig. 279.2*). It must be noted that the small amount of free fluid typically resulting from bowel perforation is not sufficient for reliable ultrasound diagnosis. Retroperitoneal injuries may not communicate with the peritoneal cavity and do not always cause hemoperitoneum. As a result, ultrasound remains unreliable in diagnosing retroperitoneal and hollow viscus injuries.

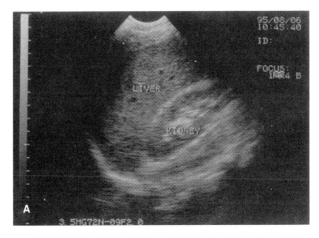

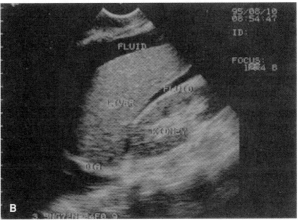

FIGURE 279.2. (A) Sagittal section of liver, kidney, and diaphragm. Normal findings. (B) Sagittal section of right upper quadrant showing blood between the liver and kidney and between the liver and diaphragm. (Reprinted with permission from Rozycki GS, Ballard RB, Feliciano DV, et al. Surgeon-performed ultrasound for the assessment of truncal injuries: lessons learned from 1540 patients. Ann Surg 1998;228(4):557–567.)

Although the FAST exam has historically been used only for blunt trauma patients, many centers have begun using ultrasound in penetrating trauma patients. Many clinicians have found that the FAST exam is helpful not only in triaging patients directly to the operating room, but also in prioritizing body cavity exploration (i.e., deciding on thoracotomy vs. laparotomy first). The overall sensitivity of FAST in penetrating trauma has been reported to be 46%, and as a result, FAST should not be used as the sole screening tool in penetrating trauma.

Although it is not a sensitive screening test in overall penetrating trauma, the FAST exam may be useful in penetrating thoracic trauma. Ultrasound is a useful screening test in the assessment of hemopericardium. With a sensitivity of 100% and a specificity of 97%, the FAST exam has become a popular adjunct in screening penetrating thoracic trauma patients. Pleural ultrasound may be as sensitive as chest x-ray in the detection of pneumothorax in the trauma population. Researchers have called for extending the FAST exam to include pleural views to diagnose both hemothorax and pneumothorax. An important limitation to the use of ultrasound in thoracic trauma is that cardiac injury cannot be effectively ruled out in the context of a fluid-filled thoracic cavity (hemothorax) because large amounts of pleural fluid can obscure a small pericardial collection and traumatic hemopericardium can decompress into the pleural space. Despite its limitations, given the ready availability of ultrasound in trauma settings, ultrasound should be used early and liberally in the evaluation of penetrating thoracic wounds.

SUGGESTED READINGS

Kirkpatrick AW, Sirois M, Laupland KB, et al. Hand-held thoracic sonography for detecting post-traumatic pneumothoraces: the extended focused assessment with sonography for trauma (EFAST). J Trauma 2004;57(2):288–295.

Meyer D, Jessen ME, Grayburn PA. The use of echocardiography to detect cardiac injury after penetrating thoracic trauma: a prospective study. J Trauma 1995;39:902–907.

Rozycki GS, Ballard RB, Feliciano DV, et al. Surgeon-performed ultrasound for the assessment of truncal injuries: lessons learned from 1540 patients. Ann Surg 1998;228(4):557–567.

Rozycki GS, Feliciano DV, Ochsner MG, et al. The role of ultrasound in patients with possible penetrating cardiac wounds: a prospective multicenter study. J Trauma 1999;46(4):543–551.

Udobi KF, Rodriguez A, Chiu WC, et al. Role of ultrasonography in penetrating abdominal trauma: a prospective clinical study. J Trauma 2001;50(3):475–479.

280

CONSIDER USING COMPUTED TOMOGRAPHY RECONSTRUCTIONS OF THE CHEST/ ABDOMEN/PELVIS TO RULE OUT THORACIC AND LUMBAR FRACTURES AND DISLOCATIONS

SUNEEL KHETARPAL, MD
BARBARA HAAS, MD

Evaluation for the presence of thoracolumbar spine injury is frequently necessary in the multiply injured patient based on clinical findings, mechanism of injury, inability to adequately assess for injury due to decreased level of consciousness, or distracting injuries. Traditionally, the thoracolumbar spine was evaluated using anteroposterior and lateral plain films, but this modality is considered less than ideal for several reasons. Because the thoracolumbar spine cannot be adequately evaluated with portable radiographs, obtaining such films requires transportation of the critically injured patient away from areas equipped for emergency resuscitation. Moreover, a significant time delay between arrival in the trauma bay and completion of these films is documented. Most important, the sensitivity of plain films has been reported to be as low as 58%, with a high proportion of films being described as technically inadequate and requiring further computed tomography (CT) imaging.

WHAT TO DO

The mechanism of injury leading to the need for thoracolumbar spine imaging frequently also requires that patients have CT imaging of the chest and abdomen, and an increasing volume of literature suggests that imaging ordered to rule out visceral injury can be used to expedite screening for thoracolumbar spine injuries. CT scans of the chest, abdomen, and pelvis were found to be more sensitive and specific for the detection of spinal injury than plain films, even if no specific spine protocol was included. In one prospective study, CT was found to have a sensitivity of 97% and a specificity of 99%. Although neither technique missed unstable fractures, CT images were more likely to detect stable fractures. Other studies reported similar results.

Published reports also suggest that the use of CT decreases the delay between arrival of the patient in the trauma bay and thoracolumbar spine clearance, which reduces demand on emergency room resources and permits the better utilization of personnel who previously were engaged in patient transport (nurses, residents, and respiratory technicians). Moreover, because patients at highest risk of thoracolumbar spine injuries are being scanned for other indications, including thoracolumbar spine reconstructions does not increase the utilization of the CT scan or expose the patient to additional radiation, and this new approach is very likely more cost effective, particularly in high-risk patients.

281

DO NOT RULE OUT CERVICAL SPINE OR SPINAL CORD INJURY ON BONY FILMS OR COMPUTED TOMOGRAPHY ALONE

MICHAEL D. GROSSMAN, MD

The incidence of cervical spine injury in blunt trauma patients varies according to the criteria used to select patients for screening, the manner in which patients are screened, and the criteria used to define injury relative to a given imaging modality. The National Emergency X-radiography Utilization Study (NEXUS) reported an incidence of 2.8% among patients evaluated in emergency departments following blunt trauma. Grossman and colleagues reported an incidence of 4.3% in more than 100,000 patients admitted to trauma centers. It has been shown that the incidence of cervical spine injury increases with injury severity, severe closed head injury, severe facial fractures, associated spinal column injury, and the use of computed tomography (CT) scanning as a screening tool. The overall clinical relevance of routine use of CT as a screening tool for cervical spine injury is not known with respect to adequate three-view cervical spine x-rays. Sensitivity for detection of bony injury is clearly better. However, treatment mandated by detection of injury that may be clinically silent has increased the use of rigid cervical collars with an unknown effect on outcomes.

It is important to note that exclusion of bony injury does not "clear" the cervical spine in every case. There is a possibility that patients without bony injury may sustain clinically significant ligamentous injury that could result in subluxation and neurologic sequelae if unrecognized. The incidence of such injuries is difficult to estimate based on considerations outlined earlier, but is most likely less than 1% in most trauma centers. Similarly the incidence of spinal cord injury without radiographic abnormality (SCIWORA) is difficult to estimate and most likely represents operational terminology prior to the widespread use of magnetic resonance imaging (MRI) to image patients with any degree of neurologic dysfunction following injury. Dysfunction includes but is not limited to anatomic syndromes (central cord, anterior cord), dysesthesias, transient symptoms (spinal "concussion"), and disc herniations. MRI has high sensitivity in detecting anatomic lesions, particularly in the presence of acquired chronic spinal stenosis or spondylolisthesis.

WATCH OUT FOR Many options exist for clearance of the cervical spine. For patients who are awake, alert, nonintoxicated, and can provide reliable physical examination, clearance through clinical exam is reasonable. Determination of "reliable physical exam" is a matter of clinical judgment informed by the clinical history. High-energy mechanism, associated lower spine fracture, advanced age, or distracting injury particularly in proximity (upper ribs, clavicle) to the cervical spine may influence the practitioner to obtain additional information.

Flexion-extension films of the cervical spine have a role in establishing stability provided adequate range of motion (30 degrees in both directions) is present and the cervicothoracic junction can be visualized. Given these considerations, this modality is most effective for awake, alert patients who can cooperate with instructions. Cervical MRI has evolved as a gold standard despite lack of specificity for injuries that are truly "unstable" (i.e., comparison to a standard that allows correlation of soft tissue findings with subluxation). However, sensitivity of MRI is good, and a normal MRI provides the clinician with the assurance that ligamentous injury has been excluded to the best degree of medical certainty.

SUGGESTED READINGS

Grossman MD, Reilly PM, Gillett T, et al. National survey of the incidence of cervical spine injury and approach to cervical spine clearance in US trauma centers. J Trauma 1999;47:684–690.

Guidelines for the Management of Cervical Spine Injury. Neurosurgery 2002;50(3):S1–S199.

Hoffman JR, Mower WR, Wolfson AB, et al. The National Emergency X-radiography Utilization Study (NEXUS) group. Validity of a set of clinical criteria to rule out injury to the cervical spine in patients with blunt trauma. N Engl J Med 2000;343:94–99.

Insko EK, Gracias VH, Gupta R, et al. Utility of flexion and extension radiographs of the cervical spine in the acute evaluation of blunt trauma. J Trauma 2002;53(3):426–429.

282

USE THE POSITION OF THE MEDIASTINUM AS A CLUE TO THE DIAGNOSIS OF A WHITE-OUT ON CHEST RADIOGRAPH

NADIA N. HANSEL, MD, MPH
NOAH LECHTZIN, MD, MHS

WATCH OUT FOR

The chest radiograph (CXR) is often the first radiologic study obtained in the evaluation of dyspnea. In the intensive care unit (ICU), portable chest radiographs are frequently ordered "STAT" to evaluate patients with new or acute onset of shortness of breath. Occasionally, there is diffuse opacification or "white-out" of a hemithorax. Though the complete differential diagnosis for "white-out" is quite large, the complete opacification of a hemithorax with no visible lung markings is usually caused by one of two main processes: atelectasis/lung collapse or massive pleural effusion, with the main types of fluids in the pleural space being serous fluid (hydrothorax), blood (hemothorax), lipid (chylothorax), and pus (pyothorax or empyema). Less common causes of white-out include a consolidative process with filling of the air spaces, such as bacterial pneumonia, soft tissue tumor, or post-pneumonectomy with the residual space filling with fluid and fibrotic material.

The prompt recognition of the correct diagnosis is important for appropriate and timely therapeutic intervention. Often, the most helpful clue to the diagnosis of white-out of a hemithorax is the position of the mediastinum. Normally, the trachea is midline; however, the mediastinum is a mobile structure and responds to differences in pressure between the two sides of the thorax. In complete lung collapse, often caused by proximal obstruction of the bronchus and post-pneumonectomy, there is loss of volume on the opacified side. The CXR reveals complete opacification of the hemithorax with shift of the mediastinum toward the collapsed side (to the side of the white-out). Other radiologic signs related to the reduction in intrapleural pressure include diaphragmatic elevation, narrowing of the intercostal spaces of the affected lung, and hyperinflation of the opposite lung.

In the case of a pleural effusion, the opacification of the thorax is usually homogeneous, and if the patient is erect, there may be a visible meniscus. In massive effusions (usually >1,000 mL), the intrapleural pressure on the affected side of the lung is increased and the mediastinum shifts to the contralateral side.

In the case of consolidation, the size of the hemithorax is often unchanged and the mediastinum remains midline. If the pneumonic consolidation is massive and the lung volume increases or if the consolidation is associated with a concomitant effusion, there may be mediastinal shift to the contralateral side. However, in the later stages of the consolidative process secretions may cause airway obstruction with associated atelectasis and volume loss, resulting in mediastinal shift to the ipsilateral side. An additional radiologic clue to the diagnosis of a consolidative process is the presence of air bronchograms.

SUGGESTED READINGS

Muller NL, Colman N, Pare PD, et al., eds. Fraser and Pare's Diagnosis of Diseases of the Chest, 4th ed. Philadelphia: WB Saunders, 1999:525–534.
Reed JC. Chest Radiology, 5th ed. Philadelphia: Mosby, 2003.

283

CONSIDER ANGIOGRAPHY FOR BLUNT SOLID-ORGAN INJURY

SUNEEL KHETARPAL, MD
BARBARA HAAS, MD

The ability to manage the majority of solid-organ injuries nonoperatively has become a cornerstone in the optimal approach to blunt trauma. Both diagnostic and therapeutic angiography is gaining increasing prominence as a technique by which this goal can be achieved.

The spleen is the most frequently injured organ following blunt abdominal trauma, with splenic injuries being present in 25% to 30% of cases. Liver injury is less frequent (15% to 20% of patients), and renal trauma is present in approximately 10% of patients. Although the circumstances in which angiography can be used in the management of these injuries are constantly evolving, a number of reports have demonstrated its value as an adjunct that can increase overall organ salvage and decrease the need for surgical intervention.

All grades of splenic injury have been successfully managed nonoperatively in hemodynamically stable patients. However, increasing grade of injury, as well as contrast extravasation or blush on admission computed tomography (which MUST be performed with intravenous contrast), has been associated with increasing likelihood of nonoperative management failure. Angioembolization has been considered useful in avoiding surgery in this subset of patients, who are most likely to fail observation in the intensive care unit. In recently published reports, between 5% and 15% of patients with splenic injuries were successfully managed with angioembolization, with success rates greater than 90% reported. The indications and technique for angioembolization in splenic trauma have been evolving rapidly and are the subject of considerable debate. Advocates of proximal splenic artery embolization theorize that this approach decreases splenic blood pressure, which prevents delayed hemorrhage and accelerates splenic healing while maintaining splenic perfusion through collateral blood flow. Others use angioembolization at the level of more distal arteries to the spleen, which requires more time and manipulation but preserves blood flow to the spleen.

WATCH OUT FOR

It is important to note that approximately 8% to 10% of patients who initially appear to have been successfully managed nonoperatively are at risk for delayed complications requiring intervention. Complications include persistent hemorrhage, delayed splenic rupture due to expanding hematoma, and splenic artery pseudoaneurysm formation. Angioembolization should be considered in the treatment of these complications, given that patients who fail nonoperative management and require delayed operative intervention have significantly worse outcomes than both patients managed nonoperatively and patients managed surgically at initial presentation.

The use of angiography and arterial embolization for hepatic injury has also undergone considerable evolution. Initially introduced as a viable therapeutic modality for hemodynamically stable patients, the technique has been shown to be a successful alternative to surgery in patients who are hemodynamically stable only with ongoing resuscitation. These are generally patients with isolated liver injuries or liver injuries associated with concomitant intra-abdominal trauma not requiring emergent laparotomy. Moreover, emphasis has been placed on the use of angioembolization in patients with high grades of injury and evidence of ongoing arterial bleeding on computed tomography in the form of contrast blush. Historically, these patients are most likely to fail nonoperative management.

A separate group of patients who benefit from hepatic artery angioembolization are severely injured patients for whom the technique is a component of postoperative stabilization and resuscitation. In particular, patients with grade IV and grade V liver injuries appear to benefit from angioembolization, although the data supporting this approach combine patients with both blunt and penetrating mechanisms of injury. Finally, angioembolization has successfully been used in the management of delayed complications in patients with hepatic injuries. Specifically, up to 5% of patients managed nonoperatively subsequently develop delayed or recurrent hemorrhage, 1% to 2% develop vascular abnormalities, such as pseudoaneurysm, and 1% develop hemobilia. In most cases of delayed vascular complications, angioembolization is the primary treatment of choice.

Angioembolization has also been used with success in the management of blunt renal injuries, although there is less experience managing this type of injury with interventional radiology. Given that 85% of renal injuries are grade III or less, these injuries are less likely to require intervention. Successful angioembolization of renal vascular injuries in patients who are hemodynamically stable has been reported by a number of groups, with emphasis being placed on highly selective embolization to attempt maximum tissue preservation and thus preserve renal function.

As with any intervention, angiography and subsequent embolization is not without risk. Angiography is associated with risk of hematoma, vessel thrombosis, and vascular injury, such as vessel dissection or pseudoaneurysm formation. Vessel embolization can be associated with tissue infarction and subsequent abscess formation, particularly when less selective techniques are used. Nevertheless, the utility of this technique in the successful nonoperative and operative management of blunt solid-organ injuries has been demonstrated in a variety of patient populations.

SUGGESTED READINGS

Haan JM, Biffl W, Knudson MM, et al. Western Trauma Association Multi-Institutional Trials Committee. Splenic embolization revisited: a multicenter review. J Trauma 2004;56(3):542–547.

Harbrecht BG. Is anything new in adult blunt splenic trauma? Am J Surg 2005; 190(2):273–278.

284

BE ALERT FOR COMPARTMENT SYNDROMES

FRANK J. FRASSICA, MD
BRETT M. CASCIO, MD
DEREK PAPP, MD

Compartment syndromes are common following trauma and other conditions in critically ill patients. Irreversible muscle and nerve injuries often occur in unrecognized compartment syndromes. Many health care providers are unfamiliar with the symptoms and signs of an incipient compartment syndrome and are unable to make an early diagnosis.

PATHOPHYSIOLOGY

Compartment syndromes are caused by a significant increase in the tissue pressure within a closed space resulting in reduced circulation to muscles and nerves. As the tissue pressure increases, the perfusion gradient decreases and muscle and nerve ischemia occurs. Working with dogs, Heckman found irreversible muscle infarction when the tissue pressure was within 10 mm Hg of the diastolic pressure. Bernot noted that muscle subjected to ischemia before an increase in compartment pressure developed hypoxic metabolic changes when the perfusion pressure was within 40 mm Hg of the mean arterial pressure. Cellular anoxia is the final common denominator of all compartment syndromes, with myoglobin released from the injured muscle cells. Patients who have compartment syndromes may experience myoglobinuria, metabolic acidosis, and hyperkalemia, which may result in renal failure, shock, hypothermia, and cardiac arrhythmias or failure.

RISK FACTORS

The most common cause of compartment syndromes is a fracture. However, virtually any condition that causes marked muscle or compartment swelling may cause a compartment syndrome, including bleeding from coagulopathies or anticoagulation; crush injuries; prolonged dependency (intravenous drug abusers, alcoholics, and stroke victims); tight casts or dressings; osteotomies; burns; reperfusion; prolonged operating room position; and military antishock trousers.

SIGNS AND SYMPTOMS

Pain out of proportion to injury is the hallmark finding in patients with a compartment syndrome. Patients note a severe, unrelenting discomfort, which is often not relieved by narcotics. Patients may explain their pain by stating that it is intolerable, or they may lay quietly with their eyes closed in an attempt to tolerate the pain. Escalating doses of narcotics are often necessary to control the pain. There is a significant risk that clinicians may prescribe sufficient narcotics to mask the compartment syndrome, leading to a significant delay in diagnosis. Patients may also describe neurologic symptoms such as paresthesias and a loss of motor function.

Pain with passive stretch of the muscles traversing the compartment, tenseness, pain on palpation of the involved compartment, and loss of motor or sensory function are the important physical examination findings. Unfortunately, tenseness and pain on palpation are not specific for compartment syndrome and are often present in patients with fractures. Patients with a compartment syndrome in the leg exhibit severe discomfort when the toes are flexed or extended; they often do not allow the examiner to repeat the test. Many patients with compartment syndrome are not able to actively flex and extend their toes.

It is very important to perform serial motor and sensory examinations. Loss of sensation is a common finding as a compartment syndrome evolves. In the leg, loss of sensation in the distribution of the deep peroneal nerve (first web space of the foot) is a very common early finding. Weakness of ankle and great toe dorsiflexion are other common early findings. Pallor, pulselessness, and paralysis are very late findings and indicate that there is complete muscle loss and possible total ischemia if there are no pulses.

PRESSURE MEASUREMENT/INDICATIONS FOR FASCIOTOMY

The measurement of compartment pressures is useful for determining whether a patient who is experiencing severe pain or the unconscious patient who has significant swelling has a compartment syndrome. When an at-risk patient has pain out of proportion to injury, a tense compartment, and pain on passive stretch, one can make the diagnosis of compartment syndrome and treat the patient with an emergency release of the fascial compartment without measuring pressures. In many patients, it can be difficult to separate the severe pain of the initial injury from that of a compartment syndrome. In this scenario measurement of the pressures assists the clinician in determining whether a compartment syndrome is present.

Intracompartmental pressures are easily measured with commercially available devices, such as the Stryker Monitor. The device has a needle with a side port, and the needle is advanced into the compartment. A small amount of saline is injected into the compartment, and tissue pressure is determined (normal pressure is 0 to 7) and then compared to the diastolic pressure. If the tissue pressure is within 30 mm Hg of the diastolic pressure, there is significant risk of muscle and nerve ischemia and fasciotomy should be performed. If the difference between the tissue pressure and the compartment pressure is greater than 30 mm Hg, a compartment syndrome is not present and the patient can be observed.

EMERGENCY FASCIOTOMY

Patients with compartment syndromes require emergency fasciotomy to reduce the tissue pressure and increase the perfusion pressure to nerves and muscle. The fasciotomies are ideally performed within 45 to 90 minutes of diagnosis. Fasciotomies are performed through standard incisions to allow complete release of the fascia. The fascia is released from the origination of the muscle to the musculotendinous junction. The skin and subcutaneous tissues are left open and either closed by delayed primary closure or skin grafts at a later date.

Occasionally, a compartment syndrome goes unrecognized for greater than 24 hours. In this scenario, patients have complete and irreversible loss of muscle and nerve function. There is no potential for recovery of function. When a compartment syndrome has been present for more than 24 hours and there is complete motor and sensory loss, there is no indication for fasciotomy. Fasciotomy may be deleterious in that there may be an increased release of myoglobin and other toxic metabolites. Even more problematic is the difficulty with attaining wound healing after fasciotomy in an extremity with an unrecognized compartment syndrome. The risk of amputation is very high.

SPECIAL CONSIDERATIONS IN THE INTENSIVE CARE UNIT

Patients are especially at risk for missed compartment syndromes in the setting of an intensive care unit because they often are unable to communicate that their limb hurts. The cardinal finding of pain out of proportion to injury may not be apparent. Careful physical examination of all extremities in the unconscious patient should be performed on a daily basis. Patients who might be especially at risk include the following:

1) In patients who have had long operations, the lateral decubitus or lithotomy position may predispose the patient to a compartment syndrome in a nontraumatized leg.

2) Patients who have reperfusion of an ischemic limb (i.e., vascular surgery) are very much at risk for the development of compartment syndrome of the leg.

3) Obese patients who are not able to turn themselves are at risk for gluteal/buttock compartment syndromes.

4) Patients who have sustained massive trauma and have been intubated at the scene of the accident or in the emergency room often have missed extremity lesions because the clinician cannot obtain a history of painful areas. Compartment syndrome may occur in the upper and lower extremities in this group of patients.

5) Patients who have had a thrombotic event or a massive intravenous infiltration are at risk secondary to swelling.

SUGGESTED READINGS

Bernot, M, Gupta, R, Dobrasz, J, et al. The effect of antecedent ischemia on the tolerance of skeletal muscle to increased interstitial pressure. J Orthop Trauma 1996;10:555–559.

Cascio BM, Buchowski JM, Frassica FJ. Well-limb compartment syndrome after prolonged lateral decubitus positioning: a report of two cases. J Bone Joint Surg 2004;86A(9):2038–2040.

Cascio BM, Wilckens JH, Ain MC, et al. Documentation of acute compartment syndrome at an academic health-care center. J Bone Joint Surg 2005;87A(2):346–350.

Heckmann MM, Whitesides TE Jr, Grewe SR, et al. Histologic determination of the ischemic threshold of muscle in the canine compartment syndrome model. J Orthop Trauma 1993;7:199–210.

285

BE ALERT FOR ACALCULOUS CHOLECYSTITIS

MEREDITH S. TINTI, MD
PATRICK K. KIM, MD

Acute acalculous cholecystitis is an inflammatory process of the gallbladder in the absence of calculi. In contrast to acute cholecystitis, in which anatomic obstruction by gallstones is the primary process, obstruction is only variably present and is not the causative process in acalculous cholecystitis. The pathophysiology of acute acalculous cholecystitis is not clearly defined but is believed to be produced by a combination of systemic mediators of inflammation, biliary stasis, and ischemia. Although 60% to 90% of all postoperative or post-trauma cases of cholecystitis are acalculous, the overall incidence of acalculous cholecystitis in the intensive care unit is only 0.2%.

SIGNS AND SYMPTOMS

Diagnosis of acalculous cholecystitis is often difficult and frequently delayed. In part, this is due to its preponderance in the difficult-to-examine critically ill patients with significant comorbidities. Early consideration of the disease and a high degree of suspicion are required to ensure prompt diagnosis. The delay in diagnosis and the ill patient population lead to a high rate of complication, such as gangrene or perforation (40% to 60%). The clinical findings are nonspecific and include fever, right upper quadrant abdominal pain, leukocytosis, and elevation of liver enzymes (LFTs) and bilirubin. Abdominal pain is the most consistent finding, but it is not always localized to the right upper quadrant; leukocytosis and elevated LFTs are present in approximately 75% of cases.

Definitive diagnosis can be made by many different tests. Abdominal ultrasonography is usually the first test performed in suspected cases of acalculous cholecystitis because it can be done at the bedside of critically ill patients and has a sensitivity and a specificity of 70%. Hepatobiliary scintigraphy (hepatobiliary iminodiacetic acid [HIDA] scan) requires transport of the patient to the nuclear medicine suite but has a sensitivity of 80% to 90% and a specificity of 90% to 100%. Computed tomography (CT) also requires transportation of the patient but is useful for evaluating other sources of abdominal signs and symptoms. CT has a specificity of 90% to 95% if certain diagnostic criteria are met.

Surgical cholecystectomy (laparoscopic or open) is the treatment of choice because the incidence of gangrene, perforation, and empyema is significantly higher than for calculous cholecystitis. However, many patients with acalculous cholecystitis have an extremely high operative mortality risk. Patients can sometimes be managed with percutaneous cholecystostomy. This procedure has a 95% to 100% technical success rate, but a clinical response of only 70% to 85%. If there is no improvement after 72 hours or if there are signs of gangrene or emphysema at the time of diagnosis, surgical cholecystectomy is required.

Following successful treatment of acalculous cholecystitis with a percutaneous cholecystostomy tube, the tube may be removed if the patient is no longer critically ill, a tract has formed over a 3- to 6-week period, the cystic and common bile ducts are demonstrated to be open, and there is no ascites present. There is no consensus in the literature as to whether cholecystectomy is mandatory following cholecystostomy; many surgeons opt to observe symptom-free patients.

SUGGESTED READINGS

Cameron J, ed. Current Surgical Therapy, 8th ed. Philadelphia: Elsevier Mosby, 2004:385–392.

Mullholland MW, Lillemoe KD, Doherty GM, et al., eds. Greenfield's Surgery: Scientific Principles and Practice, 4th ed. Philadelphia: Lippincott Williams & Wilkins, 2005:990–991.

Lane JD, Lomis N. Cholecystitis, acalculous. www.emedicine.com/RADIO/topic157.htm

286

AVOID GIVING INTRAVENOUS CONTRAST DYE MORE OFTEN THAN EVERY 48 HOURS IF POSSIBLE

AMISHA BAROCHIA, MD

Radiocontrast-induced acute renal failure is the third-leading cause of acute renal failure in hospitalized patients in the United States. More than 10 million radiocontrast studies are performed annually in the United States. Of importance, contrast-induced nephropathy, although largely preventable, is associated with 34% mortality. Radiocontrast-induced nephropathy is due to acute tubular necrosis that results from reduced renal perfusion secondary to vasoconstriction, tubular obstruction, and direct tubular toxicity from the contrast medium, which is thought to be mediated by oxygen free radicals. The definition of radiocontrast-induced nephropathy is variable, with some defining it as a greater than 25% increase from baseline serum creatinine and others defining it as an absolute increase of greater than 0.5 mg/dL of creatinine from baseline within 48 hours of exposure to contrast. Because absolute serum creatinine values are an imprecise method for measuring renal function, the calculation of estimated glomerular filtration rate is recommended before and after administration of contrast dye to evaluate for acute renal failure.

The following risk factors predispose patients to nephropathy secondary to radiocontrast agents: pre-existing chronic renal insufficiency, diabetes mellitus, reduced effective circulating volume as in patients with intravascular depletion or heart failure, and the use of large volumes of contrast dye. Most patients who develop radiocontrast-induced nephropathy recover their renal function with no lasting sequelae. The serum creatinine value usually peaks at 3 to 5 days and returns to baseline within 10 days. However, a few patients have a residual requirement for renal replacement therapy. These patients have a reported 2-year survival rate of 18%. In addition, the risk-adjusted odds ratio for death after the development of radiocontrast-induced nephropathy is nearly 5 ($p < .01$).

Of the various preventive strategies available, several studies have shown that hydration before exposure to radiocontrast material reduces the risk of nephropathy. Intravenous hydration appears to be better than oral hydration, and normal saline, if tolerated, seems to be superior to 0.45% saline. All patients should receive hydration before any study that requires the administration of intravenous radiocontrast. One recommendation is to use at least 1 cc/kg/hr for 12 hours before and after the study. One relatively small trial showed a significant benefit with use of sodium bicarbonate instead of saline 1 hour before and for 6 hours after the administration of radiocontrast, but the results have not been validated in a larger trial. In addition, medications such as metformin, aminoglycosides, angiotensin-converting enzyme inhibitors, furosemide, or nonsteroidal anti-inflammatory drugs that are likely to have an added detrimental effect on the kidneys should be stopped well before the study is undertaken. Some radiocontrast materials, such as nonosmolar and nonionic agents, appear to be less nephrotoxic. These alternatives should be considered in high-risk patients.

Many studies have investigated the role of N-acetylcysteine or sodium bicarbonate infusion in preventing radiocontrast-induced nephropathy. Another approach that needs to be validated is the use of high-dose ascorbic acid (a total of 7 g) administered in three doses before and after contrast to reduce the risk of radiocontrast-induced nephropathy. Therapies that are not recommended for preventing radiocontrast-induced nephropathy include fenoldopam, calcium-channel blockers, dopamine, atrial natriuretic peptide, mannitol, furosemide, and theophylline.

SUGGESTED READINGS

Lin J, Bonventre JV. Prevention of radiocontrast nephropathy. Curr Opin Nephrol Hypertens 2005;14:105–110.

Weisbord SD, Palevsky PM. Radiocontrast induced acute renal failure. J Intens Care Med 2005;20:63–75.

PLACE PREGNANT PATIENTS WITH RIGHT SIDE ELEVATED 15 DEGREES

GLEN TINKOFF, MD

A woman in the third trimester of pregnancy is predisposed to hypotension while in the supine or sitting position due to the hemodynamic and anatomic changes of pregnancy. The large uterus of late pregnancy can compress the inferior vena cava (IVC) such that venous return is significantly reduced. This decreased preload can lead to decreased cardiac filling and hence decreased cardiac output and hypotension. This can be especially deleterious in the usual setting of increased cardiac demand in pregnancy.

Of normovolemic pregnant patients, only 8% to 10% display supine hypotension due to adequate physiologic compensation; however, when faced with blood or other fluid losses such as in trauma or critical illness, supine hypotension of late pregnancy is more prevalent. In these instances, simple repositioning can be life saving. Establishing left uterine displacement by elevating the patient's right side greater than 15 degrees allows the uterus to be displaced off the inferior vena cava. After a traumatic injury, before this maneuver is performed assessment of the stability of the patient's spinal cord must be undertaken, and if uncertainly exists, the patient should not be moved without using formal spinal precautions.

SUGGESTED READINGS

Kinsella SM, Lohman G. Supine hypotensive syndrome. Obstet Gynecol 1994;83:774.
Ueland K, Metcafe J. Circulatory changes in pregnancy. Clin Obstet Gynecol 1975;18:41.

AVOID THE USE OF DRUGS HARMFUL TO THE FETUS IF AT ALL POSSIBLE

LEE ANN LAU, MD
HEIDI FRANKEL, MD

When treating pregnant patients, it is the physician's responsibility to treat the mother as the primary patient. Fetal considerations are secondary to ensuring maternal well-being because maternal demise will generally result in subsequent fetal death. With this in mind, however, when options for treatment exist, considering fetal effects is prudent.

Many common critical care drugs are safe in pregnancy, whereas some should be used with caution and others avoided entirely. It is also essential to remember that few drugs are extensively tested in pregnant humans, so caution should be exercised with administration of any pharmaceuticals in the pregnant woman. Consulting the *Physicians' Desk Reference* for the current safety ratings in pregnancy will ensure adherence to the most current recommendations.

WHAT TO DO

For analgesia, acetaminophen is generally considered safe when used in doses safe for the mother. Narcotics do not have reported teratogenicity; however, they can cause fetal respiratory depression if administered near the time of delivery. Aspirin should be avoided due to risks of intrauterine growth retardation and prolonged labor and bleeding. Although there is some controversy, nonsteroidal anti-inflammatory drugs are generally considered to be safe in the later part of pregnancy. Most inhalational agents and neuromuscular blockers are safe. Local anesthetics are able to cross the placenta but do not have fetal effects at common doses.

Specific antibiotics need to be assessed on an individual basis (e.g., quinolones are thought to cause tendon defects). Aminoglycosides are known to cause fetal ototoxicity, sulfonamides lead to neonatal kernicterus, tetracyclines inhibit fetal bone growth, and fluconazole is teratogenic. Penicillins, cephalosporins, vancomycin, and clindamycin are considered safe.

Hydralazine, alpha-methyldopa, and nitroglycerine are safe for the treatment of hypertension. Sodium nitroprusside can cause high cyanide levels in the fetus. Angiotensin-converting enzyme inhibitors cause fetal renal failure injury or death and should be avoided during the second and third trimesters.

For gastrointestinal prophylaxis, sucralfate, histamine-2 blockers, and pantoprazole are not associated with known fetal problems. Heparin and low-molecular-weight heparin are safe, but Coumadin causes fetal warfarin syndrome (facial dysmorphism, heart defects, growth defects). Use of anticonvulsants or sedatives is associated with some risk. Benzodiazepines, barbiturates, and propofol cause fetal respiratory depression. In addition, benzodiazepines can cause "floppy baby" syndrome and withdrawal syndromes. They are also questionably associated with cleft palate when used early. Haloperidol, phenytoin, and valproic acid are all teratogenic.

For hemodynamic instability, dobutamine is generally considered safe but is associated with decreased placental flow in some animal trials. Ephedrine preserves uterine blood flow. Phenylephrine is effective and safe for counteracting hypotension due to spinal or epidural anesthesia.

Treatment of nausea and vomiting in the pregnant patient deserves special mention. Vitamin B6 and ginger have been proven to be safe and effective; vitamin B6 may reduce the risk of congenital heart defects. Antihistamines (H1 blockers) are considered safe and generally effective. Dopamine-receptor antagonists (metoclopramide, droperidol, phenothiazines) have not been studied extensively, but limited data suggest safety and efficacy. Ondansetron has not shown toxicity in animal studies but safety and efficacy studies have not been done for human pregnancy.

SUGGESTED READINGS

Davis M. Nausea and vomiting of pregnancy: an evidence-based review. J Perinat Neonat Nurs 2004;18:312–328.

Hall JB, Schmidt GA, Wood LDH, ed. Principles of Critical Care, 3rd ed. New York: McGraw-Hill, 2005:1593–1614.

Irwin R, Rippe J, eds. Manual of Intensive Care Medicine, 5th ed. Philadelphia: Lippincott Williams & Wilkins, 2003:1751–1758.

289

Strongly Consider the Use of an Electronic Fetal Monitor in Caring for a Patient at Greater Than 24 Weeks' Gestation in the Intensive Care Unit

Robert K. Michaels, MD, MPH

It is not uncommon for a pregnant patient to be affected by critical illness. Examples of nonobstetric maladies that lead to intensive care unit admission among pregnant women are hematologic issues (venous thromboembolism and pulmonary embolus, pre-pregnancy hypercoagulable states), trauma (including motor vehicle accidents, falls, assaults, burns, etc.), asthma, valvular and congenital heart disease, and acute abdominal conditions (appendicitis, ruptured viscus associated with peptic ulcer disease, and inflammatory bowel disease).

WATCH OUT FOR

After approximately 24 weeks of gestation, most authorities consider the fetus viable, so for many pregnant patients in the intensive care unit (ICU) care must also be directed to the fetus. Although maternal life should never be jeopardized for the care of this second patient, the critical care physician should be able to recognize signs of fetal distress and collaborate with obstetric and neonatology colleagues to determine optimal therapy for both patients. Fetal distress can be caused by a host of factors; most notably, hypoxemia and hypovolemia are dangerous for the fetus. Fetal tachycardia, late fetal heart rate decelerations, and loss of heart rate variability are signs of significant fetal distress and call for immediate action. These are best identified with the use of the continuous electronic fetal monitor.

Although there is a lack of high-quality evidence, it is probably rational to use electronic fetal monitoring for any patients with estimated gestational age of 24 weeks or greater. The electronic fetal monitor consists of two probes placed on the mother's abdomen. One probe uses ultrasound (Doppler) to transmit and record the fetal heart rate. The second sensor is a pressure-sensitive device that records frequency and duration of uterine contractions. Fetal monitoring may demonstrate fetal distress, but changes in fetal heart rate are nonspecific and are often a late sign of inadequate fetal oxygen delivery. It is most accurate when performed at 32 weeks of gestation or later. The most specific indicator of fetal distress is probably fetal pH monitoring, which is performed by scalp blood sampling. However, to access the fetal scalp, cervical dilation must have begun and membranes must be ruptured, so this in not practical for many of the gravid patients in the ICU.

WHAT TO DO

If fetal distress or premature labor occurs, the first call should be to the obstetric service. Their expertise in assessment of gestational age, electronic fetal monitoring, maintenance of uterine blood flow, medication use, and the decision to perform emergency cesarean section are invaluable to the mother and child. Oxygen delivery to the fetus should be optimized by providing supplemental oxygen and restoring adequate circulating volume and cardiac function to the mother. Prevention of compression of the inferior vena cava by the gravid uterus is accomplished with placement of the mother in the left lateral decubitus position. If premature labor has commenced, tocolysis may be indicated to halt labor or delay delivery. Maternal steroid administration has been demonstrated to promote fetal lung maturity. However, delivery of the fetus may be the best option for the mother and the fetus.

SUGGESTED READINGS

Hall JB, Schmidt GA, Wood LDH, eds. Principles of Critical Care, 3rd ed. New York: McGraw-Hill, 2005:1593–1614.

290

KNOW THE NORMAL PHYSIOLOGIC CHANGES AND ASSOCIATED LABORATORY VALUES THAT OCCUR IN PREGNANCY

GLEN TINKOFF, MD

The physiologic adaptations of pregnancy occur in response to fetal development and eventual delivery. It is incumbent on the intensive care physician to have an understanding of the normal variants that occur in pregnancy to correctly interpret diagnostic tests and effectively treat clinical conditions. Some changes that occur in pregnancy include the following.

ENDOCRINE

By far the most significant physiologic changes of pregnancy are endocrinologic. Significant increases in production and serum levels of growth hormone, prolactin, thyroxin, parathyroid hormone, calcitonin, and progesterone occur in support of fetal development and parturition.

In addition, pregnancy is associated with positive nitrogen balance and postprandial hyperglycemia and hyperinsulinemia. This latter response is consistent with a pregnancy-induced state of peripheral resistance to insulin, the purpose of which is to ensure sustained supply of glucose to the fetus. Furthermore, the concentrations of plasma lipids, lipoproteins, and lipopolysaccharides increase appreciably during pregnancy and lead to central fat deposition to supply fetal demands.

CARDIOVASCULAR

Blood volume at or near term is approximately 40% above that in nonpregnancy. This hypervolemia of pregnancy meets the demands of pregnancy and protects the mother against impaired venous return and the blood loss of child birth.

Along with the increase in blood volume, left ventricular size also increases with increased contractility. Cardiac output increases as early as the fifth week of pregnancy with resting pulse rate increasing by approximately 10 beats per minute. Peripheral vascular resistance decreases. These cardiovascular changes are similar to changes occurring with moderate exercise.

HEMATOLOGIC

Although blood volume expansion occurs and results in increases in both plasma volume and erythrocyte number, more plasma is made than red cells. Thus, hemoglobin concentration and hematocrit decrease (at term hemoglobin is approximately 12.5 g/dL). Furthermore, with the increase in red cell mass, iron requirements are increased in pregnancy such that iron supplementation is necessary.

Despite the fact that pregnancy is associated with immunologic suppression to accommodate the semi-allogeneic fetus, the leukocyte count becomes elevated during late pregnancy, averaging 14,000 to 16,000. In addition, the coagulation cascade is also activated during pregnancy, with increases in most clotting factors and fibrinogen.

ELECTROLYTE

Pregnancy is marked by hypermetabolism and salt and water retention. These effects are mediated predominately through the actions of thyroxin and vasopressin. Water retention induced by increased vasopressin secretion is such that the average woman accrues an extra 6.5 L during normal pregnancy. Sodium and potassium are retained due to enhanced renal tubular resorption; however, concentrations of these electrolytes are slightly decreased as a result of the expanded plasma volume. In addition, serum magnesium levels decline during pregnancy such that pregnancy causes a state of continuous extracellular magnesium depletion.

HEPATIC

Other laboratory abnormalities that occur during pregnancy include an increase in total alkaline phosphatase, with serum levels almost doubling during normal pregnancy. Serum transaminases and bilirubin levels are usually slightly lower in pregnancy as compared with nonpregnant normal values. The concentration of serum albumin decreases during pregnancy, and therefore total calcium also decreases.

SUGGESTED READINGS

Cunningham FG, Loveno K, Bloom S, et al., eds. Williams Obstetrics, 22nd ed. New York: McGraw-Hill, 2005:121–149.

Pietzman AB, Rhodes M, Schwab CW, et al., eds. The Trauma Manual, 2nd ed. Philadelphia: Lippincott Williams & Wilkins, 2002:461–468.

291

DO NOT ADMINISTER PROPHYLACTIC ANTIMICROBIALS TO BURN PATIENTS

GARY T. MARSHALL, MD
JAMES H. HOLMES IV, MD

Despite the great strides made over the last decades in improving survival after thermal injury, infectious complications remain an important cause of morbidity and mortality. Nearly 50% of all burn deaths are related to infection. Several factors contribute to the high incidence and severity of infection in burn patients. First, a profound immune suppression is induced that is proportional to the extent of burn injury. In addition, the environment at the site of the wound is favorable for the multiplication of infecting organisms, which colonize the wound within 72 hours of injury. Despite the temptation to administer systemic antibiotics, there is *no role for prophylactic systemic antimicrobials*. This has *no impact on survival* and *leads to the emergence of resistant organisms*. Frequent exposure to antibiotics also establishes an environment favorable for yeast and fungi.

Within 3 days of injury, Gram-positive organisms colonize the wound. Gram-negative organisms then colonize the eschar, and they become dominant by the end of the first week. The typical flora of burn wounds has changed over the years. Before the advent of penicillin, β-hemolytic streptococci were the most frequent cause of burn wound and life-threatening systemic infections. Penicillin largely eliminated mortality due to streptococci, and *Staphylococcus aureus* became the more common early colonizer. As broad-spectrum antibiotics effective against *Staphylococcus* were developed, gram-negative organisms, especially *Pseudomonas aeruginosa*, became the predominant organisms. These organisms have greater invasive potential due to their production of toxins and proteolytic enzymes. The use of effective topical agents has reduced the incidence of death secondary to burn wound sepsis, but fungi have emerged as the most common cause of invasive burn wound infections.

The three most commonly used topical agents used to fight wound infections are silver sulfadiazine (SSD), mafenide acetate, and silver nitrate. SSD is the most frequently used. It has broad-spectrum activity as well as antifungal properties. SSD is limited by its inability to penetrate the burn eschar. Mafenide acetate has good eschar penetration and can suppress subeschar proliferation of bacteria. Mafenide acetate is a carbonic anhydrase inhibitor that interferes with the renal buffering. A hyperchloremic metabolic acidosis develops due to the consumption of bicarbonate and chloride retention. A compensatory respiratory alkalosis is generated by hyperventilation but is rarely of clinical significance. Silver nitrate is effective if applied before bacterial penetration into the wound. Side effects of silver nitrate include hyponatremia and methemoglobinemia.

WATCH OUT FOR

Despite these maneuvers, invasive infections still occur. Risk factors include severe injury (>30% total body surface area burn), systemic diseases such as diabetes with poor glycemic control, and delayed excision and grafting of the burn. The key to successful management of infection in the burn patient is early diagnosis. This is best accomplished by daily scheduled monitoring of the burn to identify infection at its early stages when surgical and antibiotic therapy will be most effective. Burn wound infections are classified as cellulitis, invasive infections, or burn wound impetigo. Cellulitis is diagnosed clinically based on characteristic erythema, edema, and hyperesthesia of unburned skin at the margin of the wound. Cellulitis unrelated to infection may also occur, usually peaking on the second or third day after the burn and then receding; this is rarely accompanied by systemic response. Expanding cellulitis should be treated with the application of mafenide acetate and systemic penicillin if a β-hemolytic streptococcus is involved or a broad-spectrum β-lactam if specific culture and sensitivity are not available. A local sign of invasive infection is the appearance of dark brown, black, or violaceous discoloration of the wound. Other clinical signs are the conversion of a partial-thickness injury to full thickness and necrosis of previously viable tissue in the wound bed. *Pseudomonas* may cause changes in the unburned skin at the wound margin. Infections caused by fungi display unexpected rapid eschar separation and rapid centrifugal spread of subcutaneous edema with central necrosis. Vesicular lesions appearing in healing or healed burns on the face are characteristic of herpes simplex virus type 1.

SIGNS AND SYMPTOMS

Once a burn wound infection is suspected, diagnosis is confirmed by burn wound biopsy. Surface cultures only identify the colonizing organisms present and are therefore inadequate. Quantitative bacterial counts of 10^5 or greater are suggestive of invasion but only correlate with invasive infection on histologic exam in fewer than 50% of paired samples. Histologic examination of a burn wound biopsy is the most reliable confirmatory test for invasive burn wound infection. With a scalpel, a lens-shaped sample of the eschar and unburned underlying/adjacent tissue are obtained from the area of the wound showing the most pronounced changes. On histologic exam, the presence of microorganisms in unburned tissue is diagnostic. Other findings that indicate burn wound infection are the presence of hemorrhage, small-vessel thrombosis, and necrosis in unburned tissue. After diagnosis, general supportive treatment is used, and specific systemic antibiotic therapy is initiated based on the institution's usual flora with subsequent modification as sensitivities return. Mafenide acetate should be applied to the wound twice daily. Subeschar clysis of a broad-spectrum penicillin may also be employed. Surgical excision should be performed as soon as possible. Topical clotrimazole should be applied when invasive fungi are the culprit microorganisms. Systemic treatment with amphotericin B or other, newer antifungal agents is also used when there is evidence of systemic fungemia.

Burn wound impetigo occurs after burn wound healing or grafting and is characterized by multifocal small superficial abscesses. *S. aureus* is the responsible microbe. Treatment includes unroofing of abscesses and frequent cleansing followed by application of topical antibiotics. Occasionally, systemic symptoms may be seen when the toxic shock syndrome toxin is produced. In this case intravenous vancomycin is used.

In addition to the previously described clinical situations, appropriate uses of antibiotics in the burn patient include targeted treatment of pulmonary, urinary, and catheter-related infections. In addition, perioperative prophylactic antibiotics should be administered just before wound excision. These are given based on the findings of transient bacteremia in 21% of patients following wound manipulation, although some studies have shown that bacteremia is rare when there is less than 40% total body surface area burn.

SUGGESTED READINGS

Edwards-Jones V, Greenwood JE. What's new in burn microbiology? Burns 2003;29: 15–24.

Pruitt BA Jr, McManus AT, Kim SH. Burn wound infection: current status. World J Surg 1998;22:135–145.

292

REMEMBER THAT NOT ALL FEVER IN THE BURN PATIENT IS DUE TO INFECTION

OLIVER A. VARBAN, MD
JAMES H. HOLMES IV, MD

Virtually all burn patients have elevated core body temperatures and even a leukocytosis. Thus, fever in burn patients is not a reliable indicator of infection. One study in children found that fever had no predictive value for the presence of infection and physical examination was a more reliable source of information about wound infection and sepsis. Furthermore, routine blood cultures have been shown to be of little value in working up a fever in burn patients.

WATCH OUT FOR

Mild hyperthermia in the first 24 hours following injury is almost always the result of pyrogen release. The three endogenous pyrogens that mediate fever are interleukin-1 (IL-1), tumor necrosis factor-α (TNF-α, cachetin), and interferon-γ. In addition to inducing fever, these pyrogens also modulate a large number of host defense responses. After 72 hours, burn patients develop systemic inflammatory response syndrome (SIRS), characterized by tachycardia, relative hypotension, and hyperthermia, which are the classic signs of sepsis that can occur without an infectious source. In fact, body temperature may be as high as 39°C (102.2°F) and the leukocyte count may be as high as 20,000 cells/mL during satisfactory recovery. Thus, elevation of body temperature above normal, leukocytosis, and other signs of inflammation are common among burn patients and should be expected.

The hypermetabolic response elicited by a burn injury is marked by increased energy expenditure and muscle protein catabolism. Fever further increases energy expenditure and muscle loss in burn patients. Thus, there is a theoretical metabolic benefit in attenuating fever in such patients. Mild elevation of body temperature is usually well tolerated and does not require specific treatment. However, body temperature higher than 39°C may be treated with common antipyretics (e.g., acetaminophen, aspirin, indomethacin, or ibuprofen). Burn patients also prefer warmer ambient temperature (26°C to 33°C) than do normal individuals because the fever experienced by the burn patient is an upward adjustment of the thermoregulatory center in the brain. This temperature range promotes patient comfort and reduces the physiologic demands of cold stress. Treating burn patients by surface cooling (ice packs, alcohol rubs, cooling blankets) is not uncommon but should be avoided because surface cooling creates a cold stress on an already critically ill patient.

Nonetheless, infection is a relatively common serious complication in patients with major thermal injuries. It is estimated that up to 75% of deaths following burn injury are related to infection. Immunosuppression is a universal feature of major thermal injury and burn patients are more susceptible to microbial colonization and infection. Special attention to technique during bedside procedures and the use of universal precautions are a must. In one study, up to 100% of burn patients developed an infection from one or more sources during their hospital stay. One might assume that prophylactic antibiotics, particularly against gram-positive organisms, are indicated; however, this practice has been shown to lead to the development of multidrug-resistant, gram-negative bacterial infections and fungal infections. In fact, studies have now verified that prophylactic antibiotics are not only unnecessary, but are also contraindicated in patients with thermal injuries. Exceptions to this statement are tetanus prophylaxis and perioperative antibiotics in patients who undergo excision and grafting. Otherwise, daily wound care and the application of a topical, broad-spectrum antimicrobial agent are the mainstays for the initial prevention of wound infection. Ultimately, excision and grafting is the most efficacious means of reducing the incidence of burn wound sepsis.

SUGGESTED READINGS

Bessey PQ. Metabolic response to critical illness. In: ACS Surgery: Principles and Practice. Chicago: American College of Surgeons, 2006. www.acssurgery.com

Gibran NS, Heimbach DM. Management of the patient with thermal injuries. In: ACS Surgery: Principles and Practice. Chicago: American College of Surgeons, 2006. www.acssurgery.com

Parish RA, Novack AH, Heimbach DM, et al. Fever as a predictor of infection in burned children. J Trauma 1987;27(1):69–71.

293

NEVER UNDERESTIMATE THE SEVERITY OF AN ELECTRICAL BURN

TRAVIS L. PERRY, MD
JAMES H. HOLMES IV, MD

Electrical injuries continue to be clinically and surgically challenging for surgeons and critical care physicians worldwide. Gross underestimation of the initial injury has repeatedly proven to increase morbidity and detrimental to the overall outcome.

To briefly review, electricity is the flow of electrons through a conductor via the force of voltage. Voltage is categorized into low (<1,000 volts) and high (≥1,000 volts). Alternating current (AC) and direct current (DC) are the two forms of electrical energy. Alternating current produces cyclic back and forth movement of electrons and is the common current in most households. Direct current is the flow of energy in one direction.

Severity of electrical injury is a function of three factors: (1) current source or voltage, (2) duration of contact, and (3) pathway of current flow. The clinical interplay of these factors can best be understood by Ohm's law ($I = V/R$), which states that current (I) is directly proportional to voltage (V) and inversely proportional to the resistance (R) of the conductor. Therefore, current will follow the path of least resistance. Histologically, tissues with high fluid and electrolyte contents (i.e., nerves, vessels, muscle, and mucosal membranes) have lower resistance. Therefore, the pathway of electrical current has a higher affinity for these tissues and will preferentially damage these sites. Tissues such as fat, bone, tendon, and dry skin have lower fluid and electrolyte content and therefore have higher resistance. These tissues do generate an intense amount of thermal injury, however, due to their poor ability to conduct electrical current. Because of this, the initial assessment of the severity of an electrical injury typically underestimates the extent of soft tissue injury.

It is important to note that electrical burns with alternating current, especially low-voltage current, have the propensity to produce muscle tetany due to its cyclic flow of energy. This, in turn, prolongs the duration of contact, which increases the potential of injury developing, especially from current flow through tissues with high resistance. This impeded flow of current can generate a tremendous amount of thermal injury that is often hidden in the form of coagulated necrosis of underlying subcutaneous fat, bone, and tendon.

High-voltage exposure typically produces a single violent muscle contraction leading to a shorter duration of contact due to ejection away from the primary source of current. This ejection increases the risk of fractures, dislocations, loss of consciousness, and closed-head injuries. High-voltage contact also generates severe skin burns due to arcing and flashing of the electrical current. As always, the path of current flow determines organ system involvement and overall injury severity. A flow of current parallel to the body's vertical axis increases the potential of multisystem injury. A horizontal flow of current is associated with less organ system involvement (e.g., the transfer from hand to hand).

Lightning is a form of extremely high-voltage direct current, and its strikes are fortunately rare occurrences. Lightning can strike directly or indirectly via ground or inanimate object transfer. It also has the ability to flow along the body's surface without directly entering the body. This flashing phenomenon produces a pathognomonic fern-like pattern (*Fig. 293.1*) over the body that resolves in about 24 hours.

Electrical injuries should be viewed and assessed from a multisystem perspective. Initial evaluation should proceed as in any major trauma, with primary and secondary surveys. Special attention should be given to high-voltage injury complications (e.g., extremity or digit amputation, muscle necrosis, compartment syndrome, and sepsis). Although multiple organ systems may be involved, it is damage to the major systems that may require intensive care unit evaluation and treatment.

CARDIOVASCULAR

The cardiovascular system may be affected via cellular necrosis or, more commonly, dysrhythmias. Myocardial injury could involve direct necrosis of myocytes, pacing nodes, and/or coronary vessels. Fatal dysrhythmias include ventricular fibrillation and asystole resulting from cell membrane instability, whereas a myriad of less dangerous dysrhythmias can be precipitated. Large blood vessels are susceptible to rupture or aneurysmal formation. Smaller vessels are more vulnerable to coagulation necrosis, which may lead to a compartment syndrome in the peripheral circulation. The cardiovascular system should be monitored via continuous electrocardiogram (ECG) if any dysrhythmias are detected on an initial 12-lead ECG. Cardiac enzymes should be checked and followed as clinically indicated. Physical examination and measurement of compartment pressures as needed will detect potential peripheral vascular complications.

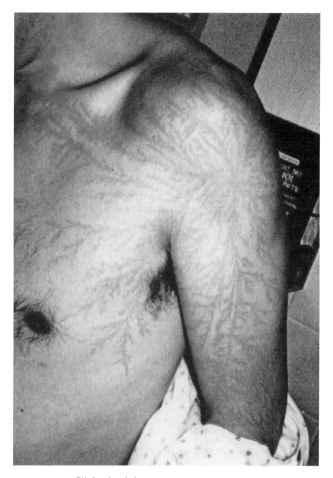

FIGURE 293.1. Lightning injury.

SKIN

Cutaneous electrical injury varies depending on voltage, contact duration, and resistance of the involved skin. Normal adult skin has a high resistance and therefore will generate underlying coagulation necrosis if prolong contact ensues. However, young children who naturally have higher water content in their skin and adults exposed to water suffer more superficial cutaneous injury due to the lowered resistance in their skin. These cutaneous burns should be approached as any burns would be. Careful resuscitation should be given to those burns that may involve subcutaneous fat, tendon, or bone necrosis. Do not under-resuscitate. However, the initial assessment of the extent and severity of an electrical burn is quite difficult and usually underestimates the amount of soft tissue involved. Thus, *multiple excisions to establish a healthy wound bed for grafting are the rule rather than the exception when excising an electrical burn*. Perioral burns from an electrical cord are the most common cutaneous electrical burns in children. These should primarily be monitored for labial artery bleeding. Special attention to potential feeding difficulties is of paramount importance in infants and warrants hospital admission until a regular feeding pattern is re-established.

PULMONARY

Respiratory arrest is related to direct injury of the brain stem respiratory center or diaphragmatic muscle tetany impeding respiratory effort. Typically, respiratory arrest from electrical injuries manifests at the scene. This is monitored for and treated symptomatically via mechanical ventilation.

OTHER

Renal dysfunction can occur directly or indirectly via exposure to hypoxemia, myoglobin, and/or creatinine phosphokinase. Serial urine myoglobin and creatinine phosphokinase should be measured as clinically indicated. Adequate resuscitation and hydration should be provided. Renal failure should be treated as indicated. Volume resuscitation should be based on a urinary output of 30 cc per hour in an adult without myoglobinuria. A minimal urine output of 100 mL/h is the goal in a patient with myoglobinuria. Central and peripheral nervous system injuries should be evaluated and recognized during the initial trauma assessment. Ophthalmologic examination should be performed on all patients suffering high-voltage injuries to assess for premorbid cataracts because cataract development is a delayed complication of high-voltage injuries.

SELECTED READINGS

Arnold B. Electrical injuries: A 20-year review. J Burn Care Rehabil 2004;25(6):479–484.

Herndon D, Muehlberger T, eds. Total Burn Care, 2nd ed. Philadelphia: WB Saunders, 2002:455–469.

Koumbourlis, AC. Electrical injuries: scientific reviews. Crit Care Med 2002; 30(11):424–430.

294

DO NOT USE HYPERBARIC OXYGEN THERAPY IN BURNS

TRAVIS L. PERRY, MD
JAMES H. HOLMES IV, MD

Hyperbaric oxygen therapy is currently used in various clinical treatment regimens. These include decompression sickness, carbon monoxide poisoning, cyanide poisoning, gas embolus, gas gangrene, resistant anaerobic infections, and threatened split-thickness skin grafts. The mechanism of action purportedly involves increasing tissue oxygenation, which increases collagen and fibroblast formation and suppresses *Clostridia* toxin production. It also enhances the killing ability of the leukocyte and capillary proliferation. This mechanism has primarily been established in animal models and limited human trials. At best, hyperbaric oxygen in the management of soft tissue infections can be promoted only as part of a coordinated medical and surgical approach.

It has been postulated that hyperbaric oxygen in burn wounds potentially exhibits some benefit by stimulating vasoconstriction and counteracting hypoxia. This theory is based on the possibility that hyperbaric oxygen may decrease acute edema, fluid requirements, and infection rates and promote re-epithialization. There have been several animal models that demonstrated varied results. However, the use and efficacy of hyperbaric oxygen in burn wound therapy is not established. Recent studies have not been able to demonstrate a statistically significant difference in the length of hospital stay, the number of operations required, and morbidity and/or mortality when comparing hyperbaric oxygen supplementation versus standard burn therapy. Thus, hyperbaric oxygen has no place in the acute management of thermal injuries.

Carbon monoxide (CO) poisoning should be suspected in virtually every fire victim. It remains one of the most frequent causes of death in smoke inhalation injuries. Hyperbaric oxygen has demonstrated value in the treatment of isolated CO poisoning. It decreases the high affinity that CO has for hemoglobin. Hyperbaric oxygen decreases the half-life of CO from about 4 hours to about 25 minutes, which leads to quicker restoration of oxygenation. Thus, hyperbaric oxygen therapy may have a place in the care for burn patients with CO poisoning. However, hyperbaric oxygen therapy in burn patients with CO poisoning is of unknown therapeutic value or efficacy and should only be used when (1) the CO bound to hemoglobin is greater than 25%, (2) a neurologic deficit exists, (3) no formal burn resuscitation is required (typically, total body surface area burned is <10% to 15%), (4) pulmonary function is stable with an intact airway, and (5) interfacility transfer does not compromise burn care.

SELECTED READINGS

Brannen LA, Law EA. Randomized prospective trial of hyperbaric oxygen in a referral burn center population. Am Surg 1997;63:205–208.

Herndon D, Traber D, eds. Total Burn Care, 2nd ed. Philadelphia: WB Saunders, 2002:221–231.

Wiseman D, Grossman RA. Hyperbaric oxygen in the treatment of burns. Crit Care Clin 1985;1(1):129–143.

295

DO NOT USE PARENTERAL NUTRITION, IF AT ALL POSSIBLE, IN BURN PATIENTS

JEREMY W. PYLE, MD
JAMES H. HOLMES IV, MD

Years of work and hundreds of studies have been performed to elucidate the best and most beneficial means of supplying nutrition to burn patients. Focus in the recent past has shifted from the overall importance of nutrition to a highly specialized and improved collection of recommendations. These include not only what and how much, but also where and when, why and how.

Burn wound pathophysiology and how it affects the body as a whole are fairly well understood, and the degree to which thermal injury alters nutrition requirements is directly related to the total body surface area (TBSA) of the burn. Burn wound derangements include grossly elevated local metabolic needs and increased systemic requirements. The battle to provide adequate nutrition in the face of this alteration has three fronts. First, a burn wound requires ramped-up repair efforts and immune support. Second, the body's response to the insult includes significant systemic derangements in neuroendocrine and cytokine-mediated processes. Finally, the gastrointestinal tract and its response to these changes are unique and important. Designing a nutrition regimen must address all three of these areas, paying special attention to the carbohydrate and protein requirements needed to avoid muscle and mucosal catabolism and avoiding a heavy reliance on lipids as a source of calories.

WHAT NOT TO DO

Postburn hypermetabolism has been shown to respond to a low-fat, high-protein enteral diet with fewer wound complications and a lower overall morbidity. Conversely, *parenteral nutrition has consistently been linked to increased mortality in the burn patient*. Burn wounds almost exclusively utilize glucose. This, coupled with the increased overall glucose requirements that come with thermal injury, means that glucose supply must be either increased in the diet or come from the catabolism of other tissues. For this reason, carbohydrates should serve as the major nonprotein source of nutrition. Doing so ensures not only that the wound will be better supplied with energy, but also that the rest of the body operates without quite so severe a demand for gluconeogenic substrates, and so protein stores can be preserved. If a patient is poorly fed, the end result of this demand in such a patient has an energy deficit that has been shown to develop very early postburn. Hence, early and aggressive feedings are recommended. They have been shown to positively affect protein requirements, energy deficiency, and insulin secretion. Because hyperglycemia and protein malnutrition are well known for their detrimental effects on wound healing, it seems reasonable to assume that increased insulin and a decreased need for endogenous gluconeogenic substrates provide a benefit. Ideal energy balance is met with 5 mg/kg/min of glucose.

The systemic effects of a burn wound, as mediated by cytokine release and neuroendocrine flux, are considerably more complex than the increased metabolism of a local wound. The altered interactions of glucagon and insulin affect blood glucose levels and protein metabolism while producing the hyperglycemia often seen in burns. Combining glucose and protein in enteral feeding provides a synergistic response that provides better nitrogen balance than either one alone. The effects of glucose are seen in decreased catabolism, and the effects of protein provide for the maintenance of amino acid stores. The importance of preburn protein levels has been delineated in studies looking at elderly patients who are protein deficient before burns, who have more complications postburn than matched, well-nourished patients. Current nutrition recommendations include 7 g/kg/day of glucose and about 2 g/kg/day of protein.

Once the basic components of nutrition are determined, attention is turned to the route and timing of administration. Research indicates that provision of enteral nutrition very early in the stay of a severely burned patient provides a benefit without sacrificing safety. Perhaps no organ benefits more from early enteral nutrition than the gut. Cell number, tissue mass, and the immunologic properties of the gastrointestinal tract are all improved by early enteral feeding, either intragastric or postpyloric. Manifestations of this benefit come in the form of fewer gastrointestinal bleeds and a decline in the incidence of the classic Curling ulcer. In fact, intragastric enteral feeding provides the equivalent of pharmacologic acid suppression. In the process of doing so, enteral feeding also increases splanchnic perfusion, thus providing better oxygen balance and decreased bacterial translocation. Preeminent among the reasons for enteral rather than parenteral nutrition is the protection that local maintenance of mucosal integrity provides against the perils of systemic infection, poor wound healing, and gut atrophy.

WHAT TO DO

Immediate institution of total enteral nutrition should be maintained for as long as a patient is in the hospital and has nutritional requirements that cannot be met by the patient taking an oral diet. This includes constant feeding, up to and throughout intraoperative periods, because both intraoperative and perioperative total enteral nutrition have been proven to be safe if postpyloric. Efforts to ensure supranormal nutrition should continue well past the immediate postburn period. That children who sustain large burn injuries can have persistent growth delay for up to 2 years supports the fact that energy needs are elevated for months to years after a burn appears to be adequately healing. Patients with large total body surface area burns can have a resting metabolic rate of 120% of normal even 9 months after the injury.

Similarly, periodic evaluation of the requirements for and overall effects of total enteral nutrition is recommended. Indirect calorimetry provides a noninvasive means of evaluating energy expenditure and a useful means of garnering caloric requirements. Urine urea nitrogen (UUN), a representative measurement of protein catabolism, can be used to determine the protein-sparing effectiveness of a particular regimen, and feeding goals should include a consistently positive nitrogen balance. Use of the visceral proteins such as prealbumin and transferrin is most helpful when viewed as a part of a trend and not as a point in time.

SUGGESTED READINGS

Magnotti LJ, Deitch EA. Burns, bacterial translocation, gut barrier function, and failure. J Burn Care Rehabil 2005;26(5):383–391.

Pereira CT, Herndon DN. The pharmacologic modulation of the hypermetabolic response to burns. Adv Surg 2005;39:245–261.

Raff T, Hartmann B, Germann G. Early intragastric feeding of seriously burned and long- term ventilated patients: a review of 55 patients. Burns 1997;23:19.

Rettmer RL, Williamson JC, Labbe RF, Heimbach DM. Laboratory monitoring of nutritional status in burn patients. Clin Chem 1992;38:334.

STRONGLY CONSIDER ESCHAROTOMY IN CIRCUMFERENTIAL BURNS

RICHARD WONG SHE, MBChB
JAMES H. HOLMES IV, MD

Eschar refers to relatively inelastic burned skin. An escharotomy is the procedure of "opening the eschar," either to restore or improve the perfusion to an extremity or to allow or improve ventilation when the torso is involved. Inflammatory mediators released in response to the burn injury, in combination with fluid resuscitation, result in generalized edema and third spacing. Unburned skin is elastic and can accommodate this increased soft tissue volume, whereas burned skin, particularly when the burn is a deep partial-thickness or full-thickness burn, is relatively inelastic and cannot. Thus, with time, ongoing tissue edema and swelling beneath the inelastic burn eschar results in decreased tissue perfusion and tissue compliance. Recognition of this evolving clinical situation requires a high index of suspicion and ongoing clinical assessment. The clinical manifestations of constricting eschar that mandate release depend on the site of involvement.

EXTREMITIES

In the extremities, the signs and symptoms are similar to those of compartment syndrome (which mandates fasciotomy) and are described by the well-known "p's": pain out of proportion, pain on passive flexion/extension, perishingly cold, palpably swollen, pallor, paresthesia, and pulselessness. Actual loss of a pulse is a late sign, whereas a diminished signal on Doppler exam is the hallmark. Treatment involves the release of the constricting, or rather limiting, envelope of tissue (the eschar).

The index of suspicion for the need for escharotomy should be raised in the patient who requires large fluid volumes for resuscitation because of the size of his or her burn and in the patient with a circumferential or near-circumferential deep partial-thickness or full-thickness burn. In this setting, clinical monitoring consists of assessment of capillary refill and pulses (either through palpation or Doppler ultrasound). Any change in the clinical examination suggestive of circulatory compromise should be investigated. Reversible causes of poor perfusion, namely hypothermia, hypovolemia, hypotension, and external causes of constriction (e.g., dressings) should be addressed. If poor perfusion remains, then escharotomy should be performed in the affected limb.

Escharotomies are made in the medial and lateral, midaxial lines with the limbs in the anatomic position, beginning a few millimeters proximal and ending a few millimeters distal to the extent of the burn. There is a tendency for the upper limbs to pronate and flex, which should be corrected prior to marking the lines for the escharotomy. Care should be taken around the medial epicondyle of the humerus and the head of the fibula for the ulnar and common peroneal nerves, respectively. Occasionally, release of the intermetacarpal (lumbrical) spaces dorsally is required for a hand burn. Digital escharotomies are of limited use due to the absence of ischemic-sensitive muscle within the finger and potential damage to the neurovascular bundles that run along the midaxial line of the digits.

TORSO

Circumferential chest wall burns decrease compliance, with resultant difficulties in ventilation. Children, who are predominantly diaphragmatic breathers, are at more risk of compromised ventilation even if just the anterior aspect of the chest and abdomen are involved. Increased peak ventilatory pressures and decreased compliance not responding to sedation or paralysis in these settings are indications for chest escharotomies. Escharotomies of the chest are made to create an independent "breast plate," much like a suit of armor. Incisions are made along the anterior axillary lines to the costal margins. Transverse incisions connecting these that run parallel to the costal margins can be added, if needed.

Patients requiring escharotomies typically have major burns and are intubated in the intensive care unit, so it is usually easy to produce satisfactory analgesia and sedation. Nonintubated patients may require a general anesthetic, even though the eschar is said to be insensate. The procedure can be done at the bedside as a clean (as opposed to sterile) procedure. A scalpel or electrocautery is used to cut through the eschar. The depth of the incision is through the entirety of the eschar to expose the underlying fat but not through the underlying fascia. Hemostasis is important because there can be significant blood loss from these incisions. Completeness of the escharotomy is confirmed by running a finger along the wound and addressing any residual bands of tissue. The effectiveness of the escharotomy is determined by the improvement in physiologic endpoints, namely perfusion in the limbs and ventilation in the torso. If there is no improvement in limb perfusion, consideration should be made for formal fasciotomies.

After escharotomy, dressings should prevent desiccation of the underlying subcutaneous tissue and not be so tight as to duplicate the original problem. Because these wounds are typically within the burn, they are most easily dressed with a topical antimicrobial and the usual gauze. Ultimately, the escharotomy wound will be excised along with the burn and resurfaced.

SELECTED READINGS

Hettiaratchy S, Papini R. ABC of burns. Initial management of a major burn: II. Assessment and resuscitation. BMJ 2004;329:101–103.
Kao CC, Garner WL. Acute burns. Plast Reconstr Surg 2000;104:2482–2500.

297

BE AWARE OF THE PITFALLS IN THE MANAGEMENT OF STEVENS-JOHNSON SYNDROME AND TOXIC EPIDERMAL NECROLYSIS

VIJAY A. SINGH, MD
STEPHEN M. MILNER, MD, FACS

There is controversy about the classification of Stevens-Johnson syndrome and toxic epidermal necrolysis. These rare but potentially debilitating dermatologic abnormalities have a mortality rate as high as 40%. The debate has centered on whether these conditions are related or separate entities. Current consensus is that they are variants of the same disease with differing severities, with the extent of epidermal detachment being the key component to its classification. A practical clinical classification considers less than 10% of the total body surface area involved to indicate Stevens-Johnson syndrome. If the epidermal detachment involves more than 30% of the total body surface area, then toxic epidermal necrolysis is the presumed diagnosis. An area between 10% and 30% is less definitive and is considered to represent Stevens-Johnson syndrome and toxic epidermal necrolysis overlap.

WATCH OUT FOR

A multitude of medications have been associated with the development of these conditions, but most commonly Dilantin, vancomycin, and sulfa drugs have been implicated. Suspicion should be raised in patients who have fever and constitutional symptoms for 2 to 3 days preceding a rash that appears following the administration of medication. Other prodromal signs and symptoms may include conjunctivitis, pharyngitis, and pruritus. The acute phase of the disease is characterized by persistent fever, mucositis, and generalized epidermal sloughing. The skin lesions begin as a painful or burning eruption, usually starting symmetrically on the face and thorax and spreading to the entire body. Denudation and erosions of the mucous membranes usually are corresponding. Mucositis can occur on conjunctival, buccal, tracheal, bronchial, pharyngeal, esophageal, nasal, anal, vaginal, and perineal mucosa. The skin involvement can be extensive. The erythematous skin lesions of toxic epidermal necrolysis exhibit the Nikolsky sign (slipping of the superficial skin layer induced by slight rubbing pressure).

Diagnosis is by definition histologic. Therefore, skin biopsy at the earliest possible stage is important in establishing an accurate diagnosis and directing specific therapeutic modalities. Consequently, early consultation with a dermatologist is recommended. Once diagnosis is made, therapy is mostly supportive together with cessation of any suspected medications used. Generally, treatment is most efficiently provided in an intensive care unit or a burn care center because these patients are or have the potential to be extremely ill and require mechanical ventilation, hemodynamic support, and specialized wound care. There is no definite treatment for the ailment. Given its autoimmune nature, immunoglobulin and/or steroid therapy has periodically been used with varying success. The outcomes of clinical controlled studies have yet to be determined.

SUGGESTED READING

Letko E. Stevens-Johnson syndrome and toxic epidermal necrolysis: a review of the literature. Ann Allergy Asthma Immunol 2005;94:419–436.

298

ADOPT A PHILOSOPHY OF EARLY EXCISION AND GRAFTING OF BURN WOUNDS

JEREMY W. PYLE, MD
JAMES H. HOLMES IV, MD

No measure has had a greater effect on the outcome for burn patients than the shift away from conservative management and toward early and aggressive surgical management. In the 1970s, the standard of care for burns was to perform dressing changes with daily debridements, with bacterial collagenase aiding in the thinning of the eschar and the development of granulation tissue. In due time, split-thickness skin grafts (STSG) would be applied, and a take of about 50% was expected. A gradual evolution has produced a new standard of care in terms of both resultant graft take and individual function. A 95% graft take is now the norm. Current practice has evolved around one principle: early excision of wounds and immediate coverage provides extraordinarily better results. No other intervention has reduced burn mortality as much.

Benefits of early excision and grafting include decreased length of stay, reduced costs, less time away from work or school, fewer debridements, fewer infectious wound complications, and reduced mortality. Furthermore, there is evidence to suggest that early excision and grafting leads to less intense complications when they do occur. Aesthetic and functional benefits are related to a less intense inflammatory response in the wound, which is reduced with early removal of eschar and provision of coverage.

WHAT TO DO

Timing of early excision and grafting is not exact. Many wounds benefit from 3 to 7 days of conservative management while the tissue in the zone of stasis declares itself as either viable or not. With the exception of wounds over a joint, if the tissue appears able to heal in less than 2 to 3 weeks, surgical management is likely unnecessary. Those wounds that do not require excision have a good vascular supply providing a pink or white and shiny base with rapid capillary refill. These are characteristics of superficial partial-thickness burns, which do well with local wound care and time. When indicated, as in obvious full-thickness burns, excision and grafting should be performed as soon as the patient is stabilized. Ideally, this is within 5 days and certainly within 1 week. Data suggest that morbidity, length of stay, local infection, and sepsis are more common if wounds needing excision are treated conservatively beyond 1 week.

Tangential and fascial excisions are the two well-accepted methods of burn wound excision. Although each has a place in current standards, tangential excisions constitute the majority of procedures. Tangential, also called sequential, excision represents a strategy that conserves as much of the native tissue as possible. Risks involved with this approach hinge on the intense blood loss that can occur. The procedure uses a hand dermatome to remove thin layers of eschar and unhealthy tissue. If removal of one layer provides an adequately vascular surface, then the excision is done. If the wound bed appears dry or gray or if thrombosed vessels are still readily apparent, excision must continue. Excision ends with the removal of all dead tissue. Hemostasis is accomplished with epinephrine (1:10,000)-soaked pads covering fresh excision sites, followed by careful electrocautery to actively bleeding vessels. Fascial excision represents the second major method of burn wound excision. Dissecting down to a fascial plane with electrocautery provides a consistent and viable wound bed for grafting. Fascial excision can significantly decrease operative blood loss while removing some of the guesswork in evaluating effective excision. Disadvantages to this technique include longer operative time, greater damage to superficial neurovascular structures and lymph passages, and inferior cosmesis that can result from obvious tissue deficits.

WHAT TO DO NEXT

Both excision techniques are immediately followed by reconstructive efforts, whenever possible. Evaluation of the wound bed and the expected overall course of the patient help to dictate where and when definitive coverage is attempted. When feasible, STSG to the entire wound is ideal. When the problem of limited donor sites arises, skin substitutes are commonly used. Most common among these are the dermal substitutes Integra, AlloDerm, and Dermagraft. Their primary purpose is to serve as a dermal replacement allowing thinner grafts to survive over them; secondarily they provide a temporary means of partially closing a wound. Using a thin STSG (<0.010 in.) allows donor sites to be more frequently reharvested. AlloDerm is cryopreserved allogeneic dermis that has been stripped of its dermal elements, thereby allowing native fibroblast infiltration and the eventual development of a stable dermis. Integra consists of a deep, porous collagen-chondroitin 6-sulfate fibrillar layer covered with a removable layer of silicone. The fibrillar layer provides scaffolding for ingress of autogenous fibroblasts and subsequent creation of a "neo-dermis." The thin silicone layer is a temporary epidermis and is extirpated after vascularization when ultimate coverage is applied. Integra is the most studied of the dermal substitutes. Dermagraft is a culture of human neonatal fibroblasts on a layer of Biobrane. Traditional wisdom has been that Alloderm can be immediately covered with graft, whereas Integra and Dermagraft should be allowed to vascularize for about 14 days before placing a graft.

Once applied, there are multiple means of securing grafts. For decades, staples/sutures with a bolster dressing has been the dressing of choice because it helps to mechanically secure the graft and inhibit seroma or hematoma formation, thereby eliminating three of the most common causes for graft failure. The advent of negative-pressure dressings (e.g., VAC ^{TM} by KCI USA, Inc., San Antonio, TX) has provided a means of limiting shear forces, fluid collections, bridging, and bacterial contamination while increasing granulation tissue formation, vascularity, oxygen tension, and thus more rapid re-epithelialization of wounds than with bolster dressings. Negative-pressure dressings are applied at the time of excision and grafting and removed 4 to 5 days later. A single layer of a nonadherent dressing is applied between the graft and the negative-pressure dressing to keep the two easily separable.

Much experimental work has been done on the use of cultured autografts for coverage of extensively burned individuals. The U.S. Food and Drug Administration has approved one cultured epithelial autograft. Epicel requires a full-thickness biopsy of a patient's skin and 2 to 3 weeks to grow. Use is significantly limited by its tremendous cost and legitimate questions of graft durability.

SUGGESTED READINGS

Atiyeh BS, Hayek SN, Gunn SW. New technologies for burn wound closure and healing. Review of the literature. Burns 2005;31(8):944–956.

Barret JP, Herndon DN. Effects of burn wound excision on bacterial colonization and invasion. Plast Reconstr Surg 2003;111(2):744–750; discussion 751–752.

Thourani VH, Ingram EL, Feliciano DV. Factors affecting success of split-thickness skin grafts in the modern burn unit. J Trauma 2003;54(3):562–568.

www.woundvac.com

BE AGGRESSIVE IN MOBILIZING BURN WOUNDS

DANA NAKAMURA, OT
JAMES H. HOLMES IV, MD

Burn patients in the intensive care unit should be seen on admission by the physical and occupational therapy team. *The key to successful rehabilitation is early intervention.* Scarring is virtually inevitable with major burns and therapy is integral to limiting its effect on patient outcomes. Initial assessments include determination of positioning and splinting needs, range of motion (ROM) and strength, prior level of functional mobility and activity independence, cognition, and ability to learn/participate in the therapy program. Early interventions include positioning and splinting, edema management, exercise, functional mobility/activity retraining, and patient/family education. Early intervention and anticipation of potential complications are critical to optimizing functional outcome. *All* members of the burn team need to be able to anticipate potential complications to be proactive and take a preventative approach to treating burn patients. Staff education with training in the roles of all team members and daily collaboration are important for smooth carryover of treatment plans.

Communication of therapy plans is vitally important so that all staff involved in the patient's care understand the techniques and procedures used and the rationale for such. Patient and family education is also important to facilitate understanding of the therapy process and build rapport for a therapeutic relationship. It is imperative to communicate that "therapy" needs to continue 24-7 because the healing and scarring process is a continuous and relentless one. Communication can occur by a number of ways such as one-on-one teaching, in-services, written information in the medical record, on-line documentation, and photos/diagrammed instructions on bedside boards.

POSITIONING AND SPLINTING

Positioning goals are to minimize edema, prevent tissue destruction, and maintain soft tissue in an elongated state to facilitate functional recovery. Likewise, splinting prevents loss of motion and deformity, promotes functional independence, protects anatomic structures, preserves skin graft integrity, and restores function. The methods used must prevent contracture and deformity but not compromise the patient's mobility and function. Individual programs are developed based on the patient's medical status, range of motion, location of burn, burn depth, and level of cooperation. It should always be stressed that the "position of comfort = position of contracture" when determining appropriate positioning and splinting programs. Frequent positioning checks and splint fit assessments are required to prevent misalignment and pressure sore complications.

EXERCISE

Frequent exercises and movement are critical. Treatment with the therapist once or twice a day for 30 to 60 minutes is not sufficient. Patients who are awake and able to participate are instructed in self-range of motion exercises to stretch the affected body part and skin. The benefits of exercise include preservation of range of motion, functional strength, endurance, and coordination; activation of the muscle pump action for edema mobilization; prevention of venous thromboembolism; endorphin release; and psychological well being including feelings of having some sense of control in a new and often chaotic medical setting.

FUNCTIONAL MOBILITY

Ambulation is critical to preserve skin flexibility, muscle strength, and tendon/ligament length. Many times, physicians automatically write admit orders for "bed rest." Nursing and therapy staff members need to assess the individual situation and question the bed rest order because being confined to bed just contributes to complications such as heterotopic ossification, venous thromboembolism, muscle wasting, and pressure sores. Ventilator-dependent patients are also mobilized in bed or to "cardiac" chairs and at some burn centers are ambulated with respiratory therapy, nursing, and occupational/physical therapy collaborating. Continued mobilization in some form is critical during ventilator support because it prevents/reduces respiratory complications.

FUNCTIONAL ACTIVITY

All self-care activities are considered exercise, especially if the hands or upper extremities are involved. Play activities for both pediatric and adult patients are also important, whether it be shooting a basketball, playing cards or a board game, bouncing a ball, or assembling a puzzle/building blocks. Many burn centers have a child life specialist or therapeutic recreation specialist who can assist with such activities. Pet therapy programs are beneficial for social visits with a therapy dog, hands-on therapy with walking the dog on a leash for balance and gait training, and brushing/grooming or playing fetch for arm range of motion.

SUGGESTED READINGS

Campbell SK, ed. Physical Therapy for Children. Philadelphia: WB. Saunders, 1994: 763–786.

Robinson LR, ed. Trauma Rehabilitation. Philadelphia: Lippincott Williams & Wilkins, 2006:181–204.

300

HAVE A LOW THRESHOLD FOR INTUBATING A PATIENT WITH AN INHALATION BURN INJURY

RICHARD WONG SHE, MBCHB
JAMES H. HOLMES IV, MD

A burn patient with an inhalation injury has twice the mortality rate of a similar burn patient without an inhalation injury. Initial presentation may be essentially asymptomatic because time (and resuscitation fluid) is required to generate the edema and alveolar damage, which will manifest as progressive airway obstruction and disturbances in pulmonary function. The mainstay of treatment for inhalation injuries involves securing the airway *prior* to obstruction and maintaining ventilation while minimizing lung damage. Inhalation injury can result from a combination of three mechanisms. First, direct thermal injury to the upper airway can be caused by superheated gases or aspiration of hot liquids. Hot liquids result in rapid edema formation and require emergent intubation if suspected. By contrast, superheated gases result in relatively gradual edema formation. Second, products of combustion can dissolve in the mucus of the lower airway, resulting in a chemical pneumonitis and alveolar damage, which develops over hours to days. Finally, systemic poisoning can result from the absorption of carbon monoxide (CO). This poisoning should be suspected in all inhalation injuries. A carboxyhemoglobin level should be measured on initial evaluation of the patient. Humidified 100% oxygen is the treatment of choice because it decreases the half-life of carboxyhemoglobin from 250 minutes on room air respiration to around 40 minutes. There is a limited role for hyperbaric oxygen. Supplemental oxygenation should continue for up to 48 h after normalization because there can be delayed release of CO from the intracellular cytochrome system.

SIGNS AND SYMPTOMS

Diagnosis of an inhalation injury requires a high index of suspicion based on a combination of the history and physical findings. A history of being trapped in a confined space with a fire is highly suggestive. By contrast, a flash fire, even when associated with singed nasal hairs, is typically not associated with an inhalation injury. Symptoms and signs of an inhalation injury include a facial burn, soot around the nose and mouth, intraoral soot or burns, singed facial and nasal hair, carbonaceous sputum, a hoarse voice, inspiratory stridor or increased work of breathing, and CO poisoning, which may present with signs as subtle as an altered level of consciousness or a decreased ratio of mean alveolar oxygen pressure to fraction of oxygen in the inspired air. Although confirmation of an inhalation injury can be achieved with nasopharyngoscopy, laryngoscopy, or bronchoscopy, these invasive diagnostic tests do not influence the outcome of an inhalation injury.

Prophylactic intubation of a suspected inhalation injury is preferable to waiting for eventual airway compromise from edema. Emergent intubation in these circumstances can be challenging. In addition, if the patient is to be transported to a regional burn center, it is better that the airway be secured before transport. A controlled extubation on arrival is better than an emergent intubation en route. During intubation, the presence of mucosal involvement and carbonaceous deposits should be noted.

With inhalation injuries, deterioration in pulmonary function can take several days to occur. The treatment of an inhalation injury is supportive. The goal is to maximize oxygenation/ventilation while minimizing alveolar damage, thus allowing the lungs to heal themselves sufficiently for extubation. Prophylactic steroids and antibiotics have no role. Bronchospasm should be treated with bronchodilators. Small airway obstruction can occur secondary to debris and slough liberated from the airways. Aggressive pulmonary toilet is essential. Nebulized heparin and N-acetyl cystine may be useful, especially in children. Subsequent pulmonary infection can occur, either as pneumonia or as a purulent tracheobronchitis. Bronchoalveolar lavage may help to quantify and identify organisms to be specifically treated. Ventilator strategies for maintaining oxygenation while minimizing airway pressures include lung-protective ventilation, permissive hypercapnia, high-frequency percussive ventilation, nitric oxide, and even extracorporeal support. Prolonging survival permits spontaneous lung recovery and finally extubation.

SELECTED READINGS

Ansermino M, Hemsley C. ABC of burns; intensive care management and control of infection. BMJ 2004;329:220–223.

Sheridan RL. Airway management and respiratory care of the burn patient. Int Anesthesiol Clin 2000;38(3):129–145.

301

DO NOT UNDER-RESUSCITATE A BURN PATIENT

OLIVER A. VARBAN, MD
JAMES H. HOLMES IV, MD

Thermal injuries result in the release of cytokines and other inflammatory mediators at the site of injury. These mediators have a systemic effect once the burn reaches about 30% of the total body surface area (TBSA). Among the cardiovascular effects, there is a loss of microvascular integrity, causing intravascular fluid to leak into the interstitial space. Peripheral and splanchnic vasoconstriction also occurs, and myocardial contractility has been shown to decrease, possibly due to a release of tumor necrosis factor-α. The end result is burn shock: systemic hypotension and end-organ hypoperfusion. The metabolic rate may also increase up to three times its basal rate, furthering the demand for tissue perfusion. In addition, a concomitant inhalation injury will typically increase resuscitation fluid requirements.

It has been shown that maintaining adequate intravascular volume is important to perfuse vital organs and may also limit the depth/extent of a burn. Use of crystalloid alone, specifically lactated Ringer's solution (LR), is a safe and effective way to resuscitate burn patients during the first 24 h after injury. Using the Parkland-Baxter formula, 4 mL LR × weight (kg) × %TBSA burn, one can estimate the total volume of lactated Ringer's solution needed in the first 24 h after thermal injury. Because the increase in capillary permeability is greatest over the first 8 h after injury, half of the volume of lactated Ringer's solution as calculated by the Parkland-Baxter formula is given over the first 8 hours *from the time of injury* and the remainder is given over the subsequent 16 hours. An accurate assessment of burn depth and %TBSA is important for the Parkland-Baxter formula to be effective. The "rule of nines" is commonly used as a quick bedside assessment to estimate TBSA: each arm is about 9% of the TBSA, each leg is about 18%, the anterior trunk is about 18%, the posterior trunk is about 18%, and the head is about 9%, with the perineum encompassing the remaining approximately 1%. Children have greater evaporative losses because they have vastly different body proportions and a greater percentage of total body water. Thus, age-appropriate diagrams (e.g., Lund-Browder or Berkow) are more accurate in determining the TBSA burned in children.

Example. A 70-kg adult with a 40% burn requires 11,200 mL (4 × 70 × 40) over 24 h from the time of injury, with 5,600 mL being given in the first 8 h from the time of injury and 5,600 mL being given in the subsequent 16 h.

It should be stressed that any resuscitation formula only provides an estimate for required fluids. Objective parameters such as urine output (0.5 cc/kg for adults and 1.0 cc/kg for children) or blood pressure should be used to adjust fluid needs. Mean arterial pressure (MAP) and urine output are considered to be the most reliable measures of adequate tissue perfusion for burn resuscitation. A MAP maintained above 60 mm Hg typically ensures adequate cerebral perfusion. Hypotension or decreased urine output should be treated by judiciously increasing the resuscitation fluid rate and not by bolusing fluids because boluses will only increase the volume of the capillary leak, resulting in worse edema. There is no consistent evidence to support the use of pulmonary arterial catheter measurements for routine resuscitation. In fact, their use may lead to over-resuscitation and subsequent complications. Nonetheless, invasive hemodynamic monitoring may be necessary in patients with significant premorbid cardiovascular, pulmonary, or renal disease.

WHAT TO DO

Delay in burn resuscitation has unequivocally been shown to increase mortality rates. Intravenous access is vital and may be obtained by placing two large-bore peripheral intravenous lines (16 to 18 gauge) or, less commonly, a central venous line. Venous cut-downs are to be avoided, given the high incidence of infection with them. Lactated Ringer's solution is the most common crystalloid solution used during resuscitation in the United States. Hypertonic saline has been advocated by some centers, but has not been shown to decrease fluid requirements. *Normal saline should never be used to resuscitate burn patients* because the volumes required will precipitate a severe hyperchloremic metabolic acidosis. Albumin is not advised in the early postburn resuscitation period because it simply passes out into the tissues, causing greater tissue edema. Glucose should be administered in children typically weighing less than 20 kg to prevent hypoglycemia because they have relatively diminished glycogen stores. This may be accomplished either intravenously in the form of weight-based dextrose-containing maintenance fluids (in addition to resuscitation lactated Ringer's volumes) or enterally in the form of total enteral nutrition.

Use of diuretics and inotropes should be avoided because they will not stop the capillary leak and may lead to ischemia of the wound, possibly resulting in conversion of a partial-thickness to a full-thickness wound or extension of the TBSA of the wound. Patients with myoglobinuria require increased volumes of fluid or mannitol to maintain urine output of 100 cc/h or greater. As the capillary leak resolves at about 24 hours after injury, the amount of fluid needed to maintain an appropriate MAP and urine output decreases. Colloids (albumin) may be used to facilitate resuscitation in a patient with persistent low urine output and/or hypotension after the first 24 hours. With colloids, the formula used is 0.3 to 0.5 cc/kg/%TBSA burned over 24 hours; 5% albumin is typically used. If the patient continues to have inadequate urine output and MAP or his or her required resuscitation volumes greatly exceed the estimated volumes, plasmapheresis may be used because there is a theoretical advantage to removing inflammatory mediators that cause vasodilation and capillary leak.

It is well known that inadequate resuscitation results in decreased tissue perfusion with subsequent multiorgan failure and increased mortality. However, over-resuscitation also exposes patients to complications. These include compartment syndromes involving the abdomen or extremities, pulmonary edema, and pleural effusions. Abdominal compartment syndrome decreases lung compliance and also impedes lung expansion, thus causing elevated airway pressures and hypoventilation. The classic presentation includes high peak airway pressures, decreased venous return, oliguria, and intra-abdominal pressures exceeding 25 mm Hg. Abdominal compartment syndrome is largely avoidable via a judicious resuscitation with close monitoring. If abdominal compartment syndrome occurs, decompressive laparotomy is the only proven effective treatment in adults, whereas children may respond to paracentesis.

WHAT TO DO NEXT

After resuscitation has been completed, ongoing fluid administration should be continued to replace insensible losses that are associated with the burn itself and the evolving hyperdynamic state. Maintenance fluid requirements in the burned patient are classically 1.5 times those of nonburned individuals. Administration of fluids may be continued intravenously; however, the preferable route is enteral. These should be in addition to and combined with total enteral nutrition support. Daily weighings can help to measure and assess ongoing insensible fluid loss or fluid retention.

SUGGESTED READINGS

Bessey PQ. Metabolic response to critical illness. In: American College of Surgeons: Principles and Practice. Chicago: American College of Surgeons, 2006: www.acssurgery.com

Gibran NS, Heimbach DM. Management of the patient with thermal injuries. In: American College of Surgeons: Principles and Practice. Chicago: American College of Surgeons, 2006: www.acssurgery.com

302

AVOID THE PITFALLS OF VASCULAR ACCESS IN BURN PATIENTS

MYRON S. POWELL, MD
JAMES H. HOLMES IV, MD

A burn patient with less than 50% total body surface area (TBSA) involved can usually begin resuscitation via two large-bore peripheral lines. With burns of greater than 50% TBSA or in patients with severe premorbid diseases, central venous access is typically needed. Vascular access should ideally be established early in the course of injury before the formation of significant edema. If resuscitation is inadequate, burn shock may lead to multiorgan dysfunction/failure syndrome, which almost invariably results in a fatal outcome.

WHAT TO DO

When obtaining vascular access on a burn patient, there are numerous options with their individual benefits, risks, and complications. Placement through unburned tissue, all things being equal, is preferable to placement through burned tissue; that is, an intravenous line should be placed through the right antecubital space in the setting of a left antecubital burn. Peripheral lines in the upper extremities are optimal; however, cut-downs are contraindicated, given the inordinate infection rate associated with them. Any line may be placed through burned tissue, if necessary, but lines through eschar should be removed within 72 hours, given the high colonization and infection rates beyond that time period. Central venous catheters are beneficial for those requiring prolonged treatments with large volumes of fluids (i.e., large burns or inhalation injury), invasive hemodynamic monitoring, total parenteral nutrition, or certain medications. Theoretically, peripherally inserted central catheters avoid some of the disadvantages of classical central lines, but their efficacy and place in the management of the severely burned patient have yet to be clinically defined.

The risks associated with placement of a vascular access device somewhat depend on the insertion site; however, they all include bleeding, infection, and injury to adjacent structures. These risks can be minimized by correcting coagulopathies, carefully maintaining sterile technique and caring for the insertion sites, and adhering to sound surgical principles. Nonetheless, an infection may still develop. Catheter-related bloodstream infection (CRBSI) risk in burn patients is theoretically less when obtaining central venous access above the diaphragm (i.e., via the internal jugular or subclavian veins). Furthermore, catheter-induced deep venous thrombosis appears to be more common with femoral lines than with other sites. About 1% of patients develop a pneumothorax from central line placement when using a vein in the chest or the neck. Changing central venous catheters on a set schedule does not reduce infection rates nor does it predict the rate of bacterial contamination of the catheter. In fact, it only exposes patients to increased complication rates. Central lines should only be changed when infection is clinically suspected.

In situations involving an inhalation injury or burns of greater than 50% TBSA, invasive hemodynamic monitoring is typically required, necessitating both venous and arterial vascular access. For serial arterial blood gas sampling, invasive blood pressure monitoring, and routine lab draws, arterial access is ideal. The radial artery is the preferred site for several reasons. It has an easily detectable pulse that lies relatively superficial to the overlying skin. Ischemic complications are low with cannulation of the radial artery secondary to collateral flow via the ulnar artery and the superficial/deep palmar arches; however, these collaterals are absent in 5% to 7% of the population. There are other sites for obtaining arterial access, but they have specific disadvantages compared with the radial artery. The femoral artery may be cannulated; however, access in the groin carries a theoretical increased risk of infection. The brachial artery is another option but often provides inaccurate readings, risk of median nerve injury, and risk of ischemia due to lack of collaterals. The axillary artery has a significant risk of injury to the brachial plexus due to its proximity.

SUGGESTED READINGS

Ramos GE, Bolgiani AN, Patino O, et al. Catheter infection risk related to the distance between insertion site and burned area. J Burn Care Rehab 2002;23(4):266–271.

Sheridan R, Nackel A, Lydon M, et al. Infradiaphragmatic central venous pressures reflect supradiaphragmatic pressures in stable burn patients. J Trauma Injury Infect Crit Care 1999;47(2):300–302.

Still JM, Law E, Thiruvaiyaru D, et al. Central line–related sepsis in acute burn patients. Am Surg 1998;64(2):165–170.

303

KNOW HOW TO ESTIMATE BURN SIZE AND DEPTH

JOHN ZANNIS, MD
JAMES H. HOLMES IV, MD

Estimating the severity of a burn is important in treating these complicated yet common injuries. Burns constitute the third-leading cause of trauma deaths in the United States and more than 2.4 million Americans are treated for burns each year. Scalding is the most common cause of thermal injury in both adults and children. House fires, although accounting for only 5% of adults treated, are responsible for greater than 40% of the adult deaths.

Careful initial evaluation and wound management is critical to the treatment of burns. Aside from patient resuscitation, proper management begins with estimating the severity of a burn, including depth and size. The ability to do this requires a basic understanding of skin anatomy and physiology.

The skin is composed of epidermis, dermis, and subcutaneous fat. The epidermal layer provides a vapor and bacterial barrier. The dermal layer provides flexibility and strength. It also contains the dermal appendages that produce oils, terminal capillaries for thermoregulation, and nerve endings. These functions are compromised after the skin suffers a burn injury. Assessing which of these layers are affected by a particular burn is often difficult to accomplish in the acute setting. Early burn depth estimates are most accurate in very deep or very superficial wounds.

SUPERFICIAL BURNS (FIRST DEGREE)

A superficial burn is limited to the epidermis. It is characterized by pain, heat, and reddening of the burned surface but does not show blistering or charring of tissue. Superficial burns heal in approximately 5 days by epidermal regeneration and do not scar. Typical superficial burns include sunburn and hot water scalds.

PARTIAL-THICKNESS BURNS (SECOND DEGREE)

The epidermis and dermis are involved in partial-thickness burns. Blistering occurs at the epidermal-dermal junction. The skin appears pink or cherry red, moist, and weepy to mottled white. These burns are typically very painful and exhibit intense swelling. Healing of superficial, partial-thickness burns occurs without scarring or contracture in 10 to 21 days.

FULL-THICKNESS BURNS (THIRD DEGREE)

Full-thickness burns extend deeply into the dermis and destroy sensory nerve endings. The tissue damage extends below hair follicles and sweat glands to subcutaneous (fat) tissue. With this degree of burn, the skin becomes charred and leathery. Initially, the skin can be bright red, waxy white, tan, or brown; there are no blisters, and massive swelling is common. Full-thickness burns are usually not painful because the injury has destroyed nerve endings. Hair pulls out easily. Skin grafting and/or other coverage options are required for treatment of a full-thickness burn.

FOURTH-DEGREE BURNS

This is a term sometimes used to describe very deep burns that involve underlying structures such as muscle, bone, tendon, and/or ligament. Surface appearance and other characteristics are similar to those of third-degree burns.

In addition to burn depth, the severity of a burn is determined by the size or body surface area affected. An accurate assessment of burn size can be made early in the patient's evaluation and is an important factor in determining resuscitative fluid administration. There are several methods that can be used to estimate the percentage of body surface area burned. The most widely used method for rapid assessment is the "rule of nines," which states that the front torso, back, and each lower extremity represents 18% total body surface area (TBSA). Each upper limb and the head represent 9% TBSA. The perineum equals 1% TBSA. Small burns or scattered wounds can also be rapidly measured using the patient's palmar surface, which represents 1% TBSA. Although the rule of nines is helpful, it is less accurate than other methods of estimating burn extent. This is particularly true with children, whose body proportions change with growth. The infant head represents 18% and the legs 14% of TBSA (in contrast to 9% and 18%, respectively, in the adult). Therefore, burn size in children is best estimated using an age-specific chart such as the Lund and Browder Chart.

Along with burn depth and size, it is important to note any circumferential components to burns of the extremities, neck, and torso. Such burns may lead to compromise of peripheral circulation and a compartment syndrome in an extremity or difficulty with ventilation in the neck or torso.

It is very difficult to predict mortality in burned patients. Age older than 60 years, full-thickness burns over 40% of TBSA, and inhalation injury are significant prognostic factors. A formula has been proposed stating that percentage mortality = age + percentage TBSA burned. However, more recent studies have shown that there is no reliable method for predicting survival on admission.

SUGGESTED READINGS

Heimbach D, Engrav L, Grube B, et al. Burn depth: a review. World J Surg 1992;16: 10–15.

Mulholland M, Lillemoe KD, Doherty GM, et al. Greenfield's Surgery: Scientific Principles and Practice, 4th ed. Philadelphia: Lippincott Williams & Wilkins, 2005.

Saffle JR, Davis B, Williams P, et al. Recent outcomes in the treatment of burn injury in the United States: a report from the American Burn Association Patient Registry. J Burn Care Rehabil 1995;16(3 Pt 1):219–232; discussion 288–289.

304

Do not talk to families about organ donation

Matthew J. Weiss, MD

Solid-organ transplantation is the therapy of choice for patients with end-organ failure. Despite numerous advances in the field, the number of individuals awaiting transplantation continues to exceed the supply of organs. One approach to increasing the supply of organs is to maximize donation rates of eligible patients. Family consent rates for donation are currently only 30% to 40%. Although families decline donation for many reasons, it is indisputable that there are myths believed to be true by families that do not aid in increasing the donation rate: patients will be prematurely declared dead to "get better organs," the organ allocation system is corrupt, and rich people "get the good organs." Particularly damaging is the perception that the physician caring for a loved one may have allegiance to a future organ recipient. This can compromise the trust necessary for increasing donation rates. Therefore, it is important that physicians caring for the potential donor do not discuss donation with the family. During the last hours of life, the physician caring for the potential donor must continue to provide aggressive care. The donor family must understand and believe that everything has been done for their loved one.

However, all families of potential donors must be approached for consent. For heart-beating donors, discussions should be initiated in a private setting as early as possible after declaration of brain death. A member of the hospital team should be present to answer medical questions after and a trained organ procurement organization (OPO) representative should approach the family. Many states have enacted legislation that requires health professionals to notify their regional OPO of potential candidates and very likely the OPO representative will be familiar with the possible donor several hours before death is declared. OPO representatives are trained to effectively communicate with donor families, and studies clearly demonstrate their success in increasing procurement rates over those of physicians on the care team. In addition, these representatives exercise innovative approaches to minority families, who are historically less likely to agree to donation.

SUGGESTED READINGS

Razek T, Olthoff K, Reilly PM. Issues in potential organ donor management. Surg Clin North Am 2000;80:1021–1032.

Siminoff LA, Gordon N, Hewlett J, et al. Factors influencing families' consent for donation of solid organs for transplantation. JAMA 2001;286(4):71–77.

305

ALERT THE TRANSPLANT TEAM EMERGENTLY IF THERE IS AN ACUTE DECREASE IN URINE OUTPUT AFTER A KIDNEY TRANSPLANT

MATTHEW J. WEISS, MD

The postoperative management of a kidney transplant recipient requires meticulous monitoring of urine output and electrolyte levels. Renal allografts will not necessarily make urine as soon as they are reperfused. Depending on the particular center, the incidence of delayed graft function ranges from 5% to 15% in cadaveric and from 0% to 5% in live donor kidney transplantation. The astute clinician will query the patient as to how much urine was produced pretransplant so as not to be lulled into a false assurance that the graft is functioning because "there is urine."

Although no physician can predict the postoperative urine output of a kidney recipient with 100% certainty, there are several factors that consistently contribute to delayed graft function. Cadaveric donors, increased age of donors, ethnicity of donors, diabetic donors, prolonged warm and cold ischemia, and ischemia/reperfusion injury are all risk factors for delayed graft failure resulting from acute tubular necrosis. It must be remembered that delayed graft function begins at the time of organ reperfusion and the urine output begins and remains low and does not change abruptly.

Acute changes in urine output in a functioning graft can be a signal that a catastrophic insult has occurred to the graft and must be reported to the transplant team immediately. Several causes of acute decreases in urine output are surgical complications and are correctable if prompt attention is appropriated. A list of technical causes of low urine output includes renal artery/vein thrombosis or kinking, ureteral obstruction, and compression of the graft by a fluid collection (hematoma, lymphocele, seroma, or urinary leak). Hypovolemia can also cause oliguria as in other postoperative patients. Vascular, urologic and lymphatic complications require prompt diagnosis and treatment to salvage the graft. The workup of decreased urine output often depends on institution and transplant team, but usually consists of ultrasound, color flow Doppler, or radionuclide imaging of the graft. An ultrasound is invaluable in this situation because it can be performed quickly at the bedside and can evaluate for both vascular compromise and fluid collections. However, the call to the transplant team must not be delayed while waiting for ultrasound results.

SUGGESTED READINGS

Halloran PF, Hunsicker LG. Delayed graft function: state of the art, November 10–11, 2000. Am J Transplant 2001;1:115–120.

Humar A, Leone JP, Matas AJ. Kidney transplantation: a brief review. Front Biosci 1997;2:41–47.

306

REMEMBER THAT CARDIAC OUTPUT IS NOT THE SAME THING AS EJECTION FRACTION

FRANK ROSEMEIER, MD

Cardiac output equals the volume of blood pumped by the heart per minute, whereas stroke volume (SV) is the amount pumped on a single beat. Cardiac output can be determined using indicator dilution methods (Fick, thermodilution), Doppler velocity data, ventricular impedance, and radionucleotide methods. Ejection fraction (EF) is measured in percent: EF (%) = (SV/EDV) × 100%; whereas SV is calculated as SV = EDV − ESV, with EDV the end-diastolic volume and ESV the end-systolic volume. Ejection fraction is typically estimated using qualitative two-dimensional echocardiography. However, the accuracy depends on the observer experience. Inadequate definition of the endocardial border and regional wall motion abnormalities with asymmetric ventricular contraction may lead to inaccuracies, which may be overcome by various yet time-consuming ventricular volume formulas.

WATCH OUT FOR

Although a satisfactory ejection fraction would suggest a similar adequate cardiac output, this relationship does not always hold true. In mitral regurgitation, ejection fraction can be excellent, yet part of the left ventricular end-diastolic volume is ejected back into the left atrium via the incompetent mitral valve during ventricular systole. In this scenario, ejection fraction can be normal, yet cardiac output is diminished. In contrast, cardiac output is supranormal in aortic incompetence, but part of the forward stroke volume regurgitates back into the left ventricle during ventricular diastole. As the disease progresses, heart failure will develop with a reduction of ejection fraction pseudonormalizing cardiac output, eventually reaching a point at which both hemodynamic parameters are severely depressed. Regurgitant volume and regurgitant fraction are used in grading the severity of these valvular lesions, adding more valuable information to the assessment of cardiac function. Temperature thermodilution methods for cardiac output determination remain accurate because these are typically measured in the pulmonary artery using a Swan-Ganz catheter and right-sided cardiac output must equal left-sided cardiac output.

SUGGESTED READINGS

Fink MP, Abrahams E, Vincent J, et al., eds. Textbook of Critical Care, 5th ed. Philadelphia: Elsevier Saunders, 2005:735–740.

Savage RM, Aronson S, eds. Comprehensive Textbook of Intraoperative Transesophageal Echocardiography. Philadelphia: Lippincott Williams & Wilkins, 2005:129–146.

307

Do not "rock the pelvis" in a fracture

J. Christopher DiGiacomo, MD

Pelvic fractures from blunt force trauma are broadly categorized as either "stable" or "unstable" based on the status of the pelvic ring. The pelvis is composed of three bones (the iliopubic bones and the sacrum), which are held together by strong ligaments: the symphysis pubis anteriorly and the anterior and posterior iliosacral ligament posterolaterally. A pelvic fracture is generally considered unstable if the ring is broken in two or more places.

The unstable pelvic fracture is sometimes identified during the secondary survey, when the pelvis is noted to "move" during either anteroposterior or lateral compression on physical examination. More commonly, today it is detected on plain radiograph or abdominal computed tomography (CT). However an unstable pelvic fracture is identified, once the diagnosis has been made, all further manual manipulation (i.e., "rocking the pelvis") must cease. Although it is tempting to use an unstable pelvic exam as a prime teaching point, the unstable pelvis should not be manipulated. Each time the damaged joint is moved, the clot may be disrupted, resulting in additional bleeding from the torn veins and bony surfaces. Consumption coagulopathy may occur as coagulation factors are used for new clot formation.

Unstable pelvic fractures include disruption of the ring anteriorly at the symphysis pubis or through a pubic bone and are broadly categorized into three types: anterior-posterior (open-book) fracture, lateral compression fracture, and vertical shear (Malgaigne) fracture.

Anterior-Posterior (Open-Book) Fracture

This type of injury typically occurs after an anterior-posterior blunt force injury to the pelvis, in which the anterior ring fracture is accompanied by disruption of the anterior iliosacral ligaments (*Fig. 307.1*). With the stability of the anterior ring lost, the pelvis opens anteriorly and laterally and the iliac bones hinge on the posterior pelvic ligaments, much as a book opens around its spine. This disrupts the iliosacral joint and the veins that lie anterior to the iliosacral joint. This results in a large amount of venous and bony bleeding into the

Anterior

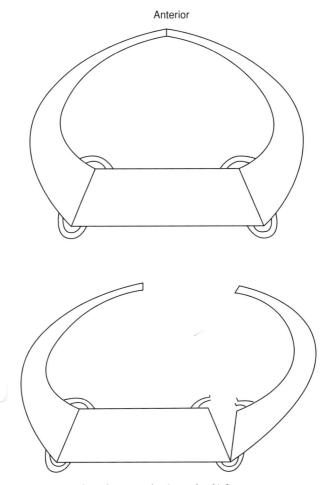

FIGURE 307.1. Anterior-posterior (open-book) fracture.

retroperitoneal space. Approximately 10% of patients have associated arterial bleeding. Initial stabilization should be in the form of external binding of the pelvis with a bed sheet tied tightly around the pelvis or a pelvic binder device.

LATERAL COMPRESSION FRACTURE

This type of injury typically occurs after lateral blunt force injury to the pelvis, such as a in a pedestrian struck by a car (*Fig. 307.2*). The

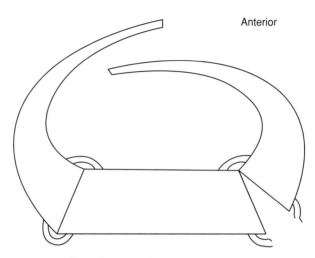

Anterior

FIGURE 307.2. Lateral compression fracture.

anterior ring fracture is accompanied by disruption of the posterior iliosacral ligaments. The iliac bones hinge on the anterior iliosacral ligaments. Venous and bony bleeding from the disrupted iliosacral joint tends to be extrapelvic. In this type of fracture, attempted stabilization with a sheet or external binder will only promote further inward collapse of the iliac bones and cause increased bleeding. External fixation of the pelvis or open reduction and internal fixation (ORIF) is preferable.

VERTICAL SHEAR (MALGAIGNE) FRACTURE

This type of injury typically occurs when a large vertical load is placed on one leg, such as in a fall from height (*Fig. 307.3*). The iliac bones are completely separated from the remainder of the pelvis by disruption of the anterior ring and both the anterior and posterior iliosacral ligaments. Venous and bony bleeding is not contained within the pelvis, and arterial bleeding must be ruled out. Initial stabilization requires traction on the injured side leg to reduce the vertical displacement, followed by external binding of the pelvis. This fracture type carries the highest mortality rate due to exsanguination.

The initial management of pelvic fractures follows the paradigm of the ABCs of trauma resuscitation. After the airway (A) and breathing (B) are considered, circulation and control of hemorrhage (C) are

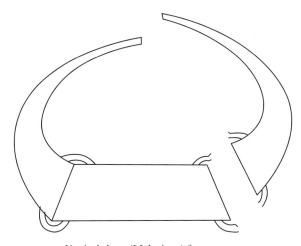

FIGURE 307.3. Vertical shear (Malgaigne) fracture.

imperative. Adequate volume resuscitation is essential, and blood should be administered early to the hemodynamically unstable or metastable patient. The pelvic x-ray will provide essential details about the bony injury that are crucial early in the resuscitation phase. Trauma and orthopedic surgical consultations should be obtained for immediate evaluation. Abdominal and pelvic CT scans with intravenous contrast are performed to assess for other injuries and further define the pelvic fracture. It is important that the pelvic portion be reviewed by the physician in attendance of the patient immediately, looking for arterial extravasation of intravenous contrast. The finding of arterial extravasation warrants immediate arteriography with therapeutic angioembolization. Operative attempts to control such bleeding are usually unsuccessful. Bleeding from other solid-organ injuries (e.g., liver, spleen, kidney) can also be addressed at the time of angiography.

If laparotomy is necessary, an external fixator should be applied prior to the abdominal procedure. The bracing arms should be directed toward the feet instead of being placed in the usual position toward the head (overlying the lower abdomen). Orthopedic surgeons will sometimes object because this interferes with the patient sitting up. However, the patient will not be sitting up in the near future, and abdominal exposure is more urgent. Definitive fixation can be accomplished by revising the bracing arms or performing internal fixation when the patient is stable.

SUGGESTED READINGS

DiGiacomo JC, Bonadies JA, Cole FJ, et al. Practice management guidelines for hemorrhage in pelvic fracture. The Eastern Association for the Surgery of Trauma. http://www.east.org/tpg.

DiGiacomo JC, McGonigal MD, Haskal ZJ, et al. Arterial bleeding diagnosed by CT in hemodynamically stable victims of blunt trauma. J Trauma 1996;40(2):249–252.

Moore EE, Feliciano DV, Mattox KL. Trauma. New York: McGraw-Hill, 2003:779–807.

CONSIDER TREATMENT FOR HETEROTOPIC OSSIFICATION AFTER TRAUMA

CONSTANTINE A. DEMETRACOPOULOS, BS
FRANK J. FRASSICA, MD

INTRODUCTION

Heterotopic ossification may occur following head or spinal cord trauma, burns, or major surgery on the musculoskeletal system. A heterotrophic bone may cause severe physical impairment by surrounding a joint such as the hip or the elbow and fixing the joint in a nonfunctional position (i.e., contracture). Heterotopic ossification is also very common following open reduction and internal fixation of acetabular fractures.

PATHOPHYSIOLOGY

Heterotopic ossification is the process of bone formation in extraskeletal soft tissue. Roberts in 1968 was first to note the association between head trauma and periarticular ectopic bone formation, and others have since demonstrated a positive correlation between the extent of head trauma and functional severity of heterotopic ossification. The pathogenesis of heterotopic ossification following head injury is uncertain. However, recent theories suggest that head trauma causes an increase in inflammatory mediators and bone morphogenic proteins, which induce soft tissue osteoprogenitor stem cells to differentiate into osteoblasts. Increased serum levels of prostaglandin E_2 after head trauma are also believed to play a role in the proliferation of differentiated osteoblasts. The osteoblasts secrete osteoid peripherally about the area of trauma within 7 to 10 days. Primitive cartilage appears after 14 days, and trabecular bone forms within 2 to 5 weeks. Mature lamellar bone in the periphery surrounding immature and undifferentiated central tissues is present by the sixth week. Plain radiographs and computerized tomography scans show a very characteristic zoning pattern of mature bone at the periphery and a lucency in the center. The lucent area represents immature musculoskeletal tissues.

CLINICAL FEATURES

The hip is the most commonly involved joint, followed by the elbow, shoulder, and knee. The incidence of heterotopic ossification of the hip following head trauma varies from 11% to 76%, with ankylosis of the joint occurring in 11% to 20% of those patients. Clinical signs that should cause one to suspect heterotopic ossification include pain and decreased range of motion at the joint, as well as inflammatory markers such as fever, erythema, swelling, and warmth at the joint. Making the diagnosis is also dependent on identifying patients who are more likely than others to develop heterotopic ossification. Risk factors include male gender, underlying systemic disorders such as ankylosing spondylitis and diffuse idiopathic skeletal hyperostosis, previous heterotopic bone formation, and limb spasticity.

The diagnosis of heterotopic ossification is typically made based on clinical suspicion and radiographic findings (*Fig. 308.1*), which appear within the first 3 to 6 weeks after injury. Brooker devised the classification system that is most frequently used to radiographically grade the amount of heterotopic ossification at the hip. Class I includes islands of bone within the soft tissue that is located about the hip. Class II consists of bone spurs from the pelvis or proximal femur leaving at least 1 cm between opposing bone surfaces. Class III allows for less than 1 cm between opposing bone surfaces, and class IV is apparent ankylosis of the hip in the anterior-posterior view. Triple-phase radionucleotide bone scan is the preferred method for early detection. It will show increased blood flow and increased concentration of the tracer within the soft tissue of the hip before any findings are apparent on radiographs. Computed tomography is most commonly used to define the areas of involvement. Although serum alkaline phosphatase does not have diagnostic or prognostic value, levels correlate with the degree of ongoing ossification, and thus it used as a marker for active disease.

TREATMENT

Nonsteroidal anti-inflammatory drugs (NSAIDS), external beam radiation, and disphosphonates have been used with varying success for prophylaxis against heterotopic ossification. In a randomized, double-blind, prospective study, 400 mg of ibuprofen three times daily administered within 48 hours of the injury and given for 8 days was found to be effective. Indomethacin has also been used for prophylaxis and is dosed at 75 to 100 mg/day for 7 to 14 days. However, patient compliance with NSAIDs is of concern because of the incidence of gastrointestinal distress. Ionizing radiation has been shown to inhibit osteogenesis. A recent meta-analysis comparing single-dose radiation with NSAIDs found radiotherapy to be more efficacious.

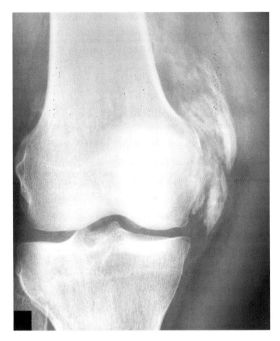

FIGURE 308.1. Characteristic radiographic appearance of heterotrophic ossification of the knee. (Reprinted with permission from Harris JH Jr. Knee. In: Harris JH Jr., Harris WH, eds. The Radiology of Emergency Medicine, 4th ed. Philadelphia: Lippincott Williams & Wilkins, 2000:836.)

A one-time dose of 700 to 800 cGy is recommended within 24 hours of trauma or 72 hours postoperatively. Although the risk of inducing malignant disease with radiotherapy exists, it is uncommon at such low doses. Finally, disphosphonates are pyrophosphate analogues that delay mineralization of osteoid by inhibiting the growth of hydroxya-patite crystals. They have not been shown to be effective and carry the risk of osteomalacia with long-term use.

Definitive treatment of heterotopic ossification once it has developed and become symptomatic is surgical excision followed by adjuvant therapy to decrease the likelihood of recurrence. Excision occurs with the intention to improve function because patients can become severely limited in their activities of daily living. However, surgery must wait until the lesion has matured. Active, ongoing ossification is an absolute contraindication. Thus, excision must await the radiographic appearance of well-defined cortex and normal serum levels of alkaline phosphatase. This typically occurs around 18 months after the injury. Other indicators for successful excision are good cognitive recovery following head trauma and good motor control of the extremity. Postoperative radiation therapy is recommended to prevent recurrence.

SUGGESTED READINGS

Garland DE, Blum CE, Waters RL. Periarticular heterotrophic ossification in head injured adults. Incidence and location. J Bone Joint Surg Am 1980;62(7):1143–1146.

Morrey BF, ed. Joint Replacement Arthroplasty. New York: Churchill Livingstone, 1991:867–876.

Sarafis KA, Karatzas GD, Yotis CL. Ankylosed hips caused by heterotrophic ossification after traumatic brain injury: a difficult problem. J Trauma 1999;46(1):104–109.

309

LOOK FOR MISSED EXTREMITY FRACTURES IN PATIENTS WITH A DIAGNOSED EXTREMITY FRACTURE

WILLIAM S. HOFF, MD

Missed injuries, commonly referred to as "the trauma surgeon's nemesis," are an expected occurrence in the management of multiply injured patients. The definition of a missed injury is institution specific. Generally speaking, however, a missed injury is an injury identified at some defined time after the initial assessment. Missed injuries are not frequently life-threatening. However, depending on the exact circumstances, a missed injury may result in long-term disability. Moreover, missed injuries may complicate the relationship between the health care provider and his or her patient.

The initial assessment of a trauma patient consists of a primary and a secondary survey. The purpose of the primary survey is to simultaneously identify and initiate treatment of immediately life-threatening conditions. The secondary survey consists of a systematic, head-to-toe physical examination. A definitive care plan is established based on injuries identified in the initial assessment. Despite a carefully performed initial assessment, the incidence of missed injury is approximately 10%. The majority of missed injuries are musculoskeletal injuries, a large proportion of which are extremity injuries. The following conditions are associated with missed injuries in trauma patients:

- Altered sensorium secondary to ethanol/drug intoxication or traumatic brain injury
- Clinical instability with more urgent treatment priorities
- Unappreciated physical findings on initial assessment
- Failure to obtain necessary radiographic studies
- Inadequately performed or misinterpreted radiographic studies

From a performance improvement perspective, the first two conditions are expected in severely injured patients in whom a reliable and complete clinical examination may not be possible. The remaining factors represent errors in judgment or management.

WHAT TO DO

The most effective way to reduce missed injuries is to perform a repeat systematic physical examination by an experienced physician. This "tertiary survey" should ideally be performed within the first 24 hours after admission or when the patient has been stabilized. During this examination, attention should be paid to any subtle areas of contusion, abrasion, swelling, or deformity. In a conscious patient, areas of tenderness should also be recorded. In the patient who is more mobile, pain with movement or ambulation is noted. Appropriate radiographic studies should be obtained based on the results of the tertiary survey. Another potential source of missed injuries may result when the trauma surgeon relies entirely on his or her interpretation of radiographic studies obtained during the initial assessment. A recent study demonstrated a 9.7% incidence of new diagnoses based on mandatory review of admission x-rays within 24 hours by a radiologist.

Because of these considerations, the experienced and skilled intensive care physician will perform his or her own thorough physical examination and independently review the images and reports of all radiology investigation in all trauma patients admitted to the intensive care unit.

SUGGESTED READINGS

Biffl WL, Harrington DT, Cioffi WG. Implementation of a tertiary trauma survey decreases missed injuries. J Trauma 2003;54:38–44.

Born CT, Ross SE, Iannocone WM, et al. Delayed identification of skeletal injury in multisystem trauma: the "missed" fracture. J Trauma 1989;29:1643–1646.

Enderson BL, Reath DB, Meadors J, et al. The tertiary trauma survey: a prospective study of missed injury. J Trauma 1990;30:666–670.

Enderson BL, Maull KI. Missed injuries—the trauma surgeon's nemesis. Surg Clin North Am 1991;71:399–418.

Hoff WS, Sicoutris CP, Lee SY, et al. Formalized radiology rounds: the final component of the tertiary survey. J Trauma 2004;56:291–295.

310

HAVE A WORKING KNOWLEDGE OF INTENSIVE CARE UNIT SCORING SYSTEMS

RON PAULDINE, MD

Severity-of-illness scoring systems are used in the intensive care unit (ICU) setting as tools to stratify risk for therapeutic trials or as predictive instruments to evaluate the performance of a specific ICU over time or in comparison to another unit. It must be noted at the outset that they have limited utility with regard to individual patient outcomes.

Intensive care unit scoring systems fall into two broad categories. Risk prediction (also called "prognostic") models are designed to assess prognosis at the time of admission to the ICU or within the first 24 hours. Organ dysfunction scores are used to quantify the burden of organ dysfunction and can be performed repeatedly throughout the ICU stay. Several generalizations can be made when comparing and contrasting the application of prognostic and organ dysfunction scoring systems. Prognostic scoring systems are concerned with predicting mortality, whereas organ dysfunction scores describe morbidity. Prognostic scores are obtained at time of admission or within the first 24 hours of the ICU stay and use a relatively complex set of calculations. Organ dysfunction measures are usually easier to use and can be obtained repeatedly. Prognostic scores reveal no information on individual organ dysfunction, whereas organ dysfunction scores are primarily concerned with individual organ function.

Risk prediction (prognostic) models are constructed from large databases obtained from patients admitted to hospitals throughout the United States and Europe. Logistic regression methods are applied to estimate the probability of mortality based on data obtained at or near the time of ICU admission. The accuracy of the system is influenced by how the criteria were derived for a specific system and how they are applied to a given patient. Patient factors, issues with data collection, and innovations in treatment over time all have an impact. The major outcomes measured by the most widely used systems are mortality and, in some cases, length of stay. The models assume that mortality is affected by physiologic derangements that occur early in the course of illness. The Acute Physiology and Chronic Health Evaluation (APACHE) was the first risk prediction model described. APACHE I included 34 physiologic variables derived from the medical

literature and expert opinion. It suffered from complexity and difficulty in application. APACHE II was designed to be more user-friendly
and included 12 physiologic variables. The score was validated in 5,815
ICU admissions at 13 different centers. Limitations include the age of
the database (outcomes are based on treatment from 1979 to 1982), lack
of applicability to individual patients, and selection bias. APACHE III
is an updated system that addresses some of these issues but is more
difficult to use and utilizes proprietary software. The Simplified Acute
Physiology Score (SAPS) was introduced in 1984 and has been updated as SAPS II. SAPS II uses data from 1991 to 1992 collected in
ICUs in the United States and Europe. Seventeen variables representing physiology, type of admission, and underlying disease comprise the
model.

Organ dysfunction scoring systems allow determination of organ
dysfunction at time of admission and at regular intervals throughout
the ICU stay. They allow assessment of the change in organ function,
and the accuracy of mortality predictions may be improved with repeat measurements. The benefit of this type of scoring system lies in
its ability to capture change. This type of assessment may be useful in
comparing a baseline level of function at time of entry into a clinical
trial or allow mortality prediction between groups of patients. Scores
typically focus on six organ systems: cardiovascular, respiratory, hematologic, central nervous system, renal, and hepatic. Two frequently
employed organ scoring systems include the Sequential Organ Failure Assessment Score (SOFA) and the Multiple Organ Dysfunction
Score (MODS). They differ mainly in the criteria used to assess the
cardiovascular system. SOFA uses the worst daily value over a representative value for the included variables and uses urine output to
assess renal function. Overall, high SOFA scores and significant increases in SOFA score correlate with mortality.

SUGGESTED READINGS

Herridge MS. Prognostication and intensive care unit outcome: the evolving role of
scoring systems. Clin Chest Med 2003;24(4):751–762.
Rosenberg AL. Recent innovations in intensive care unit risk-prediction models. Curr
Opin Crit Care 2002;8(4):321–330.
Société Française d'Anesthésie et de Réanimation. Scoring systems for ICU and surgical
patients. www.sfar.org/s/article.php3?id_article=60, 2006.

311

HAVE A WORKING KNOWLEDGE OF THE EMERGENCY MEDICAL TREATMENT AND ACTIVE LABOR ACT AS IT APPLIES TO THE INTENSIVE CARE UNIT

CHRISTIAN MERLO, MD, MPH
NADIA N. HANSEL, MD, MPH

The Emergency Medical Treatment and Active Labor Act (EMTALA) was passed by the U.S. Congress in 1986 to prevent hospitals from rejecting, refusing, or transferring patients because they are unable to pay or because they have public health insurance. The main purpose of EMTALA is to ensure nondiscriminatory patient access to emergency medical care and to prevent the transfer of uninsured patients from private to public hospitals without consideration of medical condition or clinical stability.

Although the act has historically been associated with care in the emergency department, it is important to realize that EMTALA imposes three specific legal duties on the entire hospital, including the intensive care unit (ICU). First, hospitals must perform a screening examination on any person who comes to the hospital to evaluate whether he or she has a medical emergency. Second, if an emergency medical condition exists, hospital staff must stabilize the patient to the best of their capabilities and transfer the patient to another hospital if specialized care is needed and not available at their own institution. Finally, hospitals with specialized capabilities are required to accept patient transfers if they have the capacity to care for them.

Intensive care unit management can be provided at most hospitals, but certain circumstances may necessitate specialty care (e.g., burns, trauma, neonatal ICU) that requires transfer of the patient to another institution. In this case, the referring physician is obliged to first stabilize the patient. If the medical benefits of transfer outweigh the medical risks, then the physician should effectively communicate results and treatment and transfer the patient to an accepting facility with the capability to treat the patient's condition. Although not required by EMTALA, it is often a good idea to follow up with the accepting physician after the transfer has occurred to ensure proper continuity of care.

The accepting physician in the ICU of a tertiary care center also has obligations under EMTALA rules and must have a good working knowledge of his or her specific ICU with regard to capacity (beds and staffing) and capability. A patient should not be accepted if the ICU is full. A transfer for high-frequency oscillatory ventilation, extracorporeal membrane oxygenation, or continuous renal replacement therapy should not be accepted if an ICU does not have these specific capabilities immediately available. This may sound trivial, but mistakes like these happen and compromise patient care. If beds and staffing are available and the ICU can provide for a stabilized patient requiring specialized care, then not only it is appropriate, but it is also required by law to accept the patient. Again, it is fitting to provide relevant follow-up information regarding the transfer or the patient's condition to the referring physician. Many hospital systems have a physician access line to help facilitate this process.

SUGGESTED READINGS

EMTALA.com. www.emtala.com

U.S. Department of Health and Human Services, Center for Medicare and Medicaid Services. EMTALA. www.cms.hhs.gov/EMTALA/

Williamson T, Crippen D. Do you have to accept this patient? What intensivists and hospitalists need to know about EMTALA. Cost Qual 2001;8–11.

Zibulewsky J. The Emergency Medical Treatment and Active Labor Act (EMTALA): what it is and what it means for physicians. Proc Baylor Univ Med Center 2001;4:339–346.

312

KNOW WHAT THE BASIC STATISTICAL TERMS MEAN

PETER F. CRONHOLM, MD
JOSEPH B. STRATON, MD

HOW CLINICIANS MAKE DECISIONS

To make informed, evidence-based decisions, providers need to have an understanding of several statistical concepts. The decision-making process begins by assessing information by means of a history and physical examination framed within an understanding of the relative probabilities of disease states. The next step is to determine the likelihood that the patient has the disease in question. If we have enough information at that time, no further testing is needed, and we may move on to treatment. If not, more information is needed, and further testing must be done to better determine whether the disease in question is in fact the underlying etiology. For each step of the decision-making process, we need to understand testing and disease characteristics.

Clinical decision making is based on an understanding of the incidence and prevalence of diseases considered in differential diagnoses for the types of patients considered. The prevalence of a disease tells us how many people at a given point or period of time have the disease in question. Prevalence combines people who already have the disease and those that will acquire the disease during that period of time. The incidence of a disease tells us how many new cases of a disease develop or are likely to develop over a period of time. Incidence is a measure of risk, whereas prevalence is more of a measure of the burden of disease for a given population. The process of developing a differential diagnosis is a ranking of etiologies based on our understanding of the incidence and prevalence of diseases for a given set of historical and physical data.

Decisions are made based on the likelihood of a disease for a given clinical situation. The likelihood of a disease ranges from nil (0%) to absolute (100%). There exists a range of likelihoods that vary depending on the balance of costs and benefits of provider decisions that determine what our next steps should be in terms of making choices to treat, not to treat, or to conduct diagnostic testing. Diagnostic testing should be considered when there is a difference between the likelihood that a patient has the disease and the threshold at which a provider chooses to move forward with treatment options. Two thresholds must

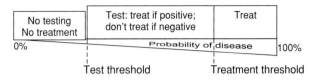

FIGURE 312.1. The threshold approach to medical decision making.

be considered that determine the range over which diagnostic testing should be considered. The first is the "testing threshold," which is the likelihood below which a provider would consider the disease sufficiently rare a cause that he or she would not empirically treat for the disorder nor test for the presence of the condition. To make treatment decisions, providers need to have some point at which they will decide to treat a patient, given the weight of the evidence with no further testing. This point is referred to as the "treatment threshold" (*Fig. 312.1*).

Shaping a differential diagnosis is a process of categorizing the probabilities of various diseases associated with the patient history and exam. The probability that a patient has the disease before any diagnostic testing is done is known as the "prior probability" of disease. Diagnostic testing increases or decreases the likelihood that a person has the disease in question. The likelihood that person has the disease after diagnostic testing is known as the "posterior probability." Diagnostic testing occurs along a continuum of likelihoods when the prior probability is lower than the treatment threshold but higher than the testing threshold (*Fig. 312.1*). If the prior probability is above the treatment threshold, one treats the patient without further testing. If the prior probability is below the treatment threshold, further testing is required, the results of which either move one away from the treatment threshold if they are negative or closer or over the treatment threshold if they are positive. A series of tests may be necessary to move the posterior probability that a patient has the disease to the point of treatment. As an illustration, if one operates on a person only if one is 70% sure that he or she has the disease, but after the history and physical one is only 40% sure, then one needs to do more testing to move the likelihood above 70%. There is no need to perform tests when one is already over the treatment threshold (although these are often done for "academic" reasons) or if the test will not provide enough evidence to move one over the treatment threshold if no other testing is linked or available. For example, if a febrile patient has tender anterior cervical anterior cervical adenopathy with an exudative pharynx and the absence of cough by history, he or she should be treated for bacterial pharyngitis without further testing.

How Clinicians Judge a Test

Sensitivity and specificity are characteristics of diagnostic tests. They inform the provider how the test will behave among people with or without disease. The sensitivity of a test is a measure of how often the test will be positive when testing people who have the disease. In contrast, the specificity of a test measures how often the test will be negative when testing patients who do not have the disease. Highly sensitive tests are used for screening because a highly sensitive test, when negative, rules the patient out for the disease (SeNsitive:OUT, or SNOUT). A highly specific test, when positive, rules the patient in for the disease (SPecific:IN, or SPIN).

As clinicians, what we really want to know is, if the test comes back positive or negative, what does this mean for the patient: do they have the disease or not? To answer this question, one needs to know the sensitivity and specificity of the tests used, but one also needs to have a sense of the prevalence of the disease among people like the person being tested so that measures known as positive and negative predictive values can be calculated. The positive predictive value of a test is the likelihood that a person has the disease if the test is positive. The negative predictive value is the likelihood that a patient does not have the disease if the test is negative. If a test comes back positive for a person who is very likely to have the disease (high prevalence), the result is likely to be a true positive. However, if the person is very unlikely to have the disease, the result is much more likely to be a false positive. Similar statements can be made for negative results for high and low prevalence conditions.

How Clinicians Know Whether Their Treatments Will Work

Measures of association are means of estimating the strength of the relationship between observed outcomes and factors that may produce the outcome. Common measures of association are the odds ratio, relative risk, absolute risk reduction, and number needed to treat. Odds ratios are used in studies in which the incidence (or true risk) of disease cannot be accurately assessed (case series, case-control studies, or some retrospective study designs). Odds ratios are determined by calculating the ratio of the odds of exposure among the cases compared with the odds of exposure among the controls. For example, if the ratio of the odds of exposure to artificial tanning lamps among cases with melanoma and controls is 3:2, the resulting odds ratio is 1.5. Relative risk specifies the risk of developing the disease in the exposed group relative to those who are not exposed and can be reported from certain prospective study designs and clinical trials. Relative risk is the best measure of the association between exposure and disease. However, odds ratios can provide robust estimates of association and can approximate relative risk for outcomes that are rare.

The absolute risk reduction (ARR) is the difference in disease rates between the exposed and unexposed groups. It is important for clinicians to understand the difference between absolute and relative risk reductions. For uncommon diseases with high relative risks or common diseases with low or moderate relative risk reductions, the absolute risk reduction of an intervention may be quite low. An intervention may have a 10-fold relative risk reduction, with rates of disease near 0.1 for those with the intervention and 1.0 for patients without it [RR = (1.0%)/(0.1%) = 10]. However, the same study findings could be described as producing an absolute risk reduction of less than 1% (ARR = 1.0% − 0.1% = 0.99%) for those patients exposed to the intervention.

A clinical use of absolute risk reduction is to take its reciprocal, which is known as the number needed to treat (NNT). The NNT for an intervention is the number of people who would need to be exposed to the intervention to produce the desired outcome for one person. For example, if the ARR is 8% when giving clopidogrel to patients getting stents placed in the setting of symptomatic coronary artery disease with the intention of reducing myocardial infarction (MI), the NNT would be 12 (NNT = 1/ARR = 1/0.08 = 12). It follows that with a NNT of 12, one would need to give clopidogrel to 12 patients to prevent 1 MI. Although 1 MI was prevented, 11 of the 12 patients received no benefit from the intervention; however, all 12 patients needed to be treated because one could not predict which one would benefit in advance. There is no single number that represents a "good" NNT. The clinical impact of NNT is based on the likelihood of the disease, the cost of the intervention (medications, procedures, harm associated with intervention), and the cost of not doing the intervention (rates and values assigned to patient morbidity and mortality associated with the disease).

When interpreting study results it is important to understand what is referred to as power as well as types of errors that may be encountered. The power of a study, usually presented as a percentage, is a measure of the probability that the null hypothesis is rejected when it

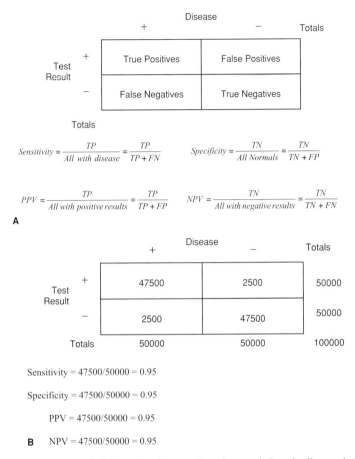

A

B

Sensitivity = 47500/50000 = 0.95

Specificity = 47500/50000 = 0.95

PPV = 47500/50000 = 0.95

NPV = 47500/50000 = 0.95

FIGURE 312.2. **A.** Measuring the operating characteristics of a diagnostic test. **B.** Of moderate-prevalence diseases. *(Continued)*

is false. That is, one will not find an association between the dependent and independent variables if there is no true relationship between them. If the measures of association (odds ratios, relative risk, etc.) of a study reach significance, then the power of the study is irrelevant and the findings stand as significant, assuming the study methods are valid. However, results may not reach significance either because there is no true relationship between the dependent and independent variables or the study did not have enough power (usually an issue of sample size) to demonstrate the relationship (*Fig. 312.2*).

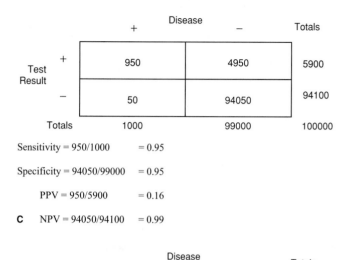

Sensitivity = 950/1000 = 0.95

Specificity = 94050/99000 = 0.95

PPV = 950/5900 = 0.16

C NPV = 94050/94100 = 0.99

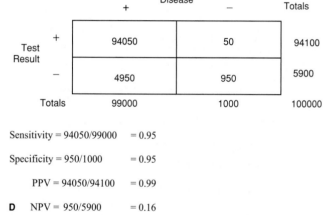

Sensitivity = 94050/99000 = 0.95

Specificity = 950/1000 = 0.95

PPV = 94050/94100 = 0.99

D NPV = 950/5900 = 0.16

FIGURE 312.2. *(Continued)* **C.** Of low-prevalence diseases. **D.** Of high-prevalence diseases. FN, false negative; FP, false positive; NPV, negative predictive value; PPV, positive predictive value; TN, true negative; TP, true positive.

Type I errors represent the chance that the null hypothesis is rejected when it is actually true, or that one finds a result that is significant by chance alone and there is no true underlying relationship between the dependent and independent variables. This is the rate of false alarms or false positives. Type I errors are the equivalent to the "significance" level reported in studies (e.g., *p* values <.05). Type II errors are the chance that one does not reject the null hypothesis when it is false. Type II errors are the complement of power (type II error rate $= 1 -$ power). Type II errors are the chance that one will miss an effect when it is really there. In other words, it is the rate of failed alarms or false negatives.

SUGGESTED READINGS

Centre for Health Evidence. Users' Guides to Evidence-Based Practice. http://www.cche.net/usersguides/main.asp

Hennekens CH, Buring JE, Mayrent SL. Epidemiology in medicine. Boston: Little, Brown, 1987.

Rothman KJ, Greenland S. Modern epidemiology, 2nd ed. Philadelphia: Lippincott-Raven, 1998.

Swinscow TDV, Campbell MJ. Statistics at square one, 10th ed. London: BMJ Books, 2002.

313

CONSIDER EMBOLI WHEN THERE IS A CHANGE IN MENTAL STATUS AFTER AN INVASIVE PROCEDURE

NIRAV G. SHAH, MD

Embolism is an uncommon complication of altered mentation after invasive procedures, but it must be placed on the list of differential diagnoses. The four most common emboli seen in the critical care patient population are air, fat, cholesterol, and blood emboli (clots).

Air embolism occurs when air enters the systemic vascular circulation during placement or removal of a central venous catheter or at other times when a central venous catheter is in use. Air can also be introduced into the systemic circulation during cardiac surgery procedures, neurosurgical procedures, and endoscopic procedures. Air that enters the venous circulation can travel to the right side of the heart and cause cardiopulmonary compromise. The clinical presentation of a venous air embolism is highly variable and depends on the amount of air entry, the speed of entry, and the patient's size and premorbid condition. Symptoms may range from mild chest discomfort to altered mentation to complete cardiovascular collapse. Alternatively, a right-to-left shunt can result in an embolus that enters the arterial circulation and causes cerebral ischemia. If a cerebral air embolus is suspected, then the head should be immediately lowered, a fraction of inspired oxygen of 1.0 should be delivered, and adequate ventilation maintained. One therapy for air embolus is hyperbaric oxygen therapy, which if desired, should be instituted within 5 h of neurologic or cardiac symptoms.

Fat emboli are most commonly the result of trauma or long-bone fracture. However, they can also present following orthopedic procedures such as spine surgery and knee and hip replacements. The classic findings include petechiae, dyspnea, and altered mental status. The symptoms usually occur 1 to 2 days after the precipitating event and are the result of a diffuse vasculitis secondary to free fatty acids. Although this entity has a classic appearance, the diagnosis is one of exclusion. The treatment of fat emboli is supportive and includes oxygen therapy and mechanical ventilation if needed.

Another uncommon cause of altered mental status, especially following cardiac catheterization or arteriography, is a cholesterol embolus. Stroke may result from the embolization of atherosclerotic material that is disturbed by the catheter during the procedure. The syndrome may present with livedo reticularis, severe limb pain, renal failure, or focal neurologic deficits. The neurologic deficits usually present acutely and are frequently reversible. If skin changes are present, the diagnosis can be confirmed with skin biopsy demonstrating cholesterol crystals. In addition, emboli to the kidney may cause renal dysfunction and emboli to the viscera may be a cause of ischemic bowel.

The most frequent embolic material after invasive procedures is blood. Clots that subsequently embolize occur secondary to intimal disruption and venous stasis from immobility. The time of onset can be variable, as can the presenting symptoms. Orthopedic surgery and neurosurgery are associated with the highest risks of venous emboli secondary to the release of tissue factor, which is a powerful trigger of blood clotting. Although deep vein thrombosis and pulmonary emboli are common in the postsurgical population, cerebrovascular accidents due to venous emboli require communication between the left and right heart via a septal defect or patent foramen ovale (the classic paradoxical emboli). The clinical manifestations of cerebral emboli depend on the specific vessel occluded and the distribution of blood from that vessel. For example, occlusion of the middle cerebral artery results in contralateral hemiparesis and sensory loss with more severe symptoms in the arms and face. Treatment of a thrombotic stroke includes thrombolytic therapy, blood pressure regulation, supportive care, and aggressive physical therapy. Multiple studies have demonstrated the effectiveness of thrombolytic therapy if instituted within the first 3 hours of symptom onset and after a noncontrast computed tomography scan excludes an intracranial hemorrhage.

SUGGESTED READINGS

Blacker DJ. In-hospital stroke. Lancet Neurol 2003;2(12):741–746.
Cramer SC. Patent foramen ovale and its relationship to stroke. Cardiol Clin 2005;23(1):7–11.

314

KNOW THE NONINFECTIOUS CAUSES OF FEVER IN THE INTENSIVE CARE UNIT

LAITH ALTAWEEL, MD

Fever in the intensive care unit (ICU) patient is a common problem that results in the performance of many diagnostics tests. This increases both the costs of medical care and the exposure of the patient to uncomfortable procedures. The astute clinician will recognize that although a common cause of fever in the ICU is infection, many cases of fever are caused by noninfectious etiologies. Proper management demands implementing a simultaneous algorithm for the workup of noninfectious causes.

Fever is thought to be a protective mechanism against infection. Many animal species are known to develop fever in response to a microbiologic organism. In humans, fever is thought to enhance several parameters of immune function and potentially enhance survival. In addition, hyperthermia also increases cardiac output, oxygen consumption, carbon dioxide production, and energy expenditure, which may be harmful to patients with low cardiopulmonary reserve or cerebrovascular injury. Maternal fever may also be a cause of fetal malformations or spontaneous abortions.

Normal body temperature is 37.0°C with circadian variation of between 0.5°C and 1.0°C. Several methods are used to measure body temperature. Taking the pulmonary artery mixed venous temperature is the most accurate method for measuring core body temperature. Infrared ear thermometry is nearly equivalent to taking pulmonary artery and brain temperatures. Rectal temperatures obtained with a mercury thermometer or electronic probe are often a few tenths of a degree higher than core body temperature. Oral temperatures can be influenced by drinking and eating or warmed air in ventilator circuits. Axillary measurements are unreliable. The Society of Critical Care Medicine defines a fever as a temperature greater than 38.3°C. Most infectious causes of fever follow a diurnal pattern.

WATCH OUT FOR

There are many noninfectious causes of fever. With the exception of drug fever and transfusion reaction, noninfectious causes of fever usually do not lead to a fever greater than 39.8°C. Most causes of noninfectious fever (*Table 314.1*) will be suggested based on a good history and

TABLE 314.1	NONINFECTIOUS CAUSES OF FEVER IN THE INTENSIVE CARE UNIT

Alcohol/drug withdrawal
Acalculous cholecystitis
Postoperative fever (48 hours postoperative)
Decubitus ulcer
Drug fever
Cerebrovascular accident/subarachnoid hemorrhage
Myocardial infarction
Pancreatitis
Ischemic bowel
Cirrhosis
Gastrointestinal bleeding
Hematoma
Aspiration pneumonitis
Acute respiratory distress syndrome (both acute and fibroproliferative phase)
Deep vein thrombosis/pulmonary embolism
Phlebitis/thrombophlebitis
Adrenal insufficiency
Intravenous contrast reactions
Neoplastic fevers

physical exam. A recent operation, chest pain with electrocardiogram (ECG) changes, and a quadriparetic patient with asymmetric lower extremity swelling or a large sacral decubitus ulcer are all commonly encountered scenarios causing fever in the ICU patient. Routine laboratory tests, such as a complete blood count to look for evidence of bleeding, leukocytosis, and eosinophilia; a liver panel and an amylase and lipase test; ECG with cardiac enzymes; and a check of lactic acid level can help to quickly rule in or rule out many of the most common noninfectious causes of fever. Imaging studies such as a chest radiograph; computed tomography of the head, chest, abdomen, and pelvis; right upper quadrant ultrasound; and lower extremity venous duplex may also be necessary to complete the workup.

Drug withdrawal fever should always be considered in a patient with a history of substance abuse. In many cases this abuse history may not be known to the clinician, so clinical suspicion should be high. Drugs are a commonly considered etiology of fever; in reality very few cases are cited in the literature. Drugs commonly associated with drug fever are the β-lactam antibiotics, procainamide, and diphenylhydantoin.

SUGGESTED READINGS

Fink M. Textbook of Critical Care, 5th ed. Philadelphia: Saunders/Elsevier, 2005:1186.
Marik P. Fever in the ICU. Chest 2000;117:855–869.

315

CARDIOVERT UNSTABLE TACHYCARDIAS (BOTH NARROW AND WIDE COMPLEX)

LAITH ALTAWEEL, MD

The assessment of a patient with a tachycardia requires a systematic approach. First, the physician must determine whether the patient is experiencing evidence of hemodynamic compromise as a result of the tachycardia, which is generally not seen until the heart rate is greater than 150 beats per minute. Unstable tachycardias can be manifested by chest pain, shortness of breath, decreased urine output, mental status changes, or hypotension. Once a patient is noted to be hemodynamically unstable, the clinician then needs to assess the type of rhythm. This is important because the rhythm dictates what further management is needed. Generally, the rhythm is classified into two broad categories: narrow complex tachycardia or wide complex tachycardia.

WHAT TO DO

Narrow complex tachycardias are rhythms with QRS duration of less than 120 ms. There are three categories of narrow complex tachycardias: junctional tachycardia, paroxysmal supraventricular tachycardia, and atrial tachycardia. In most cases of unstable narrow complex tachycardias (with the exception of junctional tachycardia) immediate synchronized cardioversion with 50 to 100 joules is warranted. In the conscious patient, premedication with a sedative or analgesic, such as diazepam, midazolam, etomidate, propofol, fentanyl, or morphine, should be attempted. Junctional tachycardia, which is rare and most frequently a sign of digitalis or theophylline toxicity, should not be cardioverted because it represents an escape rhythm. An accelerated junctional rhythm is rarely faster than 120 beats per minute and should be treated with a beta-blocker or, if the underlying ejection fraction is not known, with amiodarone withdrawal and possibly treatment of the underlying cause (e.g., digoxin).

Wide complex tachycardias (QRS >120 ms) include narrow complex tachycardias with aberrant conduction, antidromic atrioventricular nodal reentry tachycardia in patients with Wolf-Parkinson-White syndrome, and ventricular tachycardia (monomorphic or polymorphic). Immediate synchronized cardioversion with up to 360 joules (or 200 joules if biphasic defibrillation is used) should be attempted for all unstable wide complex tachycardia, with the exception of polymorphic ventricular tachycardia, which should be defibrillated with 360 joules.

SUGGESTED READING

American Heart Association in Collaboration with the International Liaison Committee on Resuscitation. Guidelines 2000 for cardiopulmonary resuscitation and emergency cardiovascular care. Part 6: Advanced cardiovascular life support: 7d: The tachycardia algorithms. Circulation 2000;102:I158.

316

BE CONCERNED ABOUT CHEST PAIN EVEN IF IT IS FOUND TO BE NONCARDIAC IN NATURE

LAITH ALTAWEEL, MD

Chest pain in the intensive care unit (ICU) is a common and potentially serious complaint. The differential diagnosis of chest pain is broad, and the physician must not be limited to cardiac etiologies, although myocardial infarction and angina must always be considered. The initial approach to chest pain requires a rapid evaluation, history, physical, electrocardiogram, chest radiograph, and the consideration of additional laboratory and radiologic tests.

The initial approach should be to ensure that the patient has hemodynamic and respiratory stability. This usually results from an assessment of the patient's vital signs and clinical condition. The patient who is bradycardic and hypotensive requires more urgent diagnosis than the patient in pain who is awake and conversant. If the condition is stable, a concise history regarding the nature of the pain should be obtained. A mnemonic that may be helpful in asking the necessary questions is OLDCAAR (*Table 316.1*). Classic symptoms of myocardial infarction or ischemia include chest pain that may be characterized as sharp, dull, pressure, tearing, or crushing or a feeling of doom. Patients may complain of radiation to the chin, left arm, or back. Associated symptoms may include nausea, vomiting, diaphoresis, and palpitations. The astute clinician should consider atypical symptoms such as "gas" or heartburn to be cardiac in etiology until proven otherwise.

A focused physical exam should be performed looking first for cardiovascular problems such as a difference in the pulses between the limbs, pulses paradoxus, pulse volume and rate, new murmurs, rubs, or gallops. It is important to note that the exam may be normal despite a cardiac etiology. Additional physical signs may provide insight to other etiologies. For example, rhonchi or rales, absent breath sounds, or hyper-resonance may point toward a pulmonary etiology, whereas abdominal tenderness, masses, absent or abnormal abdominal sounds, guarding. and rebound may provide insight into an abdominal component.

TABLE 316.1　OLDCAAR MNEMONIC

O: Onset of pain: When? What was the patient doing at the time?
L: Location of pain? Pinpoint or diffuse?
D: Duration of pain, days or seconds? Comes and goes or persists?
C: Character of pain: dull, sharp, lancinating, ripping, tearing, etc.
A: Associated symptoms such as nausea, vomiting, diaphoresis, palpitations
A: Alleviating/aggravating factors such as position, belching, deep breathing
R: Radiating to back, arm, abdomen, neck

WATCH OUT FOR

A chest radiograph should be obtained to look for a pneumothorax, widened mediastinum, effusion, new infiltrates, free subdiaphragmatic air, rib fractures, and malpositioned endotracheal, nasogastric, or chest tubes. An electrocardiogram should always be obtained. Changes suggestive of cardiac ischemia or infarction can often be seen as changes in the ST segment, T wave morphology, or the presence of Q waves, which can indicate cardiac ischemia or infarct. Cardiac serum markers such as troponin and creatinine phosphokinase MB can also identify myocardial injury. If the clinical history and ECG suggest cardiac ischemia, the treatment for acute cardiac syndromes should be initiated.

Pulmonary embolism (PE) is a constant concern for ICU patients, many of whom have at least one risk factor, which include immobilization, burns, a hypercoagulable state, and heart failure. PE can present with pleuritic chest pain, tachypnea, and dyspnea. Large PEs can result in cardiovascular collapse with hypotension from obstructive cardiogenic shock. Echocardiogram may reveal a dilated right ventricle with reduced function and a septal shift. The chest radiograph will likely be normal and a computed tomography (CT) angiogram or ventilation/perfusion scan will be necessary to confirm the clinical suspicion. The treatment for a PE in the setting of hemodynamic stability is anticoagulation.

The symptoms of aortic dissection often overlap with those of myocardial ischemic pain. The sudden onset of severe, sharp chest pain that may or may not radiate to the back is a typical symptom. A chest x-ray is usually not helpful but may reveal a widened mediastinum, the separation of intimal calcification from the aortic knob, the deviation of the trachea, or the blurring of the aortic margins. Comparison with a recent radiograph is helpful. Contrast-enhanced CT is usually the best confirmatory test. The initial management should focus on blood pressure control and be followed by surgical consultation.

A pneumothorax can occur in ICU patients secondary to iatrogenic causes such as central venous catheter placement or ventilator-associated barotrauma. Pulmonary diseases such as chronic obstructive pulmonary disease, asthma, and acute respiratory distress syndrome are risk factors. If a patient with a pneumothorax develops hypotension, jugular venous distension, absence of breath sounds, hyper-resonance to percussion, and tracheal deviation, then the development of a tension pneumothorax is likely. A tension pneumothorax is of special concern for patients on mechanical ventilation receiving positive pressure. Immediate needle decompression and chest tube placement may be life saving in this condition.

Esophageal rupture can also cause chest pain and is a life-threatening condition that can lead to lethal mediastinitis. The history may suggest ingestion of a caustic substance, forceful vomiting, or iatrogenic trauma (e.g., nasogastric tube placement, esophageal dilation). Physical examination may reveal subcutaneous emphysema or mediastinal crackling on auscultation, known as Hamman's crunch. Chest radiograph may show pneumothorax, pneumomediastinum or pneumoperitoneum, pleural effusion, or subcutaneous emphysema. A water-soluble contrast study or esophagoscopy confirms the diagnosis.

Intravenous contrast-enhanced spiral computed tomography can be helpful in evaluating for many of these conditions within the differential diagnosis of chest pain including pulmonary embolism, aortic dissection, pericardial effusion, or anterior pneumothorax. If the clinical scenario suggests one of these diagnoses but other, more fundamental testing is not definitive, contrast-enhanced spiral CT may be indicated. In addition, an echocardiogram may be useful for evaluating the patient for regional wall motion abnormalities, which may occur with coronary ischemia, left and right ventricular function, pulmonary hypertension, valvular disease, and pericardial effusion or tamponade.

SUGGESTED READINGS

Fink MP, Abraham E, Vincent JL, et al., eds. Textbook of Critical Care, 5th ed. Philadelphia: Elsevier Saunders, 2005:120–123.

Lee T. Chest discomfort and palpitations. In: Kasper D, ed. Harrison's Online, 16th edition. New York: McGraw-Hill, 2005.

KNOW THE DIFFERENCE BETWEEN mmHg AND CM H$_2$O

ANTHONY D. SLONIM, MD, DRPH

Pressure is defined as the force per unit area. It can be applied either to a solid or a liquid interface at a point perpendicular to the surface and is represented by the height of the column that exerts a pressure at its base. Depending on the fluid used, the height of a column of fluid will differ because its density and therefore the pressure it exerts will differ.

Mercury (Hg) is a very dense fluid (13.5951 g/cm^3) and is often used to calibrate pressure gradients and differentials. Normal atmospheric pressure can support 760 mm Hg. One millimeter of Hg therefore represents approximately $1/760$ of an atmosphere and is a useful measure for comparing pressures. This measure is often referred to as a Torr, after the Italian physicist Torricelli. The unit mmHg is very useful in measurements for biologic systems. It is the conventional unit used to measure blood pressure.

Water has been used as a measure of pressure for numerous physiologic parameters and remains in use. Water is less dense than mercury, and the conversion from measurements using mercury to those using water follows the relationship 1 mmHg = 1.36 cm H$_2$O. This unit is still used for measurements of central venous pressure, intracranial pressure, pressures in mechanical ventilation, and pulmonary capillary wedge pressures. It is important for the intensive care unit clinician to recognize which fluid scales are being used to correctly interpret the measurements and provide therapeutic interventions based on the numeric values. Confusion about the scales used can lead to inappropriate actions and compromise the patient's care.

SUGGESTED READINGS

Centimetre of water. Wikipedia. http://en.wikipedia.org/wiki/CmH2O
Pressure. Wikipedia. http://en.wikipedia.org/wiki/Pressure
Torr. Wikipedia. http://en.wikipedia.org/wiki/MmHg

BE ALERT FOR LUPUS FLARES

ANTHONY D. SLONIM, MD, DRPH

Systemic lupus erythematosus (SLE) is a multisystem autoimmune disease caused by autoantibodies and the deposition of immune complexes. The disease affects primarily women and has a higher prevalence among African Americans. A series of clinical findings is associated with SLE. These include a characteristic malar rash, photosensitivity, arthritis, serositis, and a discoid rash. In addition, involvement of the renal, neurologic, and hematologic systems present with system-specific symptoms. The presence of autoantibodies (e.g., anti-Sm, anti–double-stranded DNA) can also assist in making the diagnosis. When a patient exhibits four or more of these criteria the diagnosis can be made with a sensitivity and specificity of 75% and 95%, respectively.

SLE can present with an acute or subacute onset. Most patients undergo some elements of acute exacerbation and remission during the natural course of the disease. This is important because the goals of SLE treatment include mainly the control of symptoms and prevention of the worsening of organ failure. Treatment usually involves a number of systemically administered medications. For minor disease, arthritis and pain can be treated with nonsteroidal antiinflammatory medications or COX-2 inhibitors. Antimalarial agents (chloroquine, quinacrine) can also benefit patients with generalized symptoms. For severe systemic disease, the use of steroids is the mainstay of treatment. These drugs can be administered in high doses, with attempts to reduce the dose at frequent intervals once symptoms are under control. Cytotoxic agents are used for aggressive disease including renal manifestations.

It is important that intensive care unit (ICU) clinicians understand whether the presentation of a worsening clinical condition in an SLE patient in the ICU results from the adverse effects of the medications used to treat the disease, an acute lupus flare, or a separate and unrelated condition. For instance, in severe cases of SLE, the medications used for immunosuppression increase the possibility for severe sepsis and septic shock. It is important to remember that the mechanism of action of these drugs is aimed at the cellular component of the immune system and complement. Therefore, patients presenting with sepsis are likely to be infected with organisms that are usually prevented by the appropriate functioning of these systems. Broad-spectrum antimicrobials should be used to treat sepsis in these patients, but consideration of other organisms (viruses, fungi) should be considered if patients do not improve quickly.

In addition, chronic steroid use has a number of complications that may contribute to problems in the ICU patient with SLE when used. On a chronic basis, steroids are associated with hypertension, sometimes refractory to treatment. Steroids also suppress adrenal function, thereby making the patient susceptible to acute stressors like surgery or shock. This condition can manifest by refractory hypotension and needs to be addressed preoperatively and during the ICU course with maintenance steroids. Steroids lead to hyperglycemia, which has recently been shown to be an independent predictor of mortality in ICU patients; thus, strict glucose control in these patients is mandatory. Steroids also contribute to the onset of peptic ulcers in the ICU and poor wound healing. Therefore, there needs to be strict attention to both prophylaxis for ulcer disease and frequent repositioning to prevent skin breakdown and decubitus ulcer formation.

The patient with SLE may experience problems related to the disease itself when hospitalized in the ICU. The multisystem nature of the disease often creates problems that make caring for these patients difficult. Patients can exhibit pulmonary or cardiovascular disease. They can have pulmonary infiltrates, effusions, and fibrosis that necessitate mechanical ventilation. Pericarditis and valvular dysfunction can lead to shock and poor cardiac output. Patients may become hypercoagulable, making them susceptible to central neurologic thrombosis or myocardial ischemia. Renal insufficiency exacerbated by the renal stressors of the ICU may cause progressive renal failure that makes fluid and electrolyte management in the ICU difficult and may require dialysis. Bone marrow suppression may create anemia that will alter oxygen-carrying capacity or thrombocytopenia that can lead to bleeding. Both of these conditions may require ongoing transfusions.

SUGGESTED READINGS

Davidson A, Diamond B. Autoimmune diseases. N Engl J Med 2001;354:340–350.
Kasper DL, Braunwald E, Fauci AS, et al., eds. Harrison's Principles of Internal Medicine, 16th ed. New York: McGraw-Hill, 2005:1515–1518.